DIET AND HUMAN IMMUNE FUNCTION

NUTRITION ◊ AND ◊ HEALTH
Adrianne Bendich, Series Editor

Diet and Human Immune Function

Edited by

David A. Hughes, PhD, RNutr

Nutrition Division, Institute of Food Research
Norwich Research Park, Norfolk, UK

L. Gail Darlington, MD, FRCP

Epsom and St. Helier University Hospitals NHS Trust
Surrey, UK

Adrianne Bendich, PhD, FACN

GlaxoSmithKline Consumer Healthcare
Parsippany, NJ

Foreword by

William R. Beisel, MD, FACP

Professor Emeritus, The Johns Hopkins School of Hygiene
and Public Health, Baltimore, MD

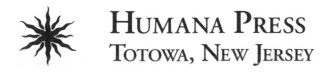

Humana Press
Totowa, New Jersey

Production Editor: Jessica Jannicelli.
Cover design by Patricia F. Cleary.

For additional copies, pricing for bulk purchases, and/or information about other Humana titles, contact Humana at the above address or at any of the following numbers: Tel.: 973-256-1699; Fax: 973-256-8341; E-mail: humana@humanapr.com; or visit our Website: www.humanapress.com

Printed in the United States of America. 10 9 8 7 6 5 4 3 2 1

e-ISBN: 1-59259-652-5

Library of Congress Cataloging-in-Publication Data

Diet and human immune function / edited by David A. Hughes, L. Gail Darlington, and Adrianne Bendich ; foreword by William R. Beisel.
       p. ; cm. -- (Nutrition and health)
Includes bibliographical references and index.
  ISBN 1-58829-206-1 (alk. paper)
  1. Immunity--Nutritional aspects.
  [DNLM: 1. Immune System--drug effects. 2. Immune System--physiology.
3. Diet--adverse effects. 4. Immunologic Diseases--diet therapy. 5.
Immunologic Diseases--etiology. 6. Nutrition--physiology. QW 504 D5645
2004]   I. Hughes, David A. II. Darlington, Gail. III. Bendich, Adrianne.
IV. Series: Nutrition and health (Totowa, N.J.)
  QR182.2.N86D53 2004
  616.07'9--dc22

                                                         2003020993

DEDICATION

D. A. H. dedicates this book with love to Jackie, his children, Emma, Sophie, Ben, Cerys, and Etholle and his parents, Mair and John, for all their love, encouragement, and support.

L. G. D. dedicates this book with love to Norman, Debbie, John, and Kelvin who have understood her love for research and have supported her through everything.

A. B. dedicates this book to Jacob Alexander Schiff, her youngest grandchild, in the hope that the information contained within this book will lead to a healthier life for everyone—including Jacob and his generation.

SERIES EDITOR'S INTRODUCTION

The *Nutrition and Health* series of books has, as an overriding mission, to provide health professionals with texts that are considered essential because each includes: (1) a synthesis of the state of the science, (2) timely, in-depth reviews by the leading researchers in their respective fields, (3) extensive, up-to-date fully annotated reference lists, (4) a detailed index, (5) relevant tables and figures, (6) identification of paradigm shifts and the consequences, (7) virtually no overlap of information between chapters, but targeted, inter-chapter referrals, (8) suggestions of areas for future research and (9) balanced, data-driven answers to patient /health professional's questions that are based on the totality of evidence rather than the findings of any single study.

The series volumes are not the outcome of a symposium. Rather, each editor(s) has the potential to examine a chosen area with a broad perspective, both in subject matter as well as in the choice of chapter authors. The international perspective, especially with regard to public health initiatives, is emphasized where appropriate. The editors, whose trainings are both research and practice oriented, have the opportunity to develop a primary objective for their book, define the scope and focus, and then invite the leading authorities from around the world to be part of their initiative. The authors are encouraged to provide an overview of the field, discuss their own research, and relate the research findings to potential human health consequences. Because each book is developed *de novo*, the chapters are coordinated so that the resulting volume imparts greater knowledge than the sum of the information contained in the individual chapters.

Diet and Human Immune Function, edited by David A. Hughes, L. Gail Darlington, and myself, clearly exemplifies the goals of the *Nutrition and Health* series. Unlike many other books in the area of nutritional immunology, this text concentrates on data from human studies, thus providing a critical assessment of the field based on recent epidemiological and clinical intervention studies. Each of the editors has extensive experience in clinical immunology and the combined experiences in academia, industry and clinical practice provide a broad perspective on the role of diet and diet modifications, nutrients, and several nonessential components of the diet on critical aspects of human immune responses.

As editors, we have chosen internationally recognized experts who are active investigators of the impact of overall diet on risks of infection, cancer, autoimmune disease, and environmental stressors in different age groups, in different countries throughout the world, and in both sexes. This important text provides practical, data-driven resources in well-organized tables and figures that assist the reader in evaluating the nutritive value of the immunomodulatory vitamins and minerals and such other dietary constituents as probiotics and long-chain fatty acids. Moreover, the critical value of nutrition for at-risk populations, including those living in poverty, those exposed to environmental extremes in the military or during athletic performance, the very young and the very old, are extensively reviewed in several unique chapters.

Diet and Human Immune Function, edited by Hughes, Darlington, and Bendich sets the benchmark for providing the most up-to-date, critical data on the role of dietary substances on immune responses. Each chapter includes an overview and historic review, examination of the literature with critical focus on comparisons between studies, discussion of the chemical composition of actives where appropriate, and conclusions and future research areas. The overarching goal of the editors is to provide fully referenced information to health professionals so they may have a balanced perspective on the value of many dietary components that are routinely consumed by patients and clients with the hope that immune responses will be enhanced. This important volume provides health professionals with balanced, data-driven answers to numerous questions about the validity of the science to date and also provides researchers with opportunities to clarify areas where many questions still exist about the effects of specific nutrients/dietary factors on human immune responses. At the end of each chapter, there is a section entitled "Take Home Messages" that summarizes the five to ten key points in the chapter readers will find exceptionally helpful.

Hughes, Darlington, and Bendich have organized the volume into five areas of focus that reflect the breadth and depth of current knowledge in the area of diet and human immune responses. In the first section, the editors have wisely included an excellent chapter that reviews the basics of human immunology so that all readers are "on the same page" before proceeding to the more detailed chapters. A second critically important chapter reviews the clinical methods used to assess immune function. Unique areas of focus include an analysis of the effects of undernutrition on immune responses in children, specific nutrients important for neonatal immune function and, at the other end of the life cycle, the significance of diet and supplement use on immune functions, such as responses to vaccines in the elderly. The second and third sections provide in-depth, separate chapters devoted to the well-recognized immunomodulatory nutrients: vitamins A, C, E, carotenoids, iron, selenium and zinc as well as a separate chapter on the immune effects of multivitamin supplements.

The fourth section on nutrition, immunity, and disease includes chapters that examine such controversial areas as probiotics, fatty acids, and elimination diets in the context of rheumatoid arthritis, HIV infection, cancer, and osteoporosis. Authors of these chapters have been particularly inclusive and objective; extensive references to the published literature are provided. Novel findings are examined in light of both national epidemiological surveys as well as well-designed clinical studies. Chapters in this section present the scientific arguments for a more broad-based approach to immune function and include an examination of the role of immune cells in the development of osteoporosis as well as in gut immunity. The final section on environmental stressors contains a chapter on the effects of exercise on cytokine production and in vivo consequences to immune responses. Another chapter looks at the effects of air pollution on the immune cells that protect the lung. There is also a unique chapter on the consequences of elite training in the US Armed Services and the effects of sleep and/or calorie deprivation in extreme environments or responses to infections. A final chapter provides an extensive overview on the immune/nutritional consequences of prescription drugs used to treat immune-mediated diseases and infections.

Understanding the complexities of the human immune system and the effects of food/ environment/age/sex/concomitant disease/drugs/stressors certainly is not simple and the interactions can often seem daunting. However, the editors and authors have focused on assisting those who are unfamiliar with this field in understanding the critical issues and important new research findings that can impact their fields of interest. Drs. Hughes, Darlington, and Bendich have carefully chosen the very best researchers from around the world who can communicate the relevance of nutrition's role in the maintenance of a healthy immune system. The authors have worked hard to make their information accessible to health professionals interested in public health, geriatrics, general medical practice, nursing, pharmacy, educators, and students, as well as nutrition-related allied health professionals. The well-referenced chapters contain tables and figures that assist the reader in understanding the information within the chapter and provide relevant citations to help readers to identify key sources of more information. Many of the tables provide health professionals with guides to assessment of vitamin/mineral contents of sources of the specific nutrient. Several chapters include unique tables of information that were not available beforehand, such as the tables on assessment of human immune responses in clinical studies, and individual tables comparing effects of specific vitamins, minerals, carotenoids, multivitamins and probiotics on human immune responses. Excellent figures clarify complex interactions between immune cells, cytokines, and other immunomodulatory molecules. The epidemiological as well as clinical study literature is extensively reviewed in each chapter. The editors have taken special care to use the same terms and abbreviations between chapters, and provide a clearly written glossary of terms as well as a list of abbreviations used throughout the volume. An extensive compilation of related books and websites is also included in the appendices

In conclusion, *Diet and Human Immune Function*, edited by David A. Hughes, L. Gail Darlington, and Adrianne Bendich provides health professionals in many areas of research and practice with the most up-to-date, well referenced and easy-to-understand volume on the importance of diet for optimal human immune function. This volume will serve the reader as the most authoritative resource in the field to date and is a very welcome addition to the *Nutrition and Health* series.

Adrianne Bendich, PhD, FACN
Series Editor

FOREWORD

Diet and Human Immune Function provides exceedingly useful information for prac-
ticing physicians. It reviews the single essential nutrients that must be included in the diet
to insure optimal function of a patient's immune system.

Other important factors, such as infancy and aging, starvation and obesity, infectious
diseases, rheumatoid arthritis, osteoporosis, and cancer, and also exercise and air pollution, are discussed in detail concerning their effects on immunity.

The relationship between diet and immunity (both innate and acquired) is a relatively
recent concern, having been studied in its broadest aspects for less than a decade. Another
book, *Nutrition and Immunology* (edited by M. E. Gershwin, L. B. German, and C. L.
Keen, published by Humana Press in 2000) discussed the basic scientific aspects of the
diet/immunology relationship, but provided less clinical information and advice.

As already noted, this present book is especial useful for physicians, in part because
each chapter concludes with two valuable specific sections: First, a clinically oriented
"Conclusions" paragraph, and second, a numerated list of "Take Home" Messages, each
of which provide clinical instructions about special nutritional problems (and their treatment) that may occur in various disease states. The list of references included after each
chapter is unbelievably long. Also, of unique importance, is an appendix that defines
hundreds of capital letter groups (e.g., AIDS, CRP, IFN, etc.) used by immunologists.
Other appendices list glossaries, related books, and key websites.

Opening chapters are meant to teach non-immunologists about immunity and its complexities, and about how human immune responses can be tested and evaluated. These
chapters also discuss the influence of infancy and old age on immune system responses
to new and previously experienced antigens. Subsequent chapters deal with the importance of individual dietary components, i.e., vitamins, minerals, carotenoids (beta-carotene, lycopene, lutein, and zeaxanthin), and ingested lipids. When tested prospectively
in elderly adults, the administration of commercial multivitamin/multimineral products
led to improvements in immune system functions.

Of note, the importance of antioxidants such as lutein and zeaxanthin has led to the
inclusion of lutein in some commercial multivitamin preparations. To date, however,
zeaxanthin (an orange-colored molecule of great importance to the optic macula) can, as
of now, only be acquired from fruits and dark green lettuces. Lack of these carotenoids,
which fill the macular rods and cones, has been implicated in the macular degeneration
experienced by many aged individuals.

Infectious illnesses, rheumatoid arthritis, osteoporosis, and some cancers are all known
to influence the immune system adversely, and each of these diseases is discussed in an
individual chapter. Similarly, exercise, military exertion, various drugs, and even air
pollution can have deleterious effects on immunity. Such negative immunologic effects
are also reviewed.

I am often asked to discuss dietary problems with groups of elderly individuals. Naturally, I emphasize the importance of a nutritionally complete, well-rounded diet, which should include a daily serving of a fruit and of some tomato product (including ketchup). But many of my listeners are eating special diets, as recommended by their own experienced dietitian. I therefore also suggest that they take a multivitamin/multimineral tablet each day along with an additional 500 mg of vitamin C, and 200 mg of vitamin E, plus (if permitted by their dietitian) a daily serving of a tomato dish, and of a dark green salad. This advice seems consistent with the recommendations outlined in this book.

William R. Beisel, MD, FACP
The Johns Hopkins School of Hygiene
and Public Health, Baltimore, MD

PREFACE

The importance of the immune system to an individual's health cannot be overstated. In recent years, the contribution of the diet to the optimal working of the immune system has become widely appreciated and the influence of different dietary components on specific aspects of immune function has been extensively studied in animals; there have also been a number of well controlled studies in individuals covering the age span from toddlers to seniors. With *Diet and Human Immune Function*, our aim is to provide a detailed, data-driven, well balanced, yet easily "dip in and out-able" review of the effects of dietary components on the immune system.

The three editors bring unique experiences and backgrounds to this volume. Dr. David Hughes is a Principal Research Scientist at the Institute of Food Research, Norwich, UK, a publicly funded Institute that undertakes independent research in nutrition, food safety, and food materials science. He has 25 years of experience as a cellular immunologist, formerly in respiratory medicine, and for the last decade in nutrition research. His main interest is in understanding the mechanisms by which dietary components modulate human immune function and translating this into dietary recommendations. He is the author of numerous peer-reviewed papers and critical reviews in this field and he is currently Honorary Secretary of the Nutritional Immunology Affinity Group of the British Society for Immunology. He is also a Registered Nutritionist with the Nutrition Society.

Dr. Gail Darlington is a senior specialist in General Internal Medicine and Rheumatology at Epsom and St. Helier University Hospitals NHS Trust in the United Kingdom, where she is also Lead Clinician for Research and heads a large clinical research team investigating rheumatoid arthritis, osteoporosis, diabetes, stroke, depression, cannabis toxicity, and Huntington's disease. Dr. Darlington was a PPP Research Fellow at Jesus College, Cambridge, and is a member of several European Research groups. She is Lead Clinician of a clinical/scientific research team in conjunction with Professor Trevor Stone of the University of Glasgow and is co-author of *Pills, Potions and Poisons*, again with Professor Stone—a book designed to make drugs understandable and more acceptable to the reader. Dr. Darlington was one of the first British specialists to undertake research into the role of dietary manipulation in the management of rheumatoid arthritis and to try to establish a dialogue between doctors (who tend to be sceptical about dietary treatment) and patients (who have tended to believe, perhaps too trustingly, in the benefits of dietary manipulation). The absence of such dialogue in the past has led to a stand-off between patients and doctors that has resulted in many patients being vulnerable to unsound advice from unscrupulous advisers. The book *Diet and Arthritis*, written by Dr. Darlington and Linda Gamlin has proved to be extremely valuable to patients needing reliable scientific advice on this subject. Dr. Darlington has a major interest in making scientific information about food available to as many people as possible and she is well known for her radio and television appearances on this subject.

Dr. Adrianne Bendich is currently a Clinical Director at GlaxoSmithKline Consumer Healthcare and is responsible for the clinical program in support of calcium and other micronutrient research. She is a pioneer in the field of nutritional immunology and was one of the first researchers to show the direct dose–response relationship between vitamin E intake and immune responses in laboratory animals; she also was a leader in exploring the roles of vitamin C and carotenoids' effects on immune function. Dr. Bendich co-chaired the seminal meeting in the field of nutritional immunology at the New York Academy of Sciences entitled: Micronutrients and Immune Functions, held in 1990. As a Director of Research at Roche Vitamins, she was involved in virtually all of the clinical studies in the field of nutritional immunology conducted around the world, providing technical expertise, clinical supplies, and funding when national and international sources were virtually unavailable. Thus, her support of this field during its infancy allowed the area to grow at a very critical point in its development.

As editors, we hope that our backgrounds, which include academic, clinical, and industrial perspectives, will provide the reader with the totality of the evidence, presented in a pragmatic, usable form for both professional and student audiences that are not well trained in nutritional immunology. Our aim is that this volume will serve as the key reference text for health professionals: physicians, nurses, pharmacists, immunologists, nutritionists, dieticians, and academics, including advanced undergraduates, and graduate, para-health professional, and medical students, as well as researchers. We have gathered together the leading international experts in the field of nutritional immunology to document the current state of knowledge on how diet influences immune function in health, in disease, and under various conditions of stress, identifying potential means of enhancing immune function by dietary means. In contrast to other textbooks covering nutritional immunology, which often tend to emphasize animal and in vitro studies, this book focuses on effects in humans. It addresses the subject in a detailed but accessible manner, which can be readily taken up by consumers who have a real interest in improving the status of their respective immunities via what they eat.

The chapters are organized so that the reader is given a broad-based introduction to the area under discussion, followed by a detailed review of clinical findings and relevant laboratory studies. All chapters use the same abbreviations and a list of these is found in the Appendices. All authors have provided the reader with a comprehensive overview of their particular speciality. Each of the authors has included detailed tables and important figures that provide added clarity to the text. Chapters are extensively referenced, including the most up-to-date review articles and research findings. At the end of each chapter there is a table listing the key "take home" messages, which provide the reader with a succinct summary of current knowledge, as well as identifying gaps in our understanding that require further research. Indeed, it will become clear to the reader that though there is now a wealth of evidence that different dietary components can modulate immune function, and a considerable understanding of the mechanisms underlying the effects of these nutrients, there is still a degree of uncertainty regarding the intakes of individual nutrients required to obtain optimal benefit. It is also clear that different groups of individuals, such as the very young and the elderly, athletes and cigaret smokers, for example, require different nutritional intakes to optimize activity of their immune system compared with the relevant control groups.

It seems increasingly likely, in the "post-genomic era," that it will be confirmed that each one of us has different nutritional needs depending on our genetic make up (genotype) and lifestyle, suggesting that, in the foreseeable future, we may be able to design individual diets tailored to meet these needs. In the meantime, this book provides the reader with the current state of our knowledge.

Diet and Human Immune Function consists of 22 chapters divided into five sections. The first section contains five chapters, providing an introduction to the human immune system, how human immune responses are measured, and overviews of the influence of diet on immune function at both ends of our lifespan. It also includes an extensive review of the important interrelationship that exists among nutrition, immunity, and infection. Section II provides comprehensive state-of-the-art critical appraisals of the known influences on the human immune system of several important vitamins, including vitamins A, C, and E, as well as the carotenoids, such as β-carotene. Although many studies have concentrated on examining the influence of single nutrients on immune response, in order to identify their functionality, there is also a need to study the effects of combinations of nutrients, to explore the potentially more beneficial results these combinations may provide. This approach is detailed in the final chapter of this section. Section III contains three chapters reviewing the current known effects of the minerals, iron, selenium, and zinc, on human immune response and, as with chapters in the proceeding section, provide details of natural sources and recommended intakes of these nutrients. Section IV describes the influence of nutrition in disease states, such as rheumatoid arthritis, osteoporosis, HIV infection, and cancer and a further chapter details our current knowledge of how probiotic intestinal bacteria may benefit health by modulating immune function. Section V provides some unique reviews of nutritional influences on immune function under three forms of stress—vigorous exercise, military conditions, and air pollution, in relation to allergic asthma. The final chapter in the section provides a much-needed overview of the nutritional consequences of drug/disease interactions and provides recommendations regarding potential nutritional interventions that could increase drug efficacy and/or reduce adverse side effects. Provided at the end of the book are a list of abbreviations, a glossary of simple descriptions for many of the terms used in the book, a listing of related books and websites, as well as a comprehensive index.

As editors, we have tried to ensure that *Diet and Human Immune Function* conveys to the reader the enormous potential ability of the diet to modulate immune function beneficially, as well as documenting the exciting recent developments in the field of nutritional immunology.

David A. Hughes, PhD, RNutr
L. Gail Darlington, MD, FRCP
Adrianne Bendich, PhD, FACN

CONTENTS

CONTRIBUTORS

RONALD ANDERSON, PhD • *Medical Research Council Unit for Inflammation and Immunity, Department of Immunology, Faculty of Health Sciences, University of Pretoria, South Africa*

JOHN R. ARTHUR, PhD • *Division of Cellular Integrity, The Rowett Research Institute, Aberdeen, UK*

MARIANNA K. BAUM, PhD, MS • *College of Health and Urban Affairs, Florida International University, Miami, FL*

GEOFFREY J. BECKETT, PhD, FRCP • *Department of Clinical Biochemistry, University of Edinburgh, Edinburgh, UK*

ADRIANNE BENDICH, PhD, FACN • *GlaxoSmithKline, Parsippany, NJ*

JEFFREY B. BLUMBERG, PhD, FACN, CNS • *Jean Mayer USDA Human Nutrition Research Center on Aging at Tufts University, Boston, MA*

JOHN D. BOGDEN, PhD • *Department of Preventive Medicine and Community Health, UMDNJ-New Jersey Medical School, Newark, NJ*

ADRIANA CAMPA, PhD, MBA, RD • *College of Health and Urban Affairs, Florida International University, Miami, FL*

SUSANNA CUNNINGHAM-RUNDLES, PhD • *The Immunology Research Laboratory, Department of Pediatrics, The New York Presbyterian Hospital—Cornell University Weill Medical College, New York, NY*

GENNARO D'AMATO, MD • *Division of Pneumology and Allergology, Department of Chest Diseases, High Specialty Hospital A. Cardarelli, Naples, Italy*

L. GAIL DARLINGTON, MD, FRCP • *Epsom and St. Helier University Hospitals NHS Trust, Epsom, Surrey, UK*

MARCO DI MONACO, MD • *Osteoporosis Research Center, Presidio Sanitario San Camillo, Torino, Italy*

KENT L. ERICKSON, PhD • *Department of Cell Biology and Human Anatomy, School of Medicine, University of California, Davis, CA*

KARL E. FRIEDL, PhD • *Military Operational Medicine Research Program, US Army Medical Research and Materiel Command, Fort Detrick, MD*

HARSHARNJIT S. GILL, PhD, MVSc • *Institute of Food Nutrition and Human Health, Massey University, Palmerston North, New Zealand*

SUNG NIM HAN, PhD, RD • *Jean Mayer USDA Human Nutrition Research Center on Aging at Tufts University, Boston, MA*

NEIL E. HUBBARD, PhD • *Department of Cell Biology and Human Anatomy, School of Medicine, University of California, Davis, CA*

DAVID A. HUGHES, PhD, RNutr • *Nutrition Division, Institute of Food Research, Norwich, Norfolk, UK*

KLAUS-HELGE IBS, PhD • *Institute of Immunology, University Hospital, Technical University of Aachen, Aachen, Germany*

DARSHAN S. KELLEY, PhD • *Western Human Nutrition Research Center, ARS, United States Department of Agriculture, Davis, CA*

DENISE KELLY, PhD • *Gut Immunology Group, The Rowett Research Institute, Aberdeen, UK*

HO-KYUNG KWAK, PhD • *Jean Mayer USDA Human Nutrition Research Center on Aging at Tufts University, Boston, MA*

DONALD B. LOURIA, MD • *Department of Preventive Medicine and Community Health, UMDNJ-New Jersey Medical School, Newark, NJ*

RODDIE C. MCKENZIE, PhD, MBA • *Laboratory for Clinical and Molecular Virology, Royal Veterinary School, University of Edinburgh, Edinburgh, UK*

SIMIN NIKBIN MEYDANI, PhD, DVM • *Jean Mayer USDA Human Nutrition Research Center on Aging at Tufts University, Boston, MA*

SUE M. MILLER, PhD • *Department of Clinical Biochemistry, University of Edinburgh, Edinburgh, UK*

KEITH E. NYE, BA, MSc, PhD • *St. Bartholomew's Hospital Medical School, London, UK*

CHRISTINE A. NORTHROP-CLEWES, DPhil, BSc, CBiol, MIBiol • *Northern Ireland Centre for Food and Health, School of Life and Health Sciences, University of Ulster, Coleraine, County Londonderry, UK*

DEBORAH O'NEIL, PhD • *Gut Immunology Group, The Rowett Research Institute, Aberdeen, UK*

BENTE K. PEDERSEN, DMSc • *The Copenhagen Muscle Research Centre and Department of Infectious Diseases, University of Copenhagen, Copenhagen, Denmark*

LOTHAR RINK, PhD • *Institute of Immunology, University Hospital, Technical University of Aachen, Aachen, Germany*

KAY J. RUTHERFURD-MARKWICK, PhD • *Institute of Food Nutrition and Human Health, Massey University, Palmerston North, New Zealand*

RICHARD D. SEMBA, MD, MPH • *Ocular Immunology Division, Department of Ophthalmology, Johns Hopkins School of Medicine, Baltimore, MD*

DAVID I. THURNHAM, PhD, BSc • *Northern Ireland Centre for Food and Health, School of Life and Health Sciences, University of Ulster, Coleraine, County Londonderry, UK*

GÜNTER WEISS, MD • *Department of Internal Medicine, University Hospital, Innsbruck, Austria*

RONIT ZILBERBOIM, PhD • *Lonzagroup, Food Applications, Annandale, NJ*

I OVERVIEW

1   The Basics of Immunology for the Non-Immunologist

Keith E. Nye

There is sound scientific evidence that the food and supplements that we ingest influence, among other functions, our immune responses. For instance, many research reports may be found using the standard scientific search engines on the effects of dietary consumption of *Bifidobacterium lactis* on natural immunity. The following chapters in this volume further enlighten the reader about current research and thinking and clarify some of the immunologic concepts for the nonimmunologist (or occasional immunologist). This volume is intentionally basic, and articles and textbooks that provide greater detail are listed in the bibliography at the end of the chapter. *Brief definitions of all italicized words can be found in the Glossary at the end of this volume.*

1. INTRODUCTION

Before going into the complexity of the immune system, it is helpful to consider what features would be required if we were to design the system from scratch. First, the host would have to recognize that the invader was not part of itself and mount an effective defense against it. Would the host need several different recognition systems and an equal number of defense mechanisms, and would they be best combined in one unit or several discrete units? Continuing with the invasion analogy, the enemy may be weak, either individually or in number, or may be an opportunist and enter through a break in the perimeter fence. Once in, the agent might hide for a considerable time and attack during a weak moment. In this analogy, we have recognition and defense and the need for either immediate defense or a timely organized counterattack, which, in the immune system, equate to *innate* or *adaptive responses*.

2. THE INNATE IMMUNE SYSTEM

The innate system is nonspecific and, in evolutionary terms, is the primal part of the immune defense. It consists of barriers, such as the skin, or other natural openings, and a system of fine hairs, such as in the nostrils, which can act as filters. These are backed up by chemical and microbiologic barriers within the mucous membranes, which may limit a pathogen's proliferation and spread within the host. Should one of the barriers break, such as when a sharp object punctures the skin, then pathogens can enter and

From: *Diet and Human Immune Function*
Edited by: D. A. Hughes, L. G. Darlington, and A. Bendich © Humana Press Inc., Totowa, NJ

multiply rapidly in the ideal condition of warm tissue. In this case, innate immune system cells are called into play, such as *monocytes* and *macrophages* (*mononuclear phagocytes*). These accumulate at the injury site within minutes, followed by *neutrophils*, which are also recruited to the infected area. These *phagocytic* cells have basic recognition molecules on their surface that are nonspecific but bind to common structures, usually lipopolysaccharides on Gram-negative bacteria, lipotechoic acid and peptidoglycans on Gram-positive bacteria, and mannans on yeast cell membranes. Phagocytosis is the ingestion of particulate material into cells for degradation and is the same process by which simple unicellular organisms, such as amoeba, ingest their nutrient. The highly conserved nature of this response, seen in even the simplest animals, confirms its importance in survival. Various serum protein components, including *complement*, may then bind to the pathogen to facilitate its phagocytosis. One characteristic of the innate system is the rapid nature of the response, which is often sufficient to destroy the invading microbes and, thus, contain the infection. A major disadvantage of this nonspecific rapid response is the indiscriminate tissue damage that occurs, which plays a major part in rheumatoid arthritis, systemic lupus erythematosus, dermatomyositis, sceleroderma, and some forms of vasculitis (often referred to as connective tissue diseases).

2.1. Anatomical Components of the Innate Immune System

2.1.1. Skin

The outer layer of dead keratinocytes that form the surface of the human body is covered at all times by many living microorganisms, but these cells can resist penetration by these organisms and act as a first-line of defense for the deeper tissues. Should penetration occur, the living keratinocytes, which constitute part of the innate immune system in the deeper layers, can, if damaged by the invader, secrete cytokines, such as interleukin (IL)-1 and IL-6 and tumor necrosis factor-α (TNF-α). These agents activate endothelial cells to express *adhesion molecules* and also prepare macrophages and neutrophils for action. On the negative side, they are also responsible for the inflammation seen after excess exposure to ultraviolet light (sunburn), where the high-energy particles penetrate the outer layer and damage the keratinocytes. The keratinocyte also secretes chemokines, such as IL-8, which, through chemotaxis, attract many cell types to the injury site. These responses are typical of the innate system in that they are rapid, but they also alert the Langerhans cells, which act as an intermediary between the innate and adaptive systems. These cells are of the *dendritic cell* lineage, which, after exposure to microorganisms in the damaged tissue, migrate to the local lymph nodes and present antigen, derived from the microorganism, to T cells that link the two systems. Although the two systems are separated by immunologists, in practice there is much interaction between them.

2.1.2. The Respiratory Tract

The respiratory tract has two distinct areas in the innate system: upper and lower. The former extends from the nose to the bronchioles, and the latter includes the terminal bronchioles and the alveoli. The mucociliary escalator provides immediate protection in the upper tract. Goblet cells in the airway secrete mucous, which creates a fine layer in the tract to physically trap microorganisms. The cilia, which are like minute motile hairs, direct the mucous toward the nose and mouth, where it is cleared by coughing and sneezing. The lower part of the respiratory tract functions as an oxygen diffusion area, and either mucous or cilia would hinder this diffusion. Here, type II pneumocytes produce surfactants that are composed of phospholipoproteins, which prevent alveoli collapse during expiration. They also contain pathogen-binding proteins, which are members of the collectin family. The globular lectin-like head recognizes sugars on the microorganism, and the long collagen tail binds to phagocytes or activates complement components. During respiratory infections, both upper and lower tract sections rely on adaptive immune system immunoglobulins for protection (*see* Section 3.3.1.).

2.1.3. THE GASTROINTESTINAL TRACT

The gastrointestinal (GI) tract has several nonspecific immune defense systems, because greater than 90% of the exposure to microorganisms occurs at the mucosal surface of the gut. Epithelial cells form a tight physical barrier, and, in the case of injury, surrounding cells quickly migrate to cover the damaged area, a process known as restitution. Concurrently, lymphocytes and macrophages migrate through pores in the basement membrane to provide temporary protection. The low pH of the gut is its major source of defense, and the normal microflora of the intestine prevents colonization by pathogenic bacteria.

2.2. Secreted Proteins of the Innate Immune System

2.2.1. INTERFERONS

A protein discovered in the 1950s by Alick Isaacs and described as a viral inhibitor was named *interferon* (IFN). Subsequent research showed that there were different types of protein with the same basic structure and that they fulfilled functions other than viral inhibition. The IFNs provide a rapid response, are produced locally at the infection site, and directly inhibit pathogen growth. They have been divided into two types, I and II. Type I IFN (IFN-α and IFN-β) has the most potent antiviral activity, whereas type II IFN (IFN-γ) is less potent as an antiviral agent but is associated with activation of the immune response. Type I IFNs are secreted by a range of cells in response to double-stranded RNA, which is not present in mammalian cells but produced by viruses as they infect cells, thus giving the IFN a specific target.

2.2.2. COLLECTINS

The collectin family includes the surfactant proteins (*see* Section 2.1.2.) and mannan-binding protein or lectin. Each is important as a pattern recognition molecule. Collectins are proteins with a globular lectin-like head and a long collagen tail. The head binds to bacterial sugars via its lectins, and this complex then binds by the collagen tail to specific receptors on phagocytic cells, which stimulates their phagocytosis. Mannan-binding protein is a specific lectin that acts identically to and through collectins. The complement component C1q (*see* Section 2.2.3.) is related to the collectins and suggests that they all evolved from a common source.

2.2.3. COMPLEMENT

The *complement* system is important in innate immunity and consists of approx 20 heat-labile serum proteins, which are activated in turn in specific sequences or cascades. Although as stated, there are approx 20 proteins in the complement system with difficult names, there are only nine fundamental components (C1–C9); the rest are regulatory, which can be triggered in three basic sequences. These three sequences or pathways, driven by the presence of a foreign antigen, are termed classical pathway, which is set in motion by antigen/antibody reactions; alternative pathway, which is activated by polysaccharides on yeasts and Gram-negative bacteria; and the mannan-binding lectin pathway, which, like the alternative pathway, joins the classical pathway at a later stage (C3).

In simple terms, there are three ways C3 can be activated:

1. The classical pathway, so named because it was the first to be described, is triggered by antigen/antibody complexes. These complexes bring together many immunoglobulin Fc portions (*see* Section 3.3.1.) and those in proximity encourage the first complement component C1 to bind to the complex. The C1 in complex then activates two further components, C2 and C4, which, in turn, activate many C3 molecules.
2. The alternative pathway really cheats and begins at C3, taking advantage of the C3 molecule's instability, which causes it to exist in low-level activation. Binding of "semi-active" C3 to cell surface polysaccharides causes complete complement cascade activation. Healthy mammalian cells express complement inhibitors on their surface, which prevents complement activation and subsequent cell destruction. Any other cell, such as an invading microorganism that does not have a surface inhibitor, will activate the C3 and, thus, the rest of the cascade, leading to destruction of the invader.
3. The lectin pathway relies on the ability of the lectin-like globular head of the mannan-binding protein to bind to bacterial carbohydrates. Although the binding protein has no enzymatic activity, the conformational change that results from binding is sufficient to trigger C2 and C4 activity, which go on to activate many C3 molecules.

It is clear that the three pathways described all reach C3 by different routes, but once C3 is activated, the final lytic sequence is common to all three pathways. This involves the sequential attachment of the complement components C5, C6, C7, C8, and C9, which results in target cell lysis. The binding of this complex to the invading microorganism's cell surface forms a transmembrane channel, which allows water and salts to pass, causing swelling and destruction of the cell. As stated, this is a much simplified version of the cascade; readers interested in the minutia should consult Janeway et al. *(1)*.

2.3. Cells Involved in the Innate Immune System

2.3.1. THE PHAGOCYTES—NEUTROPHILS, MONOCYTES, AND MACROPHAGES

Neutrophils are the most numerous white cells (*leukocytes*) in the blood stream and play a major role in the body's defense against infection. Like the monocyte–macrophage line, they develop from a common progenitor cell in the bone marrow, but, unlike macrophages, they mature and are stored in the bone marrow. They are released rapidly into the circulation in response to bacterial infection and remain in the blood stream for only a few hours before migrating into tissues, where they die within 24 to 48 h. The neutrophil's main role is to kill and degrade bacteria; the pus formed at the infection site is chiefly composed of dead neutrophils. Neutrophils contain granules that comprise several different cationic proteins, such as defensins and serprocidins, with bacteriocidal properties. These granules are often referred to as azurophil lysosomal granules. In addition, other antibacterial agents found within the cytosol include lysozyme, acid hydrolases, and myeloperoxidase.

Having all of these weapons against infective agents would be of little use if the neutrophil could not locate the infection site. To this end, the neutrophils synthesize and express receptors for *chemokines* and *cytokines* on their surface, which direct them to the inflammation site. Macrophages, which are constantly present in healthy tissue, remain in a quiescent state until stimulated by signals received at the infection site, which act on certain of their surface receptors (described below). The now-activated macrophage secretes chemokines, such as IL-8, into the circulation, which modify integrins on the neutrophil surface that enable them to adhere to, and migrate out of, blood vessels into the tissues by a process known as diapedesis. The role of the secreted chemokines is not yet finished. In concert, several different chemokines form a gradient to direct the now tissue-located neutrophils to the inflammation site. Once on site, the neutrophils ingest the microorganisms by phagocytosis, which is a form of localized endocytosis. The plasma membrane gradually envelops the microbe and buds off internally to form a compartment known as a phagosome. Some of the lysosomal granules are also taken into the vesicle to form a phagolysosome, and it is within this compartment that killing and degradation of the ingested particle occurs. In a process known as the respiratory burst, three related enzymatic pathways are activated at this stage to produce toxic molecules that assist in the destruction of ingested pathogen. Nicotinamide adenine dinucleotide phosphate (NADPH) is an energy-rich molecule that supplies "fuel" for the reduction of molecular oxygen within the phagocyte via NADPH oxidase to produce the superoxide anion. The superoxide anion is converted to hydrogen peroxide by superoxide dismutase (SOD), together with the regeneration of molecular oxygen. This nascent O_2 may be converted in neutrophils to nitric oxide (NO) by the action of NO synthase (NOS) on L-arginine in the presence of a cofactor, tetrahydrobiopterin (THBT). NO is a special molecule: it is extremely short-lived and not only is toxic to pathogens but also acts as an important signaling molecule. Thus, the neutrophil, though comparatively short-lived, is of paramount importance in the immediate response necessary for innate immunity.

Macrophages are produced in the bone marrow as immature monocytes and travel to various tissues, where they mature into macrophages and may reside for weeks to years. These tissue macrophages are heterogeneous both morphologically and in their metabolism and may travel freely within certain areas, for example, alveolar macrophages in the lung and peritoneal macrophages in the peritoneal cavity. Other macrophages are fixed within specialized tissue, such as Kupffer cells in the liver or glial cells in the brain. The major function of most macrophages is phagocytosis of invading organisms. Before the macrophage can fulfill its function, it must be made aware of the presence of the foreign antigen. This is achieved through pattern-recognition molecules, which are not specific but recognize characteristic surface markers on families of pathogens. For example, all Gram-negative bacteria have *lipopolysaccharide* (LPS) as a constituent part of their cell wall; thus, one important recognition molecule on the surface of the macrophage is for LPS. LPS is an endotoxin, which is a toxin released when bacteria die, in contrast to exotoxins, which are secreted by living bacteria. The recognition molecule for LPS is one of a family of receptors known as Toll-like receptors, whereas another Toll-like receptor recognizes peptidoglycans associated with lipotechoic acid on the surface of Gram-positive bacteria. The Toll receptor was originally identified and characterized in the late 1980s for its role in the embryonic development of the fruit fly, *Drosophila melanogaster* *(2)*. At least 10 Toll-like receptors have been identified to date, each of which can recognize a different surface marker from foreign antigens and transmit the danger signal to the macrophage's nucleus to initiate phagocytosis. The most effective triggering of this response follows opsonization of the microorganism by complement or immunoglobulin. Opsonization (from the Greek *opsonion*—victuals) is the process by which the microbe becomes coated with immunoglobulin G (IgG) or the complement component, C3b, which facilitates engulfment by phagocytic cells. Phagocytosis and killing proceed in the macrophage in much the same manner as described for the neutrophil.

2.3.2. Nonphagocytic Cells

The innate immune system has to deal with several potential pathogens; not just bacteria, viruses, and yeasts but various larger parasitic life forms. As the human race evolved, parasitic worms were a major threat. Although improved sanitation has largely removed this problem from the developed world, at least 40% of the world's population is still infested by these parasites. Some worms have complex life cycles and also have evolved strategies to evade the immune response. The majority of parasitic worms live within the gut, and, over the course of evolution, specialized cells have developed to counter this invasion. *Mast cells* and *eosinophils* are particularly adapted to respond to interluminal parasites.

Mast cells are derived from an unidentified precursor in the bone marrow. Like macrophages, they are widely distributed in the tissues and are recruited to parasitic infestation sites. When present in these sites, the mast cell produces granules that contain numerous mediators. Mast cells express a high affinity receptor for the Fc portion of immunoglobulin-E (FcεR1) and can bind IgE even when present at low levels. If this surface-bound IgE is cross-linked by antigen, possibly on the surface of a worm, then the mast cell is activated and degranulation occurs. This releases the preformed substances from the granules and also activates arachidonic acid metabolism, producing a range of fresh mediators. These include the neutral proteases, tryptase and chymase, and acid hydrolases, such as β-glucuronidase. Arachidonic acid metabolism via the cyclooxygenase pathway gives rise to *prostaglandins*, which act rapidly to cause vasodilation, increased vascular permeability, and smooth muscle constriction in the gut and bronchi. A second pathway, the lipooxygenase pathway, leads to *leukotriene* production. Though less rapid than the prostaglandins, leukotrienes synergize in contraction of the bronchial and gut smooth muscle and, probably more importantly, provide chemotactic stimuli to recruit neutrophils and eosinophils to the site. One important constituent of the preformed granules is histamine, which acts through a series of different receptors. Binding to the H_1 receptor promotes contraction of the smooth muscle tissue of the bronchi, which may have been the body's reaction to expel parasitic worms physically earlier in evolution. It is more likely to cause asthmatic-like illness now. If histamine bids to the H_2 receptor, the heart rate slows and extra hydrochloric acid is pumped into the stomach. In the brain, histamine can function as a neurotransmitter via the H_3 receptor.

Eosinophils are similar to mast cells, although two characteristics distinguish them as different. First, they are specifically recruited to inflammation sites and, second, their granules contain particularly toxic agents. Although there are always a few circulating eosinophils, their numbers increase dramatically in response to IL-3 and IL-5, which are secreted by mast cells and a subset of *helper T lymphocytes* (termed "Th2" cells) (*see* Section 3.2.2.). Eosinophils are recruited to parasitic infestation sites by the chemokine eotaxin. Unlike mast cells, eosinophils *do not* secrete histamine.

Basophils are the same size as neutrophils but even less common than eosinophils (fewer than 1% of circulating white cells). They contain dense black granules that often obscure the nucleus. Like the mast cells, basophils bind IgE on their surface and exposure to foreign antigen causes degranulation and the release of histamine, leukotrienes, and heparin.

Natural killer cells (NK cells), often known as large granular lymphocytes because they have more cytoplasm than resting T and B cells and contain one or two large azurophilic granules, are derived from the same progenitor cells as T and B cells and acquire their receptors while still in the bone marrow. Although they share some of the same surface markers as T cells (e.g., CD2), they do not undergo development within the thymus and, although employing similar killing techniques to the cytotoxic T cell, they do not have specifically rearranged T-cell receptors and are, therefore, still regarded as members of the innate immune series. They are stimulated by IFN-α, IFN-β, and IL-12, and killing is regulated via signaling through special receptors, which interact with certain carbohydrates expressed on the surface of normal cells. This binding triggers the NK cell to kill the cell to which it binds. However, the NK cell also expresses a receptor that binds to *major histocompatibility complex* (MHC) class I molecules (*see* Section 3.3.2.) present on normal cells, and this associated binding inhibits their cytotoxic activity. If a normal cell is infected by a virus, its surface expression of MHC class I molecules is altered or diminished and, thus, it becomes a target for NK cell cytotoxicity.

Antibody-mediated cellular cytotoxicity (ADCC) is an alternative method by which NK cells interact with target cells, involving the cooperation of antibodies, which first bind to the infected target cell and then link to Fc-receptors present on the NK cell surface, thus triggering an antibody-specific cytotoxic activation of the NK cell. This is a link between the *innate immune system* and the *adaptive immune system* to be described in section.

3. THE ADAPTIVE IMMUNE SYSTEM

The *adaptive* or *acquired immune response* takes over if the innate response cannot clear an infection in a short time. The "handover" is achieved through a series of messenger proteins called cytokines. The cells that participate in the adaptive response are also white cells, as in the innate response, but they are specialized because they can distinguish self from nonself antigens. The majority of cells in the adaptive system are either *T or B lymphocytes*. Although the acquired response is highly effective, it is not as rapidly active as the innate response and may take between 7 and 14 d to become fully effective. Although even the simplest unicellular animals have at least a rudimentary innate immune defense system, the adaptive response is first seen, in terms of evolution, in the vertebrates. The components that comprise this highly complex and specific immune defense network are described in the following sections.

3.1. Anatomical Components of the Adaptive Immune System

The adaptive immune system comprises a series of distinct organs and tissues that are interconnected by the blood and lymphatic systems. The primary lymphoid organs are the areas where the lymphocytes originate, whereas the secondary lymphoid organs are areas where the naïve lymphocyte meets with foreign antigens, which stimulates clonal expansion and subsequent maturation as effector cells.

3.1.1. PRIMARY LYMPHOID TISSUES

There are two primary lymphoid tissues in the adult human: the bone marrow and thymus. Most lymphopoiesis (lymphocyte production) occurs in adult life in the B-cell population in the marrow of the flat bones of the ribs, sternum and vertebrae.

Bone marrow is the major hematopoietic (red-cell production) organ in the human body. All blood cell types, except mature T lymphocytes, can be found within the extensive cavities that comprise the bone marrow. The marrow provides not only a store for progenitor cells but also the growth factors essential for differentiation and proliferation of the various blood cells. The reticular stroma of the marrow matrix contains macrophages and adipocytes that are important in the supply of cytokines that are essential for B-cell development and maturation in the bone marrow.

The *thymus* is the primary site of T-lymphocyte development. It is a bilobar organ that resides in the anterior mediastinum, with the base resting on the heart. More than 95% of the progenitor T cells that travel to the thymus die by a process of programmed cell death, known as apoptosis; the remaining cells possess the appropriate T-cell receptor repertoire to ensure the host's survival.

3.1.2. SECONDARY LYMPHOID TISSUES

In the human, the secondary lymphoid tissues comprise the spleen, lymph nodes, and *mucosa-associated lymphoid tissue (MALT)*, which lines the respiratory, GI, and reproductive tracts.

The spleen is composed of two main compartments, the red pulp and white pulp. The former contains effete red blood cells that are ready for disposal, whereas the latter is dense lymphoid tissue. The follicles and marginal zones of the white pulp contain mainly B cells; the T cells are the chief occupants of the periarteriolar sheath.

The lymph node contains two major areas within its bean-shaped structure, the medulla at the center that contains a mixture of T cells, B cells, and macrophages, surrounded by the cortex, which is predominantly a B-cell site. The B cells in the cortex organize themselves into clusters, termed follicles, which enlarge during an active immune response to form germinal centers that contain large numbers of B-lymphoblasts, surrounded by resting small B cells.

MALT includes tonsils and adenoids, Peyer's patches, the appendix, and bronchial and mammary tissue. These tissues contain many follicles, as described, for the lymph node, but the subepithelial lamina propria of the intestine, which is part of the MALT, contains many diffusely distributed lymphocytes, many of which are large granular lymphocytes. The gut also has its own variant mast cell.

3.2. Cells Involved in the Adaptive Immune System

3.2.1. B LYMPHOCYTES (B CELLS)

B cells are derived from a hematopoietic stem cell that differentiates along a pathway that can be subdivided into several developmental stages, characterized by the rearrangement status of the Ig heavy- and light-chain genes and the expression of a sequence of differential surface markers. The variety and arrangement of these genes is such that at least 10^8 different specificities can be generated. A single B cell, however, will have antigen receptors with identical combining sites. These B-cell antigen receptors, together with the secreted antibodies (discussed in Section 3.3.1.), occur as five immunoglobulin classes, known as IgM, IgG, IgA, IgE, and IgD, where the amino acid sequences of their heavy chains differ. Precursor B lymphocytes express IgM heavy chains in association with two smaller polypeptide chains, V_{pre-B} and $\lambda 5$. The IgM heavy chain, which serves as a receptor on the precursor B cell, is involved in a maturation stage where the pre-B cell produces light chains that associate with cytoplasmic μ chains, to be expressed on the surface of the immature B cell as antigen-specific surface IgM (sIgM). The signals that assist in this maturation stage are provided in the bone marrow by stromal cells, which secrete stem cell factor and IL-7. Many of the pre-B cells do not mature but undergo apoptosis either because they do not rearrange the genes that encode functional antigen receptors or they may generate receptors specific for host tissue components. Binding of these receptors to self-antigen triggers apoptosis and helps to reduce autoreactivity.

Mature unactivated B cells leave the bone marrow, expressing both IgM and IgD on their surface, together with a low level of MHC class II molecules. The B cell leaves the bloodstream and enters the T-cell-rich region of a secondary lymphoid tissue, such as the paracortex of a lymph node. If it does not encounter its target antigen, it passes through and returns to the circulation. If it meets a nonself foreign antigen for which it expresses the specific receptor, binding to this receptor will cause both the receptor and the antigen to be internalized. Once inside the B cell, the antigen is degraded and processed into a peptide-MHC class II complex, which is reexpressed on the B-cell surface. The naïve B cell is not normally activated by antigen alone but requires a costimulatory signal to initiate full activation. This may be delivered by a helper CD4-positive (CD4+) *T cell* with a T cell-antigen receptor (TCR) that recognizes the MHC class II-peptide complex on the B-cell surface. Once activated, naïve B cells enlarge and turn into lymphoblasts. Some of these lymphoblasts mature into *plasma cells*, which no longer display Ig molecules upon their surface but secrete large quantities of antibody specific for the stimulating antigen. Other B lymphoblasts return to the resting state and become *memory cells*, specific for the original stimulating antigen. If these memory cells are reexposed to the same peptide or a similar cross-reactive peptide, a rapid and more vigorous secondary response occurs.

3.2.2. T Lymphocytes (T Cells)

T-cell precursors leave the bone marrow at an early developmental stage and travel to the thymus and migrate to the outer margin of the cortex, where they are known as thymocytes. After a short time in the thymus, the thymocyte begins to express the β chain of its TCR, which associates with a polypeptide chain termed $pT\alpha$ and, like the pre-B-cell receptor, this pre-T-cell receptor plays a further part in maturation, leading to the expression of both α and β TCR chains specific for antigen and MHC. As with B cells, the variable region of the T-cell α and β chains are randomly selected from a vast pool, giving a large repertoire of specificities.

Several polypeptides, γ, δ,ε, and ζ, collectively known as CD3, associate with the TCR on the cell surface. When the T-cell receptor binds to the MHC-antigen complex on the T-cell surface, the CD3 complex passes an intracellular signal, via a series of tyrosine, threonine, and serine kinase enzymes, to the nucleus, leading to gene activation. At the thymocytic stage, each cell also bears both a *CD4* and a *CD8* surface glycoprotein molecule. Cells that survive the selection process and become mature T cells will express only one of these two molecules, normally in the ratio of 65% CD4+ T cells to 35% CD8+

B cells, although this may change in certain diseases (e.g., in HIV infection, where the numbers of CD4+ cells are drastically reduced). *CD4+ T cells always recognize antigen presented in association with MHC class II molecules, and CD8+ T cells always recognize antigen presented in association with MHC class I molecules.* The CD4 molecule interacts with the β_2 domain of MHC class II, and CD8 with the α_3 domain of MHC class I.

Mature T cells not only display different surface markers, but also have different functional properties. Some T lymphocytes are equipped to kill virally infected cells, and these are known as *cytotoxic T lymphocytes* (T_C). These are usually CD8+ T cells. Other T cells help to mount an immune response and are known as *helper T lymphocytes* (Th), and these are CD4+ T cells. The helper T cells differ in their ability to produce various cytokine combinations and, thus, will either stimulate *cell-mediated* or antibody-mediated immunity. Thus, one population, termed *Th1* cells, produce, among other cytokines, IFN-γ and IL-2. IFN-γ stimulates macrophages, and IL-2 stimulates cytotoxic T cells, both of which are cell-mediated immune responses. Another population of helper T cells, *Th2*, produce IL-4 and IL-10 that stimulate B cells to produce antibody. This is not an absolute distinction, because Th1 cells can stimulate some antibody isotypes. The progenitor of both helper types is the Th0 cell. Th1 cell production is stimulated by IL-2 derived from dendritic cells and macrophages, whereas Th2 cell production is stimulated by IL-4 derived from a subpopulation of NK cells or from $\gamma\delta$T cells. Antigens presented at high concentration or antigens with a high avidity promote Th1 cell production, whereas antigens presented at high concentration or those with low avidity promote Th2 cell production.

3.3. Proteins in the Adaptive Immune System

3.3.1. IMMUNOGLOBULINS

Immunoglobulins are produced by all vertebrates and are secreted by specialized B cells (plasma cells). Because they recognize antigens, they have also been given the alternative title of *antibodies*. A typical antibody is composed of four polypeptide chains linked by disulfide bonds. The molecule is asymmetric, having two longer chains (heavy chains) together with a shorter chain (light chain) on either side of each heavy chain, making four chains in all. The combined amino-terminal end of each heavy-light chain pair comprises the antigen-binding site; thus, there are two antigen-binding sites per Ig molecule. In any one Ig molecule, the heavy chains are identical, as are the light chains. The carboxy-terminal end of each heavy chain serves several functions when the opposite end binds its specific antigen. During early investigations of the antibody molecule, scientists used enzymes to digest parts of the chains to get smaller and, therefore, simpler examination techniques to elucidate their structure. Papain digestion yielded two fragments that still retained the ability to recognize antigen, and these were designated *Fab* fragments (fragment of antigen binding). The remaining fragment was easy to crystallize and was, therefore, termed *Fc* (fragment crystallizable). The Ig is often depicted in illustrations as a Y-shaped molecule and, in this arrangement, the Fab portion is on the two arms that point upward, with the two antigen-binding domains at the tip of each of the arms. The Fc portion is on the single upright part of the letter Y, so that the bottom of the letter would be the part of the molecule that binds to cellular Fc receptors.

Both light and heavy chains are composed of a series of globular subunits termed domains. Each domain is made up of approx 110 amino acids and is folded specially (biochemists call it a β-pleated sheet) to make a cylindric molecule. There is much similarity between the various light and heavy chain domains, with the exception of the amino-terminal domain, which shows a marked degree of variation in its amino acid residues. This region is, therefore, termed a variable domain, whereas the other domains that vary comparatively little from each other are termed constant. Light chains consist of one variable and one constant domain (V_L and C_L), and heavy chains contain one variable (V_H) and three or four constant domains (C_H1, C_H2, $C_H3 \pm C_H4$), depending on the antibody class. Within the variable domains of both the light and the heavy chains there are hypervariable regions, which, when folded, are close to each other to provide the different antigenic specificities necessary to form the antigen-binding site.

In man, there are five classes of Ig: IgG, IgA, IgM, IgD, and IgE. These show important differences between the constant regions of their heavy chains, and IgG and IgA are further subdivided into subclasses. IgG, IgD, and IgE are monomeric (that is, they are composed of only the Y-shaped molecule). IgA is often dimeric (two Ys joined tail to tail), and IgM is pentameric (five Ys joined at the tail). The heavy chains of each class are given their equivalent Greek letter; for instance, the heavy chain of IgM is termed the μ chain. There are two types of light chain, κ or λ, although the two light chains in any single Ig molecule are always the same. The immune system must be capable of recognizing a diversity of pathogens and has evolved a complex genetic system to achieve this. The light- and heavy-chain genes are carried on different chromosomes, and, as with other macromolecular systems, the genes are divided into coding segments (exons) and silent segments (introns). The heavy-chain gene is on chromosome 14 and is composed of small groups of exons coding for the constant regions of the heavy chains and several V region genes (10^3). Two small sets of exons, D and J, come between the V and C genes. Thus, if a B cell is producing IgM, one V region gene is selected and is joined to one D and J in the chromosome. The product, the V_H domain, is joined at the level of RNA processing to Cμ. The same cell could make IgG by omitting the Cμ and joining $V_H - D_J$ to Cγ. Antibody diversity is complex, and a full and lucid account may be found in Alberts et al. *(3)*.

3.3.2. CELL-SURFACE RECEPTORS

There are literally thousands of receptors on any one cell in the immune series, so this section is necessarily a compressed summary to give a general view of the concepts involved. The MHC was first recognized in the context of organ transplantation reactions. In the human, molecules of the MHC are still often referred to as the human leukocyte antigens (HLA). There are two principal classes of MHC molecules: class I and class II. They are the most polymorphic proteins known and play a crucial role in the presentation of foreign antigens. Class I presents to cytotoxic T cells (CD8+), and class II presents to helper T cells (CD4+). Class I molecules are expressed on almost all vertebrate cells, whereas class II molecules appear only on cells that interact with helper T cells, such as B cells and macrophages. The class I molecule is composed of a large α polypeptide chain and a smaller polypeptide chain known as β_2-microglobulin. The α-chain contains three domains, α1, α2, and α3; the α1 and α2 domains are distal to the cell membrane and form the antigen-binding groove. The α3 domain, together with the β_2-microglobulin, is proximal to the cell membrane, part of the α3 domain passing through the membrane into the cytosol. The MHC class II molecule is a heterodimer of α and β polypeptide chains, each containing two domains (α1,α2 and β1,β2), with α2 and β2 passing through the cell membrane. Both MHC class I and class II molecules are members of the Ig superfamily. There are three major class I molecules (HLA-A, -B and -C) and three major class II molecules (HLA-DP,-DQ and-DR). MHC restriction is a way to capturing antigens from different intracellular compartments and presenting them, in modified form, to effector cells. Endogenous antigens, such as viruses, are processed in the cytoplasm of the infected cell and transported as small peptides to the endoplasmic reticulum (ER) by shuttle proteins known as transporters associated with antigen processing (TAP-1 and TAP-2). The TAP proteins deliver the peptides to MHC class I molecules in the ER, where the peptide-MHC-complex is delivered to the cell surface for presentation to CD8+ cytotoxic T cells. Exogenous antigens are processed in endosomes and presented at the cell surface in association with MHC class II molecules to CD4+ helper T cells.

Adhesion molecules are a large and diverse family of cell-surface glycoproteins, which, as their name suggests, facilitate immune responses by mediating cell-cell adhesion or cell-extracellular matrix adhesion. Antigen presentation in the appropriate MHC molecule to the specific T-cell receptor is not sufficient to activate the immune response. The adhesion molecules can supply the coreceptor signal that is necessary to complete the activation signal sequence. There are four major families of adhesion molecule: integrins, selectins, cadherins, and members of the Ig superfamily. Although these are all structurally different, they are molecules that have come to serve the same function during the course of evolution.

Cytokine receptors gain their specificity from that part of the receptor that resides on the cell surface. Once the cytokine has attached to its specific receptor, the signal sent goes through one of two common intracellular signaling pathways to deliver either a stimulatory or an inhibitory signal to the nucleus. The cytokines include the ever-growing family of *ILs*, the *chemokines* (cytokines that induce leukocyte *chemotaxis*), the *IFNs*, and various other growth and inhibitory factors, such as TNF.

4. SUMMARY

This has been a necessarily brief review of the human immune system that occupies between 600 and 900 pages in the specialist textbooks. The summary is, therefore, even smaller, though maybe as important, for the nonspecialist reader.

We have seen that the majority of infections can be dealt with by the innate immune system, sometimes with a little help from the adaptive immune system. For some diseases, only the acquired immune mechanism is powerful enough, and even this is defeated on occasions. Vaccines stimulate parts of the adaptive system to produce immunologic memory that speeds antibody production when the infective agent invades the body. These antibodies may prevent the microbe from binding to its preferred receptor and also cause its phagocytosis through opsonization, or they may neutralize the toxins produced by the microorganism.

Hypersensitivity reactions are a common cause of disease, mediated by the immune system reacting to a range of antigens and *atopy*, which is an immediate hypersensitivity reaction to environmental antigens, mediated by IgE (Type I hypersensitivity). *Allergy*, in general, is on the increase, especially through the Th2-helper T cell, IgE, mast cell route. One theory to explain this is that this defense form evolved to fight worm infestations, which are uncommon in the developed world today. Also, because our modern lifestyle may be "too hygienic," the decline in bacterial infections has skewed the immune system in the direction of the Th2 response (*see also* Chapter 17 "Probiotics and Immunomodulation," Section 4.1.).

Autoimmunity is also a problem that is increasing. This may occur through one of three mechanisms: (1) type II hypersensitivity through the direct action of antibodies, (2) type III caused by circulating immune complexes formation, or (3) *type IV or delayed type hypersensitivity*. Autoimmunity represents the breakdown of self-tolerance. Immunodeficiency may be the result of a primary defect in the immune system or a secondary factor. The primary deficiencies are usually genetic in origin, whereas the secondary immunodeficiencies are caused by infection or certain drugs, for example, HIV-1 infection.

The immune system, both innate and acquired, despite the aberrations listed, is remarkably efficient, considering the thousands of assaults it receives each day. References *1*, *4*, and *5* supply the answers to the many gaps left by this brief review.

REFERENCES

1. Janeway CA, Travers P, Walport M, Shlomchik M. Immunobiology: The Immune System in Health and Disease. Garland Science Publishing, New York, 2001.
2. Imler JL, Hoffmann JA. Toll receptors in drosophila: a family of molecules regulating development and immunity. Curr Top Microbiol Immunol 2002;270:63–79.
3. Alberts B, Bray D, Lewis J, Raff M, Roberts K, Watson JD. Molecular Biology of the Cell (3rd ed.) Garland Science Publishing, New York, 1994, pp. 1221–1227.
4. Nairn R, Helbert M. Immunology for Medical Students. Mosby International, London, 2002.
5. MacKay I, Rosen F. Innate immunity. N Engl J Med 2000;343:338–344.

2 Assessment of Human Immune Response

Susanna Cunningham-Rundles

1. INTRODUCTION

The concept that nutrients are cofactors in the development, maintenance, and expression of immune response is based on observations in many fields, including nutrition, immunology, epidemiology, infectious disease, perinatology, geriatrics, cancer, and genetics *(1–10)*. Nutritional immunology, as a cross-disciplinary field, is emerging from widely ranging studies showing how specific nutrients regulate immune response *(11–17)*. Mechanisms of nutrient action often involve several pathways and produce a range of phenotypic effects. For example, experimental vitamin B_{12} (cobalamin) deficiency causes megaloblastic anemia in humans and also reduces complement factor C3, immunoglobulin (Ig)M, and IgG and increases IgE by causing a shift from a T helper type-1 (Th1) to a T helper type-2 (Th2) response *(2)*. Human B_{12} deficiency is associated with increased CD8+ T-cell number and natural killer (NK) activity *(18)*. Vitamins A and D have been intensively studied as critical regulators of gene expression in both growth and immune development. Vitamin A deficiency impedes retinol dependent signals during embryonic development, whereas supplementation enhances the Th2 response to viruses, as shown for influenza *(19–21)*. Vitamin D acts as a nuclear receptor for target genes and also has a regulatory influence on immune response by affecting immune cell differentiation *(12,22,23)*. Studies such as these may illustrate basic elements of experimental design for studies of nutrients' mechanisms of action on the immune system.

Key questions for the future center on whether different immune mechanisms are affected according to level of deficiency, if specific immune compartments might be differentially affected, and whether there are critical differences in mechanism of action obtained when the same nutrient is used differently, such as nutrient repletion in deficiency, nutrient supplementation in the absence of deficiency, or using nutrients in pharmacologic doses as immune modulators. Study setting will also profoundly affect the type of study design. For example, the work of Arifeen et al. has suggested that when low birth weight is caused by chronic intrauterine undernourishment, catch-up growth is limited, despite normal growth rate in the first months of life *(6)*. Thus, when studying infant growth in an environment with restricted access to food, one must consider perinatal factors, endemic infections, and other potentially interacting variables. Inequities in groups or the presence of unrecognized factors may confound interpretation and, when

From: *Diet and Human Immune Function*
Edited by: D. A. Hughes, L. G. Darlington, and A. Bendich © Humana Press Inc., Totowa, NJ

these can be clarified, prove revealing. Studies of the effects of eicosapentaenoic acid (EPA) given as a fish oil supplement on circulating levels of adhesion molecules have shown different results in different age groups *(8)*. A recent population study of risk for esophageal and gastric cancer showed that β-carotene, folate, and vitamins C and B$_6$ were associated with risk reduction among controls when compared with subjects with cancer *(24)*. However, Mayne et al. showed that this difference may result from the specific source of nutrients *(24)*. Increased intake of micronutrients from plants reduced cancer risk, whereas increased micronutrient intake from animal sources was associated with cancer, suggesting that the presence of other dietary elements, such as animal fat, might have overwhelmed protection.

Differences in large studies that evaluate the effects of dietary factors in reducing the risk of specific diseases or outcome occur for many reasons. In some cases, the difference may occur because of design elements; in other cases, secondary predisposing factors may dilute or offset protection. In most current studies, genetic differences in the host were not evaluated. Clearly, fundamental studies are needed to determine how nutrient status influences the development and expression of host genes involved in the immune response. Bendich *(25)* has proposed that immune function tests should be considered when determining the recommended dietary allowance (RDA) of certain nutrients, because the levels of several micronutrients needed to support optimal immune function may be different from those needed to support other functions. Likely settings where conventionally developed normal ranges are inadequate may include chronic illnesses that cause increased stress on immune response. Zinc is an example of such a nutrient: low, normal, or marginal range levels are associated with impaired immune function in chronic anemia, epidermolysis bullosa (a serious genetic skin disorder), and cancer *(26,27)*.

Because of technological advances in the basic study of immune response during the past 5 yr, investigators in this cross-disciplinary field will increasingly have much better tools to study these complex questions. Advances in the fundamental biology of immune responses have led to a different conception of immunity, which places major emphasis on the microenvironment, where nutrient factors are likely to exert specific effects in real time. In this chapter, key nutritional elements currently identified as central to normal immune function are discussed in terms of how experimental design and methods were used to investigate specific issues. A general survey of possible methodologic approaches is presented. Current and future studies will likely illuminate many of the controversial findings in nutritional immunology and build the foundation for the next stage of this rapidly developing field.

2. STUDY OF NUTRIENT-IMMUNE INTERACTION

Current approaches to immune evaluation typically include assessment of both in vitro immune cell differentiation and assay of in vivo immune function. The effect of nutrients on immune response can depend on the site of action, e.g., the gastrointestinal-associated lymphoid tissue (GALT), thymus, spleen, regional lymph nodes, or immune cells of the circulating blood *(28,29)*. The same nutrient may have a different mechanism of action at different sites. For example, zinc may potentiate Th1 responses systemically *(30)* and Th2 responses at the GALT level *(31)*. Investigation of nutrient-immune interaction usually begins with an observation that leads to a series of initial questions and a hypothesis. Two such events in the history of nutritional immunology are Smythe et al.'s hypothesis *(32)* that immune or "thymolymphatic" deficiency is the basic cause of susceptibility to infectious disease in protein calorie malnutrition (PCM) and hypothesis of Prasad and Sanstead's hypothesis *(33)* that conditioned zinc deficiency secondary to phytate in the diet was the central etiologic factor in a clinical syndrome of infections and growth retardation. A general approach to investigational and experimental studies of nutritional immunology is described in the following discussion.

2.1. The Human Setting

Defining the study group, setting and assessing the possible interaction of other factors, such as role of endemic infection, is essential experimental design. Clinical presentation is vital. For example, malnutrition's effect on susceptibility to infection differs in clinically distinguishable forms of PCM, such as marasmus, which is a chronic wasting condition, or kwashiorkor, which is characterized by edema and anemia *(34,35)*. Stunting has been considered as an adaptive response to limited food availability and may be associated with effective response to intracellular pathogens. Assessing risk factors for malaria in children in Papua, New Guinea, Genton et al. *(36)* found that increased height for weight at baseline (an indicator of a good nutritional state) predicted greater susceptibility to malaria during the study that correlated with lower cytokine response to malarial antigens among the better nourished children. The benefit of nutritional habilitation is affected by timing and setting. Thus, some investigators have found that refeeding in certain environments worsened malaria, whereas others have reported that well-nourished subjects were less susceptible to malaria *(37,38)*.

Consideration of study group heterogeneity is critical to determine the size of the study required to draw inferences, perform hypothesis testing, or establish fundamental relationships. Developmental stage, as well as age, has clearly emerged as a critical variable in human immune response. Neonates and infants rely primarily on innate immunity, specifically complement, maternal antibody, circulating mediators of the inflammatory response, and phagocytes, but these components of innate immunity are not as functional in young children as they are in adults *(39)*. Pathogens, such as parasitic infections or viruses, may easily compromise the innate immune system, and, when malnutrition is present, the overall development and expression of immune response is significantly impaired *(40,41)*. Studies on the deterioration of immune response involve changes in nutrient intake, metabolism, and age-related immune regulation. Aging often leads to reduced response to immunization, but this state is conditional and, perhaps, reversible, as suggested by studies demonstrating micronutrients' enhancing effects *(42,43)*.

With rare exceptions, gender differences have not been considered in nutritional immunology, but there is a growing body of evidence that endocrine differences affect both innate and adaptive immune response. Examples include response to experimental Coxsackie's B3 infection *(44)* and to shock-related cytokine release of interleukin-1β (IL-1β) and interleukin 6 (IL-6) by the human macrophage *(45)*. Endocrine regulation of immune response is affected by nutritional status, as shown in studies of changes in growth hormone levels in malnourished children during repletion *(46)*. Zamboni et al. have reported high basal growth hormone (GH) levels, but reduced GH receptors in malnourished children *(46)*. Other studies have shown that serum leptin levels and insulin-like growth factor-1 (IGF-1) are reduced in both marasmus and kwashiorkor, suggesting that nutrient deprivation may lead to decreased fat mass, insulin, and, possibly, IGF-1, suppressing leptin, which may, in turn, stimulate the hypothalamic pituitary adrenal axis to increase cortisol and GH secretion *(47)*. Because cortisol also affects cytokine secretion as part of the stress response, it is likely that gender differences do occur, by analogy, with the effects of traumatic injury *(45)*.

Whether comparisons are based upon highly stratified or relatively heterogeneous groups, questions of significance usually rest on whether the immune parameter being studied is within the normal range. Use of concurrent published data is an inadequate substitute for parallel controls during the study. Historical controls, even when studied by the same investigators, also pose problems, because presentation, treatment, or methods of evaluation may have changed. Intrasubject variation in normal human immune responses may be relatively great *(48,49)*. This variability can also be magnified by immune assays that do not adequately consider that the maximum response of normal controls to any activator may occur at different antigen concentrations. The establishment of strong laboratory methods requires that the response's kinetics be evaluated in a large group of controls over a range of concentrations so that normal ranges are sufficiently encompassing. Laboratory controls are highly informative for internal technical quality control when run in parallel with subject studies. Study controls should include fresh samples from subjects matched for age, sex, and clinical status. Cryopreserved cells from all subjects can be used for assessment of changes over the length of study for many immunologic assays. There may be changes in some cellular phenotypes that may be partly condition related. For example, thawing causes a significant loss of B cells from HIV+ donors *(50)*. Other changes that have been observed in normal donors include increased secretion of interferon gamma, apparently caused by regulatory cells that are affected by the freezing process *(51)*.

2.2. Evaluation of Immune Cell Phenotypes

Assessment of human immune response usually begins with an evaluation of immunophenotype, which measures the relative and absolute number of cells of the adaptive and innate immune system in peripheral blood at a specific time. Measurement of changes in the frequency and number of circulating lymphocyte subpopulations in the course of observation, or dietary intervention, is now so well standardized in flow cytometric procedures that permit direct comparisons with other studies. Attention should be placed on reagent choice and controls. If nonstandard reagents or combined reagents from various sources are used, titrations must be performed and antibody combinations must be compared with single-source premixes of reagents to avoid spectral interference. When using three or more colors, anchor gate selection must be unambiguous to avoid incorrect inferences. Preparation for studies should include standardized performance of immunophenotyping, correcting for purity of the gating region, quantitative recovery of the cell type, and positive identification of cellular subsets *(52)*. For human studies, a complete blood count (CBC) and differential are needed to quantify effects on absolute numbers of cells. It is essential that the baseline evaluation include parallel studies providing a CBC, hematologic analysis of hemoglobin, hematocrit, etc. on an aliquot of the same blood specimen. The parallel studies must be included because in acute conditions, there may be major shifts in the relative percentage of lymphocytes that will affect the significance of the data.

The immune system has, until recently, been viewed as two essentially separate systems responding to the evolving needs of the organism to defend against pathogens: the innate system and the adaptive systems. The innate system, which mediates an immediate immune reaction that is independent of specific antigen, recognizes microbial "nonself" through identifying conserved microbial products, pathogen-associated molecular patterns (PAMPS), and "self" via specific gene products, so that, in addition to unique microbial motifs, the infected or pathologically altered self can be identified as missing or altered self (53,54). Monoclonal antibodies can be used to distinguish innate immune system cells in depth, including monocytes, macrophages, several NK cells, and dendritic cells, as well as identify pattern recognition receptors for PAMPS (54–56).

Adaptive immunity has been divided by cell type and origin as the response of bone marrow-derived B cells belonging to the humoral immune system and thymus-derived T cells of the cellular immune system. The adaptive immune system, which develops specific responses to antigen after encounter, depends on a primary T-cell response in secondary lymphoid organs. Through antigen encounter, the T-cell polyclonal response is refined into a more restricted T-cell repertoire in a process that resembles the affinity maturation of B cells (57). Regulation of these processes is highly affected by the differentiation and activation state of the specific T-cells and antigen-presenting cells and is also modulated by innate immune cellular products. This differentiation of cell function and cell–cell interactions is determined by the local microenvironment; for example, the liver contains innate immune cells, such as NK T cells that have distinct cytokine secretion patterns (58). Significant thymic-independent T-cell differentiation also occurs in the gastrointestinal tract (GI) tract, where specialized intraepithelial lymphocytes reside (59). The complexity of these interactions can be approached experimentally through evaluation of coreceptor expression and memory phenotype, as well as emerging functional studies, which increasingly target defined cellular populations.

Lymphocyte development and differentiation are directly affected by malnutrition. Studies show that T cells from children with severe PCM are immature compared with those from well-nourished children and that the degree of immaturity is directly associated with thymic involution as measured by echoradiography (60). Although nutritional repletion improved anthropometric measurements within 1 mo, regrowth of the thymus took more time. Although this could reflect a generally greater stress sensitivity of the thymus to nutrient depletion, the investigators found that adding zinc to the repletion regimen shortened the thymus' recovery time by 50% (61). These differences were discovered through judicious use of a historical cohort group. Table 1 provides selected examples of the effects of controlled nutrient supplementation on immune cells. Comparisons of micronutrient effects in the same subjects can be especially informative. Evaluating the effects of vitamin A and zinc in a randomized double-blind four-arm trial of zinc and vitamin A in more than 100 elderly subjects, Fortes et al. (62) observed that 25 mg/d of zinc increased the number of CD4+HLA-DR+ T cells and, to a lesser degree, cytotoxic cells. In contrast, 800 µg/d of vitamin retinyl palmitate was associated with a reduction in CD4+ T cells.

2.3. Assessment of Immune Function In Vitro

Immune functional studies can now be conducted as defined studies of immune cell subsets cultured in highly standardized systems using a chosen stimulus and a range of

Table 1

Immune Methodology in Studies of Nutrient Supplementation In Vivo

Method: Assay	Specificity	Setting	Response to supplementation	Reference
Immune phenotyping: flow cytometric analysis of immune subpopulations	Monoclonal antibody detection of surface antigens	Zinc: 25 mg/d elderly	↑ CD4+ T cells	(61)
		Methyl B$_{12}$: single injection/B$_{12}$ deficient patients	↑ CD8+ T cells	(18)
		Early/late parenteral nutrition/ trauma	Early nutrient support ↑ CD4+ T-cell number (and response in vitro)	(94)
		Vitamin D$_3$: 1–2 µg/d women	↑ CD3+ CD8+ T cells	(106)
Proliferative response in vitro to activator: thymidine incor- poration	Activator (mitogen or antigen)	Vitamin E: 233 mg/d healthy persons	↑ Proliferative response to PHA	(69)
		Vitamin E: 100 mg/d elderly	No effect	(70)
		Vitamin E: 200 mg/d elderly	↑ Proliferative response to PHA	(71)
Phagocytosis: uptake of particles or bacteria	Nonspecific innate function	1 g Vitamin C + 200 mg E/d elderly women, both healthy and chronically ill	↑ Neutrophil phagocytosis (also ↑ lymphoproliferation, ↓ serum cortisol and lipid peroxides)	(77)
Cytokine production: ELISA or intracellular cytokine	Monoclonal antibody	β-carotene: 15 mg/d healthy persons	↑ Monocyte TNF-α secretion	(78)
		Enteral feed/trauma	Normalization of cytokine response	(92)
Antibody: response to immunization	Antibody titer	Zinc: 20 mg/d elderly	Zinc and selenium ↑ antibody response to influenza virus	(103)
	Microvirus neutralization	Vitamin A: 7.5–15 mg retinol equivalent/infants	No effect on antibody titer or rate of seroconversion to polio virus 1, 2, or 3	(102)
Skin-test response: delayed type hypersensitivity (DTH)	Antigen specific	Vitamin E: 60–800 mg/d elderly	Dose-related ↑ in DTH (also antibody response to hepatitis B but not diphtheria), no effect on T or B cells	(104)

PHA, phytohemagglutinin; ELISA, enzyme-linked immunosorbent assay; TNF, tumor necrosis factor.

22

endpoints. Although several tests are available, the time required to establish them appropriately is significant (63–66). A basic panel of tests is also useful to detect how the overall balance of the immune system has been affected. Newer methods have made it possible to assess the differentiation of antigen expression on peripheral blood mononuclear cells in response to activation, to study early events in the activation pathway, and to analyze gene expression. In vitro methods are especially useful in analyzing the effects of specific single nutrients under defined conditions, as illustrated by the examples in Table 2. In the mouse, Wallace et al. (67) have shown that dietary fatty acids directly influence the production of Th1 cytokines in vivo and in vitro. Studies, such as those of Hughes (68), demonstrating that n–3 polyunsaturated fatty acids regulate antigen-presenting cell function, have used in vitro methods to address related questions in humans.

The most widely applied methods to evaluate human T-lymphocyte activation have used peripheral blood mononuclear cells isolated by density gradient centrifugation and cultured with plant lectins (mitogens), bacterial or viral activators, or antigens, which elicit a secondary response that depends on previous priming or natural exposure in vivo (52). Immune activators used in the study of immune response are either specific antigens or nonspecific activators. Unless there is concurrent infection, the peripheral blood lymphocyte is a resting cell but can respond to nonspecific triggers or to previously encountered antigens in appropriately sensitive systems. The nonspecific signal is often a plant lectin, but other activators, such as certain divalent cations, calcium ionophores, or surface-reactive molecules, including monoclonal antibodies to CD3 (which binds to the T-cell receptor, TCR), can provide a strong T-lymphocyte signal.

The typical mononuclear cell culture contains a mixture of T cells, B cells, and monocytes. After several days in culture, the cells are pulse-labeled with a radioactive precursor (usually thymidine), and incorporation is measured by assessing their incorporation into DNA. The amount of incorporated tracer is closely related to the amount of DNA synthesis and ensuing cell division. The use of whole blood diluted and cultured in the presence of activators also provides a mononuclear cell response index but is fundamentally different, because the concentration of cells is not standardized, as it is when mononuclear cells are isolated from whole blood. However, the advantage of this kind of ex vivo test is that plasma proteins and soluble factors present in blood are not removed (63,69).

Functional studies should be conducted on fresh anticoagulated blood whenever possible (or on blood that has been diluted and stored at room temperature in the dark for fewer than 24 h). There may be differences between venous and arterial blood. When the blood should be drawn is important. Generally, most data have been obtained with blood that was drawn in the morning, because circadian effects on hormones and immune cell phenotypes may influence results.

Initial immune function studies usually begin with a general assessment of response in vitro to a mitogen, another nonspecific activator, or an antigen and are generally based on cell division assay at the peak of response after microtiter plate culture for several days. Culture methods profoundly affect results, and conditions must be optimized according to kinetics of response. Responses measured under most conditions favor T-cell proliferation as the most prevalent lymphocyte in peripheral blood. The elicited composite response is highly quantitative. Thus, as shown in Table 1, differences in the

Table 2
Immune Methodology in Studies of Nutrient Modulation In Vitro

Nutrient	Experimental approach	Observation	Mechanism of action	Reference
Glutamine	Transcription of early activation cytokine markers, production, proliferation, and cytotoxic function	↑ Cytokine production, proliferation, and killer cell activity but not early IL-2, IL-2 R, IL-4, or IFN-γ	Posttranscriptional immune response	(74)
N–3 PUFAs DHA and EPA	Effect on monocyte MHC class II and cytokine response	EPA but not DHA ↓ HLA-DR on monocytes, DHA ↑ HLA-DR on unstimulated monocytes, both ↓ gamma interferon response	N–3 PUFAs show differential regulation of antigen presenting cell function	(67)
β-carotene	Natural killer cell activity	Dose-related ↑ cytotoxic effect in vitro, no correlation in vivo	Local effect, immunologic significance unclear	(101)
Vitamin C	Chronic or acute HIV infection of human lymphoid cell lines	High levels of vitamin C ↓ viral replication	↑ Uptake resulting from ↑ glucose transporter, viral ↓ caused by NF-κB inhibition	(96)
Vitamin D	Effect of Vitamin D3 on cultured PBMC and oral pulse in vivo	↓ HLA-DR expression and ↑ superoxide production; also in vivo	Regulation of function through genetic expression	(73)
Vitamin E	Effects on cyclic adenosine monophosphate (cAMP) response element binding (CREB) family proteins	Vitamin E had abolished effect of prostaglandin (PG) E_2 on CREB1 and enhanced CREB2, partly reversed by PGE_2 in T lymphocytes	Reciprocal regulation of T-cell signaling	(82)
Zinc	Th1/Th2 cytokine production after zinc depletion/repletion in vivo	↓ Th1 cytokine production in depletion, ↑ with repletion	Zinc required for generation of new CD4+ T cells	(109)
Selenium	Proliferative response to PHA	Se↑ response in vitro; also correlated with PHA response after supplementation in vivo	Activation of IL-2 response	(100)
Iron	Alveolar macrophages cultured with and without iron chelators activated with lipopolysaccharides	Chelation of iron ↑ IL-1β release not TNF-α	Iron shifts affect inflammatory response	(79)

IL, Interleukin; IFN, interferon; PUFA, polyunsaturated fatty acid; DHA, docosahexaenoic acid; EPA, eicosapentaenoic acid; NF, nuclear factor.

effect of vitamin E supplementation in vivo on proliferative response in vitro may be dose related *(70–72)*. Whole blood methodology can also be used for proliferative studies *(62)*. Under appropriate culture conditions, whole blood culture can be used to detect cytokine production; correlation with parallel studies from isolated mononuclear cells has been demonstrated *(73)*. Some laboratories have replaced thymidine incorporation assays with a combination of cell-surface marker induction assays and a measurement of the percentage of cells in various phases of the cell cycle after activation. Dyes have been developed that stably integrate live lymphocytes into the membranes so that with each successive division, the amount of dye per cell is decreased. Fluorescence can be used to measure the number of cell divisions. Other whole-blood based assays measure the early responses of cells selected through adherence to magnetic beads to which monoclonal antibodies that recognize cells of particular interest are attached. Assessment is achieved by assay of ATP production by the luciferin/luciferase reaction *(69)*. Most methods may be combined with quantitative measure of specific lymphocyte subsets by flow cytometry for examination of response per cell.

In addition to assessment of surface-antigen expression for immunophenotyping, flow cytometry can be used for functional studies based on detection of activation antigen expression (e.g., CD69), or coexpression of critical molecules involved in cell-cell interaction (e.g., CD28). One of the earliest events that occurs after T-cell activation is the rapid increase in intracellular free calcium. This is followed by a change in pH and changes in the membrane potential. All of these effects can be measured by flow cytometry using functional probes. After T-cell activation via CD3/TCR (T-cell receptor) or via CD2 (the alternate T-cell activation pathway), the first measurable surface marker that is induced is CD69. This marker is a disulfide-linked homodimer that is present on some normal thymocytes but not expressed on immune cells in the circulating blood, where the T lymphocyte is a resting cell. It is apparent that CD69 induction is not part of the pathway leading to cell division, because CD69 induction can occur without subsequent cell proliferation. Other cell surface markers appear on activated T cells at variable times after activation, including CD25 (the α chain of the IL-2 receptor), CD71, both within 24–48 h, and HLA-DR after 48 h. Alteration in HLA-DR expression can be used to assess effects on antigen presentation in cells where this molecule is already expressed *(67,74)* or activation when T cells are observed. Consideration of T-cell receptor differences and memory phenotype with functional assays is often informative. For example, memory T cells produce more interferon-gamma than do naïve cells. Methods measuring early events in T-lymphocyte activation may or may not correlate with cell division, because cell division is a late event in the immune response. Therefore, it is advisable to use more than one method and to assess response at several levels (*see* Table 3).

Some nutrients, such as glutamine, may affect amplification of the immune response and not have a discernible effect on early cytokine signaling *(75)*. However, several studies show the importance of glutamine and arginine as conditionally essential amino acids in stress conditions. Using the methods described here to assess changes in immune response in complex settings, such as postoperative recovery involving loss of enteral nutrition and potential risk of infection, require particular consideration of controls for setting and entails longitudinal design to clarify relationships *(76)*.

The growth of cytokine biology has provided a valuable means to clarify the fundamental effect of nutrients on immune response. Both T cells and B cells are affected by

Table 3
Assessment Methods

Assay	Specific method	Advantages	Disadvantages	Notes/comments
Immunophenotyping	Flow cytometry/whole blood	Quantitative, rapid, specific, small-volume blood needed	Depends on accuracy of technique, good instrumentation, and choice of panel	Experience and proficiency are needed. Complete blood count and differential required for absolute counts
Subpopulation coexpression	Flow cytometry	Quantitative, fast evaluation of functional state	Need good control range information	Highly versatile, needs strong controls
Cell division/proliferation	Whole blood	Quantitative, fast, mirrors in vivo cells and plasma	Variation in cell number and soluble factors may affect results	Good choice for field studies, requires little blood. Pair with immune phenotyping to show cell relationships
Cell division/proliferation	Isolated mononuclear cells	Quantitative, well standardized, reflects intrinsic differences	Technically complex, added serum must be screened	Useful for analytic study of intrinsic functional activity
Initial activation or recognition	Neoantigen expression by flow cytometry	Reflects early events and does not require amplification, analytical	Must select population of interest, evaluate kinetics of expression	Timing is important
Circulating cytokine	Enzyme-linked immunosorbent assay (ELISA) or radio-immunoassay (RIA)	Reflects in vivo activation	Must be standardized in serum or plasma	Must check kits to avoid interaction with receptors, antibodies
Cytokine secretion	ELISA or RIA	Quantitative, specific, conditions can be controlled	Producer cell may be hard to identify	Must use an interrelated cytokine panel
Intracellular cytokine	Flow cytometry	Test for producer cell, activation requirements	Technical proficiency required	Widely used
Cytotoxic effector cells	Elispot, chromium release	Quantitative and specific	Technically difficult. If restricted response, need MHC presentation	Natural killer cytotoxicity often correlates with nutrients changes
Delayed type hypersensitivity	Skin test	Reflects in vivo immunity	Response evaluated qualitatively as positive or negative	Useful in large, well-controlled studies

nutrients, which are increasingly recognized as cofactors of immune response. Innate immune cells, such as NK and NK-T cells, monocytes, and dendritic cells, influence the cytokine production pattern by the adaptive immune system in part by direct secretion of cytokines into the microenvironment *(77)*. Innate immune responses are affected by nutrients, such as the effect of vitamin C on phagocytosis *(78)* and β-carotene on monocyte secretion of tumor necrosis factor-α (TNF-α) *(79)*. O'Brien et al. used cytokine detection to show that iron selectively affected IL-1β but not TNF-α release in alveolar macrophages *(80)*. The microenvironment effect can polarize immune response toward either a Th1 or to a Th2 response. For example, the trace element zinc supports a Th1 cytokine response in which IL-2 and interferon-gamma are produced, and vitamin A supports the secretion of Th2 cytokines IL-4, IL-5, and IL-10 *(81,82)*. Many nutrients interact with other immune regulatory molecules, such as the counterregulatory effect of vitamin E on prostaglandin E_2 (PGE_2) suppression of a cyclic adenosine monophosphate (c-AMP) response element-binding protein *(83)*.

Some of the best work in nutritional immunology centers on the cytokine response. Investigating the impact of starvation, Savendahl and Underwood *(84)* demonstrated that acute starvation directly reduces the IL-2 production of cultured peripheral blood mononuclear cells. Investigators such as Rink and Kirchner, who have focused on the effects of zinc, have concluded that zinc status is a primary modulator of cytokine response *(81)*. Current studies suggest that the Th1 or Th2 cytokine response specificity to a particular microbe is critically associated with host defense. Study designs that incorporate antigens that are encountered at the time of study or focus on the type of cytokine production, may, therefore, provide important and unique information.

Dietary elements that influence cytokine production include trace elements, vitamins, and fatty acids. The cell's activation state is a determining factor in how specific fatty acids affect immune responses, as suggested by murine studies *(67)*, which showed that n–3 fatty acids could be strongly suppressive of Th1 cytokines. This classic feeding study included measurement of fatty acid incorporation, cytokine secretion, and cytokine mRNA production. In a small but precisely designed human supplementation study, Kelley et al. found that docosahexaenoic acid lowered PGE_2 production, NK activity, and monocyte secretion of IL-1β and TNF-α *(85)*.

2.4. Evaluation of Mucosal Immune Response

Evaluation of GI immune response in humans has been largely based on experience in clinical settings, and advances in the field have occurred with the support of critical animal model studies *(86–93)*. Work in the field has shown that total parenteral nutrition suppresses immune response in the surgical patient and that glutamine becomes a conditional essential amino acid during metabolic stress *(86,94)*. These observations have led to the discovery that nutrients provide an essential stimulus for the induction, differentiation, and maintenance of the mucosal immune system. Lack of enteral dietary intake impairs mucosal IgA and secretory component production, the number of IgA containing cells, and the level of IgG, whereas enteral intake promotes mucosal growth *(14,94)*. Sacks et al. have shown that nutritional support in the early phase of traumatic injury promotes increase in CD4+T cell number, as well as improved proliferative response in vitro *(95)*. Study of how the immune system responds at the mucosal level during stress or how it may be modulated by diet continues to be an important area for future investigation.

3. CORRELATION OF IMMUNE RESPONSE IN VITRO AND IN VIVO

Malnutrition is a major cause of susceptibility to infection worldwide, and susceptibility to infection is often used as a meaningful correlate of immune deficiency in malnutrition. The interaction between infections and malnutrition is often described as a vicious cycle. However, infections also directly affect metabolism through the initiation of the acute phase response. Conversely, nutritional intervention has been used to block this cascade (96), leading to normalization of the cytokine response. Some nutrients can have direct effects on the pathogen, such as the vitamin C effect on HIV replication (97). Because of the complexity of these interactions, specific nutrient immune interactions have been difficult to evaluate in chronic infections characterized by growth abnormalities and wasting, such as HIV infection. Many studies have shown that micronutrient status is profoundly affected in HIV infection, but the etiologic significance of these changes has been difficult to demonstrate (98). The work of Campa et al. (99) is an exception. Using careful longitudinal studies and good statistical design, this group established that selenium deficiency in children with AIDS was independently associated with mortality. In less clear-cut situations where there may be interactive and multiple factors contributing to outcome, such as pregnancy-related morbidity in poor environments, longitudinal studies are often essential to demonstrate significant effects, such as the beneficial effect of vitamin A supplementation on maternal mortality (100).

In general, immune response to nutrients detected in well-standardized in vitro tests have predictive value in vivo. Examples include response to vitamin D3 (74) and the studies of Roy et al., showing that response to selenium in vitro correlated with response in vivo (101). Relationships between response in vitro and in vivo are not always clearcut and may be contradictory. For example, in a recent study, β-carotene activated NK cells in vitro, but this effect was not seen in vivo (102). Investigators often seek to strengthen inferences by inclusion of in vivo tests, such as delayed type hypersensitivity (DTH), measured by skin testing, and by assessment of the humoral immune response through assay of specific antibodies arising in response to primary or secondary (booster) immunization. Thus, antibody response to influenza was used to detect significant effects on immune response in a recent large study of zinc supplementation in the elderly (103). Similarly, Semba et al. investigated the effect of vitamin A supplementation on antibody response to oral polio vaccine. In this important investigation, virus neutralization was also used. Thus, the negative findings provide the basis for a definitive interpretation in this setting (104).

Skin test response continues to be a valid measure of the DTH response in vivo, in the hands of skilled investigators. When evaluating skin test response in elderly volunteers receiving vitamin E, Meydani et al. found a dose-related increased response (105), as well as increased response to hepatitis B vaccination. Use of skin test reactivity to detect infection, such as response to purified protein derivative (PPD) of *Mycobacterium tuberculosis* in suspected tuberculosis infection, is compromised by malnutrition. Mishra et al. (106) found impaired cellular immunity in all grades of malnutrition, except grade 1, where response to PPD could be used to assess the presence of infection.

Studies of human supplementation in healthy persons are increasing, in light of growing interest in dietary supplements. Studies such as those of Meydani et al. *(105)* and Pallast et al. *(43)* with vitamin E, Fortes et al. with zinc and vitamin A *(62)*, De Waart et al. and De la Fuente et al. with zinc *(71,72)*, and Girodon using zinc and selenium *(103)* in elderly subjects, suggest the possibilities and benefits of supplementation *(42,107)*. These studies also show significant differences, which reflect the importance of dose, for example, of vitamin E *(70–72)*. Although low doses of some micronutrients, such as vitamin E, may not produce a change in immune response, low-dose supplementation has been shown in other studies to have effects. For example, the studies of Zofkova showed an increase in T cells in women given low doses of vitamin D_3 *(108)*. The issues of health and specific micronutrients are likely to be critical variables, explaining why some studies of immune response in the elderly have not shown relationships to micronutrient intakes *(109,110)*. Some investigators have compared the effects of supplements in healthy persons with those with chronic illness, such as De la Fuente et al., who evaluated the effects of vitamins E and C in a small group of healthy women compared with a larger group of elderly subjects with age-related conditions (heart disease and depression), finding that both groups benefited from antioxidant supplementation *(78)*. As a whole, these studies can guide methodology that can reflect sensitive effects on immune response. Rare studies of depletion and repletion of single nutrients, such as zinc in healthy volunteers, are particularly valuable *(111)*. In this study, the investigators tracked the effects of zinc depletion on suppression of the Th1-type cytokine response and restoration with repletion. Studies such as these form the foundation for future investigations in nutritional immunology.

4. "TAKE-HOME" MESSAGES

1. Nutrients act as cofactors in immune response and have modulating effects that can be measured ex vivo or studied in vitro by quantitative methods.
2. Setting is important for design, e.g., malnutrition is often complicated by infection, leading to acute, phase responses and triggering the cytokine cascade.
3. Evaluating mechanism of action requires inclusion of alternative effects, i.e., measurement of both type 1 and type 2 cytokines.
4. Repletion, supplementation, and supraphysiologic levels of nutrients do not affect the immune system in the same way and require distinct experimental approaches.
5. Measurement of both innate and adaptive elements of the immune response reflects the new philosophy that immune response is integrated in the microenvironment.

REFERENCES

1. Fraker PJ, King LE, Laakko T, Vollmer TL. The dynamic link between the integrity of the immune system and zinc status. Nutrition 2000;130:1399S–1406S.
2. Funada U, Wada M, Kawata T, et al. Vitamin B-12-deficiency affects immunoglobulin production and cytokine levels in mice. Int J Vitam Nutr Res 2001;71:60–65.
3. Campbell JD, Cole M, Bunditrutavorn B, Vella AT. Ascorbic acid is a potent inhibitor of various forms of T-cell apoptosis. Cell Immunol 1999;194:1–5.
4. Cunningham-Rundles S. Nutrition and the mucosal immune system. Curr Opin Gastroenterol 2001;17:171–176.
5. Ashworth A. Effects of intrauterine growth retardation on mortality and morbidity in infants and young children. Eur J Clin Nutr 1998;52:S34–S41.

6. Arifeen SE, Black RE, Caulfield LE, et al. Infant growth patterns in the slums of Dhaka in relation to birth weight, intrauterine growth retardation, and prematurity. Am J Clin Nutr 2000;72:1010–1017.

7. Ing R, Su Z, Scott ME, Koski KG. Suppressed T helper 2 immunity and prolonged survival of a nematode parasite in protein-malnourished mice. Proc Natl Acad Sci 2000;97:7078–7083.

8. Miles EA, Thies F, Wallace FA, Powell JR, Hurst TL, Newsholme EA, Calder PC. Influence of age and dietary fish oil on plasma soluble adhesion molecule concentrations. Clin Sci 2001;100:91–100.

9. Forchielli ML, Paolucci G, Lo CW. Total parenteral nutrition and home parenteral nutrition: an effective combination to sustain malnourished children with cancer. Nutr Rev 1999;57:15–20.

10. Carroll K. Obesity as a risk factor for certain types of cancer. Lipids 1998;33:1055–1059.

11. Blanchard RK, Cousins RJ. Regulation of intestinal gene expression by dietary zinc: induction of uroguanylin mRNA by zinc deficiency. J Nutr 2000;130:1393S–1398S.

12. Cippitelli M, Santoni A. Vitamin D3: a transcriptional modulator of the interferon-gamma gene. Eur J Immunol 1998;28:3017–3030.

13. Cunningham-Rundles S, Giardina P, Grady R, Califano C, McKenzie P, DeSousa M. Immune response in iron overload: implications for host defense. J Infect Dis 2000;182:115–121.

14. Kudsk KA, Wu Y, Fukatsu K, et al. Glutamine-enriched total parenteral nutrition maintains intestinal interleukin-4 and mucosal immunoglobulin A levels. J Parenter Enteral Nutr 2000;24:270–274.

15. Lord GM, Matarese G, Howard JK, Baker RJ, Bloom SR, Lechler RI. Leptin modulates the T-cell immune response and reverses starvation-induced immunosuppression. Nature 1998;394:897–901.

16. Maddox JF, Aherne KM, Reddy CC, Sordillo LM. Increased neutrophil adherence and adhesion molecule mRNA expression in endothelial cells during selenium deficiency. J Leukoc Biol 1999;65: 658–664.

17. Semba R. Vitamin A and immunity to viral, bacterial and protozoan infections. Proc Nutr Soc 1999;58:719–727.

18. Tamura J, Kubota K, Murakami H, et al. Immunomodulation by vitamin B12: augmentation of CD8+ T lymphocytes and natural killer (NK) cell activity in vitamin B12-deficient patients by methyl-B12 treatment. Clin Exp Immunol 1999;11:28–32.

19. Ross AC, Gardner EM. The function of vitamin A in cellular growth and differentiation, and its roles during pregnancy and lactation. Adv Exp Med Biol 1994;352:187–200.

20. Batourina E, Gim S, Bello N, et al. Vitamin A controls epithelial/mesenchymal interactions through Ret expression. Nat Genet 2001;27:74–78.

21. Cui D, Moldoveanu Z, Stephensen CB. High-level dietary vitamin A enhances T-helper type 2 cytokine production and secretory immunoglobulin A response to influenza A virus infection in BALB/c mice. J Nutr 2000;130:1132–1139.

22. Freedman LP. Transcriptional targets of the vitamin D3 receptor-mediating cell cycle arrest and differentiation. J Nutr 1999;129:581S–586S.

23. Piemonti L, Monti P, Sironi M, et al. Vitamin D3 affects differentiation, maturation, and function of human monocyte-derived dendritic cells. J Immunol 2000;164:4443–4451.

24. Mayne ST, Risch HA, Dubrow R, et al. Nutrient intake and risk of subtypes of esophageal and gastric cancer. Cancer Epidemiol Biomarkers Prev 2001;10:1055–1062.

25. Bendich, A. Immunology functions to assess nutrient requirements. J Nutr Immunol 1995;3:47–56.

26. Mocchegiani E, Paolucci P, Granchi D, Cavallazzi L, Santarelli L, Fabris N. Plasma zinc level and thymic hormone activity in young cancer patients. Blood 1994;83:749–757.

27. Cunningham-Rundles S, Bockman RS, Lin A, et al. Physiological and pharmacological effects of zinc on immune response. Ann NY Acad Sci 1990;587:113–122.

28. Kudoh K, Shimizu J, Wada M, Takita T, Kanke Y, Innami S. Effect of indigestible saccharides on B lymphocyte response of intestinal mucosa and cecal fermentation in rats. J Nutr Sci Vitaminol 1998;44:103–112.

29. Fukatsu K, Lundberg AH, Hanna MK, et al. Route of nutrition influences intercellular adhesion molecule-1 expression and neutrophil accumulation in intestine. Arch Surg 1999;134:1055–1060.

30. Shankar AH, Prasad AS. Zinc and immune function: the biological basis of altered resistance to infection. Am J Clin Nutr 1998;68:447S–463S.

31. Scott ME, Koski KG. Zinc deficiency impairs immune responses against parasitic nematode infections at intestinal and systemic sites. J Nutr 2000;130:1412S–1420S.

32. Smythe PM, Schonland M, Brereton-Stiles GG, et al. Thymolymphatic deficiency and depression of cell-mediated immunity in protein-calorie malnutrition. Lancet 1971;2:939–943.

33. Sandstead HH, Prasad AS, Schulert AR, et al. Human zinc deficiency, endocrine manifestations and response to treatment. Am J Clin Nutr 1967;20:422–442.

34. Bern C, Zucker JR, Perkins BA, Otieno J, Oloo AJ, Yip R. Assessment of potential indicators for protein-energy malnutrition in the algorithm for integrated management of childhood illness. Bull World Health Organ 1997;75:87–96.

35. Choudhary RP. Anthropometric indices and nutritional deficiency signs in preschool children of the Pahariya tribe of the Rajmahal Hills, Bihar. Anthropol Anz 2001;59:61–71.

36. Genton B, Al-Yaman F, Ginny M, Taraika J, Alpers MP. Relation of anthropometry to malaria morbidity and immunity in Papua New Guinean children. Am J Clin Nutr 1998;68:734–741.

37. Murray MJ, Murray AB, Murray MB. Diet and cerebral malaria: the effect of famine and refeeding. Am J Clin Nutr 1978;31:57–61.

38. El Samani FZ, Willet WC, Ware JH. Nutritional and socio-demographic risk indicators of malaria in children under five: a cross sectional study in Sudanese rural community. J Trop Med Hyg 1987;90: 69–78.

39. Insoft RM, Sanderson IR, Walker WA. Development of immune function in the intestine and its role in neonatal diseases. Pediatr Clin North Am 1996;43:551–571.

40. Cunningham-Rundles S, Cervia JS. Malnutrition and host defense. In: Walker WA, Watkins JB (eds.). Nutrition in Pediatrics: Basic Science and Clinical Application (2nd ed.). Marcel Dekker, Europe, Inc., 1996, pp. 295–307.

41. Cunningham-Rundles S, Nesin M. Bacterial infections in the immunologically compromised host. In: Nataro J, Blaser M, Cunningham-Rundles S (eds.). Persistent Bacterial Infections. American Society of Microbiology Press, Washington, DC, 2000, pp. 145–164.

42. Lesourd BM. Nutrition and immunity in the elderly: modification of immune responses with nutritional treatments. Am J Clin Nutr 1997;66:478S–484S.

43. Pallast EG, Schouten EG, de Waart FG, et al. Effect of 50- and 100-mg vitamin E supplements on cellular immune function in noninstitutionalized elderly persons. Am J Clin Nutr 1999;69:1273–1281.

44. Huber SA, Kupperman J, Newell N. Hormonal regulation of CD4+ T-cell responses in coxsackievirus B3-induced myocarditis in mice. J Virol 1999;736:4689–4695.

45. Angele MK, Knoferl MW, Schwacha MG, et al. Sex steroids regulate pro- and anti-inflammatory cytokine release by macrophages after trauma-hemorrhage. Am J Physiol 1999;277:C35–C42.

46. Zamboni G, Dufillot D, Antoniazzi F, Valentini R, Gendrel D, Tato L. Growth hormone-binding proteins and insulin-like growth factor-binding proteins in protein-energy malnutrition, before and after nutritional rehabilitation. Pediatr Res 1996;39:410–414.

47. Soliman AT, El Zalabany MM, Salama M, Ansari BM. Serum leptin concentrations during severe protein-energy malnutrition: correlation with growth parameters and endocrine function. Metabolism 2000;49:819–825.

48. Froebel KS, Pakker NG, Aiuti F, et al. Standardization and quality of lymphocyte proliferation assays for use in the assessment of immune function. European Concerted Action on Immunological and Virological Markers of HIV Disease Progression. J Immunol Methods 1999;227:85–97.

49. Malone JL, Simms TE, Gray GC, Wagner KF, Burge JR, Burke DS. Sources of variability in repeated T-helper lymphocyte counts from human immunodeficiency virus type 1-infected patients: total lymphocyte count fluctuations and diurnal cycle are important. J Acquir Immune Defic Syndr 1990;3: 144–151.

50. Reimann KA, Chernoff M, Wilkening CL, Nickerson CE, Landay AL. Preservation of lymphocyte immunophenotype and proliferative responses in cryopreserved peripheral blood mononuclear cells from human immunodeficiency virus type 1-infected donors: implications for multicenter clinical trials. The ACTG Immunology Advanced Technology Laboratories. Clin Diagn Lab Immunol 2000;7: 352–359.

51. Venkataraman M. Effects of cryopreservation on immune responses. VIII. Enhanced secretion of interferon-gamma by frozen human peripheral blood mononuclear cells. Cryobiology 1995;32: 528–534.

52. Paxton H, Cunningham-Rundles S, O'Gorman MRG. Laboratory evaluation of the cellular immune system. In: Henry JB (ed.). Clinical Diagnosis and Management by Laboratory Methods (20th ed.). W.B. Saunders and Co., Philadelphia, 2001, pp. 850–877.

53. Medzhitov R, Janeway C. Decoding the patterns of self and nonself by the innate immune system. Science 2002;296:298–300.

54. Kopp EB, Medzhitov R. The Toll-receptor family and control of innate immunity. Curr Opin Immunol 1999;11:13–18.

55. Hajjar A, Ernst R, Tsai J, Wilson C, Miller S. Human Toll-like receptor 4 recognizes host-specific LPS modifications. Nat Immunol 2002;3:354–359.

56. Cooper MA, Fehniger TA, Turner SC, et al. Human natural killer cells: a unique innate immuno-regulatory role for the CD56 (bright) subset. Blood 2001;97:3146–3151.

57. Lanzavecchia A. Lack of fair play in the T cell response. Nat Immunol 2002;3:9–10.

58. Doherty DG, Norris S, Madrigal-Estebas L, et al. The human liver contains multiple populations of NK cells, T cells, and CD3+CD56+ natural T cells with distinct cytotoxic activities and Th1, Th2, and Th0 cytokine secretion patterns. J Immunol 1999;15:2314–2321.

59. Campbell N, Yio XY, So LP, Li Y, Mayer L. The intestinal epithelial cell: processing and presentation of antigen to the mucosal immune system. Immunol Rev 1999;172:315–324.

60. Parent G, Chevalier P, Zalles L, et al. In vitro lymphocyte-differentiating effects of thymulin (Zn-FTS) on lymphocyte subpopulations of severely malnourished children. Am J Clin Nutr 1994;60:274–278.

61. Chevalier P, Sevilla R, Sejas E, Zalles L, Belmonte G, Parent G. Immune recovery of malnourished children takes longer than nutritional recovery: implications for treatment and discharge. J Trop Pediatr 1998;44:304–307.

62. Fortes C, Forastiere F, Agabiti N, et al. The effect of zinc and vitamin A supplementation on immune response in an older population. J Am Geriatr Soc 1998;46:19–26.

63. Kramer TR, Burri BJ. Modulated mitogenic proliferative responsiveness of lymphocytes in whole-blood cultures after a low-carotene diet and mixed-carotenoid supplementation in women. Am J Clin Nutr 1997;65:871–875.

64. Jaye A, Magnusen AF, Sadiq AD, Corrah T, Whittle HC. Ex vivo analysis of cytotoxic T lymphocytes to measles antigens during infection and after vaccination in Gambian children. J Clin Invest 1998;102:1969–1977.

65. Cunningham-Rundles S. Issues in assessment of human immune function. In: Institute of Medicine's Committee on Military Nutrition Research (eds.). Military Strategies for Sustainment of Nutrition and Immune Function in the Field. Institute of Medicine National Academy Press, Washington DC, 1999, pp. 235–248.

66. Bergquist C, Mattsson-Rydberg A, Lonroth H, Svennerholm A. Development of a new method for the determination of immune responses in the human stomach. J Immunol Methods 2000;234:51–59.

67. Wallace FA, Miles EA, Evans C, Stock TE, Yaqoob P, Calder PC. Dietary fatty acids influence the production of Th1- but not Th2-type cytokines. J Leukoc Biol 2001;69:449–457.

68. Hughes DA, Pinder AC. N–3 polyunsaturated fatty acids modulate the expression of functionally associated molecules on human monocytes and inhibit antigen-presentation in vitro. Clin Exp Immunol 1997;110:516–523.

69. Sottong PR, Rosebrock JA, Britz JA, Kramer TR. Measurement of T-lymphocyte responses in whole-blood cultures using newly synthesized DNA and ATP. Clin Diagn Lab Immunol 2000;7:307–311.

70. Lee CY, Man-Fan Wan J. Vitamin E supplementation improves cell-mediated immunity and oxidative stress of Asian men and women. J Nutr 2000;130:2932–2937.

71. De Waart FG, Portengen L, Doekes G, Verwaal CJ, Kok FJ. Anti-oxidants as modulators of immune function. Immunol Cell Biol 2000;78:49–54.

72. De la Fuente M, Victor VM. Effect of 3 months vitamin E supplementation on indices of the cellular and humoral immune response in elderly subjects. Br J Nutr 1997;78:761–774.

73. Yaqoob P, Newsholme EA, Calder PC. Comparison of cytokine production in cultures of whole human blood and purified mononuclear cells. Cytokine 1999;11:600–605.

74. Tokuda N, Kano M, Meiri H, Nomoto K, Naito S. Calcitriol therapy modulates the cellular immune responses in hemodialysis patients. Am J Nephrol 2000;20:129–137.

75. Heberer M, Babst R, Juretic A, et al. Role of glutamine in the immune response in critical illness. Nutrition 1996;12:S71–S72.

76. Cunningham-Rundles C. Evaluation of the effects of nutrients on immune function. In: Calder PC, Field CJ, Gill HS (eds.). Nutrition and Immune Function. CAB International, United Kingdom, 2002, pp. 21–39.

77. Garcia VE, Uyemura K, Sieling PA, et al. IL-18 promotes type 1 cytokine production from NK cells and T cells in human intracellular infection. J Immunol 1999;162:6114–6121.

78. De la Fuente M, Victor VM. Anti-oxidants as modulators of immune function. Immunol Cell Biol 2000;78:49–54.

79. Hughes DA, Wright AJ, Finglas PM, et al. The effect of beta-carotene supplementation on the immune function of blood monocytes from healthy male non-smokers. J Lab Clin Med 1997;129:285–287.

80. O'Brien-Ladner AR, Blumer BM, Wesselius LJ. Differential regulation of human alveolar macro-phage-derived interleukin-1beta and tumor necrosis factor-alpha by iron. J Lab Clin Med 1998;132:497–506.

81. Rink L, Kirchner, H. Zinc-altered immune function and cytokine production. J Nutr 2000;130:1407S–1411S.

82. Frankenburg S, Wang X, Milner Y. Vitamin A inhibits cytokines produced by type 1 lymphocytes in vitro. Cell Immunol 1998;185:75–81.

83. Valenti A, Venza I, Venza M, Fimiani V, Teti D. Effects of vitamin E and prostaglandin E2 on expression of CREB1 and CREB2 proteins by human T lymphocytes [in process citation]. Physiol Res 2000;49:363–368.

84. Savendahl L, Underwood LE. Decreased interleukin-2 production from cultured peripheral blood mononuclear cells in human acute starvation. J Clin Endocrinol Metab 1997;82:1177–1180.

85. Kelley DS, Taylor PC, Nelson GJ, et al. Docosahexaenoic acid ingestion inhibits natural killer cell activity and production of inflammatory mediators in young healthy men. Lipids 1999;34:317–324.

86. Calder PC, Yaqoob P. Glutamine and the immune system. Amino Acids 1999;17:227–241.

87. Bengmark S. Gut microenvironment and immune function. Curr Opin Clin Nutr Metab Care 1999;2:83–85.

88. Mayer L. Mucosal immunity and gastrointestinal antigen processing. J Pediatr Gastroenterol Nutr 2000;30:S4–S12.

89. Harrison LC, Honeyman MC. Cow's milk and type 1 diabetes: the real debate is about mucosal immune function. Diabetes 1999;48:1501–1507.

90. Donnet-Hughes A, Duc N, Serrant P, Vidal K, Schiffrin EJ. Bioactive molecules in milk and their role in health and disease: the role of transforming growth factor-beta. Immunol Cell Biol 2000;78:74–79.

91. Efron D, Barbul A. Role of arginine in immunonutrition. J Gastroenterol 2000;35:S20–S23.

92. Walker WA. Role of nutrients and bacterial colonization in the development of intestinal host defense. J Pediatr Gastroenterol Nutr 2000;30:S2–S7.

93. Redmond HP, Gallagher HJ, Shou J, Daly JM. Antigen presentation in protein-energy malnutrition. Cell Immunol 1995;163:80–87.

94. Heel KA, Kong SE, McCauley RD, Erber WN, Hall J. The effect of minimum luminal nutrition on mucosal cellularity and immunity of the gut. J Gastroenterol Hepatol 1998;10:1015–1019.

95. Sacks GS, Brown RO, Teague D, Dickerson RN, Tolley EA, Kudsk KA. Early nutrition support modifies immune function in patients sustaining severe head injury. JPEN J Parenter Enteral Nutr 1995;19:387–392.

96. Jeevanandam M, Shahbazian LM, Petersen SR. Proinflammatory cytokine production by mitogen-stimulated peripheral blood mononuclear cells (PBMCs) in trauma patients fed immune-enhancing enteral diets. Nutrition 1999;15:842–847.

97. Rivas CI, Vera JC, Guaiquil VH, et al. Increased uptake and accumulation of vitamin C in human immunodeficiency virus 1-infected hematopoietic cell lines. J Biol Chem 1997;272:5814–5820.

98. Cunningham-Rundles S. Trace elements and minerals in HIV infection and AIDS: implications for host defense. In: Bogden JD, Kelvay LM (eds.). In: The Clinical Nutrition of the Essential Trace Elements and Minerals. Humana Totowa, NJ, 2000, pp. 333–351.

99. Campa A, Shor-Posner G, Indacochea F, et al. Mortality risk in selenium-deficient HIV-positive children. J Acquir Immune Defic Syndr Hum Retrovirol 1999;15:508–513.

100. West KP Jr, Katz J, Khatry SK, et al. Double blind, cluster randomized trial of low dose supplementation with vitamin A or beta carotene on mortality related to pregnancy in Nepal. The NNIPS-2 Study Group. Br Med J 1999;318:570–575.

101. Roy M, Kiremidjian-Schumacher L, Wishe HI, Cohen MW, Stotzky G. Supplementation with selenium and human immune cell functions. I. Effect on lymphocyte proliferation and interleukin 2 receptor expression [published erratum appears in Biol Trace Elem Res 1994;46:183]. Biol Trace Elem Res 1994;41:103–114.

102. Ashfaq MK, Zuberi HS, Anwar Waqar M. Vitamin E and beta-carotene affect natural killer cell function. Int J Food Sci Nutr 2000;51:S13–S20.

103. Girodon F, Galan P, Monget A, et al. Impact of trace elements and vitamin supplementation on immunity and infections in institutionalized elderly patients: a randomized controlled trial. MIN. VIT. AOX. geriatric network. Arch Intern Med 1999;159:748–754.

104. Semba RD, Muhilal, Mohgaddam NE, et al. Integration of vitamin A supplementation with the expanded program on immunization does not affect seroconversion to oral poliovirus vaccine in infants. J Nutr 1999;129:2203–2205.

105. Meydani SN, Meydani M, Blumberg JB, et al. Vitamin E supplementation and in vivo immune response in healthy elderly subjects. A randomized controlled trial. JAMA 1997;277:1380–1386.

106. Mishra OP, Agrawal S, Ali Z, Usha. Adenosine deaminase activity in protein-energy malnutrition. Acta Paediatrica 1998;87:1116–1119.

107. Bogden JD, Louria DB. Aging and the immune system: the role of micronutrient nutrition. Nutrition 1999;15:593–595.

108. Zofkova I, Kancheva RL. The effect of 1,25(OH)$_2$ vitamin D3 on CD4+/CD8+ subsets of T lymphocytes in postmenopausal women. Life Sci 1997;61:147–152.

109. Gardner EM, Bernstein ED, Popoff KA, Abrutyn E, Gross P, Murasko DM. Immune response to influenza vaccine in healthy elderly: lack of association with plasma beta-carotene, retinol, alpha-tocopherol, or zinc. Mech Ageing Dev 2000;117:29–45.

110. Santos MS, Leka LS, Ribaya-Mercado JD, et al. Short- and long-term beta-carotene supplementation do not influence T cell-mediated immunity in healthy elderly persons. Am J Clin Nutr 1997;66: 917–924.

111. Beck FW, Prasad AS, Kaplan J, Fitzgerald JT, Brewer GJ. 106 Changes in cytokine production and T cell subpopulations in experimentally induced zinc-deficient humans. Am J Physiol 1997;272:E1002–E1007.

Effects of Infection on Nutritional and Immune Status

David I. Thurnham
and Christine A. Northrop-Clewes

1. INTRODUCTION AND HISTORICAL PERSPECTIVE

1.1. Early Studies

Mankind has been aware of interactions between malnutrition and disease for centuries. Even early biblical scholars discussed the accompaniment of pestilence with famine (Ezekiel 5:12). However, detailed scientific descriptions of the effect of infection on nutrition and nutrition on infection only appeared in the early to middle parts of the last century (1,2). Early reviews suggest that although diet does not influence the frequency of infection, severity was enhanced by inadequate diets, and many studies show that experimental deficiencies of vitamins A and C lowered resistance to bacterial infection (3). During and after World War II, the taking of vitamin supplements was extolled as a way of curing and preventing disease. However, the lack of positive results led to a sharp public reaction against vitamins, and nutrition in general, as possible factors in resistance to infection (1,2,4). Nevertheless, experimental work at the time suggested that specific nutritional deficiencies retarded the development of viral and protozoan (1,2) and parasitic infections, such as malaria (4,5). Consequently, experiments attempted to relate specific nutrients to each infectious disease, and, when reviewed (2), results suggested that interactions between dietary deficiencies and bacterial and helminth infections were synergistic, whereas the relationships between nutritional disorders and viral infections were antagonistic.

By 1968, ideas had not changed greatly (1). Infectious disease was believed to adversely affect the nutritional state indirectly by loss of appetite and food intolerance, resulting in metabolic effects. It was observed that cultural factors resulted in the substitution of less nutritious diets as therapeutic measures, as well as the administration of purgatives, antibiotics, and other medicines to reduce digestion and absorption of specific nutrients. It was recognized that there was an increased loss of nitrogen and that nitrogen balance should be maintained by dietary measures during the acute phase of the infection. In addition, it was accepted that classical nutritional deficiencies were precipitated by

From: *Diet and Human Immune Function*
Edited by: D. A. Hughes, L. G. Darlington, and A. Bendich © Humana Press Inc., Totowa, NJ

infection in those with borderline nutrient depletion, including keratomalacia, scurvy, and beriberi resulting from avitaminoses A, C, or B_1, respectively. However, in well-nourished individuals, body reserves and normal dietary intake ensured that malnutrition would not result unless infection was prolonged.

1.2. Global Burden of Infection

Malnutrition and infection are the major causes of preventable deaths and disabilities worldwide, especially in the most vulnerable group, children *(6)*. Better education, health care, diet, and sanitation have resulted in marked improvements in morbidity and mortality in the developed world during the 20th century. However, the global burden of malnutrition and infection is still enormous, with more than 6 million children under 5 yr dying directly or indirectly from these problems *(7)*. The World Health Organization (WHO) estimates that 2 million children die each year from disease for which vaccines already exist. In addition, 25 million low-birth-weight babies are born each year who are particularly at risk from disease and malnutrition *(7)*. In any 2 wk, between 4% and 40% of African children under 5 yr suffer acute respiratory infections; this, together with diarrhea, account for approx 50% of mortality in children younger than 5 yr in the developing world *(8)*.

1.3. Interrelationship of Malnutrition and Infection

Malnutrition is frequently a consequence of illness, and illness is commonly the result of malnutrition. The two problems are closely interrelated *(9)*.

Infection can alter nutritional status in several ways:

- reduced nutrient intake of anorexia caused by an inflammatory response;
- reduced dietary absorption caused by intestinal damage;
- increased nutrient(s) requirements resulting from increased metabolic rate, redistribution of nutrients, or to the activation of inflammatory/immune responses; or
- loss of endogenous nutrients, perhaps caused by diarrhea.

In addition, poverty, ignorance, poor hygiene, lack of clean water, poor housing, poor health services, cultural practices, and frequent exposure to infectious agents increase the risk of poor nutrition *(6)*. Also, populations exposed to endemic malaria, HIV/AIDS, severe hookworm, schistosomiasis, and other infections common to tropical and underdeveloped areas are likely to lack the physical stamina to be efficient in agriculture or industrial labor, which impairs productivity and perpetuates poverty.

1.4. Immunity

Vertebrates respond to infection through a combination of adaptive and acquired immunity and innate or natural immunity. The principal feature of acquired immunity is the generation of receptors on B and T lymphocytes that can distinguish between self and nonself, and hence protect the organisms from infectious agents such as bacteria and viruses. By contrast, the hallmarks of innate immunity consist of physical barriers and the ability to generate a battery of cytokines in response to conserved structures on infectious agents, such as bacterial lipopolysaccharides (LPS) *(10)*. Nutritional status and innate immunity are closely linked. Undernutrition compromises the barrier function of innate immunity, allowing easier access by pathogens and a decreasing ability of the host to eliminate the invaders once they have entered the body *(6)*. Physical barriers are dependent on good nutritional status of most nutrients, especially vitamin A *(11)*. Severe malnutrition can impair the body's response to cytokine activation, and the malnourished child with kwashiorkor is much more vulnerable to severe infection than his well-nourished peer *(12)*. Likewise, vitamin A deprivation, detectable as night blindness or corneal Bitot's spots, was associated with significantly more respiratory disease and diarrhea in Indonesian infants *(13)*, and, in Nepalese pregnant women, night blindness was associated with more urinary, reproductive, and gastrointestinal (GI) illness *(14)* in comparison to control populations (*see* Chapter 6).

Innate immunity comprises many factors that are present in the body at birth and are available to give protection from challenges from those elements that are foreign or nonself, e.g., skin, mucous, cough reflex, and low stomach pH. If any of these defenses is damaged and an invading microorganism penetrates, then further protection is afforded by:

- the reticuloendothelial system (RES);
- phagocytic cells, e.g., macrophages and polymorphonuclear (PMN) leukocytes;
- a leukocytosis and migration of PMN leukocytes to the site of inflammation;
- production of cytokines, e.g., interleukin (IL)-1, interferon γ (IFN-γ), tumor necrosis factor-α (TNF-α), etc.; and
- production of acute phase proteins (APP), e.g., C-reactive protein (CRP), α-1 acid glycoprotein (AGP), α-1-antichymotrypsin (ACT), ferritin, etc.

However, as a consequence of some of these responses, the concentrations of various important blood nutrients are altered *(15,16)*. In this chapter, explanations are given for the changes that occur and why it is important to allow for infection when interpreting nutritional status biomarkers. Otherwise, assessing nutritional status in the presence of infection can be easily misinterpreted *(17,18)*.

1.5. Objective

The purpose of this chapter is to describe the influence of infection on nutritional and immune status. As indicated above, there is much evidence to suggest that the effects of infection are not unidirectional and that poor nutritional status compromises immune defenses and magnifies the consequences of infection. However, the influence of nutrition on infection is discussed in part II of this volume. In this chapter, the purpose is to describe the influence of infection on those aspects of the immune response that affect nutritional indicators and, potentially, nutritional status.

2. DETAILED OVERVIEW OF CURRENT KNOWLEDGE

2.1. Cytokine Production and Nutritional Status

The stimulation of the RES by pathogens and other foreign antigens and the metabolic effects resulting from the production of cytokines and their actions on a range of body tissues are central to many of the changes that affect the host's nutritional status.

2.2. Reticuloendothelial System

The RES can be viewed as a dispersed defense organ with a major role in activating the immune system by means of vigorous phagocytic abilities. Macrophages enter the blood as monocytes, but they eventually migrate to various tissues where they differentiate to several histologic forms that are collectively called mononuclear phagocytes, or the RES. To cause an infection, pathogens must breach normal host defenses. Hence, the wide tissue distribution of macrophages is particularly important in the body's defense at common points of entry. Macrophages are found in the skin, in the mucosal surfaces, as filtering agents within the lymphoid organs, in the lungs and pleural spaces as alveolar macrophages to protect against inhaled microorganisms, in the synovial fluid, in the peritoneum, and at inflammatory sites. Fixed macrophages within the liver, the Kupffer cells, and the spleen provide a robust form of protection against blood-borne bacterial infection. Mononuclear phagocytes also have the ability to eliminate viruses from the circulation after a blood-borne infection, and their scavenger function constitutes the first line of defense that reduces the viral load until specific immune responses become available *(19)*. In addition, irrespective of where the macrophage is located, all are capable of producing the cytokines IL-1, IL-6, and TNF-α.

2.3. Cytokines

An inflammatory stimulus, such as an invasion of tissue by bacteria, virus, or parasites, or tissue damage incurred through trauma, surgery, excessive exercise, or burns, induces IL-1, IL-6, and TNF-α production from a range of immune cells. Such cells include phagocytic macrophages and other leucocytes, T and B lymphocytes, mast cells, and nonimmune cells, such as fibroblasts and endothelial cells. Once induced, IL-1 and TNF-α induce each other's and IL-6 production, and IL-6 also potentiates IL-1 production *(20)*. Peripheral blood mononuclear (PBMN) cells or alveolar macrophages are cell types that are commonly used to assess the functional capacity to produce cytokines because of their easier accessibility. In vitro measurements of cytokine production are useful tools to assess immune capacity. However, frequently, in vitro measurements do not correlate with in vivo measurements, because cytokine upregulation also stimulates cytokine clearance mechanisms. Thus, in studies that used damaging exercise to produce an inflammatory response, plasma cytokine concentrations were greatest at 6 h, but the in vitro secretion of cytokines by PBMN was greatest at 24 h *(21)*, and there are many other examples.

Many cytokines have important functions in their own right. IL-1 is produced by mononuclear phagocytes after stimulation by almost all infectious agents. It is proinflammatory, an endogenous pyrogen, and believed to raise body temperature by influencing the prostaglandin production. IL-1 induces the liver to produce antiinflammatory acute phase reactants and activates T (producing IL-2) and B (proliferation and enhancement of antibody production) cells. TNF-α, like IL-1, is induced by LPS, a component of Gram-negative bacterial cell membranes. TNF-α is also an endogenous pyrogen; it enhances superoxide production by PMN leukocytes (i.e., granulocytes, including neutrophils, eosinophils, basophils, and mast cells) and enhances their adherence to endothelial cells. The cytokines are powerful regulators of the body's responses to invasion by microorganisms and have the potential to be lethal to the host *(22)*. Fortunately, control mechanisms are activated at the same time as stimulation to ensure that lethal effects do not usually occur *(23,24)*.

Dietary factors can influence the cytokine response. Certain fats can have a strong influence on proinflammatory cytokine production. The long-chain polyunsaturated fats (PUFA) of the omega-3 (n–3) family can significantly reduce production of proinflammatory cytokines. In vitro, fish oils (rich in n–3 PUFA) reduce the ability of monocytes to produce IL-1, TNF-α, and TNF-β in response to endotoxin, and, in vivo, inflammatory symptoms were reduced in patients with rheumatoid arthritis, Crohn's disease, psoriasis, and ulcerative colitis *(20)*.

IFN describes a family of cytokines, which is of particular importance in viral infections. The IFN system becomes operative within hours of systemic viral infection *(19)* and, contrary to most other cells in the body, macrophages can be induced by several microbial pathogens, as well as viruses to produce IFN-α and IFN-β, and cooperate with T cells in IFN-γ production. IFN-γ dramatically enhances the capacity of the macrophage to generate a respiratory burst by which reactive oxygen intermediates (ROI) are produced to destroy bacteria *(24)*. Cytokines, such as IL-1 and IFN-γ increase the expression of adhesion molecules, e.g., intercellular adhesion molecule-1 (ICAM-1, CD54) by endothelial cells and can, therefore, facilitate monocyte margination and migration to inflammation sites *(25)*.

2.4. Iron, Zinc, and Copper Status in Infection

With the onset of infection, the plasma concentrations of several nutrients fall rapidly, irrespective of nutritional status (*see* Table 1), whereas a few, e.g., copper, increase. Any detrimental consequence of these changes on nutritional status in the short term is minimal. The changes probably protect the organism from the effects of infection by either conserving nutrients or altering the serum environment to reduce its desirability or the nutritional support it provides to the invading pathogen *(15)*. However, if infection is prolonged or the patient is malnourished at the outset, then a further reduction in the concentration of a circulating nutrient caused by a pathogen may well impair tissue functions, so producing or worsening a nutritional deficiency. The resultant deficiency may also impair the body's ability to deal with the infection.

There are rapid falls in the plasma concentrations of both iron and zinc after infection onset and even before the onset of any fever. The greatest falls occur in those who subsequently develop fever *(26,27)*. Nutritional deficiencies of these minerals result in anemia and poor growth, respectively. Both anemia and poor growth are common in many developing countries where both exposure to and rates of infection are particularly high. To understand the potential role of infection in contributing to iron and zinc deficiencies, it is important to understand the purpose and possible functions of the pathological responses to infection that affect these minerals.

2.4.1. IRON

Iron affects lymphocyte activation and proliferation and how macrophages handle iron. The proliferative phase of lymphocyte activation is an iron-requiring step, because iron is essential for enzymes, such as ribonucleotide reductase, which is involved in DNA synthesis. Hence, a number of clinical studies have found reduced T-cell function in vivo as manifest by impaired skin-test reactions and reduced in vitro proliferation of T cells

Table 1
Effects of Infection on Biomarkers of Micronutrient Status[a]

Nutrient	Consequence of infection	Mechanism	Possible reason for change seen
Retinol	Reduction in plasma retinol	Reduced synthesis of retinol-binding protein	To prevent losses of essential nutrient
Vitamin C	Short-term fall in leukocyte ascorbate of 3–5 d	Leukocytosis followed by uptake of plasma ascorbate into new leukocytes	Redistribution to target tissue Protect leukocytes from oxidative damage
	Longer term fall in plasma ascorbate		Reduce concentration of a potential prooxidant in body fluids
Iron	Rapid reduction in plasma iron	Scavenged by macrophages to reduce plasma iron to storage sites within tissues	Reduce bioavailability for bacteria or parasites
	Longer term reduction in hemoglobin	Reduction in absorption of iron	Reduce concentration of a potential pro-oxidant in plasma
Zinc	Reduction in plasma zinc	Movement to tissues	Reduce losses of an essential nutrient
Riboflavin	Increase in EGR saturation—suggesting an improvement in status	Breakdown of tissue with release of flavin coenzymes into plasma	Conservation of riboflavin resources
Thiamin	Beriberi reported in patients with acute infections	Increase in thiamin requirements for energy generation	Consequence of increased energy needs in infection

[a]Modified from references (15) and (38).
EGR, erythrocyte glutathione reductase.

Table 2
Influence of Inflammation on Iron-Binding Proteins and Vitamin C in Plasma

Plasma constituent (units)	Normal range	Function	Plasma response in infection
Ceruloplasmin (g/L)	0.155–0.529	Fe^{II} to Fe^{III}	Increases 30–60%
Transferrin (g/L) (μmol/L)	1.9–2.58 25–34	Bind and transport iron	Decrease approx 30%
Lactoferrin (μg/L)	0.91–0.448	Binds iron, especially at low pH	Released from granulocytes Increases 200–500%
Ferritin (μg/L) (nmol/L)	15–250 0.034–0.562	Binds iron	Can increase 3000% (6.7 nmol/L)
Haptoglobin (g/L) (μmol/L)	0.703–3.79 7.0–37.9	Binds hemoglobin	Increases 200–500%
Ascorbate (μmol/L)	11–80	Fe^{III} to Fe^{II}	Reduction

[a]Modified from references (38) and (165).
Fe, iron.

in individuals who are iron-deficient (28). The extent to which mild anemia, a major problem in developing countries (29), impairs lymphocyte proliferation and impairs immune responses is more difficult to evaluate.

Serum iron is depressed during the incubation period of most generalized infectious processes, in some instances, several days before the onset of fever or any symptoms of clinical illness (27). In volunteers given endotoxin to induce therapeutic fever, or live attenuated virus vaccine, depression of serum iron values began within several hours, were maximum at 24 h, and were greatest in those developing severe fever (27). Administration of iron to such patients by oral or parenteral routes had little effect on serum iron or other indices of iron status, probably because iron absorption is inhibited by the inflammatory process (30), irrespective of iron status (31). The hypoferremia of inflammation does not represent a genuine iron deficiency but, rather, a redistribution of iron that can prevail in the face of normal iron stores (32). Chronic illnesses, such as cancer or rheumatoid arthritis, are frequently accompanied by an anemia of chronic infection, but many children and adults in developing countries also display mild anemia (29), which may have similar causes. Frequent exposure to endemic diseases will continuously maintain a hypoferremic state and promote anemia by impairing erythrocyte synthesis and/or a shortening red cell life span. Whether this is also accompanied by iron deficiency depends on the frequency and severity of infections and the amount and bioavailability of dietary iron.

The hypoferremia of infection is accompanied by changes in plasma concentrations of several iron-binding proteins (Table 2) that facilitate iron uptake by the RES or removal and reuse of hemoglobin from effete erythrocytes. The regulation of iron metabolism is normally under the control of iron-regulatory proteins (IRP) that bind to sequences on mRNA and protect it from degradation. As a consequence of iron deficiency, IRP binds to mRNA and promotes the expression of transferrin receptor protein, and ferritin synthesis is repressed. Hence, iron use and absorption are increased. When iron is adequate, ferritin synthesis is promoted and iron storage occurs *(33)*. However, in infection, the normal control of iron metabolism is reorganized by IL-1 and TNF-α. Plasma ferritin levels increase, despite hypoferremia, because ferritin mRNA is sensitive to both iron and cytokines. Rat hepatoma cells exposed to IL-1 and TNF-α doubled the amounts of ferritin released into the medium during 24 and 48 h *(34)*, and others have reported that TNF-α, in particular, promoted ferritin translation, resulting in increased iron storage in a human monocytic cell line *(35)*.

It was initially suggested that the hypoferremia of infection protected the host by reducing the amount of iron available for bacterial growth *(36)*. Although this may be true for some bacteria, other pathogenic bacteria have powerful siderophores, enabling them to compete successfully against the iron-binding proteins in the plasma *(37)*. The importance of the hypoferremia, therefore, may be more closely linked with its potential influence on the redox status in the tissues *(16)*. Hypoferremia may protect against the potential prooxidant properties of iron and exacerbation of tissue damage at inflammation sites *(38)*. This connection is interesting to highlight because lactoferrin is secreted by neutrophils at inflammation sites. Lactoferrin has a higher affinity for iron than transferrin and can also bind iron under acid conditions, such as those found at inflammation sites *(37)*. In addition, plasma ascorbate concentrations are reduced in infection. Vitamin C catalyses the prooxidant activity of iron (*see* Section 2.6.); therefore, the reduction of both vitamin C and iron can be considered antiinflammatory in infection.

Alternatively, in vitro studies show that hypoferremia stimulates IFN-γ effects on T helper cells and TNF-α effects in macrophages with a net effect of increasing cytotoxicity in macrophages *(39)*. In a low-iron environment, IFN-γ, TNF-α, IL-1, or LPS induce macrophage nitric oxide synthase (NOS) and NO is central to macrophage-mediated cytotoxicity *(40)*. The mechanisms involved here are complex. NO would normally be expected to increase transferrin receptor expression on macrophages and repress NOS *(41,42)*. However, recent work suggests that NO ameliorates rather than potentiates iron sequestration in stimulated macrophages. It is believed that the major source of iron uptake by stimulated macrophages is phagocytosis of effete erythrocytes, and iron acquired by the phagocytic route is released more slowly than that from transferrin *(43)*. Hence, stimulated macrophages both store iron and display enhanced NOS activity, characteristic of hypoferremia.

At the outset of this section, we indicated that iron was essential for lymphocyte proliferation, but it is also apparent that hypoferremia promotes macrophage cytotoxicity. Does mild anemia benefit the host against infection? There may be no single answer to this question, and different diseases may pose different demands on host responses. However, there are many reports of adverse consequences after both parenteral and oral iron treatment where there is also a high risk of disease, as in developing countries *(32,44,45)*, particularly in children with malnutrition *(46)* and malaria *(4)*. In our own experience, in Pakistani infants who received oral iron daily for 3 mo, there was evidence of more infection in those who received the iron, but this was most obvious in those with the lower plasma retinol concentrations *(47)*. Thus, no nutrient should be considered on its own, but, nevertheless, mild anemia in groups where there is a high risk of infection may be more of an advantage than a disadvantage, and caution should be exercised, especially before administering parenteral iron.

2.4.2. ZINC

Severe zinc deficiency, as described in the rare autosomal recessive disease acrodermatitis enterohepatica, is accompanied by thymic atrophy and a high frequency of bacterial, viral, and fungal infections if not treated (48). Furthermore, experimental data suggest that zinc deficiency depresses recruitment and chemotaxis of neutrophils, impairs natural killer (NK) cell activity, impairs phagocytosis of macrophages and neutrophils, and impairs oxidative burst generation (49). Zinc is essential for the function of more than 300 metalloenzymes, and the highly proliferative immune system is reliant on zinc-dependent proteins involved in the general cellular functions, such as replication, transcription, and signal transduction. Zinc influences all immune cell subsets. However, zinc is especially important in the maturation and function of T cells, because zinc is an essential cofactor for the thymus hormone, thymulin. T-cell activation is delicately regulated by zinc, and the physiologic zinc concentration of 12–16 µmol/L represents the concentrations for optimally balanced T-cell function (50). The normal range for plasma zinc in well-nourished adults and children is 10.5–17 µmol/L (51).

Because of zinc's widespread involvement in so many enzyme systems, it is not surprising that moderate zinc deficiency in infants and children (i.e., low plasma zinc concentrations below 10.7 µmol/L [52]) has been associated with not only reduced growth and development but also impaired immunity and increased morbidity from infectious diseases (53,54). The physiologic role of zinc during periods of rapid growth and development emphasizes its importance during gestation and fetal growth. However, at a recent workshop to evaluate the benefits of maternal zinc supplementation in eight randomized controlled studies in developing countries where low plasma zinc was common, no data emerged to support the hypothesis that maternal zinc supplementation promoted intrauterine growth (55). Nevertheless, the studies did indicate that maternal zinc supplementation had beneficial effects on neonatal immune status, early morbidity, and infant infections. Zinc metabolism has close associations with vitamin A; therefore, zinc stimulates the synthesis of retinol binding protein (56) and improves gut integrity in malnourished infants (57,58). Zinc supplements also reduced duration of acute diarrhea in Indian infants (3–36 mo) (59). However, the latter also received a daily multivitamin supplement containing vitamin A and zinc that may have improved use of vitamin A. Zinc supplements (10 mg zinc as zinc gluconate 6 d/wk for 10 mo) also reduced the prevalence of malaria (60) and, more recently (12.8 mg zinc acetate or placebo every 2–3 h while cold existed), to shorten the duration of the common cold; the latter in otherwise-healthy adults with normal zinc levels at the outset (61). The mechanism responsible for the latter effects is currently unexplained.

Zinc is another nutrient for which status is difficult to evaluate. Normal plasma zinc concentrations (10.5–17.0 µmol/L) fall rapidly after the onset of infection and by as much as 70% in a febrile illness (27). In other words, the fall in zinc is even more dramatic than that of iron, but less than 1% of body zinc is present in plasma (49), so changes in blood may mean little in overall body zinc status. Infection is also accompanied by negative zinc balance, because zinc is lost in sweat and mucosal secretions, e.g., diarrhea (62). The fall in plasma zinc concentrations is probably a consequence of monocyte stimulation by bacterial products, because IL-1 infusions into animals resulted in decreases of iron and zinc, and incubating hepatocytes with IL-1 increased metallothionine transcription (40). Metallothionine is an important metal-binding protein and provides defense against oxidative stress *(63)*. Hepatocyte metallothionine may be the destination of the zinc leaving the plasma *(49)*. Furthermore, the fall in plasma zinc may be a protective response, because fever was greater in patients on home parenteral nutrition with catheter sepsis who were given zinc supplements (30 mg/d for 3 d) compared with those given 0 or 23 mg/d *(64)*. Depressed immune response was observed in another study where patients were given 100–300 mg/d *(65)*.

Zinc is also a mitogen, capable of inducing cytokine production in PMN leukocytes, but zinc can act synergistically with bacterial LPS or phytohemagglutinin (PHA) at concentrations of plasma zinc that would not normally be mitogenic *(50)*. Hence, immunologic disadvantages of low plasma zinc concentrations at the start of infection may be overcome by the synergism with bacterial antigens. In patients with catheter sepsis, where plasma zinc concentrations were elevated by modest supplements (30 mg for the first 3 d), there was an increased febrile response *(64)*. Workers have suggested that different concentrations of zinc influence the activities of T cells and monocytes differently—T cells being stimulated by normal concentrations (12–16 µmol/L) and inhibited by higher concentrations *(50)*, whereas monocytes respond more actively to larger amounts of zinc (100 µmol/L) *(66)*. Thus, low zinc concentrations in plasma at the onset of infection may prevent too vigorous activity of the acute-phase response (APR), and this may be augmented by increased tissue levels of the antioxidant metallothionine and by the role of zinc in the antioxidant enzyme, superoxide dismutase (SOD). The role played by the movement of zinc from blood into the tissues with the onset of infection is not known. Nevertheless, it is tempting to speculate that augmentation of tissue zinc provides increased protein and DNA syntheses and general metabolism *(67)*, whereas that amount of zinc left in the plasma is still capable of optimally stimulating PMN leukocytes in conjunction with bacterial antigen.

Thus, although plasma zinc is described as "the immunologically important pool" *(49)*, there is a variable response in health benefits from supplementation where plasma zinc is low. Such results possibly suggest that the low concentrations do not represent deficiency but represent the effect of inflammation and may already be optimal. Therefore, it is important to find out why concentrations are low before supplements are given, because the latter can cause harm *(49)* (*see* Chapter 13).

2.4.3. COPPER

In general, plasma copper concentrations increase two- to threefold between 48 and 72 h postinfection in most diseases *(26)*. Most of the copper in plasma is bound to ceruloplasmin, which is a positive acute-phase protein (APP). The increase in plasma copper is a consequence of the APR, and the ferroxidase activity of ceruloplasmin (*see* Table 2) assists in iron uptake from the plasma by the RES *(38)*.

Copper, like zinc, is depleted by acute diarrhea. Workers reported there was a negative balance for both minerals in hospitalized infants (3–14 mo) during the first 5 d, and copper balance was still negative 1 wk after admission *(62)*. In 1995, the WHO estimated that 1.8 billion children died of diarrhea annually, and this constitutes approx 23% of all under-fives deaths in the developing world *(8)*. Therefore, diarrhea is a major problem in children in developing countries; hence, copper deficiency is potentially of concern. However, unfortunately, there are no good indicators of copper status; therefore, the magnitude of the problem in human populations is difficult to estimate. In ruminants, both primary and induced copper deficiency impair the innate immune response. Neutrophils are the components most affected and microbicidal activity, superoxide production, SOD activity and, *potentially*, phagocytic activity, are all reduced. Likewise, ceruloplasmin production was impaired in copper deficiency. The workers could find no evidence that copper deficiency affected macrophage or acquired immune function in ruminants *(68)*.

Both zinc and copper are components of SOD enzyme present in the cytosol. Both this and the manganese containing SOD present in mitochondria are universally distributed antioxidant enzymes in biologic tissues. SOD activity appears to be more sensitive to copper deficiency than zinc *(69)*, although other workers using a human promonocytic cell line depleted for 4 d of 62% copper, using a copper chelator, found no change in copper/zinc SOD *(70)*. Nevertheless, the copper deficiency suppressed respiratory burst and compromised phagocytic activity, and, in other cells, LPS-stimulated secretion of inflammatory mediators was decreased. Although the results suggest that immune defenses in experimental copper deficiency are compromised, their in vivo significance in man is difficult to evaluate.

2.5. Influence of the Acute-Phase Response on Vitamin A and Iodine

Hyporetinolemia is an early feature of many infections *(71–73)*. The cause is linked with reduced hepatic synthesis of retinol-binding protein (RBP) *(74)*. RBP, like transthyretin (TTR), albumin, and transferrin, is a negative acute-phase protein. The rapidity of the response suggests that the changes in RBP synthesis accompany those of the other APP initiated by cytokines IL-1 and IL-6. The rapid fall in plasma retinol associated with infection may initially result from increased capillary permeability facilitating quicker distribution of retinol to tissues where it is needed to counter the infection. Labeling studies suggest that vitamin A in the extravascular pool is only slowly (37 d) returned to the plasma *(75)*; hence, the recovery of plasma retinol after infection is dependent on a resumption of RBP synthesis and mobilization from the liver.

Iodine is necessary for the synthesis of the thyroid hormones, tri- and tetra-iodothyronine, and a lack of dietary iodine is associated with goiter and cretinism. The transport protein for the thyroid hormones is TTR, and this couples with RBP in the plasma *(76)*. There is a rapid reduction in plasma TTR concentrations and the thyroid hormones at the onset of infection or trauma *(77)*. There are also indications that goiter severity may be linked more closely to severity of infection than iodine intake *(78)*.

2.5.1. ACUTE-PHASE PROTEINS

Cytokines IL-1, TNF-α, and IL-6 typically orchestrate the inflammatory response, and this is characterized by a specific series of local and systemic effects that are collectively grouped under the name the APR *(79)*. Local events include vasodilatation, platelet aggregation, neutrophil chemotaxis, and the release of lysosomal enzymes, histamine, kinins, and oxygen radicals. The systemic events comprise such phenomena as fever, hormonal changes, such as activation of the pituitary adrenal system; leukocytosis; thrombocytosis; muscle proteolysis; alterations in carbohydrate, lipid, vitamin, and trace mineral metabolism; and changes in the hepatic synthesis of APP *(80)*. The metabolic changes in peripheral tissues and the liver provide additional nutrients like glucose and amino acids to fuel the activated immune system *(20)*. There are specific sites on the hepatocyte that respond to the cytokines IL-1 and TNF-α and others that respond to IL-6. During a 12–24 h period, the liver responds to cytokine exposure by initiating the hepatic APR with the uptake of amino acids and modulation of gluconeogenesis. IL-1 and TNF-α are also important in exerting profound effects on APR progression.

Glucocorticoid production is stimulated by TNF-α, and this both enhances hepatic APP production and diminishes IL-1 synthesis by the macrophage *(81)*. The APR is designed to facilitate both the inflammatory and the repair processes and to protect the organism against the potentially destructive action of inflammatory products *(81)*, e.g., limiting cytokine production, neutralizing ROI, inhibiting proteinases *(82)*. The APR is not just a response to infection but a broad-based response to many different types of tissue injury, e.g., allergic reaction, thermal damage, hypoxia, surgery, malignancy, and muscular damage after excessive exercise *(21)*. The functions of APP are still being revealed, but, in general, they are protective and antiinflammatory.

2.5.2. VITAMIN A

It has been widely accepted for more than 50 yr that vitamin A plays a role in infection. Vitamin A is essential for normal epithelial and mesenchymal cell maintenance and differentiation, morphogenesis, growth, vision, resistance to infection, and reproductive function, most likely after its conversion to retinoic acid. Retinoic acid, by activating nuclear receptors to modulate gene transcription, behaves as a hormone with important roles in regulating cell proliferation and differentiation *(83)*.

However, one of the earliest effects of infection on vitamin A metabolism is a reduction in plasma retinol. Plasma retinol concentrations in healthy infants, and young children have a mean of approx 1 μmol/L. This value increases gradually through childhood to reach adult values in early teenage years of approx 2.2 and 1.8 μmol/L in men and women, respectively. With the onset of infection *(71)* or physical trauma *(73)*, there is a rapid fall in plasma retinol. However, even when the retinol concentration falls to values that are associated with severe deficiency of vitamin A, e.g., plasma retinol < 0.35 μmol/L in children with severe *Shigella* dysentery, normal retinol concentrations of ≥ 1.0 μmol/L were restored on clinical recovery without any supplementary vitamin A treatment *(84)*.

Experimentally, the fall in plasma retinol is associated with a reduction in the hepatic synthesis of the messenger RNA for RBP in response to treatment with cytokines IL-1 and IL-6. At first sight, it is curious that RBP is a negative APP when evidence suggests that there may an increased need for retinol in infection, but the reduction in RBP synthesis may be to protect retinol reserves. Retinol is found in the urine, particularly in patients with fever *(85)* or after surgery *(77)*, and this may result from impaired reabsorption of retinol in the kidney during inflammation. It is estimated that 50% of plasma retinol turnover in the rat is in the kidneys and nearly all is recycled to the plasma in the healthy animal *(75)*. The degree of protection of vitamin A stores afforded by the downregulation of RBP synthesis is not known and presumably depends on frequency, duration, and severity of infection. Children who were infected with the chicken pox virus during a vitamin A-supplementation trial had lower vitamin A reserves at the end of the year when compared with those who were not affected *(86)*. Such results suggest that protection of vitamin A stores by downregulation of RBP synthesis may not be effective. However, there are reports that APP changes are not as pronounced in viral as bacterial diseases *(87)*, which may explain the greater losses of vitamin A in those children who had the chicken pox infection.

From what has been said, the fall in plasma retinol concentrations after infection is a protective response to reduce vitamin A losses. Benefits obtained by the host depend on the nutritional status of vitamin A before infection, as well as the length of infection. We showed that malaria produced a similar absolute reduction in plasma retinol concentration, irrespective of concentration at the outset. Thus, plasma retinol concentrations in adult Thai patients from rural areas were 56% lower than matched uninfected controls, and retinol values of approx 30% of the rural patients were below 0.35 μmol/L. In the urban groups, the difference between patients and controls was only 34% and there were none with retinol concentrations of <0.35 μmol/L *(71)*. That is, there was greater protection (i.e., reduction) of vitamin A in those with the lowest preinfection concentrations, but the net result was dangerously low plasma retinol concentrations. If the infection quickly resolves, then, presumably, no harm results, but if complications develop and the infection is protracted, then those organs where access to vitamin A is vital will start to fail. Vision is one of the first functions to fail in vitamin A deficiency, but the immune functions of vitamin A in preventing morbidity are also important. The outstanding success of vitamin A supplements in overcoming shortfalls in vitamin A supply and reducing morbidity and mortality in infants in many developing countries is clearly indicated in three meta-analyses *(88–90)* (*see* Chapter 6 by Semba).

2.5.3. IODINE

Iodine is necessary for the production of the thyroid hormones, triiodothyronine and tetraiodothyronine. An absence of iodine from the diet leads to an overgrowth of the thyroid gland and the production of a goiter. The thyroid hormones regulate the metabolic combustion of sugars, lipids, and proteins and are, therefore, involved in the metabolism of all cells of the organism during growth and in the development of most organs, particularly the brain. The selenoprotein, thioredoxin, also plays a role in the synthesis of throxine *(91)*, and combined deficiencies of the two nutrients may be important in the etiology of cretinism *(92)*.

Iodine deficiency is one of the major micronutrient deficiencies worldwide. However, deficiency primarily results from the loss of iodine from soils by leaching, because the deficiency is rarely found where sea fish are consumed. Nevertheless, there is some evidence that the APR may impair the metabolic functions of iodine because plasma transthyretin (TTR), the transport protein for thyroxine, is a negative APP. There is an immediate decrease in TTR in moderate or severe injury *(93)* or acute inflammation *(94)*, but the implications of this decrease on thyroxine supply are not known. Of course, TTR does couple with RBP in transporting vitamin A in human plasma *(76)*, and long-term reductions in plasma retinol are associated with higher rates of morbidity and mortality. TTR is not depressed in asymptomatic HIV *(95)*.

It has been suggested that a thyroxine deficiency depresses aldosterone activity and that diarrheal episodes may be worsened by hypothyroidism, because aldosterone regulates the passage of electrolytes and water across cell membranes *(96)*. Data from other workers also suggest that infection worsens hypothyroidism *(78)*. In a report from central Guinea, West Africa, the prevalence of the different stages of goiter were positively associated with the APPs, CRP, and AGP. CRP and AGP are useful indicators of acute and chronic infections, respectively *(97)*. Those with goiter stage 3 had the highest plasma concentrations of both CRP and AGP. At first sight, it is unlikely that the clinical measurement of goiter size should be causally linked to severity of subclinical infections, unless the decrease in thyroid hormone caused by infection, stimulated thyroid hyperplasia through some feedback mechanism. There was no difference in urinary iodine concentrations (i.e., which represents dietary intake) between those without and (the three groups) with thyroid swelling, and the prevalence of cretinism was surprisingly low (2%) for the prevalence of goiter reported (70%). There is no doubt that dietary iodine was a problem in Guinea, but endogenous infections worsened the clinical outcome.

Similar inconsistencies in thyroid swelling and iodine status were reported in a study in Bangladeshi women, where the prevalence of goiter was 99%, and 79% of women had grade-2 or grade-3 goiters. The authors suggested that urinary iodine only indicated moderate iodine deficiency and that deficiencies of vitamin A and selenium or the presence of dietary goitrogens were not a problem *(98)*. Unfortunately, markers of infection were not measured in the Bangladeshi study, but Bangladesh is a developing country, and exposure to infection is likely to be high and may have been responsible for the inconsistencies.

2.6. Vitamin C

2.6.1. THE INFLAMMATORY RESPONSE AND LEUKOCYTOSIS

Most of the cells involved in the inflammatory response are phagocytic cells. In a local response, the first cells to accumulate at the site of tissue damage (30–60 min) are mainly PMN leukocytes. If the cause of the inflammation persists for more than 5–6 h, then the area will be infiltrated by mononuclear cells, thus adding to the defensive process *(99)*. The effects result in the accumulation of fluid (edema) and leukocytic cells in the injured areas. If the cause of the inflammation is systemic, e.g., bacterial or viral disease or surgery, then a more general leukocytosis results, comprising mainly PMN leukocytes, approx 70% of which are neutrophils *(100,101)*.

A key role in the relationship between the local inflammatory reaction and the systemic APR is played by IL-1 and TNF-α *(79)*. These cytokines are the main mediators, both of the local sequelae of inflammation and for its systemic effects. Endothelial cells are induced to undergo major changes in gene regulation and surface expression of important adhesion molecules, including ICAM-1. These interact specifically with neutrophils and other circulating leukocytes to slow the rate of flow and initiate transendothelial passage out of the vessels in a process known as extravazation. At an early stage, a predominant aspect of the APR is the modification of vascular tone caused by dilation and leakage of blood vessels particularly at the postcapillary venules. These alterations are likely to be mediated by ROI and NO. Thus, activation of macrophages or aggregation of platelets can rapidly result in altered vessel permeability, allowing escape (or transfer) into tissues of important biological substances *(79)*.

2.6.2. LEUKOCYTOSIS AND VITAMIN C

Evidence for changes in leukocyte vitamin C associated with stress was first reported in the early 1970s, when rapid decreases in leukocyte ascorbate concentration was documented within 24 h of the onset of the common cold *(102)* or after surgery *(103)*. Leukocyte ascorbate concentrations normalized during the next 3–6 d, and the changes resulted from the rapid influx into the circulation of newly synthesized white cells, most of which were neutrophils and contained little vitamin C. Normalization in leukocyte ascorbate concentrations can be accompanied by lower plasma concentrations *(101)*. The leukocytosis is, of course, a feature of the APR *(99)*, and the dilution of the resident PMN leukocytes by the newly synthesized vitamin C-depleted leukocytes accounts for the apparent fall in leukocyte ascorbate concentration associated with stress conditions.

2.6.3. VITAMIN C

Plasma ascorbate concentrations are strongly linked to dietary intake and limited by a renal threshold of approx 80 µmol/L *(104)*. In patients with disease, concentrations of plasma ascorbate are frequently lower than those seen in well-nourished subjects, but, of course, this may well result from the anorexia of infection *(38)*. However, administration of therapeutic doses of IL-2 to patients with malignancies produced a profound decrease (80%) in plasma ascorbate concentrations, but the fate of the vitamin C in these patients was not known, and ascorbate returned to pretreatment values when treatment was stopped *(105)*. It is well-known that the ascorbate concentration of leukocytes is higher than that in plasma *(106)* and that vitamin C stimulates chemotaxis *(107)*. Furthermore, intracellular ascorbate can be increased tenfold in neutrophils by activation *(108)*, and this is necessary to maintain the redox integrity of the cell. Neutrophils from scorbutic guinea pigs displayed a normal in vitro phagocytic response against latex particles and hydrogen peroxide production, but supplementary vitamin C was necessary to maintain the response if the neutrophils had previously phagocytozed red cells *(109)*. That is, oxidant substances within the phagocytozed cells had upset the redox integrity of the neutrophil. The accumulation of intracellular ascorbate by neutrophils was first linked with stress factors (bacterial products and raised temperature) by Moser and Weber *(110)*.

Various workers suggest that the increased intracellular ascorbate protects the cells against bactericidal products generated during the respiratory burst *(108)*. The uptake of ascorbate by neutrophils, preferentially as dehydroascorbate, may be a necessary part of neutrophil function, because this ability is absent in the neutrophils of patients with chronic granulomatous disease. It is also suggested that both extracellular and intracellular vitamin C are necessary for optimal bacterial killing in vitro and in vivo *(108)*. The optimal plasma concentration to provide physiologic benefit is debatable. Vitamin C and E supplements (600 mg of both/d for 14 d) given to healthy volunteers *(111)* or patients with acute myocardial infarction (MI) *(112)* inhibit ROI production by PMN leukocytes. Similarly, de la Fuente *(113)* also showed that vitamin C supplements (1 g/d) and vitamin E (200 mg, both daily for 16 wk) depressed neutrophil superoxide production and lowered serum lipid peroxides and cortisol in healthy elderly women, as well as those with depressive disorders or coronary heart disease. In contrast, a smaller dose of vitamin C given without vitamin E to both young and elderly Indian men and women (200 mg/d for 90 d), significantly increased neutrophil superoxide production *(114)*. However, in the studies of de la Fuente and colleagues *(113)* and Jayachandran and colleagues *(114)*, neutrophil adherence and phagocytic capacity were increased in all groups of volunteers and was also associated with an increase in leukocyte ascorbate *(114)*. Thus, a high vitamin C concentration more than approx 600 mg/d (possibly with the additional presence of supplemental vitamin E) in plasma may be counterproductive to neutrophil free-radical generation and cytotoxicity, despite the improved ability to engulf bacteria.

However, a reduction in ROI production may benefit patients with acute MI, reducing the incidence and severity of arrhythmias and the size of the infarct *(112)*.

Large doses of vitamin C will raise blood and tissue concentrations and potentially aggravate oxidant damage within tissues *(115)*. Vitamin C can reduce iron to the ferrous form (FeII), thus potentially stimulating the formation of hydroxyl radicals (OH·) from superoxide and hydrogen peroxide *(115)*. Iron in the circulation is normally bound to transport proteins and is, thus, unavailable to react with ascorbate; however, free iron or nontransferrin-bound iron (NTBI) is detectable in damaged tissues *(116)*, various pathologies *(117)*, or tissue exudates after ischemia *(118)*. Furthermore, indirect evidence of the presence of NTBI in plasma is indicated by the rapid changes in iron and iron-binding proteins in the circulation after trauma (*see* Table 2 and section on iron). Vitamin C uptake by the neutrophil may provide a safe store for an important antioxidant and lower the risk of inflammatory reactions between ascorbate and iron at the site of trauma or bacterial attack. As indicated, neutrophils rapidly congregate at such sites, releasing lactoferrin, which also assists in removing iron. Thus, the risk of interaction between intracellular vitamin C and NTBI is minimized.

The fall in plasma ascorbate concentrations associated with infection, and trauma is clearly a consequence of the APR and should, therefore, be viewed as protective to the host. However, the widespread use of vitamin C supplements, without any obvious adverse or beneficial consequences in the general population, suggests that reduction in plasma ascorbate concentrations associated with acute infection is not of major pathologic importance in most people. Nevertheless, in certain chronic disease states, such as coronary heart disease, there are suggestions that vitamin C supplements may have beneficial effects *(112,119,120)*. Evidence suggests that vitamin C alters the redox state of arterial smooth muscle guanyl cyclase, thereby altering arterial sensitivity to NO *(121)*. In patients with coronary heart disease, flow-mediated dilation (FMD) of the brachial artery was measured before, 2 h after 2 g vitamin C, and 30 d after a further 500 mg/d. In the treatment group, FMD was significantly increased at both times posttreatment *(119)*. A progressive neutrophil leukocyte infiltration of damaged myocardium has been observed within the first 24 h after infarction. This is initially a beneficial process designed to remove damaged tissue. However, if the process continues, it may exacerbate myocardial injury owing to overproduction of ROI, and endothelial cells can be the primary target of immunologic injury, resulting in vasculopathy and organ dysfunction *(122)*. As indicated, vitamin C and E supplements increase neutrophil adherence and chemotactic and phagocytic capacity, coupled with a reduction in superoxide production *(113)*. Furthermore, 250 mg vitamin C daily for 6 wk significantly reduced monocyte adhesion to endothelial cells in subjects with low compared with high concentrations of plasma ascorbate (mean 32 and 67 μmol/L, respectively). Thus, vitamin C (+/– vitamin E) supplements in chronic disease states, such as coronary heart disease improve blood flow through damaged tissues, reduce infiltration by monocytes, and, possibly, reduce the net superoxide production from infiltrating neutrophils. That is, vitamin C supplements in the posttraumatic stage may assist the healing process by promoting endothelial function.

However, there are subgroups, particularly in developing countries, in whom vitamin C supplements can cause harm. Coma and death have resulted from excessive vitamin C intakes in patients with glucose-6-phosphate dehydrogenase (G-6-PD) deficiency

(123,124), and hemoglobinuria was increased in patients with paroxysmal nocturnal hemoglobinuria (PNH) *(125)*. G-6-PD deficiency is an enzymopathy that affects approx 1% of the world's population, although its prevalence is mainly in tropical and subtropical countries, where malaria infection is or has been of recent importance. The condition causes red cell instability, which shortens the life span of the erythrocyte and increases the risk of red cell contents in the plasma. In the reports mentioned, the death occurred in a patient with burns where 4 g of vitamin C was given for 2 d *(123)*. However, in the other, the trauma resulted after the consumption of fortified soft drinks by 2 young Indian boys, and the amount of vitamin C consumed was probably between 3 and 4 g in 4–6 h *(124)*. PNH is a rare hemolytic disease caused by a somatic mutation in a multipotential stem cell and where the hemolysis generally occurs at night. In this particular report, the patient's hemoglobin had fallen from 102 to 85 g/L after consumption of vitamin C-fortified fruit drinks *(125)*. Experimentally, the workers showed that hemolysis could occur in such patients after the consumption of 1 g vitamin C, which could temporarily raise plasma ascorbate to approx 220 µmol/L, a concentration that did not affect red cell stability in normal subjects.

It has also been suggested that persons with iron overload should not consume large amounts of vitamin C because of the risk of generating excessive ROI. Iron overload occurs in patients with thalassemia, as well as homozygote carriers of the gene for hemochromatosis. The latter only occurs in approx 1/400 people, but it is argued that 20% of Americans may be heterozygote carriers with moderate iron overload *(126)* and, therefore, at risk of iron toxicity and oversensitive to vitamin C. Although other workers believe this is an overemphasis, they also confirm that large quantities of vitamin C have been associated with fatal cardiac arrhythmias in patients with iron overload but suggest the prevalence of heterozygote carriers is only 8% and only 1% to 3% of these develop iron overload *(127)*. Among the various recommendations for such people, it is suggested that supplemental vitamin C be limited to 500 mg/d.

In conclusion, the clinical consequence of elevated vitamin C intakes in persons with unstable red cells and/or where the level of NTBI is increased indicates the potential dangers of the vitamin in patients with infection or trauma. However, the dangers of vitamin C are associated only with intakes in excess of approx 500 mg/d and such intakes would not be available to persons consuming nonfortified diets. Nevertheless, plasma vitamin C uptake by activated neutrophils may be beneficial by reducing the risk of elevated oxidative stress in the tissues or hemolysis in the blood and also by increasing the phagocytic properties of neutrophils.

2.7. Redox State, Antioxidant Micronutrients, and the Innate Immune Response

The inflammatory state is essentially an oxidative state; hence, there is considerable interest in the potential role of antioxidant nutrients in modulating disease activity, from both the protectiveness of endogenous antioxidants and the effectiveness of exogenous antioxidant treatment of disease. The major antioxidant nutrients are vitamins E and C, the minerals zinc and copper through their role together in superoxide dismutase, copper in ceruloplasmin, and selenium in glutathione peroxidase and other selenoenzymes. The degree of protection afforded by antioxidants depends also on prooxidant activity in disease; thus, iron nutrition must also be considered in the equation as previously discussed (*see* section on iron). The influence of infection on vitamin C and its possible role in PMN leukocyte metabolism has also just been discussed. In this section, the importance of overall antioxidant status is discussed, as well as some of the individual features of the other dietary antioxidants.

2.7.1. NUCLEAR FACTOR KAPPA B (NF-κB)

The ability to generate cytokines by nonspecific immune cells distributed through the body is the prime stimulatory component of innate or natural immunity. The cytokines help to mount an inflammatory response and to recruit specialized cells, such as mononuclear phagocytes, NK cells, and neutrophils, to the infection site. It is now known that the rapid induction of the synthesis of these cytokines is coordinated by a common cellular element, a transcription factor known as nuclear factor B (NF-κB).

NF-κB is critical for the inducible expression of many genes involved in the immune and inflammatory responses, including IL-1, IL-2, IL-6, IL-8, TNF-α, TNF-β, serum amyloid A protein etc. It is reported that NF-κB exists in almost all cells but that it remains in the cytoplasm bound to an inhibitory protein, inhibitory B (IκB). Exposure of cells to various inducers leads to the dissociation of the cytoplasmic complex and the translocation of the free NF-κB to the nucleus. In vitro studies have shown that phosphorylation accompanies the dissociation of the NF-κB/IκB complex, with a rapid degradation of the IκB protein. Inducers, such as TNF-α, can cause significant activation of NF-κB within minutes, allowing NF-κB to function as an effective signal transducer and rapidly connect events in the cytoplasm to response genes in the nucleus. One such response is the rapid upregulation of IκB-α synthesis, which then helps to shut down the NF-κB response and provide a uniquely suited feedback loop to sensitively control a transient inducer of responsive genes *(128)*. The rapidity of the NF-κB response to induction is similar to that shown by IFN *(19)* or the nongenomic membrane actions of steroids *(129)*. However, a unique feature of signaling through NF-κB is the diversity of signaling molecules (viruses, ROI, mitogens, cytokines, etc.) and situations that activate NF-κB and the types of genes responsive to NF-κB. Nevertheless, the common feature of the inducers is that they all signal situations of stress, infection, or injury to the organism *(128)*.

That NF-κB can be activated by ROI *(130)* and that common inducers can be inhibited by antioxidants *(131)* has made the NF-κB mechanism particularly interesting to those wishing to account for the health advantages associated with antioxidant-rich fruit and vegetable diets. ROI are produced by macrophages and granulocytes as part of the oxidative burst to kill pathogens and are also elevated in the inflammatory response *(20)*. That N-acetyl-L-cysteine, which is a precursor of the antioxidant reduced glutathione and an ROI scavenger, suppresses the activation of NF-κB by many agents, supports the idea that the redox state of the cell plays a general role in the activity of NF-κB *(128,130,131)*. However, in vitro studies with micronutrients that influence the redox state must be carefully interpreted *(132)*. In neutrophils, iron deficiencies can reduce myeloperoxidase activity *(133)*, and supplements of vitamins C and E suppress production of oxygen free radicals *(113)*, so potentially both dietary deficiency and dietary excess could impair the killing of bacteria and/or reduce tissue damage. Among the questions that remain to be answered are: is there an optimal redox state in vivo to enable efficient bacterial killing with minimal damage to surrounding tissues *(132)* and are certain antioxidant nutrients more important than others in regulating this state?

2.7.2. VITAMIN E

Vitamin E is transported in plasma mostly in the form of α-tocopherol by lipoproteins, and from an early age in industrialized countries, the concentration is approx 20–28 µmol/L *(134)*. The usual daily intake of vitamin E in these countries is approx 6–12 mg, and because the vitamin is available in vegetable oils and nuts, deficiency is unlikely, unless there are metabolic problems, e.g., fat malabsorption. It is the main antioxidant in lipoproteins (approx 6 µmol/mol LDL) and, in the same way that plasma retinol concentration is determined by its transport protein RBP, vitamin E is influenced by the lipoprotein concentration. Cholesterol is a structural component of lipoproteins and easily measured, and to assess vitamin E status, the ratio of vitamin E to cholesterol can be used. This ratio is usually fairly constant, approx 4–6 µmol/mmol cholesterol *(134)*, even in developing countries where the median plasma concentration of vitamin E may be as low as 7 µmol/L *(38)*. Thus, although plasma concentrations of vitamin E in some populations may be quite low, the ratio to cholesterol is normal. It is also interesting to note that during supplementation studies with amounts greater than 100 mg/d, plasma vitamin E concentration may double, but within 5 d of removing the supplement, the levels return to presupplementation levels *(135)*. The requirements of vitamin E are linked to the dietary intake of polyunsaturated fatty acids (PUFA). However, maintaining a suitable ratio of vitamin E to PUFA may be more important in the infant than adult, because infants are on a relatively restricted diet *(136)*.

In disease, plasma lipoproteins are influenced mainly by anorexia, which reduces liver lipoprotein synthesis; hence, vitamin E concentrations are reduced but ratios to cholesterol remain normal *(15)*. Increased vascular permeability may also lower plasma lipoprotein concentrations, but because lipoproteins are larger molecules than RBP, vascular permeability must be quite markedly increased, e.g., during malaria, to influence plasma lipoproteins *(137)*.

Tissue concentrations of vitamin E have been studied less widely than blood. Vitamin E is widely distributed in the body in cell membranes, where it is believed to protect lipids from oxidation in biologic membranes. Experimental studies suggest that the amount in tissues is more strongly related to oxygen exposure than with PUFA; thus, the molar ratio of vitamin E/PUFA is four times higher in heart and lungs than in the muscle *(138)*. Supplementation studies in man, even with doses of 300 mg/d, fail to increase tissue levels by more than two- to threefold *(139)*, even in one terminally ill patient who received the dose for more than 2 yr *(140)*. It is probable that tissue levels remain elevated for longer than those in blood after supplement withdrawal, because vitamin E turnover in man is quite slow. It is questionable whether increasing tissue concentrations of vitamin E has any physiologic advantages, for although it is suggested that vitamin E is the most important nutritional antioxidant in the tissues *(141)*, it is also efficiently regenerated *(142)*, and this may be why turnover is so slow. The resistance to increase in plasma and tissue levels even when large amounts of supplements are used and the efficient regeneration of vitamin E question the need for supplements. Vitamin E supplements, in general, have not provided any benefits against some of the major chronic diseases, such as cancer, diabetes, and cardiovascular disease *(143)*. Indeed, in a recent 15-mo study to investigate benefits of multivitamins/minerals or vitamin E (200 mg/d) on respiratory tract infections in noninstitutionalized elderly persons older than 60 yr, severity of infections was significantly worse in those receiving vitamin E and there were no advantages in either group *(144)*. Aspects of this study have been criticized by Han and Meydani (*see* Chapter 8 on vitamin E) who maintain that there may be some merit in supplementing specific groups in the population, such as the elderly, but more evidence is needed to support these suggestions, because most people are adequately nourished with vitamin E.

2.7.3. SELENIUM

Selenium status is assessed by the concentration in plasma or the activity of red cell glutathione peroxidase (GPx). The latter is the better measure of functional status, whereas plasma concentrations reflect dietary intake *(145)* and, therefore, decrease as a result of anorexia during infection.

Selenium is a constitutive component of the enzyme glutathione peroxidase. The enzyme exists in several isoforms, with slightly different functions, but is found in all tissues *(146)*. One of its main functions is to convert lipid peroxides to the hydroxy acids and hydrogen peroxide to water. Thyrodoxin is a specific selenoperoxidase found in the thyroid, where it removes peroxides. Disease and trauma are linked with increases in redox stress within tissues *(69)*, and experimental studies indicate that certain viruses can take advantage of compromised antioxidant status.

Keshan disease in China is geographically associated with selenium deficiency, but temporal fluctuations in incidence suggested that other factors were involved in its etiology. Chinese workers suspected that enteroviruses, particularly coxsackieviruses, were responsible for the cardiomyopathy, and experimental studies showed that Se-deficient mice were more susceptible than Se-supplemented mice to cardiotoxic effects of coxsackievirus B4 that had been isolated from the blood of a Keshan disease victim *(147)*. These initial observations were explored by Beck and colleagues, who found that susceptibility to these viruses was not specifically associated with Se deficiency but could also be increased by vitamin E deficiency or a combination of vitamin E deficiency and PUFA excess. Their work showed that a previously avirulent strain of coxsackievirus CVB3/0 was changed to a virulent phenotype when passed through vitamin E deficient animals *(147)*. More recently, these workers have also reported that similar observations had been made in mice given excess iron and in glutathione peroxidase-knock-out mice *(148)*. Analysis of the genomic structure of the newly developing viruses led Beck and colleagues to suggest that increased oxidative stress in disease facilitates the enhanced growth rate of the invading virus, increasing the likelihood of development of more virulent mutations *(149)*.

Of course, the experimental studies described were conducted in animals in which true dietary deficiencies were established. Experiments have not been performed to determine the extent of deficiency of the different antioxidants needed to facilitate viral growth and mutation in man. Keshan disease occurred in people living in an area deficient in selenium, but other micronutrients were probably marginal or inadequate in the same communities. The experimental studies show that deficiencies of several, if not all, the antioxidant nutrients had similar effects on viral growth, indicating that the mechanism was not specific to one antioxidant but to the overall antioxidant status.

2.8. Other Micronutrients Influenced by the Disease Process

The dietary intake of all nutrients is likely to be depressed by the anorexia of infection. This particularly affects the water-soluble vitamins, as well as carotenoids, vitamin K, and substances, such as the flavonoids and other polyphenols. Sickness may also be associated with lower exposure to sunlight; thus, vitamin D synthesis may be depressed. In general, the fat-soluble micronutrients are less affected by infection, because there are usually sufficient stores to overcome short-term restrictions. Two of these, vitamins A and E, are discussed in Sections 2.5. and 2.7. There are no specific effects of infection on vitamins D and K. In the remaining paragraphs, a few examples highlight how anorexia or other aspects of disease affect some of the B vitamins.

2.8.1. RIBOFLAVIN

As with most of the B vitamins, the majority of riboflavin present in the tissues is incorporated into functional coenzymes. Therefore, the saturation of red cell enzyme glutathione reductase (EGR) by its coenzyme, flavin adenine dinucleotide, is used as a functional index of riboflavin status. The measurement used is the activation coefficient (EGRAC).

Riboflavin first appeared in the infection literature when experimental work suggested that riboflavin deficiency protected against malaria [5], and even in human studies, red cell parasitemia (parasite count) was inversely proportional to status [150]. Status was measured by EGRAC, and, because the red cell is one of the first tissues to loose riboflavin in dietary deficiency and an adequately nourished red cell is important for parasite development, a correlation between EGRAC and parasitemia is not surprising. Later studies showed that the parasite count was not a good indicator of disease severity and riboflavin deficiency did not protect against disease [151].

Other studies using the EGRAC method to assess status gave unexpected results. There are two reports that suggest that riboflavin status improves in infection [152, 152a]. The probable explanation for this is that riboflavin is released into the blood as a result of tissue breakdown to fuel the APR. The riboflavin is taken up by apo-EGR, leading to an apparent improvement in status [151].

2.8.2. THIAMIN

Thiamin is primarily involved in carbohydrate metabolism, which increases particularly in febrile infections. A 1°C rise in body temperature increases energy requirements by 10% [153]. Thiamin is particularly important, because it is an essential cofactor in the multienzyme complex that oxidises pyruvate to acetyl-S-coenzyme A. This pyruvate dehydrogenase complex is situated strategically between glycolysis and the tricarboxylic acid (Krebs) cycle; thus, thiamin deficiency interferes with efficient production of energy from carbohydrate. The other B vitamins, riboflavin and niacin, are also involved in ATP generation, but thiamin deficiency is the most critical, because it blocks access of carbohydrate to oxidation by the Krebs cycle [154]. Therefore, infection increases the need for several nutrients but especially thiamin.

In regions or groups of people where thiamin status is marginal, infection can precipitate beriberi outbreaks, e.g., in China [155]. In addition, little to no thiamin is stored in the body, except as the functional coenzyme; thus, dietary deficiencies can produce biochemical evidence of deficiency in 2 wk [156]. Hence, anorexia may impair thiamin status quite quickly, particularly in groups where previous intake may be marginal, such as in the elderly. This may account for the high prevalence of thiamin deficiency in hospitalized elderly patients [157].

2.8.3. Folate, Cyanocobalamin (B$_{12}$), and Pyridoxine (B$_6$)

Deficiencies of all three of these vitamins can have a major effect on both innate and acquired immune mechanisms because of their important roles in nucleotide and protein intermediary metabolism. Thus, as in the case of thiamin, infection will increase requirements of the vitamins and may precipitate clinical signs of deficiency in subjects with borderline nutritional status. Of the three, folate is probably the vitamin most likely to be marginal in industrialized countries, but the initial clinical consequence of all three vitamin deficiencies is anemia—a condition that is not immediately obvious. However, recently elevated plasma homocysteine has been linked to inadequacies of all three micronutrients (158). Elevated homocysteine is a risk factor for cardiovascular disease (CVD) (159), and the prevalence of CVD is directly associated with infection (160). Indeed, the elevated oxidant stress associated with infection may initiate the disease process culminating in the thrombosis or other vascular damage. It is possible that if the increased need for the three vitamins in infection is not met in those with marginal status, then homocysteine is elevated. This scenario could, in part, explain the association of elevated homocysteine with the incidence of CVD.

3. FUTURE RESEARCH

Research is needed in the following areas:

- To obtain better ways of interpreting and assessing micronutrient status in the presence of infection and subclinical infection.
- To obtain better ways to evaluate when a protective change in micronutrient concentration produced by the acute-phase response is no longer protective.
- To understand more clearly the reasons for the hypoferremia in infection to know when it is appropriate to give iron, particularly to those who are exposed to high levels of infection.
- To understand more clearly the reasons for the hypozincemia in infection, for the same reasons.
- More studies to investigate whether the prevalence of infection does, indeed, influence the severity of goiter.
- To obtain a clearer understanding of the reasons for the intracellular/extracellular movements of vitamin C associated with infection to know if and when it is appropriate to supplement.
- To interpret and assess oxidant stress in tissues during infection.
- Ways to obtain a better understanding of the interactions between antioxidants and prooxidants in the tissues, in health, and in disease; to determine what is a most favorable redox status for optimal immune function.

4. CONCLUSIONS

Experimental studies clearly show that micronutrient deficiencies impair immune system functions in several ways (161), but intervention studies in humans give conflicting results. Much of this confusion results from the difficulties in measuring micronutrient status in the presence of infection. As described, plasma concentrations of vitamin A and C, iron, and zinc are altered rapidly with the onset of the inflammatory process, and other micronutrients are influenced to a smaller and less rapid extent by anorexia, tissue catabolism, or increases in micronutrient requirements. In the short-term, these alterations in plasma concentrations are probably protective and certainly not harmful, but in a marginally malnourished person or in the presence of severe or frequent infections, the changes may have detrimental consequences. Thus, long-term hypoferremia may lead to anemia of chronic infection, and hyporetinolemia may increase susceptibility to disease.

The effects of the APR on micronutrient concentrations in plasma complicates the measurement of micronutrient status and the likely clinical effects of providing supplements. For example, a child in the industrialized world, with a low plasma zinc concentration, may nevertheless have satisfactory zinc status and is, therefore, unlikely to benefit from supplements. However, exposure to infectious disease is enormous in the developing world and, consequently, in any survey of apparently healthy children, a large number are likely to have been recently exposed (and possibly incubating disease) or currently convalescing. Elevated APP concentrations can be used to indicate the numbers of persons in these two states. For example, serum $\alpha 1$-antichymotrypsin (ACT) concentrations rises to a maximum after infection in the first 24 to 48 h *(162)*. In contrast, serum $\alpha 1$-acid glycoprotein (AGP) concentration rises more slowly to a maximum during 2–5 d *(162)* but remain elevated for longer than ACT *(163)*. In a recent survey of 3000 apparently healthy Pakistani preschool children, these elevated APP indicated that the respective proportions of children influenced by recent infection and convalescence were 10% and 45%, respectively *(164)*, and other studies also confirm variable prevalences of subclinical infection and convalescence in children and adults in both the developing world and industrialized countries *(18)*. Such studies highlight the need for better ways to assess nutrient status in persons exposed to or currently affected by infection.

5. "TAKE-HOME" MESSAGES

1. Frequent or severe infection is likely to increase the requirement for all nutrients and, therefore, the risk of deficiency, as a result of alterations in basic metabolism, to meet the challenges posed by the infective organism.
2. The catabolic effects and major changes in intermediary metabolism that accompany infection can also interact with micronutrients, such as copper and B vitamins. These are indirect effects of metabolism rather than the protective role for the host or of the nutrient.
3. Infection depresses the plasma concentration of vitamins A and C and minerals, iron and zinc. These changes occur irrespective of nutritional status, and the resulting plasma concentrations may not reflect the current nutritional status of the patient.
4. The clinical effects of iodine deficiency, i.e., goiter, are worsened by infection.
5. Vitamin A supplements given to infants and children in developing countries have usually been beneficial.
6. Antioxidant status is important in determining the innate immune response of tissues to disease.
7. Selenium deficiency in man and various experimental antioxidant deficiencies or iron excess can increase the cardiotoxic effects of coxsackie virus in animal models.
8. Be aware that infection depresses the plasma concentrations of many important micronutrients. These are physiological responses to the infection and are probably protective in the short-term. Attempts to correct the nutrient concentrations by intervention during acute infection should be resisted, because these may result in increased severity of disease symptoms.

REFERENCES

1. Scrimshaw NS, Taylor CE, Gordon JE. Effect of infection on nutritional status. Interactions of nutrition and infection. World Health Organization, Geneva, 1968, pp. 24–59.
2. Scrimshaw NS, Taylor CE, Gordon JE. Interactions of nutrition and infection. Am J Med Sci 1959;237: 367–403.
3. Clausen SW. Nutrition and infection. J Am Med Assoc 1935;104:793–798.
4. Oppenheimer SJ. Iron and malaria. Parasitol Today 1989;5:77–79.
5. Thurnham DI. Nutrient deficiencies and malaria: a curse or a blessing. In: Taylor TG, Jenkins NK (eds.). Proceedings of the XIII International Congress of Nutrition. John Libbey, London, 1985, pp. 129–131.
6. Calder PC, Jackson AA. Undernutrition, infection and immune function. Nutr Res Rev 2002;13:3–29.
7. World Health Organization. Life in the 21st Century: A Vision for All. World Health Report. WHO, Geneva, 1998.
8. World Health Organization. Bridging the Gaps. World Health Organization, Geneva, 1995.
9. UNICEF. The State of the World's Children. US Department of Health, Education and Welfare, Atlanta, GA, 1988.
10. Colten H, Ravetch J. Curr Opin Immunol 1992;4:1–2.
11. Thurnham DI, Northrop-Clewes CA, McCullough FSW, Das BS, Lunn PG. Innate immunity, gut integrity and vitamin A in Gambian and Indian infants. J Infect Dis 2000;182:S23–S28.
12. Doherty JF, Golden MHN, Raynes JG, Griffin GE, McAdam KPWJ. Acute-phase protein response is impaired in severely malnourished children. Clin Sci 1993;84:169–175.
13. Sommer A, Katz J, Tarwotjo I. Increased risk of respiratory disease and diarrhea in children with preexisting mild vitamin A deficiency. Am J Clin Nutr 1984;40:1090–1095.
14. Christian P, Schultz K, Stoltzfus MC. Hyporetinolemia, illness symptoms and APP response in pregnant women with and without night-blindness. Am J Clin Nutr 1998;67:1237–1243.
15. Thurnham DI. Impact of disease on markers of micronutrient status. Proc Nutr Soc 1997;56:421–431.
16. Thurnham DI. Micronutrients and immune function: some recent developments. J Clin Pathol 1997;50:887–891.
17. Das BS, Thurnham DI, Das DB. Influence of malaria on markers of iron status in children: implications for interpreting iron status in malaria-endemic communities. Br J Nutr 1997;785:751–760.
18. Thurnham DI, McCabe GP, Northrop-Clewes CA. Nestel P. A meta-analysis of 15 studies to quantify the effects of sub-clinical infection on plasma retinol concentrations to assess the prevalence of vitamin A deficiency. Lancet 2003, in press.
19. Gendelman HE, Morahan PS. Macrophages in viral infections. In: Lewis CE, McGee JO (eds.). The Macrophage. Oxford University Press, Oxford, 1992, pp. 157–213.
20. Grimble RF. Dietary manipulation of the inflammatory response. Proc Nutr Soc 1992;51:285–294.
21. Cannon JG, Meydani SN, Fielding RA, et al. Acute phase response in exercise. II. Associations between vitamin E, cytokines, and muscle proteolysis. Am J Physiol 1991;260:R1235–R1240.
22. Beutler B, Cerami A. Tumour necrosis factor as two sides of the same coin. Nature 1986;320:376–387.
23. Stadnyk AW, Gauldie J. The acute phase protein response during parasitic infection. Immunoparasit Today 1991;7:A7–A12.
24. Speert DP. Macrophages in bacterial infection. In: Lewis CE, McGee JO (eds.). The Macrophage. Oxford University Press, Oxford, 1992, pp. 215–263.
25. Auger MJ, Ross JA. The biology of the macrophage. In: Lewis CE, McGee JO (eds.). The Macrophage. Oxford University Press, Oxford, 1992, pp. 1–74.
26. Pekarek RS, Burghen GA, Bartelloni PJ, Calia FM, Bostian KA, Beisel WR. The effect of live attenuated Venezuelan equine encephalomyelitis virus vaccine on serum iron, zinc, and copper concentrations in man. J Lab Clin Med 1969; 6:293–303.
27. Beisel WR. Trace elements in infectious processes. Med Clin North Am 1976;60:831–849.
28. Brock J. Iron and immunity. J Nutr Immunol 1993;2:47–106.
29. Stoltzfus RJ. Rethinking anaemia surveillance. Lancet 1997;349:1764–1766.
30. Beresford CH, Neale RJ, Brooks OG. Iron absorption and pyrexia. Lancet 1971;i:568–572.
31. Weber J, Werre JM, Julius HW, Marx JJM. Decreased iron absorption in patients with active rheumatoid arthritis, with and without iron deficiency. Ann Rheum Dis 1988;47:404–409.

32. Hershko C, Peto TEA, Weatherall DJ. Iron and infection. BMJ 1988;296:660–664.
33. Hesketh JE, Vasconcelos MH, Bermano G. Regulatory signals in messenger RNA: determinants of nutrient-gene interaction and metabolic compartmentation. Br J Nutr 1998;80:307–321.
34. Tran TN, Eubanks SK, Shaffer KJ, Zhou CYJ, Linder MC. Secretion of ferritin by rat hepatoma cells and its regulation by inflammatory cytokines and iron. Blood 1997;90:4979–4986.
35. Fahmy M, Young SP. Modulation of iron metabolism in monocyte cell line U937 by inflammatory cytokines: changes in transferrin uptake, iron handling and ferritin mRNA. Biochem J 1993;296: 175–181.
36. Weinberg ED. Iron withholding: a defense against infection and neoplasia. Physiol Rev 1984;64:65–102.
37. Bullen JJ. The significance of iron in infection. Rev Infect Dis 1981;3:1127–1138.
38. Thurnham DI. Antioxidants and prooxidants in malnourished populations. Proc Nutr Soc 1990;48: 247–259.
39. Weiss G, Wachter H, Fuchs D. Linkage of cell-mediated immunity to iron metabolism. Immunol Today 1995;16:495–500.
40. Moncada S, Palmer RMJ, Higgs EA. Nitric oxide physiology, pathophysiology and pharmacology. Pharmacol Rev 1991;43:109–142.
41. Domachowske JB, Rafferty SP, Singhania N, Mardiney M, Malech HL. Nitric oxide alters the expression of g-globulin, H-ferritin, and transferrin receptor in human K562 cells at the posttranscriptional level. Blood 1996;88:2980–2988.
42. Rouault TA, Klausner RD. Iron-sulfur clusters as biosensors of oxidants and iron. Trends in Biochem Sci 1996;21:174–177.
43. Brock J, Mulero V. Cellular and molecular aspects of iron and immune function. Proc Nutr Soc 2000;59:537–540.
44. Tomkins A, Watson F. Malnutrition and infection—a review. The Lavenham Press Ltd., Lavenham, Suffolk, 1989.
45. Murray MJ, Murray AB, Murray MB, Murray CJ. The adverse effect of iron repletion on the course of certain infections. BMJ 1978;2:1113–1115.
46. McFarlane H, Reddy S, Adcock KJ, Adeshina H, Cooke AR, Akene J. Immunity, transferrin and survival in kwashiorkor. BMJ 1970;4:268–270.
47. Northrop-Clewes CA, McCloone UJ, Paracha PI, Thurnham DI. Influence of iron supplementation on markers of infection in Pakistani infants. Proc Nutr Soc 1994;153:264A.
48. Nelder KH, Hambidge KM. Zinc therapy in acrodermatitis enteropathica. N Engl J Med 1975;292: 879–882.
49. Rink L, Gabriel P. Zinc and the immune system. Proc Nutr Soc 2000;59:541–552.
50. Wellinghausen N, Kirchner H, Rink L. The immunobiology of zinc. Immunol Today 1997;18:519–521.
51. Hambidge KM. Zinc deficiency in man: its origins and effects. Phil Trans R Soc Lond B 1981;294: 129–144.
52. Gibson RS. Assessment of trace elements. Principles of nutritional assessment. Oxford University Press, Oxford, 1990, pp. 511–576.
53. Brown KH, Peerson JM, Allen LH. Effect of zinc supplementation on childrens' growth: a meta-analysis of intervention trials. Biblthca Nutr Dieta 1998;54:76–83.
54. Zinc Investigators Collaborative Group. Prevention of diarrhea and pneumonia by zinc supplementation in children in developing countries: pooled analysis of randomized controlled trials. J Pediatr 1999;135:689–697.
55. Osendarp SJM, West CE, Black RE. Maternal zinc supplementation study group. The need for maternal zinc supplementation in developing countries: an unresolved issue. J Nutr 2003;133:817S–827S.
56. Solomons NW, Russell RM. The interaction of vitamin and zinc: implications for human nutrition. Am J Clin Nutr 1980;33:2031–2040.
57. Roy SK, Behrens RH, Haider R, Tomkins AM. Impact of zinc supplementation on intestinal permeability in Bangladeshi children with acute diarrhoea and persistent diarrhoea syndrome. J Pediatr Gastroenterol Nutr 1992;15:289–296.
58. Bates CJ, Evans PH, Dardenne M, et al. A trial of zinc supplementation in young rural Gambian children. Br J Nutr 1993;69:243–255.

59. Sazawal S, Black RE, Bhan MK, Bhandari N, Sinha A, Jalla S. Zinc supplementation in young children with acute diarrhea in India. N Engl J Med 1995;333:839–844.

60. Shankar AH, Genton B, Baisor M, et al. The influence of zinc supplementation on morbidity due to *Plasmodium falciparum*: a randomized trial in pre-school children in Papua New Guinea. Am J Trop Med Hyg 2000;626:663–669.

61. Prasad AS, Fitzgerald JT, Beck FWJ, Chandrasekar PH. Duration of symptoms and plasma cytokine levels in patients with the common cold treated with zinc acetate. Ann Intern Med 2000;133:245–252.

62. Castillo-Duran C, Vial P, Uauy R. Trace mineral balance during acute diarrhea in infants. J Pediatr 1988;113:452–457.

63. Camhi SL, Lee P, Choi AMK. The oxidative stress response. New Horizons 1995;32:170–182.

64. Braunschweig CL, Sowers M, Kovacevich DS, Hill GM, August DA. Parental zinc supplementation in adult humans during the acute phase response increases the febrile response. J Nutr 1997;127:70–74.

65. Chandra RK. Excessive intake of zinc impairs immune response. JAMA 1984;252:1443–1446.

66. Wellinghausen N, Fischer A, Kirchner H, Rink L. Interaction of zinc ions with human peripheral blood mononuclear cells. Eur J Cell Immunol 1996;171:255–261.

67. Vallee BL, Falchuk KH. The biochemical basis of zinc physiology. Physiol Rev 1993;73:79–118.

68. Minatel L, Carfagnini JC. Copper deficiency and immune response in ruminants. Nutr Res 2000;2010:1519–1529.

69. Evans P, Halliwell B. Micronutrients: oxidant/antioxidant status. Br J Nutr 2001;85:S67–S74.

70. Huang ZL, Failla ML. Copper deficiency suppresses effector activities of differentiated U937 cells. J Nutr 2000;130:1536–1542.

71. Thurnham DI, Singkamani R. The acute phase response and vitamin A status in malaria. Trans R Soc Trop Med Hyg 1991;85:194–199.

72. Reddy V, Bhaskaram P, Raghuramulu N, et al. Relationship between measles, malnutrition, and blindness: a prospective study in Indian children. Am J Clin Nutr 1986;44:924–930.

73. Louw JA, Werbeck A, Louw MEJ, Kotze TJvW, Cooper R, Labadarios D. Blood vitamin concentrations during the acute-phase response. Crit Care Med 1992;20:934–941.

74. Rosales FJ, Ritter SJ, Zolfaghari R, Smith JE, Ross AC. Effects of acute inflammation on plasma retinol, retinol-binding protein, and its messenger RNA in the liver and kidneys of vitamin A sufficient rats. J Lipid Res 1996;37:962–971.

75. Green MH, Green JB. Dynamics and control of plasma retinol. In: Blomhoff R (ed.). Vitamin A in Health & Disease. Marcel Dekker Inc., New York, 1994, pp. 119–133.

76. Smith FR, Goodman DS. The effect of diseases of the liver, thyroid and kidneys on the transport of vitamin A in human plasma. J Clin Invest 1971;50:2426–2436.

77. Ramsden DB, Prince HP, Burr WA, et al. The inter-relationship of thyroid hormones, vitamin A and their binding proteins following acute stress. Clin Endocrinol Oxf 1978;8:109–122.

78. Konde M, Ingenbleek Y, Daffe M, Sylia B, Barry O, Diallo S. Goitrous endemic in Guinea. Lancet 1994;344:1675–1678.

79. Baxendale JH, Gauldie J. The acute phase response. Immunol Today 1994;15:74–80.

80. Van Leeuwen MA, Van Rijswijk MH. Acute phase proteins in the monitoring of inflammatory disorders. Bailliere Clin Rheum 1994;83:531–554.

81. Steel DM, Whitehead AS. The major acute phase reactants: C-reactive protein, serum amyloid P component and serum amyloid A protein. Immunol Today 1994;15:81–88.

82. Tilg H, Dinarello CA, Mier JW. IL–6 and APPs: anti-inflammatory and immunosuppressive mediators. Immunol Today 1997;18:428–432.

83. IARC Working Group. Vitamin A. International Agency for Research on Cancer, Lyon, 1998.

84. Mitra AK, Alvarez JO, Wahed MA, Fuchs GJ, Stephensen CB. Predictors of serum retinol in children with shigellosis. Am J Clin Nutr 1998;68:1088–1094.

85. Stephensen CB, Alvarez JO, Kohatsu J, Hardmeier R, Kennedy JI Jr, Gammon RB Jr. Vitamin A is excreted in the urine during acute infection. Am J Clin Nutr 1994;60:388–392.

86. Campos FACS, Flores H, Underwood BA. Effect of an infection on vitamin A status of children measured by the relative dose response RDR. Am J Clin Nutr 1987;46:91–94.

87. Sann L, Bienvenu J, Lahet C, Divry P, Cotte J, Bethenod M. Serum orosomucoid concentration in newborn infants. Eur J Pediatr 1981;136:181–185.

88. Glasziou PP, Mackerras DEM. Vitamin A supplementation in infectious diseases: a meta-analysis. BMJ 1993;306:366–370.

89. Beaton GH, Martorell R, Aronson KJ. Effectiveness of vitamin A supplementation in the control of young child mortality in developing countries. United Nations Administration Committee on Coordination/Subcommittee on Nutrition, New York, 1993.

90. Fawzi WW, Chalmers TC, Herrera MG, Mosteller F. Vitamin A supplementation and child mortality. A meta-analysis. JAMA 1993;269:898–903.

91. Howie AF, Arthur JR, Nicol F, Walker SW, Beech SG, Beckett GJ. Identification of a 57-kilodalton selenoprotein in human thyrocytes as thioredoxin reductase and evidence that its expression is regulated through the calcium phosphoinositol-signalling pathway. J Clin Endocrinol Metab 1998;83:2052–2058.

92. Vanderpas JB, Contempre B, Duale NL, et al. Iodine and selenium deficiency associated with cretinism in northern Zaire. Am J Clin Nutr 1990;52:1087–1093.

93. Fleck A. Clinical and nutritional aspects of changes in acute-phase proteins during inflammation. Proc Nutr Soc 1989;48:347–354.

94. Dickson PW, Howlett GJ, Schreiber G. Metabolism of prealbumin and changes induced by acute inflammation. Eur J Biochem 1982;129:289–293.

95. Jahoor F, Gazzard B, Phillips G, et al. The acute phase response to human immunodeficiency virus infection in human subjects. Am J Physiol 1999;276:E1092–E1098.

96. Tomkins A, Behrens R, Roy SK. The role of zinc and vitamin A deficiency in diarrhoeal syndromes in developing countries. Proc Nutr Soc 1993;52:131–142.

97. Fleck A, Myers MA. Diagnostic and prognostic significance of acute phase proteins. In: Gordon AH, Koj A (eds.). The Acute Phase Response to Injury and Infection. Elsevier Scientific Publishers, Amsterdam, 1985, pp. 249–271.

98. Filteau SM, Sullivan KR, Anwar US, Anwar ZR, Tomkins AM. Iodine deficiency alone cannot account for goitre prevalence among pregnant women in Modhupur, Bangladesh. Eur J Clin Nutr 1994; 48:293–302.

99. Sipe JD. Cellular and humoral components of the early inflammatory reaction. In: Gordon AH, Koj A (eds.). The Acute Phase Response to Injury and Infection. Elsevier, London, 1985, pp. 3–21.

100. Vallance S. Platelets, leucocytes and buffy layer vitamin C after surgery. Hum Nutr Clin Nutr 1986;40C:35–41.

101. Vallance P, Hume R, Weyers E. Reassessment of changes in leucocyte and serum ascorbic acid after acute myocardial infarction. Br Heart J 1978;40:684–689.

102. Hume R, Weyers E. Changes in leucocyte ascorbic acid during the common cold. Scot Med J 1973; 18:3–7.

103. Irvin TT, Chattopadhyay K, Smythe A. Ascorbic acid requirements in postoperative patients. Surg Gynecol Obstet 1978;147:49–55.

104. Friedman GJ, Sherry S, Ralli EP. The mechanism of the excretion of vitamin C by the human kidney at low and normal plasma levels of ascorbic acid. J Clin Invest 1941;20:685–689.

105. Marcus SL, Petrylak DP, Dutcher JP, et al. Hypovitaminosis C in patients treated with high-dose interleukin 2 and lymphokine-activated killer cells. Am J Clin Nutr 1991;54:1292S–1297S.

106. Evans RM, Currie L, Campbell A. The distribution of ascorbic acid between various cellular components of the blood in normal individuals, and its relation to the plasma concentration. Br J Nutr 1982;47:473–482.

107. Dallegri F, Lanzi G, Patrone F. Effects of ascorbic acid on neutrophil locomotion. Int Arch Allergy Appl Immunol 1980;61:40–45.

108. Washko PW, Wang Y, Levine M. Ascorbic acid recycling in human neutrophils. J Biol Chem 1993;268:15531–15535.

109. Stankova L, Gerhardt NB, Nagel L, Bigley RH. Ascorbate and phagocyte function. Infect Immun 1975;12:252–256.

110. Moser U, Weber F. Uptake of ascorbic acid by human granulocytes. Int J Vit Nutr Res 1984;54:47–53.

111. Herbaczynska-Cedro K, Wartanowicz M, Panczenko-Kresowska B, Cedro K, Klosiewicz-Wasek B, Wasek W. Inhibitory effect of vitamins C and E on the oxygen free radical production of human polymorphonuclear leucocytes. Eur J Clin Invest 1994;24:316–319.

112. Herbaczynska-Cedro K, Klosiewicz-Wasek B, Cedro K, Wasek W, Panczenko-Kresowska B, Wartanowicz M. Supplementation with vitamin C and vitamin E suppresses leukocyte oxygen free radical production in patients with myocardial infarction. Eur Heart J 1995;16:1044–1049.

113. de la Fuente M, Ferrandez MD, Burgos MS, Soler A, Prieto A, Miquel J. Immune function in aged women is improved by ingestion of vitamins C and E. Can J Physiol Pharmacol 1998;76:373–380.

114. Jayachandran M, Rani PJI, Arivazhagan P, Panneerselvam C. Neutrophil phagocytic function and humoral immune response with reference to ascorbate supplementation in aging humans. J Anti-Aging Med 2000;3:37–42.

115. Stadtman ER. Ascorbic acid and oxidative inactivation of proteins. Am J Clin Nutr 1991;54:1125S–1128S.

116. Smith C, Mitchinson MJ, Aruoma OI, Halliwell B. Stimulation of lipid peroxidation and hydroxyl-radical generation by the contents of human athersclerotic lesions. Biochem J 1992;286:901–905.

117. Hider RC. Nature of non-transferrin-bound iron. Eur J Clin Invest 2002;32:50–54.

118. Chevion M, Jiang Y, Har-El R, Berenshtein E, Uretzky G, Kitrossky N. Copper and iron are mobilised following myocardial ischemia: possible predictive criteria for tissue injury. Proc Natl Acad Sci USA 1993;90:1102–1106.

119. Gokce N, Keaney JF, Frei B, et al. Long-term ascorbic acid administration reverses endothelial vaso-motor dysfunction in patients with coronary artery disease. Circulation 1999;99:3234–3240.

120. Wilkinson IB, Megson IL, MacCallum H, Sogo N, Cockroft JR, Webb DJ. Oral vitamin C reduces arterial stiffness and platelet aggregation in humans. J Cardiovasc Pharmacol 1999;34:690–693.

121. Murphy ME. Ascorbate and dehydroascorbate modulate nitric oxide-induced vasodilations of rat coronary arteries. Circulation 2002;105:1155–1157.

122. Grech ED, Dodd NJF, Jackson MJ, Morrison WL, Faragher EB, Ramsdale DR. Evidence of free-radical generation after primary percutaneous transluminal coronary angioplasty recanalization in acute myocardial infarction. Am J Cardiol 1996;77:122–127.

123. Cambell GD, Steinberg MH, Bower JD. Ascorbic acid induced haemolysis in G-6-PD deficiency. Ann Intern Med 1975;82:810.

124. Mehta JB, Singhal SB, Mehta BC. Ascorbic acid induced haemolysis in G-6-PD deficiency. Lancet 1990;335:944.

125. Iwamoto N, Kawaguchi T, Horikawa K, et al. Haemolysis induced by ascorbic acid in paroxysmal nocturnal haemoglobinuria. Lancet 1994;343:357.

126. Herbert V, Shaw S, Jayatilleke E. Vitamin C-driven free radical generation from iron. J Nutr 1996;126:1213S–1220S.

127. Barton JC, McDonnell SM, Adams PC, et al. Management of hemochromatosis. Ann Intern Med 1998;129:932–939.

128. Kopp EB, Ghosh S. NF-κB and rel proteins in innate immunity. Adv Immunol 1995;58:1–27.

129. Borski RJ. Nongenomic membrane actions of glucocorticoids in vertebrates. Trends Endocrinol Metab 2000;11:427–436.

130. Schreck R, Meier B, Maennel D, Draege W, Baeuerle PA. Dithiocarbamates as potent inhibitors of nuclear factor κB activation in intact cells. J Exp Med 1992;175:1181–1194.

131. Schreck R, Reiber P, Baeuerle PA. Reactive oxygen intermediates as apparantly widely used messengers in the activation of NF-κB transcription factor and HIV-1. EMBO J 1991;10:2247–2258.

132. Erickson KL, Medina EA, Hubbard NE. Micronutrients and innate immunity. J Infect Dis 2000;182: S5–S10.

133. Keith ME, Jeejeebhoy KN. Immunonutrition. Bailliere Clin Endocrinol Metab 1997;11:709–738.

134. Thurnham DI, Davies JA, Crump BJ, Situnayake RD, Davis M. The use of different lipids to express serum tocopherol:lipid ratios for the measurement of vitamin E status. Ann Clin Biochem 1986;23: 514–520.

135. Esterbauer H, Puhl H, Dieber-Rotheneder M, Waeg G, Rabl H. Effect of antioxidants on oxidative modification of LDL. Ann Med 1991;23:573–581.

136. Department of Health. Dietary Reference Values for Food Energy and Nutrients for the United Kingdom. Report on Health and Social Subjects, No. 41. Her Majesty's Stationary Office, London, 1991.

137. Das BS, Thurnham DI, Das DB. Plasma α-tocopherol, retinol and carotenoids in children with falciparum malaria. Am J Clin Nutr 1996;64:94–100.

138. Bieri JG, Thorpe SL, Tolliver TJ. Effect of dietary polyunsaturated fatty acids on tissue vitamin E status. J Nutr 1978;108:392–398.

139. Mickle DAG, Weisel RD, Burton GW, Ingold KU. Effect of orally administered alpha-tocopheryl acetate on human myocardial alpha-tocopherol levels. Cardiovasc Drugs Ther 1991;5:309–312.

140. Burton GW, Traber MG, Acuff RV, et al. Human plasma and tissue α-tocopherol concentrations in response to supplementation with deuterated natural and synthetic vitamin E. Am J Clin Nutr 1998;67:669–684.

141. Burton GW, Ingold KU. Autoxidation of biological molecules. 1. The antioxidant activity of vitamin E and related chain-breaking phenolic antioxidants in vitro. J Am Chem Soc 1981;103:6472–6477.

142. Chaudiere J, Ferrari-Iliou R. Intracellular antioxidants from chemical to biochemical mechanisms. Food Chem Toxicol 1999;37:949–962.

143. Heart Protection Study Group. MRC/BHF Heart protection study of antioxidant vitamin supplementation in 20536 high-risk individuals: a randomised placebo-controlled trial. Lancet 2002;360:23–33.

144. Graat JM, Schouten EG, Kok FJ. Effect of daily vitamin E and multivitamin mineral supplementation on acute respiratory tract infections in elderly persons: a randomized controlled trial. JAMA 2002;288:715–721.

145. Greenman E, Phillipich MJ, Meyer CJ, Charamella LJ, Dimitrov NV. The effect of selenium on phagocytosis in humans. Anticancer Res 1988;8:825–828.

146. Halliwell B, Gutteridge JMC. Free Radicals in Biology and Medicine. Clarendon, Oxford, 1985.

147. Beck MA, Kolbeck PC, Rohr LH, Shi Q, Morris VC, Levander OA. Vitamin E deficiency intensifies the myocardial injury of coxsackievirus B3 infection of mice. J Nutr 1994;124:345–358.

148. Beck MA. Selenium and host defence towards viruses. Proc Nutr Soc 1999;58:707–711.

149. Beck MA, Matthewes CC. Micronutrients and host resistance to viral infection. Proc Nutr Soc 2000;59:581–585.

150. Thurnham DI, Oppenheimer SJ, Bull R. Riboflavin status and malaria in infants in Papua New Guinea. Trans R Soc Trop Med Hyg 1983;77:423–424.

151. Das BS, Das DB, Satpathy RN, Patnaik JK, Bose TK. Riboflavin deficiency and severity of malaria. Eur J Clin Nutr 1988;42:277–283.

152. Bates CJ, Prentice AM, Paul AA, Sutcliffe BA, Watkinson M, Whitehead M. Riboflavin status in Gambian pregnant and lactating women and its implications for recommended dietary allowances. Am J Clin Nutr 1981;34:928–935.

152a. Banji MS, Baskalam P, Jacob CM. Urinary riboflavin excretion and erythrocyte glutathione reductase activity in pre-school children suffering from upper respiratory tract infections and measles. Ann Nutr Metab 1987;31:191–196.

153. Du Bois EF. Fever and the regulation of body temperature. Charles C Thomas, Springfield, IL, 1948.

154. Cathcart AE, Thurnham DI. Thiamin: physiology. In: Sadler MJ, Caballero B, Strain JJ (eds.). Encyclopedia of Human Nutrition. Academic Press, London, 1998, pp. 1858–1863.

155. Platt BS. Epidemiology and clinical features of endemic beriberi. Proceedings of a conference on beriberi, endemic goitre and hypervitaminosis A. Proc FASEB 1958;17(Suppl 2):3–20.

156. Brin M. Erythrocyte as a biopsy tissue for functional evaluation of thiamine adequacy. JAMA 1964;187:762–766.

157. Suter PM, Vetter W. Diuretics and vitamin B1: are diuretics a risk factor for thiamin malnutrition. Nutr Rev 2000;58:319–323.

158. Ward M. Homocysteine, folate and cardiovascular disease. Int J Vit Nutr Res 2001;71:173–178.

159. McCully KS. Micronutrients, homocysteine metabolism, and atherosclerosis. In: Bendich A, Butterworth CE (eds.). Micronutrients in Health and Disease. Dekker, New York, 1991, pp. 69–94.

160. Ferns GAA, Lamb DJ. Coronary heart disease: pathophysiological events and risk factors. Nutr Bull 2001;26:213–218.

161. Beisel WR. Single nutrients and immunity. Am J Clin Nutr 1982; 35:415–468.

162. Stuart J, Whicher JT. Tests for detecting and monitoring the acute phase response. Arch Dis Child 1988;63:115–117.

163. Thompson D, Milford-Ward A, Whicher JT. The value of acute phase protein measurements in clinical practice. Ann Clin Biochem 1992;29:123–131.

164. Paracha PI, Jamil A, Northrop-Clewes CA, Thurnham DI. Interpretation of vitamin A status in apparently-healthy Pakistani children using markers of sub-clinical infection. Am J Clin Nutr 2000;72: 1164–1169.
165. Baynes RD, Bezwoda W, Bothwell TH, Khan Q, Mansoor N. The non-immune inflammatory response: serial changes in plasma iron, iron-binding capacity, lactoferrin, ferritin and C-reactive protein. Scand J Clin Lab Invest 1986;46:695–704.

4 Neonatal Nutrition and Immunity

Deborah O'Neil and Denise Kelly

1. INTRODUCTION

The adaptive immune system is formed throughout embryonic life, and although intact in cellular content and lymphoid infrastructure *(1–6)* it is antigenically naïve at birth *(2,4,5,7–9)*. Structural components of the innate arm of the immune system are in place from the first few weeks of gestation *(2,5–7,10–14)* and provide, along with maternally derived immunoglobulins (Igs), the bulk of host protection for the otherwise susceptible infant during the first few hours, days, and months of life outside the womb (*see* Table 1). However, an absolute biological priority for the neonatal immune system is antigenic exposure and the concomitant expansion and maturation of the immune system. If the newborn is to thrive, then the developing innate and adaptive immune system must mount adequate and appropriate immune responses to both pathogenic and beneficial microbial and dietary antigens that are encountered at and immediately after birth.

Nutrition is a critical factor in facilitating the host immune response and the immune ontogenic processes that occur in the newborn. Importantly, nutrition affects health/disease status during both early and later life *(15–21)*, and the anecdotal reports that have linked health and disease susceptibility with nutritional status in infants throughout history now have a firm basis in scientific and clinical fact.

Impaired immune responses, secondary to macronutrient or micronutrient deficiencies, increase susceptibility to infectious agents but also predispose to immune dysregulation, which underpins many debilitating inflammatory and autoimmune diseases. These diverse biologic effects result from the negative effect of nutritional deficiency on several innate and adaptive immune functions, including cell-mediated immunity, complement function, phagocyte activity, and secretory antibody production and function *(15–23)*. Largely because of recent advances in nutritional immunology, the molecular mechanisms by which such nutrient-mediated immunomodulatory effects are achieved are now unraveling. In particular, the direct interaction between nutrients and immune gene expression and the relationship between nutrient bioavailability and lymphoid cell and tissue differentiation *(19,22,23)* are more completely defined.

From: *Diet and Human Immune Function*
Edited by: D. A. Hughes, L. G. Darlington, and A. Bendich © Humana Press Inc., Totowa, NJ

Table 1
Functional Components of the Neonatal Immune System at Birth

Soluble factors
- Defensins, cathelicidins, lysozyme, lactoferrin, and other broad-spectrum anti-microbial factors produced by epithelial cells and neutrophils
- Cytokines, chemokines and growth factors produced by immune and also stromal cells
- Prostaglandins, nitric oxide, and other inflammatory target gene products
- Complement proteins

Receptors
- Pattern recognition receptors against numerous microbial moieties
- Fc receptors
- Natural killer cell receptors

Cells
- Epithelial barrier cells
- Granulocytes—neutrophils, eosinophils, mast cells, and basophils
- Myeloid cells—monocytes, macrophages, and dendritic cells
- Natural killer cells
- Immature T and B cells

Antibodies
- Fetal IgA
- Maternal IgG

Ig, immunoglobulin.

2. IMMUNE ONTOGENIC PROCESSES IN THE NEONATE

Exposure to antigens derived from commensal bacteria and milk proteins at and immediately after birth drives the development of the neonatal adaptive immune response *(2,4,5,7–9)*. The functional immaturity of the neonatal cellular and secretory immune response is such that newborns can generate only limited T- and B-cell responses when challenged with pathogens, thus contributing to their immunocompromised state *(7,24–31)*. However, exposure of naïve lymphocyte populations to protein and bacterial antigens within mucosal lymph aggregates primes the activation, maturation, and expansion of the adaptive immune response, both locally and systemically *(2,5,7,8,24,27,32)*. Importantly, the neonate must mount tolerogenic rather than immunogenic responses toward inert microbial and dietary antigens if an appropriately balanced adaptive immune response is to develop *(30–36)*. One belief is that antigen-specific recognition in the neonatal immune system has an inherent T helper type 2 (Th2) bias, thereby skewing cellular mucosal immune processes toward a Th2-like, rather than an immunogenic T helper 1 (Th1)-type, response *(30,34–36)*. Such Th2 predisposition may also be linked to allergy and atopy development in children under 12 *(31,33,37–39)*.

However, a global Th2 bias does not explain how neonates can still mount, albeit weakly, immunogenic Th1-mediated cellular responses against infectious agents and vaccines. Therefore, it is not surprising that recent studies using human cord blood cells and mouse models contradict the Th2 bias hypothesis. These studies demonstrate that T-cell receptor (TCR)-stimulated neonatal cord blood CD4+ and CD8+ T cells produce levels of interferon (IFN)-γ and interleukin (IL)-4, IL-12, IL-10 and tumor necrosis factor-α (TNF-α) comparable to those of their adult counterparts, indicating that although naïve, the neonatal T-cell compartment is competent to respond to TCR-mediated stimulation and to produce both Th1 and Th2 cytokines *(32,37,40)*. IL-10, a crucial regulatory Th3 cytokine, may be of greater importance in maintaining neonatal tolerance, because it is produced by primary TCR stimulation of neonatal cord blood but not adult peripheral blood-derived naïve T cells *(40)*. Compartmentalization of Th1 vs. Th2 skewed responses in the neonate may explain why neonates have an overall Th2 or tolerogenic immuno-phenotype, while still being able to mount Th1 responses as required. Furthermore, the primary immune response in neonates is strongly dependent on the initial antigen exposure site, with antigen-specific responses initiated in neonatal lymph nodes of mixed Th1/Th2 bias, whereas those occurring in the spleen are heavily Th2 biased *(41)*.

Bacterial colonization of the gastrointestinal (GI) tract has a major impact on infants' early health and development. Establishing an optimal intestinal microbiota, particularly one rich in *Bifidobacteria*, is a vital factor that regulates both immune ontogeny and intestinal barrier integrity and prevents colonization by pathogenic microbes *(2,9)*. Premature neonates with an even more immature immune system than their term counterparts acquire intestinal organisms slowly, and the establishment of bifidobacterial flora is retarded compared with that in the healthy full-term infant gut *(42,43)*. Such delayed bacterial colonization results in the presence of a limited number of bacterial species that may contain pathogenic elements believed to be important in the development of necrotizing enterocolitis *(42–44)*. Furthermore, the gut microflora in these neonates may also predispose to the development of atopic diseases, suggesting that a "balanced" indigenous flora may represent a crucial factor in the human immunity maturation toward a nonatopic mode *(45,46)*. Because of the impact of the commensal flora on the short-term and longer term health of the neonate, the use of biotherapeutic agents, such as prebiotics and probiotics, to promote the development of a more beneficial microbiotia may become a routine form of dietary modulation in the newborn *(47–51)*.

3. PROTEIN AND AMINO ACID INTAKE AND IMMUNITY

Although rare in term babies born in developed countries, protein malnutrition contributes to a significant immunosuppression in neonates in developing countries. Protein deficiency in the newborn limits substrate availability for the biomanufacture of immunoproteins, such as Igs, granulocytes, complement proteins, enzymes, cytokines, and chemokines, thereby exerting immunosuppressive effects on both the existing innate host defense mechanisms and immune ontogenic processes. In fact, protein malnutrition is the most common form of secondary or acquired immunodeficiency in the developing world, most often presenting as recurrent infections in the neonate *(16,52)*. Even in developed industrialized nations, a marked correlation exists between immune function and birth weight, with many malnourished or small-for-gestational age infants being immunocompromised to a much greater extent than larger babies of the same developmental age *(15–17,19,52)*. In preterm neonates, the immunodeficiency is more severe and prolonged and is associated with a higher incidence of infections and sepsis.

Immunologic impairment may persist in such infants for several months or even years *(53)*. Reduced neutrophil granule antimicrobial protein content is a common feature in the neonate and accounts, in part, for neonates' increased susceptibility to Gram-negative sepsis *(54)*. Limited biomanufacture of the hematopoietic growth factors and cytokines that drive the production, differentiation, and function of innate and adaptive cellular components, combined with the immaturity of the neonatal hematopoietic system, results in a clinically relevant cytopenia and neutropenia, conditions that are more apparent in low-birth-weight and premature babies *(16,30,25,53,55–59)*. To combat malnutrition-related hindrance of hematopoiesis, several cytokines and growth factors have already been applied as therapies in neonates *(56,60)*.

Arginine, glutamine, and S amino acids are particularly important building blocks for the production of many key immunoproteins involved in neonatal immunity *(20,21,61)*. In addition to facilitating general growth and development *(22)*, glutamine also regulates lymphocyte proliferation *(62)* and the inflammatory immune response in the neonate *(63)*. It is an essential nutrient during rapid tissue turnover, used as both a primary fuel source and a carbon and nitrogen donor for nucleotide precursor synthesis and is particularly important for monocyte, lymphocyte, and neutrophil function. Glutamine supplementation also reduces infectious morbidity *(63)*, particularly by decreasing the incidence of sepsis in low-birth-weight infants *(21)*. In addition to its immuno-regulatory activity, the protective effect of both glutamine and N-acetylcysteine may be derived from their indirect actions on antioxidant status *(62)*. Furthermore, L-arginine, a precursor of nitric oxide, polyamines, and other biologically important molecules, is an essential amino acid for the neonate. L-arginine supplementation is also beneficial in improving both GI and immune functions by facilitating wound healing *(64)*, reducing complications associated with infectious diseases, and lowering mortality *(21)*.

4. MICRONUTRIENT AFFECTS HOST DEFENSE

Micronutrients, including zinc, selenium, iron, copper, and vitamin A, can influence several components of both innate and adaptive immunity *(17,65,66)* (as described in Chapters 6–13). Vitamin A deficiency increases the incidence and severity of infections during childhood *(16)*. Vitamin A is required to maintain epithelial barrier function of mucosal surfaces, such as the developing and maturing GI, respiratory, and urogenital tract of neonates *(68,69)*. Vitamin A is a key mediator of innate immunity and is required for neutrophil, macrophages, and natural killer (NK) cell function *(16,17)*. Vitamin A also promotes adaptive immunity, particularly humoral immunity, with effects on CD4+ Th cells and B-cell development. Vitamin A deficiency inhibits Th2 CD4+ T cell function and, therefore, antibody-mediated responses. Some aspects of Th1-mediated immunity are also diminished in children who have vitamin A deficiency *(68)*. The cumulative effects on mucosal epithelial regeneration and immune function most probably account for the increased morbidity and even mortality seen in neonates who have a vitamin A deficiency. Vitamin A supplementation reverses, in part, the immunosuppression in neonates who are undernourished *(69)* and results in significant reductions in mortality among even apparently healthy infants *(70)*. In particular, vitamin A supplements reduce the severity of measles infections and also reduce the severity of diarrhea in neonates and infants *(70,71)*, probably because of promoting intestinal epithelial barrier integrity.

Deficiencies in the biometallic micronutrients zinc, iron, and copper also have numerous immunosuppressive consequences *(15,16,20,22)*. Zinc, particularly, is a micronutrient with great nutritional and immunologic importance. It is particularly important during periods of rapid growth and development in the neonate owing to its intervention in cellular replication. Zinc deficiency in neonates results in impaired function of both innate and adaptive immune responses and consequently leads to an increased susceptibility to bacterial, viral, and fungal infections *(72)*. Immunologic defects are not only seen in pronounced deficiency but also in marginal and moderate zinc deficiency. The biorequirement for zinc begins in utero during the first stages of immune ontogeny. Gestational zinc deficiency is a common problem worldwide for all demographics, and the immune defects that are observed in the neonate *(73)*, such as lower antibody levels and mitogen lymphocyte proliferation rates, impaired neutrophil adhesion, and depressed NK cell function *(17,73,74)*, may even persist in subsequent generations and are not fully reversible by postnatal zinc administration *(73)*. However, reports exist in which neonates and infants have responded to zinc supplementation with significantly higher linear growth rates and with concomitant increases in immune function, such as enhanced mitogen-induced lymphoproliferative responses and increased salivary IgA concentrations *(74,75)*, suggesting that supplementation can reverse, to some extent, the immunosuppressive phenotype of at least some malnourished and previously zinc-deficient neonates.

5. POLYUNSATURATED FATTY ACIDS AND IMMUNE MODULATION

Dietary lipids and their metabolites are of major importance for the growth, body composition, development, and long-term health of children. Lipids are the major source of energy in early childhood, also facilitating the supply of essential lipid-soluble vitamins and polyunsaturated fatty acids (PUFA) during early growth *(20,22,76,78)*. Deficiencies in essential fatty acids (EFA) in the neonatal diet often manifest as decreased prostaglandin biosynthesis and turnover *(77)*. N–3 PUFA, such as those found in fish, algal, starflower, and borage oils, are the lipid source from which the antiinflammatory prostaglandins, PGE_1 and PGE_3 are biosynthesized. PGE_3 is a powerful inhibitor of arachidonic acid release and its conversion to the inflammatory prostaglandin, PGE_2. This is one mechanism by which n–3 PUFAs directly modulate the inflammatory process *(20,21,61,77)*. PUFA also have ontogenic effects, driving antigen-specific neonatal T-cell maturation and expansion. Feeding babies with formula containing the n–3 PUFA, docosahex-aenoic acid (DHA), has increased the proportion of CD45RO+ CD4+ cells (memory T-cell phenotype), increased IL-10 production, and reduced IL-2 production levels. These processes could be important in the context of oral tolerance *(78)*.

Dietary supplementation with essential lipids alleviates EFA deficiency symptoms *(77)*, but the balance between beneficial vs. harmful immunomodulatory effects of EFAs is a fine one and is dose dependent. N–3 and n–6 PUFA levels in breast milk, infant formulas, and parenteral fat emulsion often exceed the optimal PUFA intake, and early studies suggest that an excessive intake of these substrates can be immunosuppressive, inhibiting both prostaglandin biosynthesis and also NK cell function *(16,77)*. Furthermore, both n–3 and n–6 PUFA induce apoptosis of neonatal cord blood monocytes in vitro in a dose-dependent fashion, with DHA being the most effective lipid in promoting neonatal monocyte-programmed cell death *(79)*. Taken together, these reports suggest that although PUFAs are certainly an essential dietary component for the neonate, exposure to unnecessarily high levels should be avoided.

6. NUCLEOTIDES AND NEONATAL HOST DEFENSE

Nucleotides and their related metabolic products are central factors in most biochemical pathways and, as such, play key roles in many biologic processes. Because they are synthesized endogenously, nucleotides and their metabolites are considered as semi-essential or conditionally essential but not essential nutrients for the neonate *(80,81)*. However, bioavailability can be limited because of the huge biologic requirement during neonatal growth and tissue turnover. In this context, dietary nucleotides provide an important supplementary source to that derived by *de novo* synthesis by acting as an additional source for the rapidly dividing tissues of the maturing immune system and the GI tract *(82–85)*. Exogenous nucleotides, derived either from breast milk or nucleotide-supplemented formula, promote humoral immune responses to T-dependent antigens and increase total antibody titers, improve immune responses to vaccines, and increase tolerance to dietary antigens *(86,87)*. Enhanced cellular immunity and the consequent increase in resistance to infection *(21,88)*, inhibition of T-cell proliferation *(61)* and NK-mediated killing *(89,90)* are also reported, sometimes conflicting immunomodulatory effects of nucleotides. Nucleotides and nucleosides also affect neonatal immunity indirectly by facilitating the bioavailability of other immunomodulatory nutrients, for example in promoting the absorption of iron across the gut and in enhancing the desaturation and elongation of PUFAs during their synthesis *(87)*.

7. IMMUNE POTENTIATION THROUGH BREASTFEEDING

Breastfeeding provides important back-up for neonatal innate host defenses in the face of an immature adaptive neonatal immune system. The array of anti-infectious and immunomodulatory factors contained in human breast milk (*see* Table 2) provide both passive and specific active protection of the newborn against several infections and diseases, including gastroenteritis, septicemia, otitis media, urinary tract infection, encephalitis, pneumonia, and necrotizing enterocolitis *(91,92)*. Although more controversial, breastfeeding of infants has also been associated with a decreased risk of developing allergic diseases *(31,33,93)*. The antibody content in breast milk seemingly contributes not only to the immediate but also to the longer-term protection of the infant by providing both resistance to infection and by facilitating the development of immunological tolerance toward harmless environmental antigens. Colostral milk contains IgM, IgA, and IgG antibodies specific against several pathogenic microbial moieties, including endotoxin, thereby providing an additional source of maternal antibody protection to that transferred during intrauterine development *(91,93–95)*. In addition, milk also contains active antimicrobial factors, such as defensins, and lactoferrin, and also oligosaccharides, which function as decoy microbial receptors by preventing mucosal attachment of pathogenic bacteria, a prerequisite step in most infections *(92,93)*. There are also clear differences in mucosal colonization pattern in the breastfed infant vs. the formula-fed infant. Breastfed infants have a less virulent intestinal microflora and a

Table 2
Immune Protective Properties of Breast Milk

Bystander immune protection provided by breast milk derived factors	Immunomodulatory protection provided by breast milk derived factors
Humoral protection from maternal IgG, IgA, and IgM	Antiinflammatory regulation from interleukin-10 (IL-10) and transforming growth factor-β (TGF-β)
Broad-spectrum antimicrobial protection from the antibiotic peptides human β-defensin 1, lactoferrin, lysozyme, and milk lipids	Promotion of the selective growth of beneficial rather than pathogenic enteric bacteria from bifidus factor
Prevention of intestinal attachment of enteropathogens from oligosaccharides and glycoconjugates, which act as receptor homologues	Promotion of intestinal epithelial cell maturation by growth factors and nucleotides
	Regulation of T-cell and neutrophil function and monocyte survival by polyunsaturated fatty acids

decreased microbial translocation and hence derive less antigenic stimulation for the gut immune system, resulting in, for example, lower salivary IgA antibody titers (95).

In addition to providing passive immune protection, breast milk also contains a rich source of biologically active factors, including hormones, growth factors, cytokines, and other immunomodulatory molecules (93,96) that drive both the development and the function of the immune and GI systems. These factors interact and synergize to influence the growth, development, and immune status of the newborn infant (92,93,96,98). Bioactive transforming growth factor-β (TGF-β), present in significant levels in breast milk, drives two essential neonatal mucosal immune processes, IgA production and oral tolerance induction. TGF-β derived through this route may also prevent the development of immune dysregulation and atopic disease and also promote specific IgA production in the intestinal mucosa (99).

The immunoregulatory effects of breast milk factors are demonstrated in studies in which distinct immune cell phenotype and function have been described in formula vs breastfed neonates. Formula-fed babies have significantly higher phagocyte function, which also coincides with the higher expression of FcγRI-, Fcα-, and CR3 receptors (all of which aid the binding of bacteria to phagocytic cells) on neutrophils compared with that of exclusively breastfed infants (100). Breastfed infants have higher numbers of circulating CD3–/CD16++ CD56+ NK cells and a lower CD4:CD8 ratio (91,101) and demonstrate significantly higher levels of soluble lCAM-1 and L-selectin for the first few days of life, compared with those fed with formula (102), indicating that immunological priming and education differs between the two groups of infants.

Developmental differences in breastfed and formula-fed infants probably reflect qualitative and quantitative differences in biologically active factors in breast milk vs.

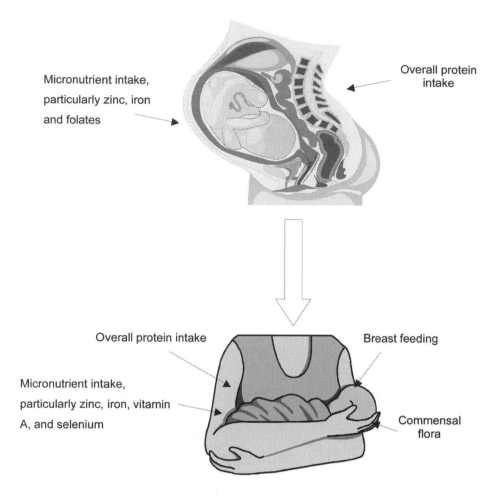

Fig. 1. The effect of nutrition on neonatal immunity: schematic summary of the dietary factors that combine to shape immune status in the newborn.

formula. Breast milk contains nucleotides in the form of nucleic acids, nucleosides, nucleotides, and related metabolic products *(86,103)*. The nucleotide content of human milk is significantly higher than that found in most bovine milk-based infant formulae. Due to the widely reported health and developmental enhancing properties of nucleotides and nucleosides, formulae have been supplemented with these factors for the past 30 yr *(21,86–90)*. Breastfed infants also differ markedly from formula-fed infants in the potentially immunoregulatory fatty acid pattern of their diet, because human milk contains long-chain n–3 and n–6 PUFA, comprising roughly 2% of total fatty acids and which have been essentially absent in formula milk until recently *(104–106)*.

8. CONCLUSIONS

The causal relationship between nutrition, immunity, health, and development in the neonate is now beyond doubt *(see* Fig. 1). Several nutritional factors are required to optimize the innate host defense systems present at birth and also to promote immune ontogenic processes that drive the development and specificity of the adaptive immune system. Overall protein intake, glutamine, arginine, S-amino acids, PUFAs, zinc, and vitamin A are particularly important in the neonate. Breastfeeding provides much in the way of antimicrobial protection in the susceptible neonate and also promotes the growth and development of the immune and GI systems. There are indications that for some beneficial effects, dietary supplementation in neonates, particularly low-birth-weight, premature, and undernourished babies, can promote developmental and functional immunity. Such dietary factors include antioxidant vitamins, trace elements, fatty acids, arginine, glutamine, and nucleotides. Finally, infant foods with altered antigen contents, including novel substrates and conditionally essential nutrients (e.g., growth factors, amino acids, and PUFAs) may be made available in the future to enhance and optimize immune development and its function in the longer term.

9. "TAKE-HOME" MESSAGES

1. Maternal nutrition (macronutrient and micronutrient status) is vitally important for immune development in utero.
2. Structurally, the immune system is intact at birth but is functionally/antigenically naïve. The newborn relies on innate systems of immune defense (evolutionarily conserved and lacking memory) and passive protection (maternal colostrum/milk).
3. Antigen exposure is essential to drive the maturation and expansion of cells of the innate and adaptive mucosal and systemic immune system.
4. Microbial antigens play a vital role in the appropriate education of the immune system and represent an important factor in the predisposition to allergic, inflammatory, and autoimmune diseases in later life.
5. Dietary factors, both macronutrient and micronutrients play an important role in immune ontogeny and immune function. Nucleotides and PUFAs are important dietary constituents for immune function, and fortification of infant foods provides immunological benefits.
6. Identification of natural antimicrobials in human breast milk may also provide functional foods that minimize infection risk of formula-fed infants but may also significantly protect the antiinflammatory status of the developing gut immune system.
7. Breast feeding provides the infant with developmental advantages that importantly include, but also extend beyond, the immune system.

REFERENCES

1. Raveche ES. Possible immunoregulatory role for CD5+ B cells. Clin Immunol Immunopathol 1990;56:135–150.
2. Smith DJ, Taubman MA. Ontogeny of immunity to oral microbiota in humans. Crit Rev Oral Biol Med 1992;3:109–133.
3. Thilaganathan B, Nicolaides KH, Mansur CA, Levinsky RJ, Morgan G. Fetal B lymphocyte subpopulations in normal pregnancies. Fetal Diagn Ther 1993;8:15–22.
4. Silverstein AM. From the forehead of Zeus: the ontogeny of the immune response. Eye 1995;9:147–151.
5. Noia G, Romano D, De Santis M, et al. Ontogeny of the fetal immune system: study on pregnancies with Rh-isoimmunization and nonimmune fetal hydrops. Clin Immunol 1999;90:115–118.
6. Gurevich P, Ben-Hur H, Moldavsky M, Szvalb S, Shperling I, Zusman I. An immunohistochemical study of the secretory immune system in human fetal endocrine glands and their precursors. Early Pregnancy 2001;5:191–200.
7. Garcia AM, Fadel SA, Cao S, Sarzotti M. T cell immunity in neonates. Immunol Res 2000;22:177–190.

8. Cummins AG, Thompson FM. Postnatal changes in mucosal immune response: a physiological perspective of breast feeding and weaning. Immunol Cell Biol 1997;75:419–429.

9. Walker WA. Role of nutrients and bacterial colonization in the development of intestinal host defense. J Pediatr Gastroenterol Nutr 2000;30(Suppl 2):S2–S7.

10. Thrane PS, Rognum TO, Brandtzaeg P. Ontogenesis of the secretory immune system and innate defense factors in human parotid glands. Clin Exp Immunol 1991;86:342–348.

11. Thilaganathan B, Abbas A, Nicolaides KH. Fetal blood natural killer cells in human pregnancy. Fetal Diagn Ther 1993;8:149–153.

12. Mallow EB, Harris A, Salzman N, et al. Human enteric defensins. Gene structure and developmental expression. J Biol Chem 1996;23:4038–4045.

13. Fusunyan RD, Nanthakumar NN, Baldeon ME, Walker WA. Evidence for an innate immune response in the immature human intestine: toll-like receptors on fetal enterocytes. Pediatr Res 2001;49:589–593.

14. Steinborn A, Sohn C, Sayehli C, Niederhut A, Schmitt E, Kaufmann M. Preeclampsia, a pregnancy-specific disease, is associated with fetal monocyte activation. Clin Immunol 2001;100:305–313.

15. Chandra RK. Nutrition and immune responses. Can J Physiol Pharmacol 1983;61:290–294.

16. Chandra S, Chandra RK. Nutrition, immune response, and outcome. Prog Food Nutr Sci 1986;10:1–65.

17. Erickson KL, Medina EA, Hubbard NE. Micronutrients and innate immunity. J Infect Dis 2000;182 (Suppl 1):S5–S10.

18. McDade TW, Beck MA, Kuzawa CW, Adair LS. Prenatal undernutrition and postnatal growth are associated with adolescent thymic function. J Nutr 2001;131:1225–1231.

19. Meydani SN, Erickson KL. Nutrients as regulators of immune function: introduction. FASEB J 2001;15:2555.

20. Field CJ, Johnson IR, Schley PD. Nutrients and their role in host resistance to infection. J Leukoc Biol 2002;71:16–32.

21. Singh R, Gopalan S, Sibal A. Immunonutrition. Indian J Pediatr 2002;69:417–419.

22. Koletzko B, Aggett PJ, Bindels JG, et al. Growth, development and differentiation: a functional food science approach. Br J Nutr 1998;80(Suppl 1):S5–S45.

23. Sanderson IR. Dietary regulation of genes expressed in the developing intestinal epithelium. Am J Clin Nutr 1998;68:999–1005.

24. Paronen J, Vaarala O, Savilahti E, Saukkonen T, Akerblom HK. Soluble adhesion molecules and oral antigen feeding in infants. Pediatr Res 1996;40:276–279.

25. Suen Y, Lee SM, Qian J, van de Ven C, Cairo MS. Dysregulation of lymphokine production in the neonate and its impact on neonatal cell mediated immunity. Vaccine 1998;16:1369–1377.

26. Elliott SR, Roberton DM, Zola H, Macardle PJ. Expression of the costimulator molecules, CD40 and CD154, on lymphocytes from neonates and young children. Human Immunol 2000;61:378–388.

27. Fadel S, Sarzotti M. Cellular immune responses in neonates. Int Rev Immunol 2000;19:173–193.

28. Giannaki G, Rizos D, Xyni K, et al. Serum soluble E- and L-selectin in the very early neonatal period. Early Human Dev 2000;60:149–155.

29. Press JL. Neonatal immunity and somatic mutation. Int Rev Immunol 2000;19:265–287.

30. Liu E, Tu W, Law HK, Lau YL. Decreased yield, phenotypic expression and function of immature monocyte-derived dendritic cells in cord blood. Br J Haematol 2001;113:240–243.

31. Brandtzaeg PE. Current understanding of gastrointestinal immunoregulation and its relation to food allergy. Ann NY Acad Sci 2002;964:13–45.

32. Delespesse G, Yang LP, Ohshima Y, et al. Maturation of human neonatal CD4+ and CD8+ T lymphocytes into Th1/Th2 effectors. Vaccine 1998;16:1415–1419.

33. Husby S. Sensitization and tolerance. Curr Opin Allergy Clin Immunol 2001;1:237–241.

34. Ganschow R, Broering DC, Nolkemper D, et al. Th2 cytokine profile in infants predisposes to improved graft acceptance after liver transplantation. Transplantation 2001;15;72:929–934.

35. Langrish CL, Buddle JC, Thrasher AJ, Goldblatt D. Neonatal dendritic cells are intrinsically biased against Th-1 immune responses. Clin Exp Immunol 2002;128:118–123.

36. Marodi L. Down-regulation of Th1 responses in human neonates. Clin Exp Immunol 2002;128:1–2.

37. Chipeta J, Komada Y, Zhang XL, Azuma E, Yamamoto H, Sakurai M. Neonatal (cord blood) T cells can competently raise type 1 and 2 immune responses upon polyclonal activation. Cell Immunol 2000;205:110–119.

38. Field CJ, Clandinin MT, Van Aerde JE. Polyunsaturated fatty acids and T-cell function: implications for the neonate. Lipids 2001;36:1025–1032.
39. Herz U, Ahrens B, Scheffold A, Joachim R, Radbruch A, Renz H. Impact of in utero Th2 immunity on T cell deviation and subsequent immediate-type hypersensitivity in the neonate. Eur J Immunol 2000;30:714–718.
40. Rainsford E, Reen DJ. Interleukin 10, produced in abundance by human newborn T cells, may be the regulator of increased tolerance associated with cord blood stem cell transplantation. Br J Haematol 2002;116:702–709.
41. Adkins B, Bu Y, Cepero E, Perez R. Exclusive Th2 primary effector function in spleens but mixed Th1/Th2 function in lymph nodes of murine neonates. J Immunol 2000;164:2347–2353.
42. Duffy LC, Zielezny MA, Carrion V, et al. Bacterial toxins and enteral feeding of premature infants at risk for necrotizing enterocolitis. Adv Exp Med Biol 2001;501:519–527.
43. Butel MJ, Waligora-Dupriet AJ, Szylit O. Oligofructose and experimental model of neonatal necrotising enterocolitis. Br J Nutr 2002;87(Suppl 2):S213–S219.
44. Claud EC, Walker WA. Hypothesis: inappropriate colonization of the premature intestine can cause neonatal necrotizing enterocolitis. FASEB J 2001;15:1398–1403.
45. Kirjavainen PV, Gibson GR. Healthy gut microflora and allergy: factors influencing development of the microbiota. Ann Med 1999;31:288–292.
46. Kalliomaki M, Kirjavainen P, Eerola E, Kero P, Salminen S, Isolauri E. Distinct patterns of neonatal gut microflora in infants in whom atopy was and was not developing. J Allergy Clin Immunol 2001;107:129–134.
47. Hoyos AB. Reduced incidence of necrotizing enterocolitis associated with enteral administration of *Lactobacillus acidophilus* and *Bifidobacterium infantis* to neonates in an intensive care unit. Int J Infect Dis 1999;3:197–202.
48. Dai D, Walker WA. Protective nutrients and bacterial colonization in the immature human gut. Adv Pediatr 1999;46:353–382.
49. Caplan MS, Jilling T. Neonatal necrotizing enterocolitis: possible role of probiotic supplementation. J Pediatr Gastroenterol Nutr 2000;30(Suppl 2):S18–S22.
50. Bengmark S, Garcia de Lorenzo A, Culebras JM. Use of pro-, pre- and synbiotics in the ICU—future options. Nutr Hosp 2001;16:239–256.
51. Pickering LK. Biotherapeutic agents and disease in infants. Adv Exp Med Biol 2001;501:365–373.
52. Nelson M. Childhood nutrition and poverty. Proc Nutr Soc 2000;59:307–315.
53. Chandra RK. Interactions between early nutrition and the immune system. Ciba Found Symp 1991;156:77–89; discussion 89–92.
54. Levy O, Martin S, Eichenwald E, et al. Pediatrics impaired innate immunity in the newborn: newborn neutrophils are deficient in bactericidal/permeability-increasing protein. 1999;104:1327–1333.
55. Rondini G, Chirico G. Haematopoietic growth factor levels in term and preterm infants. Curr Opin Hematol 1999;6:192–197.
56. Nesin M, Cunningham-Rundles S. Cytokines and neonates. Am J Perinatol 2000;17:393–404.
57. Cohen SB, Dominguez E, Lowdell M, Madrigal JA. The immunological properties of cord blood: overview of current research presented at the 2nd EUROCORD workshop. Bone Marrow Transplant 1998;22(Suppl 1):S22–S25.
58. Dominguez E, Madrigal JA, Lavrisse Z, Cohen SB. Fetal natural killer cell function is suppressed. Immunology 1998;94:109–114.
59. Kallman J, Schollin J, Schalen C, Erlandsson A, Kihlstrom E. Impaired phagocytosis and opsonisation towards group B streptococci in preterm neonates. Arch Dis Child Fetal Neonatal Ed 1998;78:F46–F50.
60. Nesin M, Cunningham-Rundles S. Cytokines and neonates. Am J Perinatol 2000;17:393–404.
61. Hodge S, Hodge G, Flower R, Han P. Cord blood leucocyte expression of functionally significant molecules involved in the regulation of cellular immunity. Scand J Immunol 2001;53:72–78.
62. Grimble RF. Nutritional modulation of immune function. Proc Nutr Soc 2001;60:389–397.
63. Pierro A. Metabolism and nutritional support in the surgical neonate. J Pediatr Surg 2002;37:811–822.
64. Andrews FJ, Griffiths R. Glutamine: essential for immune nutrition in the critically ill. Br J Nutr 2002;87(Suppl 1):S3–S8.

65. Wu G, Meininger CJ, Knabe DA, Bazer FW, Rhoads JM. Arginine nutrition in development, health and disease. Curr Opin Clin Nutr Metab Care 2000;3:59–66.

66. Delvin EE, Salle BL, Reygrobellet B, Mellier G, Claris O. Vitamin A and E supplementation in breast-fed newborns. J Pediatr Gastroenterol Nutr 2000;31:562–565.

67. Oppenheimer SJ. Iron and its relation to immunity and infectious disease. J Nutr 2001;131:616s–633s.

68. Thurnham DI, Northrop-Clewes CA, McCullough FS, Das BS, Lunn PG. Innate immunity, gut integrity, and vitamin A in Gambian and Indian infants. J Infect Dis 2000;182(Suppl 1):S23–S28.

69. Stephensen CB. Vitamin A, infection, and immune function. Annu Rev Nutr 2001;21:167–192.

70. Fawzi WW, Mbise R, Spiegelman D, Fataki M, Hertzmark E, Ndossi G. Vitamin A supplements and diarrheal and respiratory tract infections among children in Dar es Salaam, Tanzania. J Pediatr 2000;137:660–667.

71. Villamor E, Fawzi WW. Vitamin A supplementation: implications for morbidity and mortality in children. J Infect Dis 2000;182(Suppl 1):S122–S133.

72. Lie C, Ying C, Wang EL, Brun T, Geissler C. Impact of large-dose vitamin A supplementation on childhood diarrhoea, respiratory disease and growth. Eur J Clin Nutr 1993;47:88–96.

73. Valdes-Ramos R. Zinc: a perinatal point of view. Prog Food Nutr Sci 1992;16:279–306.

74. Wellinghausen N. Immunobiology of gestational zinc deficiency. Br J Nutr 2001;85(Suppl 2):S81–S86.

75. Fan PC, Teng RJ, Chou CC, Wu TJ, Tsou Yau KI, Hsieh KH. Impaired immune function in a premature infant with zinc deficiency after total parenteral nutrition. Zhonghua Min Guo Xiao Er Ke Yi Xue Hui Za Zhi 1996;37:364–369.

76. Schlesinger L, Arevalo M, Arredondo S, Diaz M, Lonnerdal B, Stekel A. Effect of a zinc-fortified formula on immunocompetence and growth of malnourished infants. Am J Clin Nutr 1992;56:491–498.

77. Koletzko B, Demmelmair H, Socha P. Nutritional support of infants and children: supply and metabolism of lipids. Baillieres Clin Gastroenterol 1998;12:671–696.

78. Friedman Z. Polyunsaturated fatty acids in the low-birth-weight infant. Semin Perinatol 1979;3:341–361.

79. Field CJ, Clandinin MT, Van Aerde JE. Polyunsaturated fatty acids and T-cell function: implications for the neonate. Lipids 2001;36:1025–1032.

80. Sweeney B, Puri P, Reen DJ. Polyunsaturated fatty acids influence neonatal monocyte survival. Pediatr Surg Int 2001;17:254–258.

81. Van Buren CT, Rudolph F. Dietary nucleotides: a conditional requirement. Nutrition 1997;13:470–472.

82. Sanchez-Pozoz A, Gill A. Nucleotides as semiessential nutritional components. Br J Nutr 2002;87(Suppl 1):S135–S137.

83. Yamamoto S, Wang MF, Adiei AA, Amecho CK. Role of nucleosides and nucleotides in the immune system, gut reparation after injury, and brain function. Nutrition 1997;13:372–374.

84. Cosgrove M. Perinatal and infant nutrition. Nucleotides. Nutrition 1998;14:748–751.

85. Carver JD. Dietary nucleotides: effects on the immune and gastrointestinal systems. Acta Paediatr Suppl 1999;88:83–88.

86. Lerner A, Shamir R. Nucleotides in infant nutrition: a must or an option. Isr Med Assoc J 2000;2:772–774.

87. Schlimme E, Martin D, Meisel H. Nucleosides and nucleotides: natural bioactive substances in milk and colostrum. Br J Nutr 2000;84(Suppl 1):S59–S68.

88. Maldonado J, Navarro J, Narbona E, Gil A. The influence of dietary nucleotides on humoral and cell immunity in the neonate and lactating infant. Early Human Dev 2001;65(Suppl):S69–S74.

89. Grimble GK, Westwood OM. Nucleotides as immunomodulators in clinical nutrition. Curr Opin Clin Nutr Metab Care 2001;4:57–64.

90. Krishnaraj R. Negative modulation of human NK cell activity by purinoceptors. 1. Effect of exogenous adenosine triphosphate. Cell Immunol 1992;141:306–322.

91. Alarcon B, Redondo JM, Bugany H, Carrasco L, Fresno M. Inhibition of natural killer cytotoxicity by extracellular ppp(A2'p5')nA oligonucleotides. Int J Immunopharmacol 1988;10:73–80.

92. Telemo E, Hanson LA. Antibodies in milk. J Mammary Gland Biol Neoplasia 1996;1:243–249.

93. Oddy WH. Breastfeeding protects against illness and infection in infants and children: a review of the evidence. Breastfeed Rev 2001;9:11–18.

94. Hanson LA, Korotkova M, Haversen L, et al. Breast-feeding, a complex support system for the offspring. Pediatr Int 2002;44:347–352.
95. Nagao AT, Friedlander-Del Nero D, Arslanian C, Carneiro-Sampaio MM. Elevated levels and different repertoire profile of colostral anti-LPS antibodies may have a significant role in compensating newborn immunity. Scand J Immunol 2001;53:602–609.
96. Wold AE, Adlerberth I. Breast feeding and the intestinal microflora of the infant—implications for protection against infectious diseases. Adv Exp Med Biol 2000;478:77–93.
97. Hawkes JS, Gibson RA. Lymphocyte subpopulations in breast-fed and formula-fed infants at six months of age. Adv Exp Med Biol 2001;501:497–504.
98. Rondini G, Chirico G. Haematopoietic growth factor levels in term and pre-term infants. Curr Opin Hematol 1999;6:192–197.
99. Donnet-Hughes A, Duc N, Serrant P, Vidal K, Schiffrin EJ. Bioactive molecules in milk and their role in health and disease: the role of transforming growth factor-beta. Immunol Cell Biol 2000;78:74–79.
100. Kalliomaki M, Ouwehand A, Arvilommi H, Kero P, Isolauri E. Transforming growth factor-beta in breast milk: a potential regulator of atopic disease at an early age. J Allergy Clin Immunol 1999;104:1251–1257.
101. Gronlund MM, Nuutila J, Pelto L, et al. Mode of delivery directs the phagocyte functions of infants for the first 6 months of life. Clin Exp Immunol 1999;116:521–526.
102. Dahlgren UI, Hanson LA, Telemo E. Maturation of immunocompetence in breast-fed vs. formula-fed infants. Adv Nutr Res 2001;10:311–325.
103. Xyni K, Rizos D, Giannaki G, Sarandakou A, Phocas I, Creatsas G. Soluble form of ICAM–1, VCAM–1, E- and L-selectin in human milk. Mediators Inflamm 2000;9:133–140.
104. Hamosh M. Bioactive factors in human milk. Pediatr Clin North Am 2001;48:69–86.
105. Putnam JD, Carlson SE, De Voe PW, Barness LA. The effect of variations in dietary fatty acids on the fatty acid composition of erythrocyte phosphatidylcholine and phosphatidylethanolamine in human infants. Am J Clin Nutr 1982;36:106–114.
106. Pita ML, Fernandez MR, De-Lucchi C, et al. Changes in the fatty acids pattern of red blood cell phospholipids induced by type of milk, dietary nucleotide supplementation, and postnatal age in pre-term infants. J Pediatr Gastroenterol Nutr 1988;7:740–747.
107. Farquharson J, Cockburn F, Patrick WA, Jamieson EC, Logan RW. Infant cerebral cortex phospholipid fatty acid composition and diet. Lancet 1992;340:810–813.

5 Nutrition and Immunity in the Elderly

John D. Bogden and Donald B. Louria

1. INTRODUCTION

Within the past few years, a considerable amount of new information on the role of nutrition in the aging immune response has been published. This chapter is an update and expansion in scope of a chapter written by us and published in 2001 *(1)*.

Aging has been described as a group of processes that promote vulnerability to challenges, thereby increasing the likelihood of death. Because there is evidence that depressed immunity can increase the risk of death, it is likely that changes in immunity with age are key factors in the aging process.

Theories of aging include the free-radical, programmed senescence, and immunological theories *(2)*. Evidence for the immunological theory of aging is based largely on the well-described changes that occur with age in various species that have been studied, including man, and on observations from cross-sectional studies that demonstrate an association between maintenance of good immune function and longevity *(1,2)*. A limitation of this theory is that it lacks the universality of other theories, such as the free-radical theory of aging, because it is not applicable to lower organisms that do not have well-developed immune systems. Of course, the complexity of aging may require the use of more than one theory to understand it, and the various theories are not necessarily independent of one another. For example, there is evidence that demonstrates that antioxidant nutrients that reduce free-radical damage can improve immunity in older people *(3)*, suggesting that the free-radical and immunological theories may be complementary.

2. AGING AND IMMUNITY

2.1. General Changes in Immunity with Aging

It is useful to distinguish between primary changes that develop because of the age-dependent intrinsic decline of immunity and secondary changes that result from "environmental" factors, such as prescription and nonprescription drug use, physical activity, and diet. In fact, Lesourd and Mazari *(4)* have suggested that secondary, rather than primary, changes in immunity with age are more likely to explain the increased incidence and severity of infectious diseases in older people.

From: *Diet and Human Immune Function*
Edited by: D. A. Hughes, L. G. Darlington, and A. Bendich © Humana Press Inc., Totowa, NJ

Table 1
Some Specific Changes in Immunity with Aging

Involution of the thymus
Decreased thymic hormone concentrations
Decreased delayed type hypersensitivity (DTH) skin-test responses
Decreased interleukin-2 (IL-2) secretion
Decreased lymphocyte proliferative responses to mitogens
Lower antibody titers after vaccination
Increased serum autoantibodies
Increased soluble IL-2 receptors
Reduced phagocytosis by polymorphonuclear leukocytes
Reduced intracellular killing by polymorphonuclear leukocytes

---

Changes in immunity with aging include inhibited T-lymphocyte functions, decreased antibody production and responses, increased autoimmune activity with compromised self-nonself discrimination, and greater heterogeneity in immunological responses *(5–9)*. Concerning the latter, depressed T-cell function is the most common and may begin as early as the sixth decade. However, T-cell dysfunction is neither inevitable nor predictable. For example, we *(8)* measured delayed hypersensitivity skin-test responses in 100 people aged 60–89 yr. We found that although 41% were anergic to a panel of seven skin-test antigens and an additional 29% were "relatively anergic," responding to only 1 of the 7 antigens, the remaining 30% were reactive, responding to 2 or more of the skin-test antigens, often with sizable reactions.

2.2. Specific Changes in Immunity with Aging

2.2.1. INVOLUTION OF THE THYMUS

The most striking changes in immunity with increasing age are inhibited T-cell functions (*see* Table 1). These are likely related to the well-known involution of the thymus *(10)*. The differentiation process by which stem cells become T lymphocytes occurs in this organ. It is a two-lobed structure in mammals, located in the thorax above the heart.

There are several stages in the process by which immature stem cells (pre-T cells) become mature T cells. These include migration to the thymus, where some cells are stimulated to grow and others die; differentiation, in which the mature phenotype of T cells develops in the thymus, including surface expression of accessory molecules; positive selection, in which self major histocompatibility complex (MHC)-restricted T cells are selected and other cells rejected; and negative selection, which ensures that surviving mature T cells are self-tolerant. The selective survival or death of cells results in a self-MHC-restricted self-antigen-tolerant mature T-cell population *(10)*.

The thymus is the principal site of T-cell maturation. Involution with age occurs soon after puberty. Because some T-cell maturation continues throughout adult life, it is likely that a remnant of the thymus or some other tissue continues to effect T-cell maturation *(10)*. However, because memory T cells have a long life span (20 yr or more) *(10)*, the involution of the thymus does not cause compromised immunity in young adults but is likely to contribute to depressed immunity with age, because the time since thymic involution becomes longer.

The involution of the thymus before the peak reproductive years suggests that this process may provide an evolutionary advantage. One hypothesis is that involution provides a net benefit, because it reduces the risk of autoimmune reactions *(11)*. According to this theory, the increased risk of cancer or infectious diseases resulting from depressed cellular immunity is a detriment that is offset by a reduced risk of autoimmune disease that accompanies thymic involution. Although attractive, this theory of immunological "trade-offs" as an adaptation to aging requires additional supporting evidence.

An alternative hypothesis has been proposed by Siskind *(12)*, who suggests that adaptation to environmental pathogens occurs early in life and, thereafter, relative constancy of immune function, rather than adaptability, may be most beneficial. He further speculates that efforts to modify cellular immunity in later life, e.g., by pharmacological or nutritional means, may do more harm than good. Although interesting, this hypothesis is not widely supported and not consistent with the known association between good cellular immunity and reduced morbidity and mortality in older people.

2.2.2. T-Lymphocyte Functions

Changes in T lymphocytes with aging include a shift in relative percentages of subpopulations and qualitative changes in individual cell-surface receptors *(13)*. When compared with T cells from younger people, cells of the elderly are deficient in in vitro production of certain T-cell growth factors, such as interleukin (IL)-2 and have a decreased ability to bind and respond to it *(14–17)*. McMurray *(15)* has outlined evidence that implicates nutrient-mediated effects at virtually every step in the development and expression of T-cell immunity, from direct effects on the thymus and thymic hormone production to T cell maturation and distribution, antigen reactivity, lymphokine production, and even composition of the T-cell membrane.

Delayed type hypersensitivity (DTH) skin-test responses involve T-lymphocyte proliferation, production of IL-2 and other lymphokines, and infiltration of the test site with mononuclear cells, resulting 24–72 h later in induration and erythema; it is the T-cell parameter that is most consistently and profoundly affected by nutritional status *(15)*. Reduced DTH is also the immune parameter in older people most consistently associated with increased infectious disease morbidity and mortality from all causes, according to Meakins et al. *(18)* and Christou et al. *(19)* for surgery patients and Wayne et al. *(20)* and Roberts-Thomson et al. *(21)* for initially healthy people age 60 yr or older.

In their investigation, Christou et al. *(19)* studied the relationship between presurgery DTH responses and postsurgical sepsis-related death in 245 subjects with a median age of 67 yr and a range of 24 to 98 yr. Initially, anergic subjects experienced significantly more postsurgical mortality than those who were reactive. Because all the subjects had gastrointestinal (GI) cancers that prompted the decision to operate, it can be argued that the initial severity of the disease increased both the incidence of anergy and the risk of dying after surgery. Thus, initial disease severity could explain the apparent strong relationship between preoperative DTH responses and postsurgical mortality. However, Wayne et al. *(20)* did not have this confounder, because they looked prospectively at healthy adults during a 10-yr period. In this investigation, the authors followed 273 initially healthy subjects age 60 yr or older with no history of serious medical problems. DTH responses were measured at enrollment. Anergy (failure to respond to any of four skin-test antigens) at enrollment in the study was associated with a significantly increased risk of dying in the 10-yr follow-up period. For example, at the end of 10 yr, 89% of the initially reactive subjects were still alive, but 22% of the anergic subjects had died. The study demonstrates that anergy to skin-test antigens, even when present in healthy older people, is associated with subsequent increased all-cause mortality. The authors also found a 2.5-fold increase in cancer mortality in the initially anergic group in comparison to the reactive group. However, this was not statistically significant, probably because of the relatively small number of cancer deaths observed.

Evidence for the decline in T-cell function with age includes a considerable number of studies that demonstrate reduced lymphocyte proliferative responses (LPR) to mitogens or antigens, as well as depressed delayed hypersensitivity responses to recall antigens (7,16–23). Indeed, these two measures of T-cell function have been the most widely studied functional tests performed in conjunction with assessment of the effects of nutritional intervention on immunity. A problem with LPR to mitogens is the considerable variability of these assays, even in laboratories with rigid quality control procedures.

There is some evidence for changes in T lymphocyte subsets with aging, particularly decreases in CD4+, increases in CD8+ cells, and decreases in the CD4+/CD8+ ratio (9). There is also evidence that lymphocyte subsets are altered in older people who are ill. For example, Markewitz et al. (24) have found that immunosuppression in cardiopulmonary bypass surgery patients age 55 yr or older is associated with decreased CD4+ T cells and increases in CD8+ T cells. Higa et al. (25) have found that increases in CD8+ T cells predict a longer period of recovery after onset of acute herpetic pain during herpes zoster infection. The increased incidence of this disease in older people is believed to result from the depressed cellular immunity that occurs with age (14).

Measurement of lymphocyte subsets is a key component in immune function evaluation (26,27). Knowledge of lymphocyte subset numbers (cells/mL and percentage of total) allows determination of relationships between immune functions and the number and percentage of cells responsible for these functions. This can allow one to distinguish between effects owing to increased numbers of a particular subgroup of cells and enhanced activity by the same number of cells. The latter could be related to antigen-binding capacity per cell. Indeed, changes in antigen-binding capacity per cell could be a mechanism by which nutrition influences immune functions. However, the importance of changes in antigen-binding capacity per cell in declining immunity with age is largely unexplored.

2.2.3. Other Immune System Changes with Aging

There is some evidence for a decline in B-cell functions with age, although it is likely related, at least in part, to the T-cell dependence of B-cell functions. Older people vaccinated with tetanus toxoid, varicella-zoster, or hepatitis B antigens demonstrate reduced antibody production, as well as a greater percentage of nonresponders than young adults. This may also be true after pneumococcal and influenza virus immunization, although the evidence is not as convincing (28).

Perskin and Cronstein (29) have reported that aging produces alterations in neutrophil plasma membrane viscosity that may result in compromised neutrophil function and increased susceptibility to infection with specific pyogenic bacteria. This is consistent with studies of Nagel et al. (30), Shoham-Kessary and Gershon (31), and Corberand et al. (32) that suggest compromised in vitro activity of neutrophils from older people.

Depending on the microorganism studied, the depressed neutrophil activity was phagocytosis or intracellular killing.

A review by Makinodan et al. *(33)* suggests that although antigen-responsive cells, such as B cells, monocytes, and killer cells, are vulnerable to aging, T cells are clearly the most vulnerable. This is why most nutrition, immunity, and aging studies have focused on T-cell functions.

Sen et al. *(28)* have published an insightful review that distinguishes between an increased incidence vs. greater severity of infectious diseases in older people. For example, they report an increased case-fatality ratio for bacterial meningitis and pneumococcal pneumonia in older people and an increased incidence of diseases, such as urinary tract infections and varicella zoster. Other diseases, such as influenza virus infection and Gram-negative sepsis, are both more frequent and more severe in older people. They suggest that in addition to changes in immunity with age, local urinary tract, respiratory tract, and neurologic changes may contribute to the increase in infectious disease morbidity and mortality in older people.

Relationships among the ILs, their receptors, and immunity have been recently widely discussed. Particularly interesting in the elderly is IL-2, because its production is decreased in older people *(9)*. Interestingly, soluble IL-2R levels are higher in older than in younger adults *(34)*, and it has been suggested that this may be a factor in the decline of cellular immunity with age, because high serum concentrations of soluble IL-2R may compete with and decrease IL-2 binding to T-cell IL-2 receptors and, thereby, compromise immunity *(35,36)*. We have previously found that serum IL-2R concentrations are relatively lower in physically active older people compared with sedentary seniors and that exercise/physical activity habits and multivitamin supplementation may interact to influence soluble serum IL-2R concentrations *(37)*. We have also verified the higher levels of soluble IL-2R in older people (unpublished data).

There may be a "survivor" aspect to the relationship between advanced age and immune capacity. The oldest people, including centenarians studied by Sansoni et al. *(38)*, have well-preserved immune functions, such as natural killer (NK) cell activity, that are often better than those age 50–80 yr. In addition, those older than 90 yr have lower serum autoantibody concentrations than those in the 60–80-yr range *(14,39)*. Thus, enhanced immunity and reduced autoimmunity are associated with the ability to live to age 90 and beyond.

3. NUTRITION AND IMMUNITY

3.1. Nutrition, Immunity, and Aging

Scrimshaw and SanGiovanni *(40)* have noted that infections, no matter how mild, can adversely affect nutritional status, which, in turn, can compromise immunity and exacerbate the effects of infection. They discuss evidence for the effects of various micronutrient deficiencies on immunity, including beta-carotene; pyridoxine; folic acid; pantothenate; vitamins A, B_{12}, C, D, and E; the trace elements iron, zinc, and copper; and magnesium. In general, cell-mediated and nonspecific immune functions are more sensitive to single micronutrient deficiencies than humoral immunity.

Fraker *(41)* has noted that the immune system is a large "organ," comprised of the blood, spleen, lymphatic system, thymus, and other components. In addition, millions of new immune system cells are produced daily. Its large size and high cellular turnover combine to make the immune system a major nutrient user. Thus, it is not surprising that some aspects of immunity are sensitive to nutritional deficiencies.

One key question is whether the decline in immunity with aging is, at least in part, owing to nutritional deficiencies and/or increased requirements. Another possibility is that micronutrient supplementation might improve immunity even in the absence of an underlying "deficiency," defined by factors such as low circulating nutrient concentrations or consistently low intakes.

Human studies of protein-calorie malnutrition (PCM) in underdeveloped countries or in adults who are hospitalized demonstrate a causal association between undernutrition and secondary immunodepression that results in diminished resistance to infectious diseases *(14,15,42,43)*. This association is consistent enough to permit the use of DTH in medical and surgical patients as a predictor of clinical prognosis *(19)*. Thus, there is little doubt that severe malnutrition has a major effect on resistance to disease that is mediated, in part, through the immune system. There is also evidence that moderate to marginal undernutrition may compromise immunity *(44,45)*.

McMurray *(15)* has noted that both moderate and severe dietary deficiencies of specific nutrients profoundly alter cell-mediated immune responses in humans and experimental animals. Diets with inadequate contents of calories, protein, vitamin A, pyridoxine, biotin, or zinc can result in depressed production of thymic hormones critical for T-lymphocyte differentiation. Reduced numbers and depressed in vitro function of T cells have also been reported in experimental deficiencies of zinc, copper, iron, and vitamins A and E. Depressed DTH responses are a consistent result of dietary inadequacies of protein, pyridoxine, iron, zinc, and vitamins A and C.

The classic review by Beisel *(46)* extensively examined the literature up to 1982 on single nutrients and immunity. The water-soluble vitamins that are most critical for maintaining immunity are vitamin B_6, folate, vitamin B_{12}, and vitamin C. Among the lipid-soluble micronutrients, vitamins A and E exert the most significant impacts. Recent studies have shown that vitamin D is also an important immune modulator. Trace metals also exert substantial influences on immune functions *(15,46)*, the effects of which are described in detail in Chapters 11–13.

Because the variability in immune responses increases with aging, subgroups that have impaired immunity because of nutrient deficiencies are more likely to be observed in the elderly than in other age groups. In addition, when episodes of nutritional vulnerability overlap with suboptimal immune function, an adverse synergistic interaction is possible *(15)*. These factors make it more rewarding to study nutrition/immunity relationships in older rather than in younger adults. Beisel *(47)* has noted that individual studies of immunity in humans have not been systematic or comprehensive. This is no doubt related to the considerable expense that would be incurred in studying multiple immune responses in a sizeable number of older people.

It can be useful to compare relationships between nutrition and immunity in older people with those of diseases in which immune functions are compromised. In the case of HIV infection, we *(48)* have found that compromised nutritional and antioxidant status begins early in the course of infection and may contribute to disease progression. This observation can be compared with the decline in cellular immunity that begins in many older people in the fifth or sixth decade and eventually is associated with a reduced life span *(2,5,20)*.

3.2. Cross-Sectional Studies on Micronutrient Nutrition and Immunity

Goodwin and Garry *(49)* compared immunologic functions of healthy elderly New Mexico residents consuming higher than Recommended Dietary Allowance (RDA) levels (five times RDA or greater) of micronutrients with similar individuals not taking supplements. Vitamins A, C, D, and E; the B vitamins; iron; calcium; and zinc were evaluated. There was no significant difference between the two groups in DTH responses or in vitro LPR to mitogens. The authors suggested that the immune-enhancing properties of high doses of vitamins might be the result of a nonspecific adjuvant effect that does not persist with time.

More recently, the same authors *(50)* studied 230 healthy older men and women to determine if subclinical micronutrient deficiencies contribute to the depressed immunity found in many of the elderly. Immune functions studied included DTH responses, in vitro LPR to phytohemagglutinin (PHA), lymphocyte counts, and serum autoantibody levels. Spearman correlation coefficients were calculated to assess associations between blood micronutrient concentrations and selected immune functions. The authors also compared subjects with the lowest responses to those with the highest. There were no significant associations between low serum micronutrient concentrations and immune functions, and the authors suggested that subtle nutrient differences did not contribute to the immunodeficiency of aging. However, the population sample studied was relatively affluent, and people taking prescription drugs or daily over-the-counter medications, as well as those with a serious medical problem, were excluded. Thus, the study may have excluded those subjects who might benefit most from micronutrient supplements.

Kawakami et al. *(51)* studied 155 healthy subjects aged 20–99 yr and suggested that cell-mediated immunity was reduced as a result of malnutrition.

In a recent study *(52)*, we examined relationships between immunity and dietary and serum antioxidants, B vitamins, essential trace metals, and serum homocysteine in 65 older men and women aged 53–86 yr. Subjects who had used vitamin or mineral supplements in the preceding 3 mo were excluded. Soluble serum IL-2 receptor (sIL-2R) concentrations were positively associated with body mass index (BMI) and serum concentrations of homocysteine and vitamin B_6 and negatively associated with serum β-carotene and dietary lycopene. In a multiple regression model, these five factors explained 52% of the variability in sIL-2R. The percentage of subjects with anergy to a panel of seven recall skin antigens was 25%, and these responses were negatively associated with T helper cell (CD4+) number, suggesting the reduced numbers of the latter as a factor that may have contributed to the anergy of the subjects. T helper cell numbers were positively associated with serum copper, and NK cell numbers were positively associated with dietary folate and vitamin B_6. The results document relationships between nutrition and immunity and suggest that IL-2 may be influenced by dietary antioxidants and B vitamins, including those that modify homocysteine metabolism.

The studies mentioned were not attempts to intervene by provision of micronutrient supplements but were assessments of associations between the subjects' usual intakes or blood concentrations and selected immune functions. Variables that cannot be controlled in cross-sectional studies may mask associations between nutritional factors and immunity, especially because immunity is likely to be dependent on several factors, only one of which is nutritional status. Such studies are valuable in identifying nutrients for more intensive study but can only provide statistical associations that may not be cause-and-effect relationships. The latter can be assessed by standard placebo-controlled double-blind clinical trials.

3.3. Clinical Trials of Single Nutrients

Several clinical trials have been conducted in recent years. These have included depletion/repletion studies in young volunteers and provision of micronutrient supplements to older people who did not have preexisting deficiencies.

Jacob et al. *(53)* studied the effects of moderate ascorbate depletion on immunity and other factors in young adult males confined to a metabolic ward. Ascorbate depletion was achieved using daily doses of 5–20 mg/d, whereas repletion was achieved with doses of 60 (the RDA at that time) to 250 mg/d. Although LPR to mitogens were not affected by ascorbate depletion/repletion, DTH responses to a panel of seven recall antigens were markedly depressed by ascorbate depletion. Repletion for 28 d at either 60 or 250 mg/d did not restore the mean antigen score to the predepletion level, although there was some improvement in induration in 3 of the 8 men studied. These results suggest that DTH is more sensitive to ascorbate depletion than mitogen responses. They further suggest that the length of the repletion period was insufficient to produce a return of DTH to baseline levels and/or the repletion doses were not large enough.

Fuller et al. *(54)* studied the effect of β-carotene supplementation on the ultraviolet (UV)-radiation induced photosuppression of DTH in 24 young adult males, aged 19–39 yr. They found that exposure to a UV-A/B light source for a 16-d period significantly reduced DTH responses in a control (placebo) group to 39% of the initial values but did not induce significant reductions in a group given 30 mg β-carotene per day. Because young men were studied, it was not known if these results would occur in young women or in older men and women. This group repeated the study in an elderly population and found similar UV-suppression effects that were prevented with β-carotene supplementation, although there was more variability in DTH responses in the older people compared to young adults *(55,56)*.

Watson et al. *(57)* investigated the effects of β-carotene on lymphocyte subpopulations in male and female subjects with a mean age of 56 yr. Beta-carotene was given at doses of 15, 30, 45, or 60 mg/d for 2 mo. Using monoclonal antibodies to identify lymphocyte subsets, they found that the percentages of T helper and NK cells, as well as cells with IL-2 and transferrin receptors, were increased in a dose-related fashion. There were no significant effects of β-carotene on T-suppressor cells. However, the number of subjects in each treatment group was only 3–5; thus, further investigation is needed to confirm these findings.

Santos et al. *(58)* found that men participating in the Physicians' Health Study who consumed 50 mg of β-carotene on alternate days for an average of 12 yr had significantly greater NK cell activity than controls given placebos. Surveillance by NK cells is protective against the development of cancer. However, two large intervention trials have found an association between high doses of β-carotene and the development of lung cancer in cigarette smokers *(59,60)*. The role of the immune system in leading to the development of lung cancer in these studies is not known, but the results suggest that there are risks associated with the long-term use of high doses of β-carotene supplements in smokers.

Talbott et al. *(61)* in a pilot study investigated the impact of pyridoxine supplementation on lymphocyte responses in 15 older (aged 65–81 yr) mostly female subjects and found that administration of 50 mg/d of pyridoxine hydrochloride significantly increased in vitro lymphocyte proliferative responses to PHA, pokeweed mitogen, and *Staphylococcus aureus*.

Meydani et al. *(62)* have reported that vitamin B_6 deficiency impairs IL-2 production and lymphocyte proliferation in older adults. Each of these measurements was reduced by approx 50% by depletion, whereas repletion with near RDA levels of B_6 eventually increased values to about the baseline levels. Although only 8 subjects were studied, this well-designed investigation supports several other studies that suggest that vitamin B_6 may play a key role in immune responses *(63)*.

In another study, Meydani et al. *(64)* gave older people 50, 200, or 800 mg of vitamin E daily for 4–5 mo. This resulted in improved antibody titers to hepatitis B vaccine and enhanced DTH responses, especially in the group consuming 200 mg of vitamin E per day. This suggests 200 mg as a recommended dose, although lower doses may be equally effective when administered for longer time periods. In a more recent study, Pallast et al. *(65)* investigated the effects of 6 mo of supplementation of healthy older men (aged 65–80 yr) with vitamin E at doses of 50 and 100 mg/d for 6 mo. There was a dose-related trend of increased DTH responses, especially in those subjects with initially low responses, suggesting that there are subgroups of older people who might benefit most from vitamin E supplements.

There has been considerable interest in the potential for zinc to improve immune functions in older people. It is clear that severe zinc deficiency in animals and people, e.g., as found in the disease acrodermatitis enteropathica, can greatly compromise cellular immunity and lead to the development of life-threatening opportunistic infections *(66)*. There are also reports of significant associations between plasma or cellular zinc concentrations and immune functions, such as DTH responses, in older people *(8,67)*. However, recent studies of the effect of zinc supplementation on immunity in older people have not been encouraging. They have demonstrated either no beneficial effect of zinc supplements on immunity or an adverse effect, even when the supplements contained modest doses of zinc in the range of 15–25 mg/d *(68,69)*. In the absence of an underlying deficiency, use of zinc supplements by older people, especially at doses that exceed 15 mg/d, is more likely to adversely affect immunity than improve it.

Doherty et al. *(70)* studied the effect of low (1.5 mg/kg) vs. higher (6.0 mg/kg) zinc supplementation on mortality in 141 young children in Bangladesh with protein-energy malnutrition and weight-for-age z scores of approx –4.6. Mortality was significantly greater in the high-dose group, with sepsis frequently contributing to death. The results suggest that high-dose zinc supplementation may contribute to increased mortality and risk of sepsis in children who are severely malnourished. Although this study involved only young children, aged 6 mo to 3 yr, it suggests caution in the use of high-dose zinc supplements by any age group.

3.4. Clinical Trials of Micronutrient Combinations

The studies discussed here focused on the effects of relatively large doses of individual micronutrients on immune functions. There have been only a limited number of published placebo-controlled trials of the effects of multivitamin/mineral supplements on immune functions in older people.

In the first of these studies, we investigated the effects of zinc given in combination with a multivitamin on immune functions in 63 older people *(71)*. All subjects received a standard multivitamin/mineral supplement that contained all the essential micronutrients, except zinc. In addition, subjects received 15 or 100 mg of zinc or a placebo. Daily consumption of the multivitamin/mineral supplement for 1 yr was associated with enhanced DTH and mitogen responses, but these effects were reduced and delayed by ingestion of 15 and especially 100 mg of zinc each day. These data suggest that interactions among micronutrients may influence their effects on immunity and that some individual micronutrients, even at modest doses, may have unexpected adverse effects. The adverse effect of zinc is consistent with other previously cited recent studies that indicate that zinc supplements in healthy older people either do not improve immunity or adversely affect it *(68,69)*.

The second multivitamin intervention trial is the study of Chandra *(72)*, who reported the results of 12 mo of daily supplementation of a group of healthy subjects aged 65 yr or older, with a micronutrient formulation containing relatively low doses of nine vitamins and five trace elements and higher levels of the antioxidants vitamin C, vitamin E, and β-carotene. Chandra found that when compared with a placebo group, the micronutrient group had higher numbers of some T-cell subsets and NK cells, enhanced lymphocyte proliferation to mitogens, increased in vitro IL-2 production, higher antibody responses to influenza vaccine, and greater NK cell activity. In addition, subjects who received supplements experienced significantly fewer days (23 ± 5) of illness per year because of infectious diseases than subjects in the placebo group (48 ± 7 d). These results are consistent with the hypothesis presented in our article published in 1990 *(71)* that an RDA-level micronutrient supplement could improve immune functions in older people. The results of Chandra further suggest that there may be beneficial clinical effects, i.e., a reduced prevalence of infectious diseases, as a result of micronutrient supplementation.

Presupplementation plasma concentrations of retinol, β-carotene, vitamin C, and vitamin B_6 were low in some subjects in Chandra's study, with the percentage of subjects with initially low concentrations of each between 12.5% and 22.9%. Most of the low concentrations were corrected by supplementation, so that the percentage of subjects with low values of the above concentrations decreased to 0–4.4%, and this was accompanied by enhanced immune functions. However, this observation does not prove that the decrease in the percentage of subjects with low concentrations was responsible for the improved immune functions that were found.

Limitations of the study of Chandra include the absence of an assessment of dietary micronutrients from food and the assessment of immune functions at only baseline and after 1 yr of supplementation. In addition, the occurrence of infectious diseases was reported as the number of days on which subjects were infected per year. The latter is the product of the incidence of infectious diseases and their duration. Thus, a single infection persisting for 30 d is equivalent to six infections of 5 d duration each. It is important to know the effects of micronutrient supplementation on the incidence of new infections, as well as the nature and duration of each type of infection.

Penn et al. *(73)* studied the effects on immune functions of a supplement containing vitamin C (100 mg), vitamin A (8000 IU), and vitamin E (50 mg); it was given for 28 d to 50% of the 30 elderly subjects. All were patients who had been hospitalized for at least 3 mo. The number and percentage of CD4+ and CD8+ T cells were significantly increased in the group receiving supplements but not in the group receiving placebo. Proliferative responses of lymphocytes to the mitogen PHA were also significantly increased in the group receiving supplements by 64%–283% but were not affected by the placebo. There was biochemical evidence of deficiencies of vitamins A, C, and/or E in 5% to 47% of the subjects receiving the supplements at study enrollment. Thus, it is possible that the improvement in cellular immunity in these subjects with short-term administration of vitamins A, C, and E resulted from correction of underlying deficiencies that are more likely to be present in hospitalized than in independently living older people. These results suggest that this group of micronutrients may be particularly important for immune response enhancement in older people.

In another study, Chavance et al. *(74)* enrolled 218 subjects aged 60 yr or older who were living independently and had not used any vitamin supplements for at least the previous 3 mo. They were given a low-dose multivitamin or placebo for 4 mo. No clinical or laboratory assessments of immune function were conducted. The authors found no significant effects of supplementation on the incidence of infections; however, effects on the duration of each infection or the total number of days of infection were not assessed. As suggested by the authors, the failure to find any significant effects on the incidence of infections may be result from the short duration of supplementation. This is consistent with our results and those of Chandra *(72)*, which suggest that periods of supplementation of approx 12 mo are required before improvements in immune functions occur in older people.

We also conducted a randomized placebo-controlled double-blind trial of the effects of RDA-level micronutrient supplementation on plasma vitamin and trace metal concentrations and immune functions in independently living healthy older subjects *(75)*. The over-the-counter micronutrient supplement used in the study contained RDA levels of each of the essential vitamins and low to moderate doses of minerals.

Of the 65 subjects enrolled, 56 (86%) completed the 1-yr study. Approximately 2/3 were women. As expected, there were no statistically significant effects of the placebo on plasma micronutrient concentrations. In contrast, the data for the micronutrient supplement group show statistically significant increases at 6 and/or 12 mo for plasma concentrations of ascorbate, β-carotene, folate, vitamin B_6, and α-tocopherol. These data verify that supplementation with RDA levels of the latter micronutrients can increase their plasma concentrations in older people.

Table 2 contains the DTH data for all study subjects combined and for men and women separately. For induration in the placebo group, there were no statistically significant differences between the 0- and 6-mo results, 0- and 12-mo results, or 6- and 12-mo data. Similar results were obtained for the analyses of the data for the placebo group on the number of positive responses.

For the micronutrient supplement group, there was also no significant difference for the data on induration at 0 and 6 mo. However, there was a statistically significant difference between the 0- and 12-mo induration results ($p = .005$). There was an increase in induration between 6 and 12 mo, but this did not achieve statistical significance ($p = 0.056$). Similar trends were observed for the individual skin-test antigens.

Similar results were also obtained for the number of positive responses in the micronutrient treatment group. The mean number of positive responses in the placebo group

Table 2
Delayed Type Hypersensitivity Skin-Test Responses in Placebo and Micronutrient Groups[a]

Subgroup and response type	Placebo group			Micronutrient group		
	0 mo	6 mo	12 mo	0 mo	6 mo	12 mo
All subjects						
Positive responses	1.65 ± 0.30	1.42 ± 0.25	1.73 ± 0.29	1.45 ± 0.25^b	$1.76 \pm 0.27^{b,c}$	2.38 ± 0.33^c
Total induration (mm)	5.37 ± 1.02	4.76 ± 0.93	5.80 ± 0.95	5.21 ± 0.98^b	$5.73 \pm 0.94^{b,c}$	8.40 ± 1.25^c
Males						
Positive responses	2.93 ± 0.60	1.93 ± 0.30	2.50 ± 0.78	1.64 ± 0.33^b	$2.59 \pm 0.43^{b,c}$	2.86 ± 0.53^c
Total induration (mm)	8.86 ± 1.91	6.36 ± 1.29	8.88 ± 2.51	6.23 ± 1.15	8.85 ± 1.58	10.91 ± 2.08
Females						
Positive responses	1.18 ± 0.29	1.24 ± 0.31	1.45 ± 0.27	1.33 ± 0.36^b	$1.25 \pm 0.29^{b,c}$	2.08 ± 0.42^c
Total induration (mm)	4.08 ± 1.09	4.17 ± 1.16	4.67 ± 0.83	4.58 ± 1.41^b	3.83 ± 0.95^b	6.86 ± 1.49^c

[a]Mean ± SE; $n = 26$ for placebo group (7 men, 19 women), $n = 29$ for micronutrient group (11 men, 18 women). Positive responses are the mean number of antigens eliciting a response from a total of seven antigens. Total induration is the sum of the indurations of all positive responses. Within groups, values in the same row with different letter superscripts are significantly different, $p < 0.05$ (Wilcoxon signed-rank test).

increased by only 4.8% between 0 and 12 mo, and induration by 8.0%. In contrast, in the micronutrient supplement group, the mean number of positive responses increased by 64% and induration by 61% between 0 and 12 mo. These data provide strong evidence for DTH enhancement after 1 yr of micronutrient supplementation.

The results also suggest that some DTH response enhancement occurred sooner (at 6 mo) in the male subjects than in the females (Table 2). The male subjects had significantly greater DTH responses than the women at enrollment; this is consistent with previous data that suggest that DTH responses in men may differ from those in women (76). The diets of the male subjects differed from the females; they were higher in energy intake, as well as individual micronutrients intake, and it is possible that this factor may have interacted with micronutrient supplementation to influence DTH responses.

There was an increase between 0 and 12 mo in the number of subjects in the placebo group with low blood concentrations of some of the micronutrients measured, specifically β-carotene, retinol, folate, and vitamin B_6. This trend differed significantly from the micronutrient group, for which the number of low values changed little between 0 and 12 mo. Thus, the improvement in skin-test responses in the micronutrient group does not result from the correction of underlying micronutrient deficiencies for the 9 micronutrient concentrations that we determined in blood, at least as defined by current guidelines for low circulating concentrations. The increased number of low values in the placebo group suggests that older people who do not take vitamin supplements for 1 yr may have an increased risk of developing one or more low concentrations, particularly for vitamin B_6, folate, and β-carotene.

Our data and Chandra's data (72) suggest that immune function enhancement in older subjects by low-dose micronutrient supplementation takes approx 1 yr. These results also suggest that older people's diets are inadequate in one or more micronutrients and/or that the current RDAs for one or more micronutrients may be too low to support optimal immunity in older adults. For optimal responses, they required the RDA level of the vitamins in the supplement, as well as the levels found in their food choices.

It can be argued that a 60% increase in DTH responses during a 1-yr period is only a mean increase of approx 5% per month. However, this increase far exceeds the decline in DTH responses per year that occurs with aging and, thus, may completely prevent it. These results suggest that older subjects who take a one-a-day-type multivitamin supplement faithfully for at least 6–12 mo may experience a substantial improvement in measures of cellular immunity, such as DTH responses. It is possible that more rapid and/or larger increases in DTH responses would occur if higher doses of micronutrients were used.

More recently, Girodon et al. (77) studied the effects of trace element and vitamin supplementation on immunity and infections in institutionalized subjects aged 65 yr and older in France. Subjects ($n = 725$) received daily for 2 yr a placebo; a trace element supplement containing 20 mg zinc and 100 µg selenium; a vitamin supplement with 120 mg vitamin C, 6 mg β-carotene, and 15 mg of vitamin E; or both the vitamin and the trace element supplements. DTH responses were not significantly influenced by any treatment, but antibody responses to influenza vaccine were improved in the groups given zinc and selenium, and the incidence of respiratory tract infection was marginally lower ($p = .06$) in these groups. The vitamin and trace element supplements also reduced the prevalence of underlying deficiencies of these nutrients. Because these subjects were institutionalized and had a high frequency of low blood micronutrient concentrations, the applicability of these results to healthy independently living people is uncertain. Nevertheless, this large study provides the first evidence that selenium may be a key nutrient in immunity maintenance in older people.

3.5. Limitations of Current Knowledge

The studies mentioned that focus on the effects of multivitamins on immune functions, in combination with the short-term higher dose single nutrient studies, such as those of Meydani et al. *(62,64)*, Watson *(57)*, and Talbott et al. *(61)*, provide solid evidence that micronutrient supplements can enhance immune functions in older people, but data on effects on the incidence and prevalence of infectious diseases are limited. Despite the evidence provided by these studies, we do not know if long-term daily use of multivitamin/mineral supplements enhances immune functions and reduces the incidence and severity of infectious diseases in older people beyond the 1–2-yr duration of the longest studies done to date. This is an unfortunate gap in our knowledge, because millions of older Americans currently consume a multivitamin/mineral supplement daily, either alone or in combination with one or more single nutrients at higher doses *(78,79)*. This situation is in part the result of the limited objectives of all previously completed studies. All of the single-nutrient studies have been short-term, usually using high doses of one micronutrient, given to a relatively small number of subjects. Most of these studies have not assessed the effect of single-nutrient supplementation on the incidence of infectious diseases, a limitation related to the small number of subjects enrolled in these studies and their short duration, with a consequent lack of statistical power to assess disease incidence. The studies on multivitamin and/or trace element supplements also have limitations:

1. Chavance et al.'s study *(74)* was only 4 mo long. Although, this study assessed the effect of multivitamin supplementation on infectious diseases incidence, it did not include any measures of immune function.
2. Penn et al.'s study *(73)* was only 1 mo long and included only older people who had been hospitalized for at least 3 mo.
3. Our studies *(71,75)* assessed DTH responses, LPR to mitogens, and NK cell activity, but we could not examine other measures of immunity or clinical outcomes, and the period of supplementation was limited to 1 yr.
4. Chandra et al.'s study *(72)* was also 1 yr long, did not include dietary micronutrient assessment, did not distinguish between the incidence and duration of infectious illnesses, and assessed selected immune functions only once after initiating supplementation.
5. Girodon et al.'s 2-yr study *(77)*, although promising, included only institutionalized subjects.

Thus, additional studies of micronutrient/immunity/disease relationships are required, particularly studies that focus on clinical outcomes.

4. FACTORS THAT CAN INFLUENCE NUTRITION-IMMUNITY RELATIONSHIPS

Factors that may influence micronutrient/immunity relationships in older people include gender, stress, disease, physical activity and exercise, obesity, and food choices.

In our recent study *(75)* of the effects of low-dose micronutrient supplements on immunity in older people, improvements in DTH responses occurred sooner in the men than the women. Although the reason for this is not known, one possibility is that the higher intake of micronutrients from food in the men results in a larger total micronutrient intake. As mentioned, this effect may be a consequence of the generally greater energy and micronutrient intakes of males.

There are a considerable number of reports that psychological and physiological stress in experimental animals and people can depress cellular immune functions *(80,81)*, although it is beyond the scope of this review to assess these studies in any detail. As an example, death of a spouse has been associated with depressed immune functions *(81)*. However, virtually all studies of relationships between stress and immunity have not adequately assessed nutritional factors that may be altered by stress and, in most cases, have completely ignored nutrition. Physical and psychological stress can modify food intake in animals and people, and, thus, studies of stress/immunity relationships are usually confounded by nutritional factors that have not been adequately evaluated.

There is considerable evidence that physical activity/exercise patterns can influence immunity *(82–86)*. In general, the data suggest that strenuous exercise can acutely depress immunity. For example, various studies have found that marathon participants have a significantly increased risk of respiratory infections in the 1–2 wk period after the race *(85,86)*. Chronic overtraining has also been associated with depressed immunity *(84)*. In contrast, regular moderate exercise enhances immune functions *(84)*. One hypothesis is that regular exercise contributes to muscle mass maintenance, and muscle is the source of a key nutrient, glutamine, that is required by lymphocytes *(87)*. In addition, alterations in cytokine levels as a result of regular exercise may also be a factor *(88,89)*.

In a review, Nieman *(90)* concluded that infection risk after intensive exercise is likely related to acute nonpersistent changes in immunity. However, unless the athlete exceeds his or her usual training limits, an immunocompromised state is unlikely, although further research is needed to confirm this conclusion. In general, studies of macronutrient or micronutrient supplements in combination with exercise have shown no effects on immunity, with the exception of attenuated humoral and cellular immune responses associated with carbohydrate consumption. For example, in a randomized trial of 112 elderly (mean = 79.2 ± 5.9 yr) men and women, Paw et al. *(91)* reported that exercising twice per week improved DTH skin-test responses to recall antigens, but consumption of micronutrient enriched foods (25–100% of the RDA for various micronutrients) did not enhance the effect of exercise.

Stallone *(92)* has outlined studies that indicate that excess body weight in humans or experimental animals is associated with impairments in host defense mechanisms. Definitive studies have not been done, but there are data suggesting both beneficial and detrimental effects of weight loss on immunity. In experimental animals, it is well-known that chronically reduced energy intake without malnutrition can profoundly ameliorate the detrimental effects of aging on immunity and can increase mean and maximum life span *(93)*.

The well-established importance of some micronutrients, such as zinc, in immune function maintenance suggests that choices of foods high in these micronutrients may be beneficial, but this has not been validated in well-controlled studies.

In recognition of the evolutionary development of humans as hunter-gatherers who consumed foods but not supplements, it has been argued that appropriate food choices are sufficient to achieve optimal health, including optimal immunity. There is a substantial body of evidence that supports wise food choices, including diets high in fruit and vegetable intake and low in saturated fat, as key factors preventing some chronic diseases. However, arguments based on evolution are compromised by two factors: first, that evolution has programmed humans and other species to live through our peak reproductive years, but not necessarily beyond them, and second, that our pre-agricultural ancestors had intakes of some nutrients (e.g., calcium, iron, and zinc) much higher than those of modern humans *(94)*. Olshansky et al. *(95)* have used the term "manufactured time" to describe use of prescription drugs and other methods to increase the odds of living beyond our reproductive years. Thus, it is not surprising that micronutrient supplements may be particularly beneficial to the immune and other organ systems of older people.

Goodwin *(96)* has suggested that the relationship between depressed cellular immune function and subsequently increased mortality may result from compromised immunity being a marker for clinically latent diseases or poor overall physiologic function. However, impaired immunity may also contribute to a reduced ability to defend against infections, cancers, and, perhaps, cardiovascular heart disease.

5. RESEARCH NEEDED ON NUTRITION AND IMMUNITY IN THE ELDERLY

Several cross-sectional studies that assess relationships between micronutrient nutrition and immunity have been conducted in the past 12 yr *(49,50)*, as discussed. Generally, significant associations between serum micronutrient concentrations or use of micronutrient supplements and various measures of immunity were found in some studies but not others *(49–52)*. However, these studies compared micronutrient supplement users with nonusers but did not evaluate use of specific supplements, and it is likely that some individual or combinations of micronutrients can improve immunity, whereas others cannot.

The micronutrient supplementation and immunity clinical trials performed to date have usually involved healthy older subjects consuming their usual diets. In the case of some single-nutrient studies, subjects lived in metabolic units and consumed standardized meals that contained approximately the RDA of all essential micronutrients. It is possible that the improvements in immunity found in some studies result from correcting underlying deficiencies. However, it is also likely that micronutrient supplements enhance immunity even in the absence of underlying deficiencies, at least based on current concepts of "deficiency." This is not surprising, because optimal immune function was not a factor in establishing the current Dietary Reference Intakes or in defining laboratory normal ranges for circulating micronutrient concentrations. In fact, daily intakes that optimize immunity may differ from both the current Dietary Reference Intakes and intakes that may prevent chronic diseases. For example, the current RDA for vitamin E (15 mg α-tocopherol equivalents for adult women and men) is substantially lower than amounts that optimize immune functions or are associated in some studies with a reduced risk of cardiovascular heart disease *(64,65,97,98)*. Similarly, the current RDA for vitamin C is adequate to prevent development of scorbutic lesions but is less than the intake that could optimize immunity or provide other health benefits *(4,99)*. Recommendations for an optimal intake of any micronutrient must balance the effect of that nutrient on various health outcomes, as well as consider possible adverse effects of relatively high doses.

Future studies that focus on clinical outcomes and have considerable statistical power are especially needed. An example is the recent investigation of Graat et al. *(100)*. They conducted a randomized double-blind placebo-controlled trial in 652 Dutch men and women over age 60 yr who were given a placebo, a multivitamin/mineral supplement, 200 mg of vitamin E as α-tocopherol, or both supplements. The multivitamin/mineral supplement included 24 essential micronutrients and 1 possibly essential trace element–silicon. The primary outcome measures were the incidence and severity of acute respiratory tract infections. The mean duration of participation was 441 d, and the percentage of subjects who complied with the protocol was 84%. The incidence of acute respiratory tract infections did not differ significantly among treatment groups. Surprisingly, infection severity, measured as duration of infection, restriction of activities, number of symptoms, and presence of fever, was increased significantly ($p = .03$ to .009) in the groups ingesting vitamin E supplements. This study focused on a clinical outcome but did not include laboratory evaluation of immunity. Thus, immune system assays that might explain the study results were not available. Only 0.2% of study subjects had low plasma α-tocopherol concentrations at enrollment, and this may have precluded a beneficial effect of vitamin E supplements. The adverse effects on infection severity may result from the long duration of high-dose supplementation in a cohort with normal plasma α-tocopherol concentrations at enrollment and is consistent with previously cited *(59,60)* studies on β-carotene that demonstrate adverse effects after long-term high-dose supplementation. The results of this study are discussed further in Chapter 8 on vitamin E. These studies suggest caution in the long-term use of high-dose single micronutrients.

There is considerable evidence that patterns of physical activity and exercise can influence immunity both acutely and chronically, but few studies have addressed interactions among physical activity, immunity, and micronutrient nutrition.

It should be emphasized that the potential of micronutrient supplements to improve immunity or exert other beneficial effects must be considered in relation to their consumption from food. This is especially true for low- to moderate-dose supplements, for which the intake from food and supplements may be similar. Clearly, supplement use should be encouraged in conjunction with a sound diet that emphasizes fruits, vegetables, whole grains, and other sources of micronutrients and limits saturated fat intake. However, it is likely that beneficial intakes of some nutrients, such as vitamin E, may not be possible from a relatively low-fat diet in the absence of supplement use.

The promising but variable results of studies conducted to date suggest continued research on nutrition and immunity in older people. Such efforts should include:

1. A focus on long-term placebo-controlled double-blind clinical trials and prospective epidemiologic studies that have sufficient statistical power.
2. Study of interactions among physical activity/exercise patterns, immunity, and nutrition.
3. Evaluation of effects of nutrition on both humoral (e.g., antibody responses to vaccination) and cellular (e.g., DTH responses) immunity using clinically relevant assays and on clinical outcomes, e.g., infectious disease incidence, duration, and severity.

4. Evaluation of dietary modification alone or in combination with low doses of supplemental micronutrients. Studies of older people consuming their usual diets are also needed.
5. Long-term studies that address the persistence of the effects of micronutrients on immunity both during and after micronutrient supplementation.
6. Use of appropriate inclusion and exclusion criteria in identifying subjects for study.
7. Study of both single micronutrients and multivitamin/minerals, with a focus on the antioxidant micronutrients and other widely used single or multiple micronutrient supplements.
8. Identification of host-specific factors (e.g., gender and age range) that influence micronutrient/immunity interactions and the basis for these effects.
9. Identification of the molecular mechanisms and genes that determine the effects of micronutrients on immunity. This will become increasingly important when new genes that influence aging are identified.

Nearly 100 million Americans (approx 40% of the population) take multivitamin/ mineral supplements, either alone or in combination with higher doses of the antioxidant vitamins *(78,79)*. Well-designed studies that assess the health effects of this practice are urgently needed and should include evaluation of effects on the immune system.

6. RECOMMENDATIONS

Physicians and other health care providers should advise their patients to eat diets low in saturated fat and high in fruits and vegetables. This can ensure consumption of significant quantities of the micronutrients (and other phytochemicals) that can favorably affect immunity. In addition, older subjects, especially those with poor diets, should be encouraged to take a low-dose multivitamin/mineral supplement. Higher daily doses of the antioxidant micronutrients vitamin C (200–500 mg) and vitamin E (200–400 IU) may also be appropriate for some, but not all, older people. Taking high supplemental doses of other micronutrients that can adversely affect immunity, for example, zinc should be persuasively discouraged. High doses of supplemental β-carotene are not recommended for current and former smokers because of their association with the development of lung cancer and also are unwise for other people as recently stated by the US Preventive Services Task Force *(101)*.

The favorable effects of regular exercise on immunity should also be mentioned to patients. Most of this advice (low-fat diet, high fruit and vegetable intake, regular exercise, and supplemental vitamins) not only may promote optimal immunity but also is likely to reduce the risk of cardiovascular heart disease and some cancers.

In a widely publicized article, Fairfield and Fletcher *(102)* recently reviewed the health effects of vitamin supplements and concluded that "all adults (should) take one multivitamin daily." They base this recommendation on beneficial health effects other than effects on immunity. The likely effect on immunity in older people is an additional benefit that further supports this recommendation.

7. "TAKE-HOME" MESSAGES

We still have much to learn about the effects of nutrition on immunity. Nevertheless, the results of studies done to date suggest that:

1. Placebo-controlled clinical trials, despite their limitations, are the best approach for studying effects of micronutrients on immunity;
2. high doses of some single nutrients may improve immunity in relatively short-time periods—weeks to months—but persistence of these effects is not currently known. High doses of other micronutrients may adversely affect immunity;
3. some micronutrients may interfere with the beneficial effects of other micronutrients on immunity; this effect depends on relative doses;
4. low- to moderate-dose multivitamin/mineral supplements may require considerable time (6 mo to 1 yr or more) before they enhance immune functions and reduce susceptibility to infectious diseases, and the timing of their effects may differ in men and women;
5. high- and even low-dose micronutrient supplements may enhance immunity, even in the absence of evidence of underlying deficiencies;
6. micronutrient supplements are not a substitute for a good diet and regular exercise but rather are a complementary measure; and
7. long-term ingestion of single-nutrient supplements, especially at high doses, may have beneficial and/or adverse effects on immunity and other outcomes.

REFERENCES

1. Bogden JD, Louria DB. Micronutrients and immunity in older people. In: Bendich A, Deckelbaum RJ (eds.). Preventive Nutrition: The Comprehensive Guide for Health Professionals (2nd ed.). Humana Press, Totowa, NJ, 2001, pp. 307–327.
2. Warner HR, Butler RN, Sprott RL, Schneider EL. Modern Biological Theories of Aging. Raven Press, New York, 1987.
3. Bendich A. Antioxidant micronutrients and immune responses. Ann NY Acad Sci 1990;587:168–180.
4. Lesourd B, Mazari L. Nutrition and immunity in the elderly. Proc Nutr Soc 1999;58:685— 695.
5. Ben-Yehuda A, Weksler ME. Immune senescence: mechanisms and clinical implications. Cancer Invest 1992;10:525–531.
6. Makinodan T. Patterns of age-related immunologic changes. Nutr Rev 1995;53:S27–S34.
7. Effros RB, Walford RL. Infection and immunity in relation to aging. In: Goidl EA (ed.). Aging and the Immune Response. Marcel-Dekker, New York, 1987, pp. 45–65.
8. Bogden JD, Oleske JM, Munves EM, et al. Zinc and immunocompetence in the elderly: baseline data on zinc nutriture and immunity in unsupplemented subjects. Am J Clin Nutr 1987;45:101–109.
9. Kuvibidilia S, Yu L, Ode D, Warrier RP. The immune response in protein-energy malnutrition and single nutrient deficiencies. In: Klurfeld DM (ed.). Nutrition and Immunology. Plenum Press, New York, 1993, pp. 121–155.
10. Abbas AK, Lichtman AH, Pober JS. Cellular and Molecular Immunology. WB Saunders, Philadelphia, 1994, pp. 166–186.
11. Aronson M. Involution of the thymus revisited: immunological trade-offs as an adaptation to aging. Mech Ageing Dev 1993;72:49–55.
12. Siskind GW. Aging and the immune system. In: Warner HR, Butler RN, Sprott RL, Schneider EL (eds.). Modern Biological Theories of Aging. Raven Press, New York, 1987, pp. 235–242.
13. Makinodan T, Kay MB. Age influence on the immune system. Adv Immunol 1980;29:287–330.
14. Weksler ME. The senescence of the immune system. Hosp Prac 1981:53–64.
15. McMurray DN. Cell-mediated immunity in nutritional deficiency. Prog Food Nutr Sci 1984;8:193–228.
16. Schwab R, Weksler ME. Cell biology of the impaired proliferation of T cells from elderly humans. In: Goidl EA (ed.). Aging and the Immune Response. Marcel Dekker, New York, 1987, pp. 67–80.
17. James SJ, Makinodan T. Nutritional intervention during immunologic aging: past and present. In: Armbrecht HJ, Prendergast JM, Coe RM (eds.). Nutritional Intervention in the Aging Process. Springer-Verlag, New York, 1984, pp. 209–227.
18. Meakins JL, Pietsch JB, Bubenick O, et al. Delayed hypersensitivity: indicator of acquired failure of host defenses in sepsis and trauma. Ann Surg 1977;186:241–250.

19. Christou NV, Tellado-Rodriguez J, Chartrand L, et al. Estimating mortality risk in preoperative patients using immunologic, nutritional, and acute-phase response variables. Ann Surg 1989;210:69–77.

20. Wayne SJ, Rhyne RL, Garry PJ, Goodwin JS. Cell-mediated immunity as a predictor of morbidity and mortality in subjects over 60. J Gerontol 1990;45:M45–M48.

21. Roberts-Thomson IC, Whittingham S, Youngchaiyud U, McKay IR. Aging, immune response, and mortality. Lancet 1974;2:368–370.

22. Hicks MJ, Jones JF, Thies AC, Weigle KA, Minnich LL. Age-related changes in mitogen-induced lymphocyte function from birth to old age. Am J Clin Pathol 1983;80:159–163.

23. Murasko DM, Nelson BJ, Silver R, Matour D, Kaye D. Immunologic response in an elderly population with a mean age of 85. Am J Med 1986;81:612–618.

24. Markewitz A, Faist E, Lang S, et al. Successful restoration of cell-mediated immune response after cardiopulmonary bypass by immunomodulation. J Thorac Cardiovasc Surg 1993;105:15–24.

25. Higa K, Noda B, Manabe H, Sato S, Dan K. T-lymphocyte subsets in otherwise healthy patients with herpes zoster and relationships to the duration of acute herpetic pain. Pain 1992;51:111–118.

26. Stites DP. Clinical laboratory methods for detection of cellular immunity. In: Stites DP, Terr AI (eds.). Basic and Clinical Immunology (7th ed.). Appleton & Lange, Norwalk, CT, 1991, pp. 263–283.

27. Giorgi JV. Lymphocyte subset measurements: significance in clinical medicine. In: Rose NR, Friedman H, Fahey JL (eds.). Manual of Clinical Laboratory Immunology (3rd ed.). American Society for Microbiology, Washington, DC, 1986, pp. 236–246.

28. Sen P, Middleton JR, Perez G, et al. Host defense abnormalities and infection in older persons. Infect Med 1994;11:364–370.

29. Perskin MH, Cornstein BN. Age-related changes in neutrophil structure and function. Mech Ageing Dev 1992;64:303–313.

30. Nagel JE, Han K, Coon PJ, Adler WH, Bender BS. Age differences in phagocytosis by polymorphonuclear leukocytes measured by flow cytometry. J Leukoc Biol 1986;39:399–407.

31. Shoham-Kessary H, Gershon H. Impaired reactivity to inflammatory stimuli of neutrophils from elderly donors. Aging Immunol Infect Dis 1992;3:169–183.

32. Corberand J, Ngyen F, Laharrague P, et al. Polymorphonuclear functions and aging in humans. J Am Geriatr Soc 1981;29:391–397.

33. Makinodan T, Lubinski J, Fong TC. Cellular, biochemical, and molecular basis of T-cell senescence. Arch Pathol Lab Med 1987;111:910–914.

34. Rubin LA, Nelson DL. The soluble interleukin-2 receptor: biology, function, and clinical application. Ann Intern Med 1990;113:619–627.

35. Manoussakis MN, Papadopoulos GK, Drosos AA, Moutsopoulos HM. Soluble interleukin-2 receptor molecules in the serum of patients with autoimmune diseases. Clin Immunol Immunopathol 1989;50:321–332.

36. Lahat N, Shtiller R, Zlotnick AY, Merin G. Early IL-2/sIL-2R surge following surgery leads to temporary immune refractoriness. Clin Exp Immunol 1993;92:482–486.

37. Bogden JD, Kemp FW, Liberatore BL, et al. Serum interleukin-2 receptor concentrations, physical activity, and micronutrient nutrition in older people. J Cell Biochem 1993;17B:86.

38. Sansoni P, Brianti V, Fagnoni F. NK cell activity and T-lymphocyte proliferation in healthy centenarians. Ann NY Acad Sci 1992;663:505–507.

39. Mariotti S, Sansoni P, Barbesino G, et al. Thyroid and other organ-specific autoantibodies in healthy centenarians. Lancet 1992;339:1506–1508.

40. Scrimshaw NS, SanGiovanni JP. Synergism of nutrition, infection, and immunity: an overview. Am J Clin Nutr 1997;66:464S–477S.

41. Fraker P. Nutritional immunology: methodological considerations. J Nutr Immunol 1994;2:87–92.

42. Chandra RK. Nutrition and immunity. Contemp Nutrition 1986;11:1–4.

43. Chandra RK. Immunodeficiency in undernutrition and overnutrition. Nutr Rev 1981;39:225–231.

44. McMurray DN, Loomis SA, Casazza LJ, Rey H, Miranda R. Development of impaired cell-mediated immunity in mild and moderate malnutrition. Am J Clin Nutr 1981;34:68–77.

45. Dowd PS, Heatley RV. The influence of undernutrition on immunity. Clin Sci 1984;66:241–248.

46. Beisel WR. Single nutrients and immunity. Am J Clin Nutr 1982;35:417–468.
47. Beisel WR. Nutrition and infection. In: Linder MC (ed.). Nutritional Biochemistry and Metabolism. Elsevier, New York, 1985, pp. 369–394.
48. Bogden JD, Kemp FW, Han S, et al. Status of selected nutrients and progression of human immunodeficiency virus type 1 infection. Am J Clin Nutr 2000;72:809–815.
49. Goodwin JS, Garry PJ. Relationships between megadose vitamin supplementation and immunological function in a healthy elderly population. Clin Exp Immunol 1983;51:647–653.
50. Goodwin JS, Garry PJ. Lack of correlation between indices of nutritional status and immunologic function in elderly humans. J Gerontol 1988;43:M46–M49.
51. Kawakami K, Kadota J, Iida K, et al. Reduced immune function and malnutrition in the elderly. Tohoku J Exper Med 1999;187:157–171.
52. Kemp FW, DeCandia J, Li W, et al. Relationships between immunity and dietary and serum antioxidants, B vitamins, and homocysteine in elderly men and women. Nutr Res 2002;22:45–53.
53. Jacob RA, Kelley DS, Pianalto FS, et al. Immunocompetence and oxidant defense during ascorbate depletion of healthy men. Am J Clin Nutr 1991;54:1302S–1309S.
54. Fuller CJ, Faulkner H, Bendich A, Parker RS, Roe DA. Effect of beta-carotene supplementation on photosuppression of delayed-type hypersensitivity in normal young men. Am J Clin Nutr 1992;56: 684–690.
55. Herraiz L, Rahman A, Paker R, Roe D. The role of beta-carotene supplementation in prevention of photosuppression of cellular immunity in elderly men. FASEB J 1994;8:A423.
56. Herraiz LA, Hsieh WC, Parker RS, et al. Effect of UV exposure and b-carotene supplementation on delayed-type hypersensitivity response in healthy older men. J Am Coll Nutr 1998;17:617–624.
57. Watson RR, Prabhala RH, Plezia PM, Alberts DS. Effect of beta-carotene on lymphocyte subpopulations in elderly humans: evidence for a dose-response relationship. Am J Clin Nutr 1991;53:90–94.
58. Santos MS, Meydani SN, Leka L, et al. Natural killer cell activity in elderly men is enhanced by β-carotene supplementation. Am J Clin Nutr 1996;64:772–777.
59. Omenn GS, Goodman GE, Thornquist MD, et al. Risk factors for lung cancer and for intervention effects in CARET, the Beta-Carotene and Retinol Efficacy Trial. J Natl Cancer Instit 1996;88:1550–1559.
60. Albanes D, Heinonen OP, Taylor PR, et al. Alpha-tocopherol and beta-carotene supplements and lung cancer incidence in the alpha-tocopherol, beta-carotene cancer prevention study: effects of baseline characteristics and study compliance. J Natl Cancer Inst 1996;88:1560–1570.
61. Talbott MC, Miller LT, Kerkvliet NI. Pyridoxine supplementation: effect on lymphocyte responses in elderly persons. Am J Clin Nutr 1987;46:659–664.
62. Meydani SN, Ribaya-Mercado JD, Russell RN, et al. Vitamin B-6 deficiency impairs interleukin 2 production and lymphocyte proliferation in elderly adults. Am J Clin Nutr 1991;53:1275–1280.
63. Rall LC, Meydani SN. Vitamin B6 and immune competence. Nutr Rev 1993;51:217–225.
64. Meydani SN, Meydani M, Blumberg JB, et al. Vitamin E supplementation and the in vivo immune response in healthy elderly subjects. JAMA 1997;277:1380–1386.
65. Pallast EG, Schouten EG, de Waart FG, et al. Effect of 50- and 100-mg vitamin E supplements on cellular immune function in noninstitutionalized elderly persons. Am J Clin Nutr 1999;69:1273–1281.
66. Oleske JM, Westphal ML, Shore S, et al. Correction with zinc therapy of depressed cellular immunity in acrodermatitis enteropathica. Am J Dis Child 1979;133:915–918.
67. Fraker PJ, Gershwin ME, Good RA, Prasad A. Interrelationships between zinc and immune function. Fed Proc 1986;45:1474–1479.
68. Bogden JD, Oleske JM, Lavenhar MA, et al. Zinc and immunocompetence in elderly people: effects of zinc supplementation for 3 months. Am J Clin Nutr 1988;48:655–663.
69. Chandra RK, Hambreaus L, Puri S, Au B, Kutty KM. Immune responses of healthy volunteers given supplements of zinc or selenium. FASEB J 1993;7:A723.
70. Doherty CP, Kashein MA, Shakur MS, et al. Zinc and rehabilitation from severe protein-energy malnutrition: higher-dose regimens are associated with increased mortality. Am J Clin Nutr 1998; 68:742–748.
71. Bogden JD, Oleske JM, Lavenhar MA, et al. Effects of one year of supplementation with zinc and other micronutrients on cellular immunity in the elderly. J Am College Nutr 1990;9:214–225.

72. Chandra RK. Effect of vitamin and trace-element supplementation on immune responses and infection in elderly subjects. Lancet 1992;340:1124–1127.

73. Penn ND, Purkins L, Kelleher J, et al. The effect of dietary supplementation with vitamins A, C, and E on cell-mediated immune function in elderly long-stay patients: a randomized controlled trial. Age Ageing 1991;20:169–174.

74. Chavance M, Herbeth B, Lemoine A, Zhu BP. Does multivitamin supplementation prevent infections in healthy elderly subjects? A controlled trial. Intl J Vit Nutr Res 1993;63:11–16.

75. Bogden JD, Bendich A, Kemp FW, et al. Daily micronutrient supplements enhance delayed-hypersensitivity skin test responses in older people. Am J Clin Nutr 1994;60:437–447.

76. Kniker WT, Anderson CT, McBryde JL, Roumiantzeff M, Lesourd B. Multitest CMI for standardized measurement of delayed cutaneous hypersensitivity and cell-mediated immunity. Normal values and proposed scoring system for healthy adults in the USA. Ann Allergy 1984;52:75–82.

77. Girodon F, Galan P, Monget AL, et al. Impact of trace elements and vitamin supplementation on immunity and infections in institutionalized elderly patients. Arch Intern Med 1999;159:748–754.

78. Park YK, Kim I, Yetley EA. Characteristics of vitamin and mineral supplement products in the United States. Am J Clin Nutr 1991;54:750–759.

79. Block G, Cox C, Madans J, et al. Vitamin supplement use, by demographic characteristics. Am J Epidemiol 1988;127:297–309.

80. Cooper EL. Stress, Immunity, and Aging. Marcel-Dekker, New York, 1984.

81. Solomon GF. Emotions, immunity, and disease. In: Copper EL (ed.). Stress, Immunity and Aging. Marcel Dekker, New York, 1984, pp. 1–10.

82. Watson RR, Eisinger M. Exercise and Disease. CRC, Boca Raton, FL, 1992, pp. 71–178.

83. Keast D, Cameron K, Morton AR. Exercise and the immune response. Sports Med 1988;5:248–267.

84. Fry RW, Morton AR, Keast D. Overtraining in athletes. Sports Med 1991;12:32–65.

85. Nieman DC, Johanssen LM, Lee JW, Arabatzis K. Infectious episodes in runners before and after the Los Angeles marathon. J Sports Med Phys Fitness 1990;30:316–328.

86. Peters EM, Bateman ED. Ultramarathon running and upper respiratory tract infections. S Africa Med J 1983;64:582–584.

87. Barry-Billings M, Blomstrand E, McAndrew N, Newsholme EA. A communication link between skeletal muscle, brain, and cells of the immune system. Int J Sports Med 1990;11:S122–S128.

88. Rubenoff R, Rall LC. Humoral mediation of changing body composition during aging and chronic inflammation. Nutr Rev 1993;51:1–11.

89. Meydani S. Dietary modulation of cytokine production and biologic functions. Nutr Rev 1990;48: 361–368.

90. Nieman DC. Exercise immunology: future directions for research related to athletics, nutrition, and the elderly. Int J Sports Med 2000;21(Suppl 1):S61–S68.

91. Paw MJ, deJong N, Pallast EG, et al. Immunity in frail elderly: a randomized controlled trial of exercise and enriched foods. Med Sci Sports Exer 2000;32:2005–2011.

92. Stallone DD. The influence of obesity and its treatment on the immune system. Nutr Rev 1994;52: 37–50.

93. Spear-Hartley A, Sherman AR. Food restriction and the immune system. J Nutr Immunol 1994;3: 27–50.

94. Eaton SB, Eaton SB III, Konner MJ, Shostak M. An evolutionary perspective enhances understanding of human nutritional requirements. J Nutr 1996;126:1732–1740.

95. Olshansky SJ, Carnes BA, Grahn D. Confronting the boundaries of human longevity. Am Scientist 1998;86:52–61.

96. Goodwin JS. Decreased immunity and increased morbidity in the elderly. Nutr Rev 1995;53:S41–S46.

97. Rimm EB, Stampfer MJ, Ascherio A, et al. Vitamin E consumption and the risk of coronary heart disease in men. N Engl J Med 1993;328:1450–1456.

98. Stampfer MJ, Hennekens CB, Manson JE, et al. Vitamin E consumption and the risk of coronary disease in women. N Engl J Med 1993;328:1444–1449.

99. Bendich A, Langseth L. Health effects of vitamin C supplementation: a review. J Am Coll Nutr 1995; 14:124–136.

100. Graat JM, Sohouten EG, Kok FJ. Effect of daily vitamin E and multivitamin-mineral supplementation on acute respiratory tract infections in elderly persons. JAMA 2002;288:715–721.
101. US Preventive Services Task Force. Routine vitamin supplementation to prevent cancer and cardiovascular disease: recommendations and rationale. Ann Intern Med 2003;139:51–55.
102. Fairfield KM, Fletcher RH. Vitamins for chronic disease prevention in adults. JAMA 2002;287: 3116–3129.

II VITAMINS AND IMMUNE RESPONSES

6 Vitamin A

Richard D. Semba

1. INTRODUCTION

Vitamin A deficiency is one of the leading causes of immunodeficiency among infants, children, and women worldwide. The consequences of vitamin A deficiency include higher morbidity and mortality from many infectious diseases. In developing countries, an estimated 253 million children are at risk for vitamin A deficiency *(1)* and an estimated 6 million women have clinical manifestations of vitamin A deficiency during pregnancy *(2)*. Vitamin A deficiency also causes night blindness, xerophthalmia, growth retardation, impaired reproductive capacity, and anemia, and it permanently blinds an estimated 350,000 children worldwide each year *(3)*. The constellation of adverse health problems ascribed to vitamin A deficiency has been termed the vitamin A deficiency disorders (VADD) *(4)*. Among all the micronutrients, the role of vitamin A in immune function has probably been the most extensively characterized, and these studies show a multifaceted role of vitamin A in many functional aspects of immunity. Vitamin A plays a role in the maintenance of mucosal surfaces, the generation of antibody responses, normal hematopoiesis, and the function of T and B lymphocytes, natural killer (NK) cells, monocyte/ macrophages, and neutrophils. The essential nature of vitamin A to different aspects of immune function is likely attributed to the action of vitamin A and related metabolites as modulators of gene transcription on the molecular level. The purpose of this chapter is to provide a current overview of the role that vitamin A plays in immune function and resistance to infectious diseases and to highlight knowledge gaps and future areas for investigation. Other aspects of vitamin A deficiency have recently been covered elsewhere in a comprehensive monograph *(4)*.

2. HISTORICAL PERSPECTIVE

2.1. The Characterization of Vitamin A

The idea that vitamin A reduces morbidity and mortality was established as early as the mid-nineteenth century. Physicians at the Brompton Hospital in London found that cod-liver oil could reduce mortality in patients with tuberculosis *(5)*. The active agent in cod-liver oil was not known at the time, but it was widely concluded from empiric use that cod-liver oil was effective. Vitamin A's existence can be seen in a period that spans more than 130 yr. François Magendie found that dogs raised on sugar and water alone

From: *Diet and Human Immune Function*
Edited by: D. A. Hughes, L. G. Darlington, and A. Bendich © Humana Press Inc., Totowa, NJ

Table 1
Early Landmark Animal Studies Relating Vitamin A to Immunity and Survival

Date	Observation	Reference
1816	Dogs fed sugar and water developed corneal ulcers and died	(6)
1881	Mice fed purified fat, protein, carbohydrate, and mineral salts died but survived if milk was added to diet	(7)
1891	Mice fed purified fat, protein, carbohydrate, and mineral salts died but survived if egg yolk was added to diet	(8)
1905	Mice fed purified basal diet could survive if milk was added to diet	(9)
1909–1911	Lipid substances present in milk and soluble in alcohol-ether were essential to support the growth and survival of mice	(11)
1909	Rats fed purified diet developed corneal ulcers and died	(20)
1912	Mice fed purified basal diet survived if milk was added to diet	(10)
1913	Lipid substances present in butter fat and soluble in ether were essential to support the growth and survival of rats	(13)
1913	Butter fat alleviates infections in nutritionally deprived animals	(15)
1928	Vitamin A-deficient rats show extensive evidence of infections	(21)
1930	Vitamin A-deficient rats more susceptible to experimental infection with paratyphoid bacteria	(22)

developed corneal ulcers and died *(6)*. Nicolai Lunin and C. A. Socin at the University of Dorpat showed that mice could not survive on purified protein, fat, carbohydrate, and mineral salts alone but were able to survive if supplemented with milk or egg yolk *(7,8)*. Cornelis Pekelharing and Frederick Hopkins both conducted studies that also suggested there was something essential in milk that supported life *(9,10)*. Wilhelm Stepp extracted lipids from milk with alcohol-ether that contained the active substance *(11,12)*, and Elmer McCollum and Marguerite Davis, working at the University of Wisconsin, used ether to extract these lipids from cod-liver oil *(13)*. At Yale University, Thomas Osborne and Lafayette Mendel made the seminal observation that infectious diseases in vitamin A-deficient animals were quickly alleviated by introduction of butterfat in the diet *(14,15)*. In 1916, this growth-promoting and antiinfectious substance was termed "fat-soluble A" *(16)*. The structure of vitamin A was deduced in 1931 by Paul Karrer *(17,18)*, and vitamin A was crystallized in 1937 *(19)*. During many of these studies, it was commonly observed that the growth and survival of animals was linked to vitamin A in the diet, findings that paved the way for investigations of vitamin A's effects on immunity and survival in humans (*see* Table 1) *(6–11,13,20–22)*.

2.2. Early Work on Vitamin A, Immunity, and Mortality

Vitamin A was long suspected to be an essential factor in lymphoid system development and for the maintenance of mucosal surfaces of the gastrointestinal (GI), respiratory, and genitourinary tracts *(23,24)*. By the 1920s, high childhood morbidity and mortality in Europe and the United States—comparable to those found in many developing countries today—were ascribed by many investigators and clinicians to vitamin A deficiency. Carl Edvard Bloch, a pediatrician in Copenhagen, clearly attributed the increased susceptibility to infection and mortality in infants and young children to lack of vitamin A, and he advocated the use of milk, cream, and butter for children to reduce their infections (25,26). Based upon the observations in Denmark and animal studies, Erik Widmark concluded in 1924 that "there must be in a population in which xerophthalmia occurs a much larger number of cases in which the deficiency in vitamin A, without producing the eye disease, is the cause of a diminished resistance to infections, of general debility, and of malnutrition" (27). A state of subclinical vitamin A deficiency was acknowledged as "the borderline between health and disease," where a child would appear healthy but, when faced with an infection, would do less well because of an underlying vitamin deficiency *(28)*. The emphasis shifted from treating children with xerophthalmia only to improving vitamin A status of children in populations.

Vitamin A became known as the "anti-infective" vitamin and, from 1920 to 1940, underwent considerable evaluation in at least 30 therapeutic trials, from dental caries to pneumonia to measles. These studies were conducted during a period when there was an increased awareness of the infant and child mortality problem in Europe and the United States *(29,30)*. In the first 50 yr of the twentieth century, public health efforts focused on eradicating vitamin A deficiency because of its known association with reduced resistance to infection. Major health organizations, including the League of Nations Health Committee, the Women's Foundation for Health, the Council of British Societies for Relief Abroad, and the Medical Research Council of Great Britain, emphasized the importance of ensuring adequate vitamin A intake to reduce morbidity and mortality from infectious diseases *(31)*. These concerns were reflected in the widespread use of cod-liver oil for children, institution of milk programs in schools, fortification of milk with vitamin A, and promotion of home gardening. With improvements in hygiene, nutrition, and socioeconomic standards, vitamin A deficiency largely disappeared from Europe and the United States, and, after World War II, more attention was paid to combating vitamin A deficiency in developing countries *(29,31)*.

3. BIOCHEMISTRY AND METABOLISM OF VITAMIN A

3.1. Dietary Sources and Metabolism of Vitamin A

Vitamin A is available in dietary sources as either preformed vitamin A or provitamin A carotenoids. Rich dietary sources of preformed vitamin A include egg yolk, liver, butter, cheese, whole milk, and cod-liver oil. In many developing countries, the consumption of foods containing preformed vitamin A is limited and provitamin A carotenoids often comprise the major dietary source of vitamin A *(32)*. The major provitamin A carotenoids consist of α-carotene and β-carotene, found in foods such as dark-green leafy vegetables, carrots, sweet potatoes, mangoes, and papayas, and β-cryptoxanthin, found in foods, such as oranges and tangerines. Recent studies show that the bioavailability of provitamin A carotenoids is probably lower than previously believed *(33,34)*.

Digested foods that contain preformed vitamin A are emulsified with bile salts and lipids in the small intestine. Retinol is esterified in the intestinal mucosa, packaged into chylomicra, and carried to the liver via the lymphatic circulation. Provitamin A carotenoids, such as β-carotene, may be converted to retinaldehyde through cleavage by carotenoid-15,15'-dioxygenase or by an asymmetric cleavage pathway. The bioavailability of provitamin A carotenoids is less than preformed vitamin A because of several factors, including differences in efficacy of absorption and biochemical conversion *(33,34)*. Approximately 90% of the body's vitamin A is stored in the liver as retinyl esters, and the liver has the capacity to store enough vitamin A to last for several months, with a longer storage capacity in adults than children. Retinol is released from the liver in combination with plasma retinol-binding protein (RBP) and transthyretin (TTR). Retinol is poorly soluble in water and is carried in the blood sequestered inside the carrier proteins, RBP and TTR. Retinol enters cells via specific receptors, although it is unclear whether all cells contain these receptors.

3.2. Retinoic Acid Receptors and Gene Regulation

Vitamin A exerts its effects via retinoic acid and retinoid receptors, which are found in the nucleus of the cell. Retinol is converted to all-*trans*-retinoic acid and 9-*cis* retinoic acid in the cytoplasm. Retinoic acid influences gene activation through specific receptors, which belong to the superfamily of thyroid and steroid receptors *(35)*. Retinoic acid receptors (RARs) act as transcriptional activators for many specific target genes. The RAR is expressed as isoforms, referred to as RAR α, β, and γ, and retinoid X receptor (RXR) is also expressed as isoforms, referred to as RXR α, β, and γ *(36)*. All-*trans* retinoic acid is a ligand for RARs, whereas 9-*cis* retinoic acid is a ligand for both RARs and RXRs. 9-*cis*-retinoic acid is functionally distinct from all-*trans*-retinoic acid, and interconversion may exist between the two isomers. Each RAR and RXR has a specific DNA-binding domain by which these nuclear receptors may effect transcriptional activity.

The DNA sequences that interact with RAR and RXR are known as retinoic acid response elements (RAREs). RAR and RXR receptors form heterodimers, which bind to DNA and control gene expression. In addition, RXR receptors also can form heterodimers with the thyroid hormone receptor, vitamin D_3 receptor, peroxisome proliferator-activated receptors, and several newly described "orphan receptors." Most RAREs occur in the regulatory region of genes. In the presence of 9-*cis* retinoic acid, RXR/RXR homodimers may form and recognize a subset of RAREs or inhibit the formation of certain heterodimers. Orphan receptors, such as chicken ovalbumin upstream promoter transcription factor (COUP-TF) *(37)*, apolipoprotein AI regulatory protein 1 (ARP-1), transforming growth factor-beta-activating kinase 1 (TAK1) *(38)*, retinoid V receptor (RVR) *(39)*, retinoid Z receptor (RZR) *(40)*, and thymus orphan receptor (TOR) *(41)*, may repress or modulate the induction of genes by retinoic acid. The three-dimensional structure of several different DNA-binding RXR complexes have recently been elucidated *(42–44)*. RARs and RXRs may interact with multiple transcriptional mediators and/or corepressors, adding an enormous level of complexity to retinoic acid response regulation. Other vitamin A metabolites in the retroretinoid family may support biologic functions via a pathway that is distinct from the retinoic acid pathway. 14-hydroxy-4,14-*retro* retinol supports cell growth, whereas anhydroretinol inhibits cell growth *(45,46)*. In addition, the oxoretinoids may play a role as retinoic acid receptor ligands *(47)*. Recently described nuclear receptor-associated proteins, such as SMRT/N-CoR, Sin3, and histone deacetylases (HDAC-1 and 2) and histone acetylases (CBP/p300 and P/CAF), function as transcription corepressors and coactivators. A binary paradigm has emerged as an attempt to explain how these proteins work. Unligated receptors bind to response elements of target genes and repress transcription through recruitment of a repressor complex containing corepressors. Ligand binding causes the dissociation of corepressor proteins and promotes the association of coactivators with liganded receptors. The formation of these regulatory complexes may prove to be critical in determining which signaling pathway is followed at a given time *(48)*.

Table 2
Effects of Vitamin A Deficiency on Immune Function

Abnormal expression of keratins and mucins in the respiratory tract, genitourinary tract, and
    ocular surface
Loss of cilia from respiratory epithelium
Loss of microvilli from small intestine
Decrease in goblet cells and mucin production in mucosal epithelia
Impaired neutrophil function
Impaired natural killer (NK) cell function and decreased number of NK cells
Impaired aspects of hematopoiesis
Shift toward Th1-like immune responses
Decrease in number and function of B lymphocytes
Impaired antibody responses to T cell-dependent and T cell-independent type 2 antigens

---

4. ROLE OF VITAMIN A IN IMMUNE FUNCTION

Vitamin A modulates many different aspects of immune function, both nonspecific (innate) immunity, i.e., maintenance of mucosal surfaces, NK cell activity, phagocytosis, and specific (adaptive) immunity, i.e., generation of antibody responses. Some aspects of immunity are not affected by vitamin A deficiency. Much of our knowledge of vitamin A and immune function is based on experimental animal studies involving mice, rats, and chickens, and from in vitro studies involving modulation of specific cell lines with retinoids. The effects of vitamin A deficiency on immune function are summarized in Table 2.

4.1. Mucosal Immunity

The mucosal surfaces of the body include the respiratory, GI, and genitourinary tracts, as well as the cornea and conjunctiva. There are at least seven known mechanisms by which vitamin A deficiency impairs mucosal immunity: (1) loss of cilia in the respiratory tract; (2) loss of microvilli in the GI tract; (3) loss of mucin and goblet cells in the respiratory, GI, and genitourinary tracts; (4) squamous metaplasia with abnormal keratinization in the respiratory tract; (5) alterations in antigen-specific secretory immunoglobulin (Ig) A concentrations; (6) impairment of alveolar monocyte/macrophage function; and (7) decreased gut integrity. In early vitamin A deficiency autopsy studies of humans and experimental animals, the findings included widespread pathologic alterations in the respiratory, GI, and genitourinary tracts (49–51). In vitamin A deficiency, there is loss of mucin and goblet cells from the conjunctiva and squamous metaplasia of the conjunctiva and cornea (52,53) and impaired wound healing (54). Vitamin A is involved in the expression of both mucins (55,56) and keratins (57–59). Lactoferrin, an iron-binding glycoprotein involved in immunity to bacteria, viruses, and fungi, is modulated in the tear film of children by vitamin A supplementation (60). Loss of mucin and alterations in keratins in vitamin A deficiency may increase susceptibility to experimental ocular infection with pathogens such as *Herpes simplex* virus (61) and *Pseudomonas* (62,63). Other corneal alterations in experimental vitamin A deficiency include high levels of interleukin (IL)-1 after injury (64) and structural abnormalities of the epithelial basement membrane complex (65).

In the respiratory tract, pathogens are constantly trapped and removed by the mucociliary elevator in the normal tracheobronchial tree. Vitamin A-deficient animals show loss of ciliated epithelial cells and mucus and replacement by stratified keratinized epithelium (66–68). The terminal differentiation of keratins is modulated by vitamin A (69,70), and mucin gene expression is regulated by all-*trans* retinoic acid (71,72). Such broad pathologic changes in the tracheobronchial tree may be reflected in the observation that vitamin A-deficient mice are more susceptible to ozone-induced lung inflammation (73).

Vitamin A deficiency is associated with morphological and function alterations in the gut that may predispose individuals to more severe diarrheal disease. Vitamin A deficiency in rats is associated with a large reduction in goblet cells in duodenal crypts (74) and impaired biliary secretion of total secretory IgA (75). Reduced villus height was observed in the jejunum of vitamin A-deficient rats that were not challenged with any GI pathogens (76). Vitamin A-deficient mice were more susceptible to the destruction of duodenal villi after experimental challenge with rotavirus (77). The genitourinary tract is also adversely affected by vitamin A deficiency, with replacement of normal transitional epithelium with stratified squamous epithelium and expression of distinct types of keratins (78). Changes in the genitourinary epithelia may contribute to increased urinary tract infections in children who are vitamin A deficient (79).

Vitamin A deficiency may affect both the concentrations of secretory IgA on mucosal surfaces and specific IgA responses in the gut. In vitamin A-deficient chickens, the concentrations of total IgA were lower in the gut than in control animals (80). Vitamin A-deficient Balb/c mice that were challenged with influenza A had a lower influenza-specific IgA response than control mice (81). Vitamin A-deficient mice had significantly lower serum antibody responses against epizootic diarrhea of infant mice (EDIM) rotavirus infection compared with pair-fed control mice (82). An impaired ability to respond with IgA antibodies to oral cholera vaccine was demonstrated in vitamin A-deficient rats (83). Vitamin A treatment prevented the decline in IgA in the intestinal mucosa of protein-malnourished mice (84). Recent studies in IL-5 receptor-knockout mice suggest that IL-5 may play an important role in vitamin A-induced modulation of mucosal IgA (85). In vitro studies with HT-29 cells, a human intestinal epithelial cell line, indicate that vitamin A may be involved in the regulation of polymeric immunoglobulin receptor by IL-4 and interferon-γ (86). These data suggest that vitamin A is involved in IgA transport regulation in response to mucosal infections. Human and animal studies suggest that vitamin A status may also influence gut integrity and healing. Using the urinary lactulose/mannitol excretion test, increased gut permeability was found in infants, and the gut integrity improved after vitamin A supplementation (87). Vitamin A-deficient rats had impaired healing of surgically induced anastamoses of the colon compared with control rats (88).

4.2. Natural Killer Cells

NK cells play a role in antiviral and antitumor immunity that is not major histocompatibility complex (MHC)-restricted, and NK cells also are involved in immune response regulation. Vitamin A deficiency reduces both the number and the activity of NK cells. In experimental animal models, vitamin A deficiency reduced the number of NK cells in the spleen (89,90) and peripheral blood (91). The NK cells' cytolytic activity is reduced by vitamin A deficiency *(90,91)*. In aging Lewis rats, marginal vitamin A status reduced the number of NK cells in peripheral blood and NK cells' cytolytic activity *(92)*. There have been few studies of vitamin A status and NK cells in humans. Children with AIDS who received two doses of oral vitamin A, 60 mg retinol equivalents (200,000 IU), had large increases in circulating NK cells compared with children who received a placebo *(93)*. A synthetic retinoid, N-(4-hydroxyphenyl)-retinamide, increased NK cells' cytolytic activity in a rat model *(94)*.

4.3. Neutrophils

Neutrophils play an important role in nonspecific immunity because they phagocytize and kill bacteria, parasites, virus-infected cells, and tumor cells. Neutrophils' function is impaired during vitamin A deficiency. Retinoic acid plays an important role in the normal neutrophils' maturation *(95)*. Experimental animal studies show widespread defects in neutrophil function, including impaired chemotaxis, adhesion, phagocytosis, and ability to generate active oxidant molecules during vitamin A deficiency *(96,97)*. In rats challenged with *Staphylococcus aureus*, impaired phagocytosis and decreased complement lysis activity were found in vitamin A-deficient rats compared with controls rats *(98)*. Vitamin A treatment increased superoxide production by neutrophils of Holstein calves *(99)*. During vitamin A deficiency, an increase in circulating neutrophils has been observed in some experimental animal studies *(100)* and the increase in neutrophils has been attributed, in part, to impaired myeloid cell apoptosis *(101)*.

4.4. Hematopoiesis

Vitamin A deficiency impairs hematopoiesis of some lineages, such as CD4+ lymphocytes, NK cells, and erythrocytes. In humans, clinical vitamin A deficiency has been characterized by lower total lymphocyte counts and decreased CD4+ lymphocytes in peripheral blood, and CD4+ lymphocyte counts or percentage increased after vitamin A supplementation *(93,102)*. Vitamin A supplementation does not have any long-term effect on CD4+ or CD8+ lymphocyte subsets among infants without clinical vitamin A deficiency *(103)*. In the vitamin A-deficient rat, lower NK-cell, B-cell, and CD4+ lymphocyte counts were found in peripheral blood, and these counts responded to retinoic acid supplementation *(100)*. Retinoids have been implicated in the maturation of pluripotent stem cells to cell lineages that produce different hematopoietic cell lines, such as lymphocytes, granulocytes, and megakaryocytes. Retinoids also play a role in the maturation of differentiation of pluripotent stem cells into multipotent (colony-forming unit granulocyte erythroid macrophage mixed [CFU-GEMM]) cells and differentiation and commitment of CFU-GEMM into erythroid burst-forming units (BFU-E) and then into erythroid colony-forming units (CFU-E) *(104–106)*.

In vitro studies show that all-*trans* retinoic acid stimulates human BFU-E colony formation, suggesting a role for retinoids in erythropoiesis *(107)*. All-*trans* retinol does not enhance growth of erythroid progenitors in this culture system involving fetal calf serum, a rich source of vitamin A *(107)*. Subsequent studies using progenitor cells from human peripheral mononuclear cells in serum-free media show that both retinyl acetate and all-*trans* retinoic acid stimulated d16 (early) erythroid colonies, and a synergism was noted between retinoids, erythropoietin, and insulin-like growth factor-I (IGF-I) *(108)*. The effect of retinoids on erythropoiesis is complex and depends on the stage of erythrocyte development *(105)*. Retinoids regulate apoptosis, or programmed cell death, in erythropoietic progenitor cells, but the nature of this interaction may be bidirectional *(109)*. All-*trans* retinoic acid stimulates the survival of purified CD34+ cells obtained from midtrimester fetal blood *(110)*. In CD34+ hematopoietic progenitor cells isolated from normal adult human bone marrow, all-*trans* retinoic acid-induced apoptosis of CD34+ cells and CD34+CD71+ cells stimulated with erythropoietin *(111)*. By using selective ligand agonists, it was noted that both RARs and RXRs were involved in retinoic acid-mediated apoptosis of erythroid progenitor cells. The effects of retinoids on hematopoiesis are complex and depend on culture conditions, maturation stage of the cells, and cytokines used for stimulation. Whether vitamin A deficiency in humans has any influence on apoptosis of erythropoietic progenitor cells has not been determined. The effects of vitamin A deficiency and supplementation on hematopoiesis has recently been elsewhere reviewed in detail *(112)*.

4.5. Monocytes/Macrophages

Macrophages are involved in the inflammatory response and in the phagocytosis of viruses, bacteria, protozoa, fungi, and tumor cells. Macrophages secrete several cytokines, including tumor necrosis factor-α (TNF-α), IL-1β, IL-6, and IL-12. The effect of retinoids on monocyte differentiation has been studied in leukemic myelomonocytic cell lines, such as HL-60, U-937, and THP-1 *(113–115)*. Retinoids influence both the number and the activity of macrophages *(116,117)*. Vitamin A-deficient animals may have increased numbers of macrophages in lymphoid tissues *(118)*. In vitro studies suggest that all-*trans* retinoic acid decreases TNF-α production in a murine macrophage cell line *(119)* and regulates IL-1β expression by human monocytes *(120)* and human alveolar macrophages *(121)*. All-*trans* retinoic acid inhibited IL-12 production in activated murine macrophages *(122)* and caused a twofold increase in phagocytosis in murine macrophages *(123)*. IL-1 expression may be modified by retinoids in murine macrophages *(123,124)*. In the rat model, vitamin A deficiency was associated with reduced phagocytic function of macrophages *(98)*. In experimental *Salmonella* infection in the rat, vitamin A supplementation improved phagocytosis by macrophages *(125)*.

4.6. Langerhans Cells

Langerhans cells serve as antigen-presenting cells in the skin. Dietary vitamin A increases contact sensitivity to several chemical agents in the murine model, and this observation may be related to vitamin A-related modulation of the numbers and function of Langerhans cells *(126,127)*. Retinoic acid treatment in vivo increases the ability of human Langerhans cells to present alloantigens to T lymphocytes and is associated with increases in surface expression of HLA-DR and CD11c, two molecules involved in antigen presentation *(128)*.

4.7. T Lymphocytes

Vitamin A deficiency may influence T-lymphocyte-related immunocompetence through mechanisms such as a decrease in numbers or distribution, changes in phenotype, alterations in cytokine production, or decreased expression or function of cell-surface molecules involved in T-cell signaling *(92,129)*. There is some evidence that each of these mechanisms may play a role in the immunosuppression associated with vitamin A deficiency. The effects of vitamin A deficiency on lymphopoiesis were discussed in Section 4.4. In preschool children with clinical and subclinical vitamin A deficiency in Indonesia, high-dose vitamin A supplementation was associated with an increase in the proportion of circulating CD4+CD45RA+, or naive CD4+ lymphocytes, suggesting that vitamin A influences lymphopoiesis *(102)*. T-lymphocyte activation requires retinol *(130)*. In human peripheral mononuclear cells, retinol is a cofactor in CD3-induced T-lymphocyte activation *(131)*. All-*trans* retinoic acid increases antigen-specific T-lymphocyte proliferation *(132)* and expression of IL-2 receptors *(133)*. In a trial in Bangladesh, vitamin A supplementation improved responses to delayed type hypersensitivity (DTH) skin testing among infants who were supplemented to higher vitamin A levels *(134)*.

Vitamin A modulates the balance between T helper type 1 (Th1)-like responses and T helper type 2 (Th2)-like responses in experimental animal studies, and this has been the prevailing paradigm for the last decade, as reviewed in detail elsewhere *(135)*. According to this model, vitamin A deficiency causes a shift toward Th1-like responses, whereas vitamin A supplementation causes a shift toward Th2-like responses. There is little evidence to support this model for human vitamin A deficiency, and, in fact, clinical observations are not consistent with this model. Vitamin A supplementation enhances immunity to several infections, such as tuberculosis, measles, malaria, HIV infection, and diarrheal diseases, where the specific immune protective immune responses have been characterized as either Th1-like or Th2-like responses.

In mice, *Trichinella spiralis* infection usually stimulates a strong Th2-like response, characterized by strong parasite-specific IgG responses and a cytokine profile dominated by IL-4, IL-5, and IL-10 production. However, in vitamin A-deficient mice, *T. spiralis* infection results in low production of parasite-specific IgG and a cytokine profile dominated by interferon (IFN)-γ and IL-12 production *(136–138)*. Lymphocyte stimulation to concanavalin A or β-lactoglobulin was higher and IL-2 and IFN-γ production was higher in lymphocyte supernatants from vitamin A-deficient rats compared with control rats, suggesting that vitamin A deficiency modulates a shift toward Th1-like responses in rats *(139)*. Vitamin A inhibits IFN-γ, IL-2, and granulocyte-macrophage colony-stimulating factor (GM-CSF) by Th1-type lymphocytes in vitro *(140)*. The effect of high-level dietary vitamin A on the shift to Th2-like responses in Balb/c mice has been used to explain the apparent lack of benefit of vitamin A supplementation for acute lower respiratory infections in humans *(141)*. The enhancement of Th2-like responses by vitamin A may be modulated via 9-*cis* retinoic acid and RXR *(142)*. Vitamin A-deficient mice show IFN-γ overproduction *(143)* and both retinol and retinoic acid downregulate IFN-γ expression and transcription *(144,145)*.

4.8. B Lymphocytes

Vitamin A deficiency impairs B lymphocyte growth, activation, and function. Activated B lymphocytes depend on retinol but not retinoic acid *(146–148)*. B lymphocytes use a metabolite of retinol, 14-hydroxy-4,14-*retro*-retinol, instead of retinoic acid, as a mediator for growth *(45)*. The effects of retinol and all-*trans* retinoic acid on Ig synthesis by B lymphocytes has been examined in human cord blood and adult peripheral mononuclear cells *(149–152)*. A T cell-dependent antigen was used to induce differentiation of human B lymphocytes into Ig-secreting cells, and all-*trans* retinoic acid increased the synthesis of IgM and IgG by these cells. Highly purified T lymphocytes incubated with retinoic acid enhanced IgM synthesis by cord blood B lymphocytes, suggesting that retinoic acid modulates T cell help through cytokine production *(152)*. B-lymphocyte apoptosis is mediated via RAR *(153)*. In common variable immunodeficiency, a B-cell deficiency syndrome characterized by defective antibody production, T-cell and monocyte dysfunction, and recurrent infections, vitamin A supplementation was associated with enhanced anti-CD40-stimulated IgG production, serum IgA concentrations, and lymphocyte proliferation to phytohemagglutinin (PHA) *(154)*.

4.9. Antibody Responses

The hallmark of vitamin A deficiency is an impaired capacity to generate an antibody response to T cell-dependent antigens *(139,155)*, including tetanus toxoid *(156,157)* and diphtheria antigens in humans *(158)*, tetanus toxoid and other antigens in animal models *(159–161)*, and T cell-independent type 2 antigens, such as pneumococcal polysaccharide *(162)*. Antibody responses are involved in protective immunity to many types of infections and are the basis for immunological protection for many vaccines. Depressed antibody responses to tetanus toxoid have been observed in children who are vitamin A deficient *(156)* and in vitamin A-deficient animals *(163,164)*. Vitamin A deficiency impairs the generation of primary antibody responses to tetanus toxoid, but if animals are repleted with vitamin A before to a second immunization, the secondary antibody responses to tetanus toxoid are comparable to control animals *(160)*. These findings suggest that formation of immunologic memory and class switching are intact during vitamin A deficiency, despite an impaired IgM and IgG response to primary immunization. Human peripheral blood lymphocytes from subjects previously immunized against tetanus toxoid were used to reconstitute control and vitamin A-deficient mice with severe combined immunodeficiency (SCID). After challenge with tetanus toxoid, vitamin A-deficient SCID mice had a 2.9-fold increase in human antitetanus toxoid antibody, compared with a 74-fold increase in control SCID mice *(165)*. In healthy children without vitamin A deficiency, vitamin A supplementation did not enhance antibody responses to tetanus toxoid *(166)*. These findings suggest that vitamin A supplementation is unlikely to enhance antibody responses in subjects who are not vitamin A deficient. Other evidence that vitamin A is needed for the generation of antibody responses has been noted in retinol-binding protein knockout mice, where serum vitamin A concentrations are extremely low and associated with circulating Ig concentrations *(167)*.

5. ROLE OF VITAMIN A IN RESISTANCE TO INFECTIOUS DISEASES

5.1. Experimental Animal Models

Vitamin A deficiency increases susceptibility to some types of infections, and there is currently an extensive literature regarding vitamin A deficiency and infection in experimental animal models, as reviewed elsewhere *(23,24,168–171)*. In the 1960s, it was noted that vitamin A-deficient animals had short survival unless they were raised in a germ-free environment *(172)*. Vitamin A-deficient animals are more susceptible to experimental infection with several pathogens *(89,96,173,174)* and, conversely, vitamin A-supplemented animals are less susceptible to experimental infection *(125,175,176)*.

Table 3
Some Notable Trials of Vitamin A and Infectious Diseases

Location	Date	Subjects	Observation	Reference
London[a]	1871	Adults	Reduced tuberculosis mortality	(5)
Sheffield[a]	1931	Women	Reduced morbidity of puerperal sepsis	(239)
London[a]	1932	Children	Reduced measles mortality	(180)
Indonesia	1986	Children	Reduced diarrheal disease mortality	(197)
South Africa	1990	Children	Reduced measles mortality	(182)
Papua New Guinea	1999	Children	Reduced malaria morbidity	(222)
Nepal	1999	Women	Reduced pregnancy-related mortality	(238)
Uganda	2001	Children	Reduced mortality during HIV/AIDS	(226)

[a]Vitamin A in the form of cod-liver oil.

5.2. Human Studies

After an extensive global survey of vitamin A deficiency, H. A. P. C. Oomen, Donald McLaren, and Humberto Escapini recognized in 1964 that there was a vicious cycle of vitamin A deficiency and infection: "Not only may deficiency of vitamin A itself play an important role in lowering the resistance to infection . . . but infectious diseases themselves predispose to and actually precipitate xerophthalmia" *(177)*. There have been more than 100 vitamin A clinical trials conducted in humans, and these studies show that vitamin A supplementation reduces the morbidity and mortality of measles and diarrheal disease, the morbidity of *Plasmodium falciparum* malaria, and maternal morbidity and mortality related to pregnancy. Vitamin A supplementation does not reduce morbidity and mortality from acute lower respiratory infections or reduce mother-to-child transmission of HIV type 1. The effects of vitamin A supplementation on infectious disease morbidity and mortality are summarized in Table 3.

5.3. Measles

Vitamin A supplementation reduces the morbidity and mortality from acute measles in infants and children in developing countries. Measles is a morbillivirus of the *Paramyxoviridae*, and measles is spread from person to person via the respiratory route. Viral replication occurs in macrophages in the lymphoid tissue of the respiratory mucosa and lungs *(178)*. A viremia allows measles virus to spread to multiple organs, including the skin, liver, and conjunctiva, and a prodrome of fever, cough, and conjunctivitis occurs approx 14 d after infection. Antibody responses against measles virus proteins are detectable at the onset of the rash. Infants are protected against measles virus infection by passively acquired maternal antibody to measles, and this is probably the strongest evidence that antibody is involved in protective immunity to measles virus. T cell-driven cellular immune responses, including activation of CD4+ and CD8+ lymphocytes, occur during measles *(178)*. DTH skin-test responses and in vitro proliferation of lymphocytes to viral antigens are often minimal or absent in measles infection *(178)*. Immune suppression often accompanies measles infection and is believed to increase the susceptibility to secondary infections. The immune response to measles is believed to be consistent with Th2-like immune responses in which antibody responses predominate and are driven by

IL-4, IL-6, and IL-10. In children with measles, low circulating vitamin A concentrations are associated with higher mortality *(179)*.

The first trial to demonstrate that vitamin A supplementation could reduce mortality of children with measles was conducted in London by Joseph Bramhall Ellison in 1932 *(30,180)*. Ellison's discovery was partially confirmed in trial conducted in Tanzania *(181)* and definitively corroborated with a trial in Cape Town, South Africa *(182)*. Other studies have provided further evidence that vitamin A supplementation reduces morbidity of acute measles *(183,184)*. The trial in Cape Town showed that during acute complicated measles, high-dose vitamin A supplementation (60 mg retinol equivalent [RE] on admission and the following day) reduced mortality by up to 80% *(182)*. Vitamin A supplementation reduces the infectious complications associated with measles immune suppression, such as pneumonia and diarrheal disease.

Vitamin A supplementation modulates antibody responses to measles and increases total lymphocyte counts. Children with acute measles infection who received high-dose vitamin A supplementation (60 mg retinol equivalent [RE] upon admission and the following day) had significantly higher IgG responses to measles virus and higher circulating lymphocyte counts during follow-up compared with children who received placebo *(185)*. When vitamin A supplementation is given simultaneously with live measles vaccine, there is an effect of vitamin A on antibody titers to measles if maternal antibodies are present. In 6-mo-old infants in Indonesia, vitamin A administration (30 mg RE) at the time of immunization with standard titer Schwarz measles vaccine interfered with seroconversion to measles in infants who had maternal antibody present and significantly reduced the incidence of measles vaccine-associated rash *(186)*. A separate clinical trial also showed that vitamin A (30 mg RE) reduced antibody responses to measles virus in 9-mo-old infants who had maternal antibody present but did not interfere with overall seroconversion rates to measles *(187)*.

In Guinea-Bissau, vitamin A supplementation (30 mg RE) enhanced geometric mean titers to measles when given simultaneously with standard titer Schwarz measles vaccine in 9-mo-old infants *(188)*. In a two-dose measles immunization schedule at ages 6 and 9 mo, simultaneous vitamin A supplementation did not interfere with seroconversion to measles when measured at 18 mo of age *(188)*. It was not possible to determine whether vitamin A supplementation interfered with seroconversion rates after measles vaccine in 6-mo-old infants in the study in Guinea-Bissau as with the study in Indonesia, because antibody titers were not measured until after two doses of measles vaccine. Although the results of the studies involving 6-mo-old infants in Indonesia and Guinea-Bissau have been viewed as contradictory *(188,189)*, the differences in the design of measles vaccine studies lends little validity to directly comparing these two studies, and the findings may be complementary. Another trial in India shows that vitamin A supplementation with measles immunization at 9 mo of age had no effect overall on antibody titers to measles but enhanced the antibody response in malnourished infants *(190)*. A smaller study in India suggests that vitamin A supplementation enhanced antibody responses to measles *(191)*. Long-term follow-up of children in the study in Guinea Bissau showed that those who received vitamin A supplementation with measles immunization at 9 mo of age had higher geometric mean antibody concentrations against measles at age 6–8 yr *(192)*.

5.4. Diarrheal Diseases

Vitamin A supplementation or fortification reduces the morbidity and mortality of diarrheal diseases in preschool children in developing countries. The reduction in diarrheal disease mortality accounts for most of the reduction in overall mortality when vitamin A is given through fortification or supplementation on a community level. The main causes of diarrheal diseases among children in developing countries are rotavirus, *E. coli*, *Shigella*, *Vibrio cholerae*, *Salmonella*, and *Entamoeba histolytica*. The epidemiology, clinical features, immunology, and pathogenesis of diarrhea may differ according to characteristics of the pathogen, such as production of toxins, tissue invasion, fluid and electrolyte loss, and location of infection. In general, host defenses in the gut include gastric acidity, the presence of normal microflora, gut motility, mucus production, microvilli integrity, local secretion of antibody, and cell-mediated immunity, and vitamin A deficiency may impair some of these host defenses.

Clinical vitamin A deficiency is associated with diarrheal disease in children *(193–196)*. A community-based controlled trial showed that periodic vitamin A supplementation reduced mortality in preschool children *(197)*, but causes of death were not addressed. Subsequent large community-based clinical trials of vitamin A supplementation in Tamil Nadu, Nepal, and Ghana showed that vitamin A supplementation reduced mortality from diarrheal disease but not pneumonia in preschool children *(198,199)*. The severity of diarrheal disease was reduced by vitamin A supplementation in a clinical trial in Brazil *(200)*. One of the mechanisms by which vitamin A may improve clinical outcomes in diarrheal disease is through restoration of gut integrity *(87,201)*. Urinary losses of vitamin A during diarrhea may be substantial in some children *(202,203)*, and persistent diarrhea may reduce the bioavailability of vitamin A *(204)*. Vitamin A supplementation (60 mg RE) reduces morbidity in children with acute shigellosis *(205)*, but the effects of vitamin A supplementation on other specific diarrheal pathogens has not been completely clarified.

5.5. Acute Lower Respiratory Infections

Acute lower respiratory infections are a major cause of death in children in developing countries, and major causes of acute lower respiratoryinfections include respiratory syncytial virus infection, parainfluenza, *Haemophilus influenzae*, *Streptococcus pneumoniae*, and *Bordetella pertussis*. Secondary bacterial infection with high case fatality may follow a primary viral infection in the lungs. Important components of the immune response in the respiratory tract that are affected by vitamin A deficiency include number and function of cilia, mucin production, and alveolar macrophage activity. Vitamin A supplementation reduces the morbidity of pneumonia in acute complicated measles *(182–184)* but does not have an effect on other types of acute lower respiratory infections *(199)*. Hospital-based studies show that high-dose vitamin A supplementation has no therapeutic effect on the morbidity of acute lower respiratory infections in children *(206–208)*. In Chile and the United States, hospital-based trials showed that vitamin A supplementation had little impact on respiratory syncytial virus (RSV) infection in infants and young children *(209–211)*.

High-dose vitamin A supplementation has been associated with adverse consequences for some children who are not malnourished *(212,213)*. In a study conducted in Dar Es Salaam, Tanzania, hospitalized children with pneumonia received high-dose vitamin A supplementation, and after discharge, they were monitored for diarrheal and respiratory disease. Vitamin A supplementation was associated with a higher rate of diarrheal disease among children who were better nourished, whereas a reduction in diarrheal morbidity was noted in wasted children. This apparent bidirectional effect has been termed the "vitamin A paradox" *(214)*. A recent controlled clinical trial conducted in Quito, Ecuador, also suggested that weekly vitamin A supplementation to children aged 6–36 mo significantly reduced the incidence of acute lower respiratory infections in underweight (weight-for-age Z score <–2) children but significantly increased the incidence of acute lower respiratory infections in normal weight children (weight-for-age Z score >–1) compared with placebo *(213)*. If further investigations confirm that high-dose vitamin A supplementation exacerbates morbidity in children who are not vitamin A deficient, then it would be reasonable to reassess community-based mass treatment programs of high-dose vitamin A capsule distribution, especially in developing countries that are undergoing rapid economic development.

Although vitamin A status is related to the severity of acute respiratory infection in children *(215)*, it is unclear why vitamin A therapy has no apparent effect in some trials on the morbidity of acute respiratory infections in preschool children. Young age might be one contributing factor to the lack of an effect, because large community-based studies suggest that vitamin A supplementation has little effect on infants' morbidity and mortality *(216–218)*. Studies also have been conducted in populations where vitamin A deficiency is not considered a public health problem. In the recent clinical trials involving RSV infection, the apparent lack of effect of vitamin A supplementation on RSV infection might result from the young age of the subjects and the lack of vitamin A deficiency in the population.

5.6. Malaria

Vitamin A supplementation may reduce the morbidity of *P. falciparum* malaria. *P. falciparum* causes an estimated 1–2 million deaths worldwide each year. Natural history studies have suggested an association between indicators of poor vitamin A status and malaria *(219–221)*. A recent randomized placebo-controlled clinical trial was conducted in Papua New Guinea, to examine the effects of vitamin A supplementation, 60 mg RE every 3 mo, on malarial morbidity in preschool children *(222)*. Children between 6 and 60 mo of age were randomly allocated to receive vitamin A or placebo every 3 mo. A weekly morbidity surveillance and clinic-based surveillance were established for monitoring acute malaria, and children were followed for 1 yr. Vitamin A significantly reduced the incidence of malaria attacks by approx 20–50% for all except extremely high levels of parasitemia. Similarly, vitamin A supplementation reduced clinic-based malaria attacks, which consisted of self-solicited visits to the clinic by mothers who believed that their children should be seen because of fever. Vitamin A supplementation had little effect in children under age 12 mo and greatest effect from 13 to 36 mo of age.

5.7. Human Immunodeficiency Virus Infection

Vitamin A supplementation may have some benefit for HIV-infected children and pregnant women in developing countries. Plasma or serum concentrations of vitamin A or vitamin A intake has been associated with increased disease progression, mortality, and higher mother-to-child HIV transmission *(273)*. Periodic high-dose vitamin A supplementation reduces morbidity in children born to HIV-infected mothers *(224)* and diarrheal disease morbidity in HIV-infected children after discharge from the hospital for acute lower respiratory infection *(225).* A recent controlled clinical trial in Uganda shows that periodic high-dose vitamin A supplementation, 30 RE every 3 mo, reduces morbidity and mortality of HIV-infected children *(226).* Vitamin A supplementation has no effect on mother-to-child HIV transmission *(227,228)* but may reduce the incidence of preterm birth *(228),* low birth weight, and anemia in infants *(229).* Recently, more long-term follow-up was reported from a controlled clinical trial in Tanzania *(227)* in which "vitamin A" (consisting of vitamin A, 5000 IU, plus high-dose β-carotene, 25 mg/d) supplementation for 2 yr after delivery was associated with increased risk of mother-to-child HIV transmission *(230).* A study in Malawi that used vitamin A supplementation, 10,000 IU/d, found no increased risk of mother-to-child HIV transmission, and, in fact, the results suggested that vitamin A was protective against late mother-to-child HIV transmission through breast-feeding *(229).* Vitamin A supplementation does not influence HIV load in the blood *(231).* A study from Cape Town, South Africa, suggests that vitamin A supplementation modulates lymphopoiesis in children with AIDS *(93).*

5.8. Tuberculosis

Although malnutrition and vitamin A deficiency are major risk factors for the progression of tuberculosis, clinical management usually involves chemoprophylaxis and chemotherapy alone. Cod-liver oil, a rich source of vitamins A and D, has been a standard treatment for tuberculosis in the past *(5).* The role of nutrition and tuberculosis remains a major area of neglect, despite the promise that micronutrients have shown as therapy for other types of infections and the long record of the use of vitamins A and D for treatment of pulmonary and miliary tuberculosis in both Europe and the United States. High-dose vitamin A supplementation may reduce the morbidity of tuberculosis in children *(232).* A recent placebo-controlled trial conducted in Indonesia suggests that daily supplements of vitamin A and zinc given to adults with pulmonary tuberculosis improves the lesion area observed on chest radiograph after 2 mo of tuberculosis chemotherapy but not at 6 mo follow-up *(233).* Vitamin A and zinc were associated with earlier clearance of tubercle bacilli from sputum, but no effects were observed on the number of cavities, the surface area of cavities, hemoglobin concentrations, or different anthropometric indicators of nutritional status *(233).* Studies that address the use of multivitamins and minerals or vitamins A and D as adjunct therapy for tuberculosis have not been conducted.

5.9. Infections in Pregnant and Lactating Women

Recent data from Nepal suggest that pregnant women with clinical vitamin A deficiency, i.e., night blindness, are at high risk of infectious disease morbidity *(234,235)* and mortality *(236).* Weekly vitamin A or β-carotene supplementation reduced the risk of infectious disease morbidity and mortality in pregnant women in Nepal, suggesting that vitamin A status may be important in pregnancy-related morbidity and mortality *(237,238).* Vitamin A or β-carotene reduced all-cause mortality, and further work is needed to both replicate these findings and determine the types of infections that might be reduced through improving vitamin A status during pregnancy. The recent trial in

Table 4
Controlled Studies of Vitamin A and Aspects of Immunity in Humans

Location	n	Subjects and intervention	Effects of supplementation	References
Indonesia	236	Preschool children; 30 mg RE vs placebo	Enhanced immunoglobulin (Ig) response to tetanus toxoid; increase in proportion of circulating CD4+ lymphocytes	(102,156,157)
Indonesia	336	6-mo-old infants, 15 mg RE with measles immunization	Reduced antibody titers to measles at 7 and 12 mo age	(186)
Indonesia	394	9-mo-old infants; 15 mg RE with measles immunization	No impact of vitamin A on antibody titers to measles at 10 and 15 mo age	(187)
Guinea Bissau	312	9-mo-old infants; 15 mg RE with measles immunization	Enhanced antibody titers to measles at 18 mo age; higher antibody titers at 6–8 yr	(188)
Guinea Bissau	150	6-mo-old infants; 15 mg RE with measles immunization; repeat vaccination at 9 mo	Higher antibody titers in vitamin A group after second immunization	(192)
India	100	9-mo-old infants; 15 mg RE with measles immunization	Enhanced antibody titers to measles at 10 mo	(191)
India	618	9-mo-old infants; 15 mg RE with measles immunization	No impact of vitamin A on antibody titers to measles at 12 mo age; vitamin A-enhanced antibody response in subgroup of malnourished infants	(190)
India	56	Infants; 15 mg RE vs placebo with diphtheria-pertussis-tetanus (DPT) immunization	Enhanced IgG response to diphtheria toxoid	(158)
India	120	Infants; 15 mg RE/mo with DPT immunization	Increased skin-test responses among those supplemented to higher vitamin A levels	(134)
Norway	6	Adults with common variable immunodeficiency; 6 patients selected from 20 patients on basis of lowest plasma vitamin A concentrations; 6500 IU per d for 6 mo	Decrease in circulating TNF-α and neopterin and increase in interleukin (IL)-10; increased IgG and enhanced lymphocyte proliferation to mitogen	(154)
India[a]	144	Hospitalized infants, 60 mg RE (1) at admission, (2) at discharge or (3) placebo at discharge	Decrease in L/M ratio in groups 1 and 2 compared with group 3	(87)
India[a]	80	Infants, 16,700 IU/wk vs placebo	No significant effect on L/M ratio	(87)
South Africa	238	Infants; 1.5 mg RE and 30 mg β-carotene/d to mothers during pregnancy	Improved gut integrity in infants	(201)

[a]L/M is the lactulose/mannitol ratio.
TNF-α, tumor necrosis factor.

120

Nepal corroborates earlier trials from England that showed vitamin A supplementation reduced the morbidity of puerperal sepsis *(239,240)*.

6. "TAKE-HOME" MESSAGES

1. Vitamin A has been used as either disease-targeted or prophylactic therapy to reduce morbidity and mortality from infectious diseases for hundreds of years, first as empirical therapy in the form of cod-liver oil and later in the form of vitamin A supplements or fortification.
2. Vitamin A plays an important role in hematopoiesis, the maintenance of mucosal surfaces, the function of T and B lymphocytes, NK cells, and neutrophils, and in the generation of antibody responses to T cell-dependent antigens and T cell-independent type II antigens.
3. Studies conducted in humans have shown an effect of vitamin A supplementation on T-cell subsets, antibody responses to protein antigens, DTH, and gut integrity (*see* Table 4).
4. Vitamin A reduces the severity but not the incidence of certain types of infections: measles, diarrheal diseases, malaria, HIV infection, and, possibly, pregnancy-related infections.
5. Vitamin A does not reduce the morbidity and mortality from acute lower respiratory infections, except for pneumonia-complicating measles infection.
6. As a general rule, there is little value in vitamin A supplementation in populations that are already relatively well-nourished; thus, clinical investigation of immune modulation and vitamin A should focus on populations at high risk of vitamin A deficiency.
7. Although tremendous advances have been made in our understanding of the role that vitamin A plays in immune function, many research questions remain regarding the relationship between vitamin A deficiency in humans and the function of immune cells, such as neutrophils, macrophages, NK cells, and cytotoxic T cells; the effect of vitamin A on T-cell development in the thymus; the relationship between vitamin A status and gut integrity at the molecular level; the relationship between vitamin A status and cytokine expression; and the effect of vitamin A on immune modulation by breast milk.

ACKNOWLEDGMENTS

This work was supported by the National Institute of Child Health and Human Development (HD32247, HD30042), the National Institute of Allergy and Infectious Diseases (AI41956), and the Fogarty International Center, the National Institutes of Health, and the United States Agency for International Development (Cooperative Agreement HRN A-0097-00015-00).

REFERENCES

1. World Health Organization/UNICEF. Global Prevalence of Vitamin A Deficiency. Micronutrient Deficiency Information System Working Paper 2. World Health Organization, Geneva, 1995.
2. International Vitamin A Consultative Group. Maternal night blindness: a new indicator of vitamin A deficiency. International Vitamin A Consultative Group (IVACG) Statement, IVACG Secretariat, International Life Sciences Research Foundation, Washington, DC, 2002.
3. Whitcher JP, Srinivasan M, Upadhyay MP. Corneal blindness: a global perspective. Bull World Health Organ 2001;79:214–221.

4. McLaren DS, Frigg M. Sight and Life Manual on Vitamin A Deficiency Disorders (VADD) (2nd ed.). Task Force Sight and Life, Basel, Switzerland, 2001.

5. Williams CJB, Williams CT. Pulmonary Consumption: Its Nature, Varieties, and Treatment with an Analysis of One Thousand Cases to Exemplify its Duration. Henry C. Lea, Philadelphia, 1871.

6. Magendie F. Mémoire sur les propriétés nutritives des substances qui ne contiennent pas d'azote. Bull Sci Soc Phil Paris 1816;4:137–138.

7. Lunin N. Über die Bedeutung der anorganischen Salze für die Ernährung des Thieres. Zeitschr Physiol Chem 1881;5:31–39.

8. Socin CA. In welcher Form wird das Eisen resorbirt? Zeitschr Physiol Chem 1891;15:93–139.

9. Pekelharing CA. Over onze kennis van de waarde der voedingsmiddelen uit chemische fabrieken. Nederl Tijdschr Geneesk 1905;41:111–124.

10. Hopkins FG. Feeding experiments illustrating the importance of accessory factors in normal dietaries. J Physiol 1912;44:425–460.

11. Stepp W. Experimentelle untersuchungen über die bedeutung der lipoide für die ernährung. Zeitschr Biol 1911;57:136–170.

12. Wolf G, Carpenter KJ. Early research into the vitamins: the work of Wilhelm Stepp. J Nutr 1997;127:1255–1259.

13. McCollum EV, Davis M. The necessity of certain lipids in the diet during growth. J Biol Chem 1913;15:167–175.

14. Osborne TB, Mendel LB. Feeding Experiments with Isolated Food Substances. Publication 156. Carnegie Institute of Washington, Washington, DC, 1911.

15. Osborne TB, Mendel LB. The relationship of growth to the chemical constituents of the diet. J Biol Chem 1913;15:311–326.

16. McCollum EV, Kennedy C. The dietary factors operating in the production of polyneuritis. J Biol Chem 1916;24:491–502.

17. Karrer P, Morf R, Schöpp K. Zur kenntnis des vitamins-A aus fischtranen. Helv Chim Acta 1931;14:1036–1040.

18. Karrer P, Morf R, Schöpp K. Zur kenntnis des vitamins-A aus fischtranen II. Helv Chim Acta 1931;14:1431–1436.

19. Holmes HN, Corbet RE. The isolation of crystalline vitamin A. J Am Chem Soc 1937;59:2042–2047.

20. Knapp P. Experimenteller beitrag zur ernährung von ratten mit künstlicher nahrung und zum zusammenhang von ernährungsstörungen mit erkrankungen der conjunctiva. Zeitschr Exp Pathol Ther 1909;5:147–169.

21. Green HN, Mellanby E. Vitamin A as an anti-infective agent. Br Med J 1928;2:691–696.

22. Lassen HCA. Vitamin A deficiency and resistance against a specific infection. Preliminary report. J Hyg 1930;30:300–310.

23. Robertson EC. The vitamins and resistance to infection. Medicine 1934;13:123–206.

24. Clausen SW. The influence of nutrition upon resistance to infection. Physiol Rev 1934;14:309–350.

25. Bloch CE. Blindness and other diseases in children arising from deficient nutrition (lack of fat soluble A factor). Am J Dis Child 1924;27:139–148.

26. Semba RD. The vitamin A and mortality paradigm: past, present, and future. Scand J Nutr 2001;45:46–50.

27. Widmark E. Vitamin A deficiency in Denmark and its results. Lancet 1924;1:1206–1209.

28. Cramer W. An address on vitamins and the borderland between health and disease. Lancet 1924;1:633–640.

29. Semba RD. Vitamin A as "anti-infective" therapy, 1920–1940. J Nutr 1999;129:783–791.

30. Semba RD. On Joseph Bramhall Ellison's discovery that vitamin A reduces measles mortality. Nutrition 2003;19:390–394.

31. Semba RD. Nutrition and development—a historical perspective. In: Semba RD, Bloem MW (eds.). Nutrition and Health in Developing Countries. Humana, Totowa, NJ, 2001, pp. 1–30.

32. Bloem MW, Huq N, Gorstein J, et al. Production of fruits and vegetables at the homestead is an important source of vitamin A among women in rural Bangladesh. Eur J Clin Nutr 1996;50:S62–S67.

33. De Pee S, West CE, Muhilal, Karyadi D, Hautvast JG. Lack of improvement in vitamin A status with increased consumption of dark-green leafy vegetables. Lancet 1995;346:75–81.

34. West CE. Meeting requirements for vitamin A. Nutr Rev 2000;58:341–345.
35. Chambon P. A decade of molecular biology of retinoic acid receptors. FASEB J 1996;10:940–954.
36. Kliewer SA, Umesono K, Mangelsdorf DJ, Evans RM. Retinoid X receptor interacts with nuclear receptors in retinoic acid, thyroid hormone and vitamin D_3 signaling. Nature 1992;355:446–449.
37. Tran P, Zhang XK, Salbert G, Hermann T, Lehmann JM, Pfahl M. COUP orphan receptors are negative regulators of retinoic acid response pathways. Mol Cell Biol 1992;12:4666–4676.
38. Hirose T, Apfel R, Pfahl M, Jetten AM. The orphan receptor TAK1 acts as a repressor of RAR-, RXR- and T_3R-mediated signaling pathways. Biochem Biophys Res Comm 1995;211:83–91.
39. Retnakaran R, Flock G, Giguère V. Identification of RVR, a novel orphan nuclear receptor that acts as a negative transcriptional regulator. Mol Endocrinol 1994;8:1234–1244.
40. Carlberg C, van Huijsduijnen RH, Staple JK, DeLamarter JF, Becker-André M. RZRs, a new family of retinoid-related orphan receptors that function as both monomers and homodimers. Mol Endocrinol 1994;8:757–770.
41. Ortiz MA, Piedrafita FJ, Pfahl M, Maki R. TOR: a new orphan receptor expressed in the thymus that can modulate retinoid and thyroid hormone signals. Mol Endocrinol 1995;9:1679–1691.
42. Zhao Q, Chasse SA, Devarakonda S, Sierk ML, Ahvazi B, Rastinejad F. Structural basis of RXR-DNA interactions. J Mol Biol 2000;296;509–520.
43. Rastinejad F, Wagner T, Zhao Q, Khorasanizadeh S. Structure of the RXR-RAR DNA-binding complex on the retinoic acid response element DR1. EMBO J 2000;19:1045–1054.
44. Rastinejad F. Retinoid X receptor and its partners in the nuclear receptor family. Curr Opin Struct Biol 2001;11:33–38.
45. Buck J, Derguini F, Levi E, Nakanishi K, Hämmerling U. Intracellular signaling by 14-hydroxy-4,14-*retro* retinol. Science 1991;254:1654–1655.
46. Buck J, Grün F, Kimura S, Noy N, Derguini F, Hämmerling U. Anhydroretinol: a naturally occurring inhibitor of lymphocyte physiology. J Exp Med 1993;178:675.
47. Blumberg B, Bolado J Jr, Derguini F, et al. Novel retinoic acid receptor ligands in *Xenopus* embryos. Proc Natl Acad Sci USA 1996;93:4873–4878.
48. Nagy L, Thomazy VA, Heyman RA, Davies PJA. Retinoid-induced apoptosis in normal and neoplastic tissues. Cell Death Differ 1998;5:11–19.
49. Wolbach SB, Howe PR. Tissue changes following deprivation of fat-soluble A vitamin. J Exp Med 1925;42:753–778.
50. Blackfan KD, Wolbach SB. Vitamin A deficiency in infants. A clinical and pathological study. J Pediatr 1933;3:679–706.
51. Sweet KL, K'ang HJ. Clinical and anatomic study of avitaminosis A among the Chinese. Am J Dis Child 1935;50:699–734.
52. McLaren DS. Malnutrition and the Eye. Academic Press, New York, 1963.
53. Sommer A. Nutritional Blindness: Xerophthalmia and Keratomalacia. Oxford University Press, New York, 1982.
54. Hayashi K, Frangieh G, Hannien LA, Wolf G, Kenyon KR. Stromal degradation in vitamin A-deficient rat cornea. Comparison of epithelial abrasion and stromal incision. Cornea 1990;9:253–265.
55. Koo JS, Jetten AM, Belloni P, et al. Role of retinoid receptors in the regulation of mucin gene expression by retinoic acid in human tracheobronchial epithelial cells. Biochem J 1999;338:351–357.
56. Tei M, Spurr-Michaud SJ, Tisdale AS, Gipson IK. Vitamin A deficiency alters the expression of mucin genes by the rat ocular surface epithelium. Invest Ophthalmol Vis Sci 2000;41:82–88.
57. Tseng SCG, Hatchell D, Tierney N, Huang AJ, Sun TT. Expression of specific keratin markers by rabbit corneal, conjunctival, and esophageal epithelia during vitamin A deficiency. J Cell Biol 1984;99:2279–2286.
58. Gijbels MJJ, van der Harn F, van Bennekum AM, Hendriks HF, Roholl RJ. Alterations in cytokeratin expression precede histological changes in epithelia of vitamin A-deficient rats. Cell Tissue Res 1992;268:197–203.
59. Darwiche N, Celli G, Sly L, Lancillotti F, DeLuca LM. Retinoid status controls the appearance of reserve cells and keratin expression in mouse cervical epithelium. Cancer Res 1993;53(Suppl 20):2287–2299.
60. Van Agtmaal EJ. Vitamin A and protein in tear fluid: a nutritional field survey on preschool children in northeast Thailand [thesis]. University of Amsterdam, Amsterdam, 1989.

61. Nauss KM, Anderson CA, Conner MW, Newberne PM. Ocular infection with herpes simplex virus (HSV-1) in vitamin A-deficient and control rats. J Nutr 1985;115:1300–1315.

62. DeCarlo JD, Van Horn DL, Hyndiuk RA, Davis SD. Increased susceptibility to infection in experimental xerophthalmia. Arch Ophthalmol 1981;99:1614–1617.

63. Twining SS, Zhou X, Schulte DP, Wilson PM, Fish B, Moulder J. Effect of vitamin A deficiency on the early response to experimental *Pseudomonas* keratitis. Invest Ophthalmol Vis Sci 1996;37:511–522.

64. Shams NB, Reddy CV, Watanabe K, Elgebaly SA, Hanninen LA, Kenyon KR. Increased interleukin–1 activity in the injured vitamin A-deficient cornea. Cornea 1994;13:156–166.

65. Shams NB, Hanninen LA, Chaves HV, et al. Effect of vitamin A deficiency on the adhesion of rat corneal epithelium and the basement membrane complex. Invest Ophthalmol Vis Sci 1993;34:2646–2654.

66. Wilhelm DL. Regeneration of the tracheal epithelium in the vitamin-A-deficient rat. J Pathol Bact 1954;67:361–365.

67. Wong YC, Buck RC. An electron microscopic study of metaplasia of the rat tracheal epithelium in vitamin A deficiency. Lab Invest 1971;24:55–66.

68. McDowell EM, Keenan KP, Huang M. Effects of vitamin A-deprivation on hamster tracheal epithelium: a quantitative morphologic study. Virchows Arch B 1984;45:197–219.

69. Fuchs E, Green H. Regulation of terminal differentiation of cultured human keratinocytes by vitamin A. Cell 1981;25:617–625.

70. Eckert Rl, Green H. Cloning of cDNAs specifying vitamin A-responsive human keratins. Proc Natl Acad Sci USA 1984;81:4321–4325.

71. Manna B, Lund M, Ashbaugh P, Kaufman B, Bhattacharyya SN. Effect of retinoic acid on mucin gene expression in rat airways in vitro. Biochem J 1994;297:309–313.

72. Manna B, Ashbaugh P, Bhattacharyya SN. Retinoic-acid regulated cellular differentiation and mucin gene expression in isolated rabbit tracheal epithelial cells in culture. Inflammation 1995;19:489–502.

73. Paquette NC, Zhang LY, Ellis WA, Scott AL, Kleeberger SR. Vitamin A deficiency enhances ozone-induced lung injury. Am J Physiol 1996;270:L475–L482.

74. Rojanapo W, Lamb AJ, Olson JA. The prevalence, metabolism and migration of goblet cells in rat intestine following the induction of rapid. synchronous vitamin A deficiency. J Nutr 1980;110:178–180.

75. Puengtomwatanakul S, Sirisinha S. Impaired biliary secretion of immunoglobulin A in vitamin A-deficient rats. Proc Soc Exp Biol Med 1986;182:437–442.

76. Warden RA, Strazzari MJ, Dunkley PR, O'Loughlin EV. Vitamin A-deficient rats have only mild changes in jejunal structure and function. J Nutr 1996;126:1817–1826.

77. Ahmed F, Jones DB, Jackson AA. The interaction of vitamin A deficiency and rotavirus infection in the mouse. Br J Nutr 1990;63:363–373.

78. Molloy CL, Laskin JD. Effect of retinoid deficiency on keratin expression in mouse bladder. Exp Mol Pathol 1988;49:128–140.

79. Brown KH, Gaffar A, Alamgir SM. Xerophthalmia, protein-calorie malnutrition, and infections in children. J Pediatr 1979;95:651–656.

80. Rombout JH, Sijtsma SR, West CE, et al. Effect of vitamin A deficiency and Newcastle disease virus infection on IgA and IgM secretion in chickens. Br J Nutr 1992;68:753–763.

81. Gangopadhyay NN, Moldoveanu Z, Stephensen CB. Vitamin A deficiency has different effects on immunoglobulin A production and transport during influenza A infection in BALB/c mice. J Nutr 1996;126:2960–2967.

82. Ahmed F, Jones DB, Jackson AA. Effect of vitamin A deficiency on the immune response to epizootic diarrhoea of infant mice (EDIM) rotavirus infection in mice. Br J Nutr 1991;65:475–485.

83. Wiedermann U, Hanson LA, Holmgren J, Kahu H, Dahlgren UI. Impaired mucosal antibody response to cholera toxin in vitamin A-deficient rats immunized with oral cholera vaccine. Infect Immunol 1993;61:3952–3957.

84. Nikawa T, Odahara K, Koizumi H, et al. Vitamin A prevents the decline in immunoglobulin A and Th2 cytokine levels in small intestinal mucosa of protein-malnourished mice. J Nutr 1999;129:934–941.

85. Nikawa T, Ikemoto M, Kano M, et al. Impaired vitamin A-mediated mucosal IgA response in IL–5 receptor-knockout mice. Biochem Biophys Res Comm 2001;285:546–549.

86. Sarkar J, Gangopadhyay NN, Moldoveanu Z, Mestecky J, Stephensen CB. Vitamin A is required for regulation of polymeric immunoglobulin receptor (pIgR) expression by interleukin-4 and interferon-γ in a human intestinal epithelial cell line. J Nutr 1998;128:1063–1069.

87. Thurnham DI, Northrup-Clewes CA, McCullough FS, Das BS, Lunn PG. Innate immunity, gut integrity, and vitamin A in Gambian and Indian infants. J Infect Dis 2000;182(Suppl 1):S23–S28.

88. Okada M, Bothin C, Blomhoff R, Kanazawa K, Midtvedt T. Vitamin A deficiency impairs colonic healing but not adhesion formation in germ-free and conventional rats. J Invest Surg 1999;12:319–325.

89. Nauss KM, Newberne PM. Local and regional immune function of vitamin A-deficient rats with ocular herpes simplex virus (HSV) infections. J Nutr 1985;115:1316–1324.

90. Bowman TA, Goonewardene IM, Pasatiempo AMG, Ross AC. Vitamin A deficiency decreases natural killer cell activity and interferon production in rats. J Nutr 1990;120:1264–1273.

91. Zhao Z, Murasko DM, Ross AC. The role of vitamin A in natural killer cell cytotoxicity, number and activation in the rat. Natural Immunity 1994;13:29–41.

92. Dawson HD, Li NQ, DeCicco KL, Nibert JA, Ross AC. Chronic marginal vitamin A status reduces natural killer cell number and function in aging Lewis rats. J Nutr 1999;129:1510–1517.

93. Hussey G, Hughes J, Potgieter S, et al. Vitamin A status and supplementation and its effects on immunity in children with AIDS. Abstracts of the XVII International Vitamin A Consultative Group Meeting, Guatemala City. International Life Sciences Institute, Washington, DC, 1996, p. 6.

94. Zhao Z, Matsuura T, Popoff K, Ross AC. Effects of N-(4-hydroxyphenyl)-retinamide on the number and cytotoxicity of natural killer cells in vitamin-A-sufficient and-deficient rats. Nat Immunol 1994;13:280–288.

95. Lawson ND, Berliner N. Neutrophil maturation and the role of retinoic acid. Exp Hematol 1999:27: 1355–1367.

96. Ongsakul M, Sirisinha S, Lamb A. Impaired blood clearance of bacteria and phagocytic activity in vitamin A-deficient rats. Proc Soc Exp Biol Med 1985;178:204–208.

97. Twining SS, Schulte DP, Wilson PM, Fish BL, Moulder JE. Vitamin A deficiency alters rat neutrophil function. J Nutr 1996;127:558–565.

98. Wiedermann U, Tarkowski A, Bremell T, Hanson LA, Kahu H, Dahlgren UI. Vitamin A deficiency predisposes to Staphylococcus aureus infection. Infect Immunol 1996;64:209–214.

99. Higuchi H, Nagahata H. Effects of vitamins A and E on superoxide production and intracellular signaling of neutrophils in Holstein calves. Can J Vet Res 2000;64:69–75.

100. Zhao Z, Ross AC. Retinoic acid repletion restores the number of leukocytes and their subsets and stimulates natural cytotoxicity in vitamin A-deficient rats. J Nutr 1995;125:2064–2073.

101. Kuwata T, Wang IM, Tamura T, et al. Vitamin A defciency in mice causes a systemic expansion of myeloid cells. Blood 2000;95:3349–3356.

102. Semba RD, Muhilal, Ward BJ, et al. Abnormal T-cell subset proportions in vitamin A-deficient children. Lancet 1993;341:5–8.

103. Benn CS, Lisse IM, Bale C, et al. No strong long-term effect of vitamin A supplementation in infancy on CD4 and CD8 T-cell subsets. A community study from Guinea-Bissau, West Africa. Ann Trop Paediatr 2000;20:259–264.

104. Van Schravendijk MR, Handunnetti SM, Barnwell JW, Howard RJ. Normal human erythrocytes express CD36, an adhesion molecule of monocytes, platelets, and endothelial cells. Blood 1992;80:2105–2114.

105. Perrin MC, Blanchet JP, Mouchiroud G. Modulation of human and mouse erythropoiesis by thyroid hormone and retinoic acid: evidence for specific effects at different steps of the erythroid pathway. Hematol Cell Ther 1997;39:19–26.

106. Zermati Y, Fichelson S, Valensi F, et al. Transforming growth factor inhibits erythropoiesis by blocking proliferation of accelerating differentiation of erythroid progenitors. Exp Hematol 2000;28:885–894.

107. Douer D, Koeffler HP. Retinoic acid enhances growth of human early erythroid progenitor cells in vitro. J Clin Invest 1982;69:1039–1041.

108. Correa PN, Axelrad AA. Retinyl acetate and all-trans-retinoic acid enhance erythroid colony formation in vitro by circulating human progenitors in an improved serum-free medium. Int J Cell Cloning 1992;10:286–291.

109. Rusten LS, Dybedal I, Blomhoff HK, Blomhoff R, Smeland EB, Jacobsen SE. The RAR-RXR as well as the RXR-RXR pathway is involved in signaling growth inhibition of CD34+ erythroid progenitor cells. Blood 1996;87:1728–1736.

110. Zauli G, Visani G, Vitale M, Gibellini D, Bertolaso L, Capitani S. All-trans retinoic acid shows multiple effects on the survival, proliferation and differentiation of human fetal CD34+ haemopoietic progenitor cells. Br J Haematol 1995;90:274–282.

111. Josefsen D, Blomhoff HK, Lømo J, Blystad AK, Smeland EB. Retinoic acid induces apoptosis of human CD34[+] hematopoietic progenitor cells: involvement of retinoic acid receptors and retinoid X receptors depends on lineage commitment of the hematopoietic progenitor cells. Exp Hematol 1999:27:642–653.

112. Semba RD, Bloem MW. The anemia of vitamin A deficiency: epidemiology and pathogenesis. Eur J Clin Nutr 2002;56:271–281.

113. Breitman TR, Selonick SE, Collins SJ. Induction of differentiation of the human promyelocytic leukemia cell line (HL-60) by retinoic acid. Proc Natl Acad Sci USA 1980;77:2936–2940.

114. Öberg F, Botling J, Nilsson K. Functional antagonism between vitamin D_3 and retinoic acid in the regulation of CD14 and CD23 expression during monocytic differentiation of U-937 cells. J Immunol 1993;150:3487–3495.

115. Hemmi H, Breitman TR. Induction of functional differentiation of human monocytic leukemia cell line (THP-1) by retinoic acid and cholera toxin. Jpn J Canc Res 1985;76:345–351.

116. Katz DR, Drzymala M, Turton JA, et al. Regulation of accessory cell function by retinoids in murine immune responses. Br J Exp Pathol 1987;68:343–350.

117. Katz DR, Mukherjee S, Malsey J, et al. Vitamin A acetate as a regulator of accessory cell function in delayed-type hypersensitivity responses. Int Arch Allergy Appl Immunol 1987;82:53–56.

118. Smith SM, Levy NS, Hayes CE. Impaired immunity in vitamin A-deficient mice. J Nutr 1987;117:857–865.

119. Mathew JS, Sharma RP. Effect of all-*trans*-retinoic acid on cytokine production in a murine macrophage cell line. Int J Immunopharm 2000;22:693–706.

120. Matikainen S, Serkkola E, Hurme M. Retinoic acid enhances IL-1β expression in myeloid leukemia cells and in human monocytes. J Immunol 1991;147:162–167.

121. Hashimoto S, Hayashi S, Yoshida S, et al. Retinoic acid differentially regulates interleukin-1β and interleukin-1 receptor antagonist production by human alveolar macrophages. Leukemia Res 1998;22:1057–1061.

122. Na SY, Kang BY, Chung SW, et al. Retinoids inhibit interleukin-12 production in macrophages through physical associations of retinoid X receptor and NFκB. J Biol Chem 1999;274:7674–7680.

123. Dillehay DL, Walla AS, Lamon EW. Effects of retinoids on macrophage function and IL-1 activity. J Leuk Biol 1988;44:353–360.

124. Trechsel U, Evêquoz V, Fleisch H. Stimulation of interleukin 1 and 3 production by retinoid acid in vitro. Biochem J 1985;230:339–344.

125. Hatchigian EA, Santos JI, Broitman SA, Vitale JJ. Vitamin A supplementation improves macrophage function and bacterial clearance during experimental *Salmonella* infection. Proc Soc Exp Biol Med 1989;191:47–54.

126. Maisey J, Miller K. Assessment of the ability of mice fed on vitamin A supplemented diet to respond to a variety of potential contact sensitizers. Contact Dermatitis 1986;15:17–23.

127. Sailstad DM, Krishnan SD, Tepper JS, Doerfler DL, Selgrade MK. Dietary vitamin A enhances sensitivity of the local lymph node assay. Toxicology 1995;96:157–163.

128. Meunier L, Bohjanen K, Voorhees JJ, et al. Retinoic acid upregulates human Langerhans cell antigen presentation and surface expression of HLA-DR and CD11c, a β2 integrin integrally involved in T-cell activation. J Invest Dermatol 1994;103:775–779.

129. Göttgens B, Green AR. Retinoic acid and the differentiation of lymphohemapoietic stem cells. Bio Assays 1995;17:187–189.

130. Garbe A, Buck J, Hämmerling U. Retinoids are important cofactors in T cell activation. J Exp Med 1992;176:109–117.

131. Allende LM, Corell A, Madrono A, et al. Retinol (vitamin A) is a cofactor in CD3-induced human T-lymphocyte activation. Immunology 1997;90:388–396.

132. Friedman A, Halevy O, Schrift M, et al. Retinoic acid promotes proliferation and induces expression of retinoic acid receptor-α gene in murine T lymphocytes. Cell Immunol 1993;152:240–248.

133. Sidell N, Chang B, Bhatti L. Upregulation by retinoic acid of interleukin-2-receptor mRNA in human T lymphocytes. Cell Immunol 1993;146:28–37.

134. Rahman MM, Mahalanabis D, Alvarez JO, et al. Effect of early vitamin A supplementation on cell-mediated immunity in infants younger than 6 mo. Am J Clin Nutr 1997;65:144–148.

135. Stephensen CB. Vitamin A, infection, and immune function. Annu Rev Nutr 2001;21:167–192.

136. Carman JA, Pond L, Nashold F, Wassom DL, Hayes CE. Immunity to *Trichinella spiralis* infection in vitamin A-deficient mice. J Exp Med 1992;175:111–120.
137. Cantorna MT, Nashold FE, Hayes CE. In vitamin A deficiency multiple mechanisms establish a regulatory T helper cell imbalance with excess Th1 and insufficient Th2 function. J Immunol 1994;152:1515–1522.
138. Cantorna MT, Nashold FE, Hayes CE. Vitamin A deficiency results in a priming environment conductive for Th1 cell development. Eur J Immunol 1995;25:1673–1679.
139. Wiedermann U, Hanson LA, Kahu H, Dahlgren UI. Aberrant T-cell function in vitro and impaired T-cell dependent antibody response in vivo in vitamin A-deficient rats. Immunology 1993;80:581–586.
140. Frankenburg S, Wang X, Milner Y. Vitamin A inhibits cytokines produced by type 1 lymphocytes *in vitro*. Cell Immunol 1998;185:75–81.
141. Cui D, Moldoveanu Z, Stephensen CB. High-level dietary vitamin A enhances T-helper type 2 cytokine production and secretory immunoglobulin A response to influenza A virus infection in BALB/c mice. J Nutr 2000;130:1322–1329.
142. Stephensen CB, Rasoly R, Jiang X, et al. Vitamin A enhances in vitro Th2 development via retinoid X receptor pathway. J Immunol 2002;168:4495–4503.
143. Carman JA, Hayes CE. Abnormal regulation of IFN-γ secretion in vitamin A deficiency. J Immunol 1991;147:1247–1252.
144. Cantorna MT, Nashold FE, Chun TY, Hayes CE. Vitamin A down-regulation of IFN-γ synthesis in cloned mouse Th1 lymphocytes depends on the CD28 costimulatory pathway. J Immunol 1996;156:2674–2679.
145. Cippitelli M, Ye J, Viggiano V, et al. Retinoic acid-induced transcriptional modulation of the human interferon-gamma promoter. J Biol Chem 1996;271:26783–26793.
146. Buck J, Ritter G, Dannecker L, et al. Retinol is essential for growth of activated human B cells. J Exp Med 1990;171:1613–1624.
147. Blomhoff HK, Smeland EB, Erikstein B, et al. Vitamin A is a key regulator for cell growth, cytokine production, and differentiation in normal B cells. J Biol Chem 1992;267:23988–23992.
148. Buck J, Myc A, Garbe A, Cathomas G. Differences in the action and metabolism between retinol and retinoic acid in B lymphocytes. J Cell Biol 1991;115:851–859.
149. Israel H, Odziemiec C, Ballow M. The effects of retinoic acid on immunoglobulin synthesis by human cord blood mononuclear cells. Clin Immunol Immunopathol 1991;59:417–425.
150. Wang W, Ballow M. The effects of retinoic acid on in vitro immunoglobulin synthesis by cord blood and adult peripheral blood mononuclear cells. Cell Immunol 1993;148:291–300.
151. Wang W, Napoli JL, Ballow M. The effects of retinol on in vitro immunoglobulin synthesis by cord blood and adult peripheral blood mononuclear cells. Clin Exp Immunol 1993;92:164–168.
152. Ballow M, Wang W, Xiang S. Modulation of B-cell immunoglobulin synthesis by retinoic acid. Clin Immunol Immunopathol 1996;80:S73–S81.
153. Lømo J, Smeland EB, Ulven S, et al. RAR, not RXR, ligands inhibit cell activation and prevent apoptosis in B-lymphocytes. J Cell Physiol 1998;175:68–77.
154. Aukrust P, Müller F, Ueland T, Svardal AM, Berge RK, Frøland SS. Decreased vitamin A levels in common variable immunodeficiency: vitamin A supplementation *in vivo* enhances immunoglobulin production and downregulates inflammatory responses. Eur J Clin Invest 2000;30:252–259.
155. Smith SM, Hayes CE. Contrasting impairments in IgM and IgG responses of vitamin A-deficient mice. Proc Natl Acad Sci USA 1987;84:5878–5882.
156. Semba RD, Muhilal, Scott AL, et al. Depressed immune response to tetanus in children with vitamin A deficiency. J Nutr 1992;122:101–107.
157. Semba RD, Muhilal, Scott AL, Natadisastra G, West KP Jr, Sommer A. Effect of vitamin A supplementation on IgG subclass responses to tetanus toxoid in children. Clin Diagn Lab Immunol 1994;1:172–175.
158. Rahman MM, Mahalanabis D, Hossain S, et al. Simultaneous vitamin A administration at routine immunization contact enhances antibody response to diphtheria vaccine in infants younger than six months. J Nutr 1999;129:2192–2195.
159. Friedman A, Sklan D. Antigen-specific immune response impairment in the chick as influenced by dietary vitamin A. J Nutr 1989;119:790–795.
160. Kinoshita M, Pasatiempo AMG, Taylor CE, Ross AC. Immunological memory to tetanus toxoid is established and maintained in the vitamin A-depleted rat. FASEB J 1991;5:2473–2481.

161. Arora D, Ross AC. Antibody response against tetanus toxoid is enhanced by lipopolysaccharide or tumor necrosis factor-alpha in vitamin A-sufficient and deficient rats. Am J Clin Nutr 1994;59:922–928.

162. Pasatiempo AMG, Bowman TA, Taylor CE, Ross AC. Vitamin A depletion and repletion: effects on antibody response to the capsular polysaccharide of *Streptococcus pneumoniae,* type III (SSS-III). Am J Clin Nutr 1989;49:501–510.

163. Lavasa S, Kumar L, Chakravarti RN, Kumar M. Early humoral immune response in vitamin A deficiency—an experimental study. Indian J Exp Biol 1988:26:431–435.

164. Pasatiempo AMG, Kinoshita M, Taylor CE, Ross AC. Antibody production in vitamin A-depleted rats is impaired after immunization with bacterial polysaccharide or protein antigens. FASEB J 1990;4:2518–2527.

165. Molrine DC, Polk DB, Ciamarra A, Phillips N, Ambrosino DM. Impaired human responses to tetanus toxoid in vitamin A-deficient SCID mice reconstituted with human peripheral blood lymphocytes. Infect Immunol 1995;63:2867–2872.

166. Kutukculer N, Akil T, Egemen A, et al. Adequate immune response to tetanus toxoid and failure of vitamin A and E supplementation to enhance antibody response in healthy children. Vaccine 2000;18:2979–2984.

167. Quadro L, Gamble MV, Vogel S, et al. Retinol and retinol-binding protein: gut integrity and circulating immunoglobulins. J Infect Dis 2000;182(Suppl):S97–S102.

168. Scrimshaw NS, Taylor CE, Gordon JE. Interactions of Nutrition and Infection. World Health Organization, Geneva, 1968.

169. Beisel WR. Single nutrients and immunity. Am J Clin Nutr 1982;35(2 Suppl):417–468.

170. Nauss KM. Influence of vitamin A status on the immune system. In: Bauernfeind JC (ed.). Vitamin A Deficiency and Its Control. Academic, Orlando, FL, 1986, pp. 207–243.

171. Semba RD. Vitamin A, immunity, and infection. Clin Infect Dis 1994;19:489–499.

172. Bieri JG, McDaniel EG, Rogers WE Jr. Survival of germfree rats without vitamin A. Science 1969;163:574–575.

173. Krishnan S, Krishnan AD, Mustafa AS, Talwar GP, Ramalingaswami V. Effect of vitamin A and undernutrition on the susceptibility of rodents to a malrial parasite *Plasmodium berghei.* J Nutr 1976;106:784–791.

174. Sijtsma SR, West CE, Rombout JHWM, van der Zijpp AJ. The interaction between vitamin A status and Newcastle disease virus infection in chickens. J Nutr 1989;119:932–939.

175. Cohen BE, Elin RJ. Vitamin A-induced nonspecific resistance to infection. J Infect Dis 1974;129: 597–600.

176. Cohen BE, Elin RJ. Enhanced resistance to certain infections in vitamin A-treated mice. Plast Reconstr Surg 1974;54:192–194.

177. Oomen HAPC, McLaren DS, Escapini H. Epidemiology and public health aspects of hypovitaminosis A. Trop Geogr Med 1964;4:271–315.

178. Griffin DE. Immune responses during measles virus infection. Curr Top Microbiol Immunol 1995;191:117–134.

179. Markowitz L, Nzilambi N, Driskell WJ, et al. Vitamin A levels and mortality among hospitalized measles patients, Kinshasa, Zaire. J Trop Pediatr 1989;35:109–112.

180. Ellison JB. Intensive vitamin therapy in measles. Br Med J 1932;2:708–711.

181. Barclay AJG, Foster A, Sommer A. Vitamin A supplements and mortality related to measles: a randomised clinical trial. Br Med J 1987;294:294–296.

182. Hussey GD, Klein M. A randomized, controlled trial of vitamin A in children with severe measles. N Engl J Med 1990;323:160–164.

183. Coutsoudis A, Broughton M, Coovadia HM. Vitamin A supplementation reduces measles morbidity in young African children: a randomized, placebo-controlled, double-blind trial. Am J Clin Nutr 1991;54:890–895.

184. Ogaro FO, Orinda VA, Onyango FE, Black RE. Effect of vitamin A on diarrhoeal and respiratory complications of measles. Trop Geogr Med 1993;45:283–286.

185. Coutsoudis A, Kiepiela P, Coovadia HM, Broughton M. Vitamin A supplementation enhances specific IgG antibody levels and total lymphocyte numbers while improving morbidity in measles. Pediatr Infect Dis J 1992;11:203–209.

186. Semba RD, Munasir Z, Beeler J, et al. Reduced seroconversion to measles in infants given vitamin A with measles vaccination. Lancet 1995;345:1330–1332.

187. Semba RD, Akib A, Beeler J, et al. Effect of vitamin A supplementation on measles vaccination in nine-month-old infants. Public Health 1997;111:245–247.

188. Benn CS, Aaby P, Balé C, et al. Randomised trial of effect of vitamin A supplementation on antibody response to measles vaccine in Guinea-Bissau, West Africa. Lancet 1997;350:101–105.

189. Ross DA, Cutts FT. Vindication of policy of vitamin A with measles vaccination. Lancet 1997;350: 81–82.

190. Bahl R, Kumar R, Bhandari N, Kant S, Srivastava R, Bhan MK. Vitamin A administered with measles vaccine to nine-month-old infants does not reduce vaccine immunogenicity. J Nutr 1999;129:1569–1573.

191. Bhaskaram P, Rao KV. Enhancement in seroconversion to measles vaccine with simultaneous adminstration of vitamin A in 9-month-old Indian infants. Indian J Pediatr 1997;64:503–509.

192. Benn CS, Balde A, George E, et al. Effect of vitamin A supplementation on measles-specific antibody levels in Guinea-Bissau. Lancet 2002;359:1313–1314.

193. Brilliant LB, Pokhrel RP, Grasset NC, et al. Epidemiology of blindness in Nepal. Bull World Health Organ 1985;63:375–386.

194. DeSole G, Belay Y, Zegeye B. Vitamin A deficiency in southern Ethiopia. Am J Clin Nutr 1987;45: 780–784.

195. Sommer A, Katz J, Tarwotjo I. Increased risk of respiratory disease and diarrhea in children with preexisting mild vitamin A deficiency. Am J Clin Nutr 1984;40:1090–1095.

196. Schaumberg DA, O'Connor J, Semba RD. Risk factors for xerophthalmia in the Republic of Kiribati. Eur J Clin Nutr 1996;50:761–764.

197. Sommer A, Tarwotjo I, Djunaedi E, et al. Impact of vitamin A supplementation on childhood mortality: a randomized controlled community trial. Lancet 1986;1:1169–1173.

198. Beaton GH, Martorell R, L'Abbe KA, et al. Effectiveness of Vitamin A Supplementation in the Control of Young Child Morbidity and Mortality in Developing Countries. ACC/SCN State-of-the-Art Nutrition Policy Discussion Paper No. 13, United Nations, New York, NY, 1993.

199. The Vitamin A and Pneumonia Working Group. Potential interventions for the prevention of childhood pneumonia in developing countries: a meta-analysis of data from field trials to assess the impact of vitamin A supplementation on pneumonia morbidity and mortality. Bull World Health Organ 1995:73:609–619.

200. Barreto ML, Santos LMP, Assis AMO, et al. Effect of vitamin A supplementation on diarrhoea and acute lower-respiratory-tract infections in young children in Brazil. Lancet 1994;344:228–231.

201. Filteau SM, Rollins NC, Coutsoudis A, Sullivan KR, Willumsen JF, Tomkins AM. The effect of antenatal vitamin A and beta-carotene supplementation on gut integrity of infants of HIV-infected South African women. J Pediatr Gastroenterol Nutr 2001;32:464–470.

202. Alvarez JO, Salazar-Lindo E, Kohatsu J, Miranda P, Stephensen CB. Urinary excretion of retinol in children with acute diarrhea. Am J Clin Nutr 1995;61:1273–1276.

203. Mitra AK, Alvarez JO, Guay-Woodford L, et al. Urinary retinol excretion and kidney function in children with shigellosis. Am J Clin Nutr 1998;68:1095–1103.

204. Kelly P, Musuku J, Kafwembe E, et al. Impaired bioavailability of vitamin A in adults and children with persistent diarrhoea in Zambia. Aliment Pharmacol Ther 2001;15:973–979.

205. Hossain S, Biswas R, Kabir I, et al. Single dose vitamin A treatment in acute shigellosis in Bangladeshi children: randomised double blind controlled trial. Br Med J 1998;316:422–426.

206. Kjolhede CL, Chew FJ, Gadomski AM, Marroquin DP. Clinical trial of vitamin A as adjuvant treatment for lower respiratory tract infections. J Pediatr 1995;126:807–812.

207. Nacul LC, Kirkwood BR, Arthur P, Morris SS, Magalhães M, Fink MCDS. Randomised, double blind, placebo controlled clinical trial of efficacy of vitamin A treatment in non-measles childhood pneumonia. Br Med J 1997;315:505–510.

208. Fawzi WW, Mbise RL, Fataki MR, et al. Vitamin A supplementation and severity of pneumonia in children admitted to the hospital in Dar es Salaam, Tanzania. Am J Clin Nutr 1998;68:187–192.

209. Dowell SF, Papic Z, Bresee JS, et al. Treatment of respiratory syncytial virus infection with vitamin A: a randomized, placebo-controlled trial in Santiago, Chile. Pediatr Infect Dis J 1996;15:782–786.

210. Bresee JS, Fischer M, Dowell SF, et al. Vitamin A therapy for children with respiratory syncytial virus infection: a multicenter trial in the United States. Pediatr Infect Dis J 1996;15:777–782.

211. Quinlan KP, Hayani KC. Vitamin A and respiratory syncytial virus infection. Serum levels and supplementation trial. Arch Pediatr Adolesc Med 1996;150:25–30.

212. Fawzi WW, Mbise R, Spiegelman D, Fataki M, Hertzmark E, Ndossi G. Vitamin A supplements and diarrheal and respiratory tract infections among children in Dar es Salaam, Tanzania. J Pediatr 2000;137:660–667.

213. Sempertegui F, Estrella B, Camaniero V, et al. The beneficial effects of weekly low-dose vitamin A supplementation on acute lower respiratory infections and diarrhea in Ecuadorian children. Pediatrics 1999;104:e1.

214. Griffiths JK. The vitamin A paradox. J Pediatr 2000;137:604–607.

215. Dudley L, Hussey G, Huskissen J, Kessow G. Vitamin A status, other risk factors and acute respiratory infection morbidity in children. South Africa Med J 1997;87:65–70.

216. West KP Jr, Katz J, Shrestha SR, et al. Mortality of infants <6 mo of age supplemented with vitamin A: a randomized, double-masked trial in Nepal. Am J Clin Nutr 1995;62:143–148.

217. WHO/CHD Immunisation-Linked Vitamin A Supplementation Study Group. Randomised trial to assess benefits and safety of vitamin A supplementation linked to immunisation in early infancy. Lancet 1998;352:1257–1263.

218. Semba RD, Munasir Z, Akib A, et al. Integration of vitamin A supplementation with the Expanded Programme on Immunization: lack of impact on morbidity or infant growth. Acta Paediatr 2001;90:1107–1111.

219. Stürchler D, Tanner M, Hanck A, et al. A longitudinal study on relations of retinol with parasitic infections and the immune response in children of Kikwawila village, Tanzania. Acta Tropica 1987;44:213–227.

220. Galan P, Samba C, Luzeau R, Amedee-Manesme O. Vitamin A deficiency in pre-school age Congolese children during malaria attacks. Part 2: impact of parasitic disease on vitamin A status. Int J Vit Nutr Res 1990;60:224–228.

221. Friis H, Mwaniki D, Omondi B, et al. Serum retinol concentrations and *Schistosoma mansoni* intestinal helminths, and malarial parasitemia: a cross-sectional study in Kenyan preschool and primary school children. Am J Clin Nutr 1997;66:665–671.

222. Shankar AH, Genton B, Semba RD, et al. Effect of vitamin A supplementation on morbidity due to *Plasmodium falciparum* in young children in Papua New Guinea: a randomised trial. Lancet 1999;354:203–209.

223. Kennedy CM, Kuhn L, Stein Z. Vitamin A and HIV infection: disease progression, mortality, and transmission. Nutr Rev 2000;58:291–303.

224. Coutsoudis A, Bobat RA, Coovadia HM, Kuhn L, Tsai WY, Stein ZA. The effects of vitamin A supplementation on the morbidity of children born to HIV-infected women. Am J Pub Health 1995;85:1076–1081.

225. Fawzi WW, Mbise RL, Hertzmark E, et al. A randomized trial of vitamin A supplements in relation to mortality among human immunodeficiency virus-infected and uninfected children in Tanzania. Pediatr Infect Dis J 1999;18:127–133.

226. Semba RD, Ndugwa C, Perry RO, et al. Effect of vitamin A on morbidity and mortality of HIV-infected children. Abstracts of the 23rd International Congress of Pediatrics, Beijing, China, September 9–14, 2001, abstract 0A-F2-2.

227. Fawzi WW, Msamanga G, Hunter D, et al. Randomized trial of vitamin supplements in relation to vertical transmission of HIV-1 in Tanzania. J Acquired Immun Syndr 2000;23:246–254.

228. Coutsoudis A, Pillay K, Spooner E, Kuhn L, Coovadia HM. Randomized trial testing the effect of vitamin A supplementation on pregnancy outcomes and early mother-to-child transmission in Durban, South Africa. AIDS 1999;13:1517–1524.

229. Kumwenda N, Miotti PG, Taha TE, et al. Antenatal vitamin A supplementation increases birthweight and decreases anemia, but does not prevent HIV transmission or decrease mortality in infants born to HIV-infected women in Malawi. Clin Infect Dis 2002;35:618–624.

230. Fawzi WW, Msamanga GI, Hunter D, et al. Randomized trial of vitamin supplements in relation to transmission of HIV-1 through breastfeeding and early child mortality. AIDS 2002;16:1935–1944.

231. Semba RD, Lyles CM, Margolick JB, et al. Vitamin A supplementation and human immunodeficiency virus load in injection drug users. J Infect Dis 1998;177: 611–616.

232. Hanekom WA, Potgieter S, Hughes EJ, Malan H, Kessow G, Hussey GD. Vitamin A status and therapy in childhood pulmonary tuberculosis. J Pediatr 1997;131:925–927.

233. Karyadi E, West CE, Schultink W, et al. A double-blind, placebo-controlled study of vitamin A and zinc supplementation in persons with tuberculosis in Indonesia: effects on clinical response and nutritional status. Am J Clin Nutr 2002;75:720–727.

234. Christian P, Schulze K, Stoltzfus RJ, West KP Jr. Hyporetinolemia, illness symptoms, and acute phase protein response in pregnant women with and without night blindness. Am J Clin Nutr 1998;67: 1237–1243.

235. Christian P, West KP Jr, Khatry SK, et al. Night blindness of pregnancy in rural Nepal—nutritional and health risks. Int J Epidemiol 1998;27:231–237.

236. Christian P, West KP Jr, Khatry SK, et al. Night blindness during pregnancy and subsequent mortality among women in Nepal: effects of vitamin A and beta-carotene supplementation. Am J Epidemiol 2000;152:542–547.

237. Christian P, West KP Jr, Khatry SK, et al. Vitamin A or beta-carotene supplementation reduces symptoms of illness in pregnant or lactating Nepali women. J Nutr 2000;130:2675–2682.

238. West KP Jr, Katz J, Khatry SK, et al. Double blind, cluster randomised trial of low dose supplementation with vitamin A or beta carotene on mortality related to pregnancy in Nepal. Br Med J 1999;318: 570–575.

239. Green HN, Pindar D, Davis G, Mellanby E. Diet as a prophylactic agent against puerperal sepsis. Br Med J 1931;2:595–598.

240. Cameron SJ. An aid in the prevention of puerperal sepsis. Trans Edinburgh Obstet Soc 1931;52:93–103.

7 Vitamin C

Ronald Anderson

1. INTRODUCTION

Vitamin C (VC) was first isolated by Szent Györgyi (1930) and subsequently identified as an essential cofactor for prolyl and lysyl hydroxylases in collagen biosynthesis, a component of connective tissue *(1)*. The vitamin is also essential for the optimum functioning of several other enzymes, including those involved in the biosynthesis of carnitine *(2)* and norepinephrine *(3)*, as well as those involved in tyrosine metabolism *(4)*.

Notwithstanding its primary function in the maintenance of the structural integrity of connective tissue through promoting collagen biosynthesis, VC was studied in several well-publicized studies, conducted in the 1960s and 1970s, that focused on its alternative properties, particularly its potential in the chemoprophylaxis, or treatment, of commonly occurring conditions, such as the common cold and cancer (reviewed in refs. *[5]* and *[6]*, respectively). Although VC confers moderate protection against the common cold by ameliorating disease symptoms and duration *(5)* and may also be important in preventing certain types of inflammation-related cancers, such as gastric carcinoma *(7)*, it is only recently that compelling evidence for the existence of alternative activities of VC, which are important in the maintenance of optimum health, has been found. Foremost among these are VC's antioxidative properties *(8)*, which are involved in maintaining optimum function of organs, such as the stomach *(7)*, lungs *(9–11)*, liver *(12)*, and pancreas *(13)*, as well as the circulatory *(14–16)*, skeletal *(17)*, and immune systems *(18,19)*, emphasizing VC's contribution to sustaining good health and longevity *(20)*. This contention is convincingly underscored by the observations that a murine ascorbic acid transporter deficiency results in the death of newborn mice within a few minutes resulting from brain hemorrhage and respiratory failure *(21)*.

Although this review focuses on VC and the immune system, this interaction should not be viewed in isolation. This is because efficient eradication of microbial and viral pathogens by host immunodefenses in the setting of VC-mediated attenuation of oxidant-inflicted damage to bystander cells and tissues may retard the loss of pulmonary, hepatic, pancreatic, and gastric function secondary to repeated and/or chronic inflammation.

From: *Diet and Human Immune Function*
Edited by: D. A. Hughes, L. G. Darlington, and A. Bendich © Humana Press Inc., Totowa, NJ

2. VITAMIN C AND IMMUNE FUNCTIONS

Because interactions of VC with the immune system have been the subject of several recent reviews *(18,19,22,23)*, this review focuses, for the most part, on recent contributions, including both human- and animal-based studies, which have provided insights into VC-mediated immunomodulatory activity targets and mechanisms.

2.1. Vitamin C and Neutrophil Functions

Human neutrophils have relatively high intracellular VC concentrations in comparison with those of circulating monocytes and lymphocytes *(24)*. These high intracellular VC concentrations in neutrophils are necessary to counteract the extremely high levels of oxidative stress to which these cells are exposed after receptor-mediated activation of the membrane-associated superoxide-generating complex, nicotinamide adenine dinucleotide phosphate (NADPH) oxidase (also known as the respiratory-burst enzyme) by chemoattractants, cytokines, and opsonized microbial pathogens. Although the NADPH oxidase activation is a crucial event in generating antimicrobial reactive oxidants by these and other types of phagocyte, as well as the restoration of calcium homeostasis to these cells *(25)*, these same oxidants, which are indiscriminate to biological targets, present the potential threat of oxidant-inflicted damage to the neutrophils. If production is excessive, these oxidants are cytotoxic, whereas at lower concentrations, they cause autooxidative inhibition of neutrophil functions, with chemotaxis and antimicrobial activity, the latter somewhat paradoxically, being particularly sensitive *(18,19)*. Autooxidative inhibition of antimicrobial activity is a consequence of the vulnerability of NADPH oxidase to oxidative inactivation *(18,19)*.

In neutrophils, it is well-accepted that VC availability, as well as the availability of other cytoprotective antioxidants, such as glutathione, is a determinant of the sustainability of the functions of these cells after receptor-mediated activation of NADPH oxidase *(18,19,26)*. The potentiating effects of high-dose supplementation with the vitamin on the ex vivo chemotactic, phagocytic, and antimicrobial functions of neutrophils that are isolated from humans, as well as from animals (fish, guinea pigs, cattle and horses), are well-documented, as are those of coincubation of isolated neutrophils with the vitamin in vitro *(18,19,26)*.

In addition to the plethora of earlier reports, Mulero and colleagues have reported that coincubation with VC of head/kidney phagocytic leukocytes, isolated from gilthead seabream, caused significant dose-related augmentation of the migratory, phagocytic, and antimicrobial functions of these cells in vitro *(27)*. Similar effects were also observed with vitamin E (VE), whereas exposure of the cells to the combination of VC and VE resulted in synergistic enhancement of the respiratory burst *(27)*. Similar findings have been reported by Delrio, Ruedas, and Medina et al., who observed that exposure of isolated murine macrophages to VC in vitro was accompanied by enhancement of chemotaxis, phagocytosis, and superoxide production by the cells *(28)*. These VC effects were mimicked by other antioxidants, such as VE, glutathione, *N*-acetylcysteine, thioproline, and thiazolidine-4-carboxylic acid, underscoring the lack of specificity of the antioxidative interactions of VC and phagocytes *(28)*. Nevertheless, the ease of administration of VC, as well as its compartmentalization at intracellular sites at which it can perform its antioxidative functions most efficiently, underpin the biologic role of this vitamin in neutrophil function modulation.

Intracellular concentrations of ascorbate in human leukocytes decline with advancing age, as do those of another important intracellular antioxidant, glutathione *(29,30)*. This age-associated deficiency of intracellular ascorbate has recently been reported to be accompanied by neutrophil function impairment, as well as with decreased total circulating concentrations of immunoglobulins (Ig) G and M *(30)*. Leukocyte ascorbate deficiency was corrected by oral administration of the vitamin and was accompanied by improved neutrophil functions and serum Ig levels *(30)*. The authors conclude that the age-related VC deficiency contributes to both impaired neutrophil functions and humoral immune responses and plays a role in the increased risk of illness in old age *(30)*.

The findings of Jayachandran and colleagues *(30)* support those of an earlier study conducted by de la Fuente and coworkers *(31)*. These investigators reported that administration of 1 g VC combined with 200 mg VE daily for 16 wk to healthy elderly women or to elderly women suffering from major depression disorders or coronary heart disease was accompanied by enhancement of neutrophil chemotaxis and phagocytic activity *(31)*. Interestingly, improved neutrophil functions were observed in both study groups and were accompanied by significant decreases in serum lipid peroxide and cortisol concentrations. Although the decreases in circulating lipid peroxides are indicative of improved resistance to oxidative stress, the relevance of decreased circulating cortisol levels to enhancement of neutrophil function is unclear, because these cells are believed to be fairly resistant to the antiinflammatory/immunosuppressive actions of corticosteroids *(32,33)* (*see* also discussion in Section 2.6.3 in Chapter 3). The depressive effects of VC supplementation on circulating cortisol concentrations, which have been reported in several studies, are, nevertheless, potentially important in the interaction of the vitamin with other cellular components of the immune system and are considered in greater detail in Section 3.3.

The aforementioned reports clearly support the substantial body of earlier literature documenting VC involvement, predominantly, if not exclusively, by antioxidative mechanisms, in the maintenance of optimum phagocyte functions. Exceptions to these do, however, exist. For example, in a recent study, VC administration (2 g/d for 1 wk) to a small group of well-trained biathlon athletes failed to attenuate the impairment of neutrophil phagocytic and antimicrobial activity secondary to the oxidative stress that accompanied participation in the biathlon event *(34)*. Although this observation may be difficult to reconcile with the proposed dependence of neutrophil function on VC status, it is noteworthy that biologic antioxidant defenses (both by enzymatic and oxidant-scavenging mechanisms) are upregulated in well-trained athletes *(35)*, which may negate the effects of VC supplementation. If this contention is correct, then the enhancing effects of the vitamin on neutrophil functions may be most evident in individuals with a sedentary lifestyle, as well as in the elderly.

Phagocyte functions that are protected/augmented by VC are shown in Table 1.

2.2. Vitamin C and Lymphocyte Functions

As with phagocytic cells, VC also modulates lymphocyte functions. However, there are several important distinctions concerning the effects of the vitamin on the functions of these two cell types. First, it is the proliferative responses of lymphocytes that are primarily affected by the vitamin (as opposed to chemotaxis and antimicrobial activity in phagocytes), and, second, several different, possibly interacting, biochemical mechanisms contribute to VC-mediated enhancement of lymphocyte functions.

Table 1
Phagocyte Functions That Are Sustained by Vitamin C

Cell type	Functions enhanced by vitamin C	References
Neutrophils (from humans, animals, and fish)	Chemotaxis, phagocytosis, superoxide production, and antimicrobial activity	(18,19,26,27,30)
Macrophages (murine)	Chemotaxis, phagocytosis, and superoxide production	(28)

Although the data from animal studies are reasonably consistent with a potentiating effect of VC on lymphocyte functions, the situation is somewhat less clear-cut in relation to the effects of the vitamin on the proliferative responses of human lymphocytes (18,19,22,23).

With respect to recent studies in animals, Schwager and Schulze have reported on the effects of ascorbic acid supplementation or deprivation on the B- and T-lymphocyte functions of pigs with a hereditary deficiency of ascorbate synthesis (36). These authors reported that the proliferative responses of peripheral blood mononuclear leukocytes activated with either B- or T-cell mitogens were greater in VC-supplemented animals relative to the corresponding responses of cells isolated from animals that had been deprived of the vitamin (36). The decrease in mitogen-activated lymphocyte proliferation resulted from an inability of the cells to respond to the growth factors interleukin-2 (IL-2; B and T cells) and interleukin-6 (IL-6; B cells), as opposed to decreased production and/ or release of these cytokines.

These observations are supported by studies performed on poultry and rats. Puthpongsiriporn and colleagues reported that oral administration of VC (1000 parts per million in drinking water) to laying hens that were subjected to heat stress was accompanied by significantly improved lymphocyte responsiveness to both B- and T-cell mitogens ex vivo, and that this could be further potentiated by the addition of VE (65 mg/ kg) to VC (37). These observations are supported by the findings of Amakye-Anim et al. who reported that VC supplementation at the same dose administered before vaccination and for 10 d after immunization of specific pathogen-free chickens with infectious bursal disease virus was accompanied by significantly higher titers of specific antibodies to the infectious agent measured after vaccination (38). Moreover, VC-supplemented nonvaccinated chickens did not exhibit clinical signs or mortality after challenge with the virus in comparison with 100% and 30% cumulative morbidity and mortality, respectively, in the corresponding unsupplemented nonvaccinated control group. VC supplementation was also associated with higher body weight and decreased serum corticosterone concentrations (38).

Campbell, in a study widely reported in the lay press (Associated Press, 23 August 1999), but to my knowledge not yet in the medical/scientific press, reported that oral administration of VC to stressed (physically immobilized) rats was accompanied by less weight loss, less thymus involution, and less depletion of adrenal ascorbic acid compared to those animals that were stressed and not provided with VC. Moreover, VC supplementation significantly attenuated the corticosterone response to stress and increased IgG levels in both stressed and unstressed animals, implying, yet again, a possible relationship between decreased cortisol levels and VC-mediated enhancement of immune function (Campbell S, University of Alabama, personal communication).

Table 2
Lymphocyte Functions That Are Sustained by Vitamin C

Cell type	Functions enhanced by vitamin C	References
Human T lymphocytes	Mitogen-activated proliferation	(31)
Porcine B and T lymphocytes	Mitogen-activated proliferation	(36)
Avian B and T lymphocytes	Mitogen-activated proliferation and antibody production	(37,38)
Murine B and T lymphocytes	Antibody production, antiapoptotic actions	(40,41)

Conclusions based on the data generated by ex vivo/in vivo immunologic studies performed on experimental animals after VC administration are reinforced by observations from in vitro studies. In the first of these, the addition of the vitamin to murine T cell-depleted splenocytes upregulated the production of antigen-specific IgM antibodies in a cytokine-dependent manner (39), whereas in the second, the vitamin prolonged murine T lymphocyte lifespan by antagonizing various pathways of apoptosis (40). These included corticosteroid-induced cell death, suggesting that the vitamin not only antagonizes the synthesis and/or release of cortisol but also interferes with its apoptosis-inducing interactions with T lymphocytes (40).

With respect to human lymphocytes, de la Fuente and colleagues investigated the effects of oral administration of VC (1 g/d) in combination with VE (200 mg/d) for 16 wk on the mitogen-activated proliferative responses of lymphocytes from elderly female subjects ex vivo (31). They observed a significant increase in lymphoproliferative capacity and decreased serum concentrations of lipid peroxides and cortisol (31). Administration of high-dose VC (≥ 1 g/d), together with either VE (800 mg/d) or N-acetylcysteine, improves oxidative stress parameters and causes modest decreases and increases, respectively, in circulating HIV RNA and $CD4^+$ lymphocytes, as well as enhanced lymphocyte proliferation in patients with advanced immunodeficiency (41,42).

Notwithstanding the limited data on humans, these reports, which are summarized in Table 2, underscore not only the potentiating effects of VC on immune functions but also the anti-infective properties of the vitamin, the latter based on data from animal models of experimental infection.

3. MECHANISMS BY WHICH VITAMIN C POTENTIATES PHAGOCYTE AND LYMPHOCYTE FUNCTIONS

There are several potential mechanisms by which VC may augment phagocyte and lymphocyte functions. Some of these are attributed to the antioxidative properties of the vitamin, whereas others are not.

3.1. Preservation of Cellular Energy Metabolism

As mentioned, phagocyte respiratory burst activation is accompanied by autooxidative inactivation of the protective functions of these cells, with chemotaxis and antimicrobial activity being the most sensitive (18). This primarily results from interference with glycolysis and resultant decreased synthesis of adenosine triphosphate (ATP) and failure to sustain ATP-dependent phagocyte functions. Hydrogen peroxide (H_2O_2) and hypochlorous acid (HOCl) in particular, both of which are produced in large amounts by activated phagocytes, are the primary offenders. These reactive oxidants target a critical cysteine residue (Cys-149) on the active site of the glycolytic enzyme, glyceraldehyde-3-phosphate dehydrogenase, causing inhibition of ATP production and loss of phagocyte functions (18,19). Because they possess few mitochondria and are consequently almost totally dependent on glycolysis to provide their energy requirements, neutrophils are particularly sensitive to premature functional inactivation by this mechanism (18,19).

VC availability, both extracellular and intracellular, is a primary determinant of the sensitivity of phagocytes to oxidative inactivation of cellular energy metabolism and function. Addition of the vitamin to human neutrophils in vitro protects glyceraldehyde-3-phosphate dehydrogenase against oxidative inactivation with resultant enhancement of neutrophil functions, a mechanism that probably also underlies the enhancement of these cells' functions observed after oral supplementation with the vitamin (18,26,43).

VC is the most efficient biological antioxidant in providing defense against HOCl (44). However, the vitamin does not scavenge H_2O_2 (18). Despite this inability to neutralize H_2O_2, VC protects various cell types, including an immature neutrophil cell line, as well as lymphocytes, against the cytotoxic actions of this relatively stable cell-permeant reactive oxidant (29,45). In this setting, VC's cytoprotective effects are mediated indirectly by augmentation of intracellular glutathione levels, glutathione being an efficient scavenger of H_2O_2 (29,45).

Lymphocytes are also vulnerable to oxidative functional inhibition with the proliferative activities of these cells, as well as the cytotoxic functions of natural killer (NK) cells being particularly sensitive (18). Although lymphocytes per se are not major producers of reactive oxidants, these cells must function in proximity to activated phagocytes and are, therefore, exposed to oxidants released extracellularly by these cells at immune and inflammatory reaction sites. As with phagocytes, the glycolytic pathway is prone to oxidative inhibition in lymphocytes exposed to HOCl, whereas several enzymes involved in the Kreb's cycle are also prone to oxidative inactivation. Oxidative inactivation of cellular energy metabolism in lymphocytes is accompanied by loss of the protective functions of these cells and can be prevented by VC in vitro (18).

Unlike neutrophils, however, lymphocytes are particularly sensitive to H_2O_2, largely as a result of the DNA-damaging effects of this reactive oxidant (18). In this setting, H_2O_2 interacts with ferrous iron in proximity to DNA, resulting in the formation of hydroxyl radical, which causes DNA strand breaks, as well as oxidative damage to DNA bases (46). Oxidative damage to DNA, in turn, results in activation of the DNA repair enzyme, poly-ADP ribose polymerase, resulting in consumption and depletion of nicotinamide adenine dinucleotide (NAD), which is also an essential cofactor for several enzymes involved in cellular energy metabolism. This results in decreased ATP production and interference with cellular immune functions (46). This mechanism, which does not involve direct oxidative inactivation of enzymes involved in cellular energy metabolism, has no relevance for neutrophils, because these are nonproliferating end-cells that do not possess poly-ADP ribose polymerase.

VC administration (1 g/d for 6 wk) to young healthy adult humans significantly attenuated the level of DNA damage after exposure of isolated peripheral blood lymphocytes from these individuals to H_2O_2 ex vivo (47). VC supplementation-mediated enhancement of resistance to the DNA damaging effects of H_2O_2 was accompanied by decreased activities of the antioxidative enzymes superoxide dismutase and glutathione peroxidase, compatible with an overall reduction in the endogenous oxidative stress level during administration of the vitamin *(47)*. Using human vascular endothelial cells, Furumoto and colleagues have reported that treatment of human vascular endothelial cells with an oxidation-resistant form of VC in vitro resulted in suppression of intracellular oxidative stress, retardation of the age-dependent shortening of telomeric DNA, and increased cellular lifespan (48). It is probable that these effects were mediated through enhancement of the glutathione-dependent intracellular antioxidant defense system and justify the conclusion of Brennan et al. that supplementation (with VC or other antioxidants) may be used to limit the possible adverse effects of reactive oxygen species, including those produced during an immune response, on lymphocytes in vivo, and so help maintain their functional capacity *(47)*.

Enthusiasm for the use of high-dose VC supplementation as a strategy to reinforce lymphocytes against oxidative damage to DNA and accompanying inactivation of immune responses must, however, be viewed against the backdrop of the report of Podmore and colleagues *(49)*. These investigators reported that administration of VC at 500 mg/d for 6 wk to healthy adult human volunteers was accompanied by an increase in 8-oxo-deoxyadenosine in lymphocyte DNA, compatible with a prooxidative DNA-damaging effect of the vitamin *(49)*. Although these findings have been challenged by others who have reported that oral VC administration at doses varying from 500 to 5000 mg/d for 2 wk has an exclusively antioxidative effect on lymphocytes *(50)*, they have generated concerns regarding the use of VC supplementation as a cytoprotective strategy to sustain lymphocyte function in vivo.

3.2. Regeneration of Vitamin E

As with the involvement of VC in maintaining intracellular glutathione in the reduced state, another indirect antioxidative function of this vitamin is achieved through VE regeneration by reducing the α-tocopherol radical *(51)*. Because VE possesses immunorestorative properties that are particularly important in preventing age-related deterioration in lymphocyte functions *(52)*, regeneration of this vitamin represents an important mechanism of VC-mediated maintenance of optimum immune functions. Although VE, like VC, can function through reinforcement of intracellular antioxidative defenses to prevent oxidative damage to DNA and loss of cellular functions *(47)*, it also inhibits the synthesis of immunosuppressive E series prostaglandins *(52)*. Acting through prostaglandin E receptors on lymphocytes, these prostaglandins cause adenylate cyclase activation with an accompanying increase in intracellular cyclic adenosine monophosphate (cAMP) that negatively regulates lymphocyte proliferation and cytokine production *(53)*.

3.3. Interference with Cortisol Production and Actions

VC regulates cortisol synthesis and/or release, and, interestingly, an association between increased dietary intake of VC and a reduction in stress-related (although in some cases in the absence of a stressor) increases in circulating concentrations of the hormone have been reported in several studies. Investigations performed on animals, including poultry *(38,54–57)*, guinea pigs *(58–60)*, rats (Campbell, personal communication), and fish *(61)*, report the relationship between increased dietary intake of VC and decreased serum cortisol levels, and this relationship has also been described in humans, such as patients undergoing surgery *(62)*, sedentary elderly women *(31)*, and ultra-marathon athletes *(63,64)*; Liakakos et al. also reported that VC administration to children was associated with a reduction in serum cortisol levels after administration of adrenocorticotrophic hormone (ACTH) *(65)*. Moreover, cell culture work on isolated porcine adrenal cells has demonstrated that VC concentration in the cell culture medium is a determinant of the magnitude of cortisol release from the cells after exposure to ACTH *(66,67)*. However, the exact mechanism by which the vitamin modulates cortisol release from adrenocortical cells is not yet established. The vitamin may act at any of several stages, including intracellular signaling events initiated by the cortisol-mobilizing stimulus, enzymatic steps involved in the biosynthesis of cortisol, or mechanisms involved in the hormone release. Irrespective of the molecular/biochemical mechanisms by which VC modulates cortisol release, it is unlikely to be coincidental that the adrenals, the site of cortisol synthesis, are also the major VC storage site.

The relationship between VC status and serum cortisol is also supported by some *(63,64)*, but not all *(68)*, studies on the effects of supplementation with the vitamin (500–1500 mg/d) on the systemic cortisol and cytokine response to intensive exercise *viz* participation in a 90 km ultramarathon event. In their studies, Peters et al. reported that intensive exercise was accompanied by elevations in the circulating levels of VC, presumably resulting from mobilization from the adrenals and other body storage sites, as well as by considerable increases in serum cortisol and those of the antiinflammatory polypeptides IL-10 and the IL-1 receptor antagonist in the placebo group *(63,64)*. In the VC-supplemented groups, the prerace serum concentrations of the vitamin, as expected, were higher than those of the placebo group. However, supplementation with the vitamin either partially (500-mg group) or completely (1000- and 1500-mg groups) attenuated the exercise-associated mobilization of the vitamin and resulted in significant reductions in serum cortisol (1000- and 1500-mg groups), as well as the antiinflammatory components IL-10 and the IL-1 receptor antagonist *(63,64)*. Using a model of acute muscle injury induced by eccentric exercise in humans, Childs et al. measured the effects of VC administration (12.5 mg/kg body weight for 7 d) immediately after induction of injury on alterations in objective serological parameters of muscle damage and inflammatory response *(69)*. VC supplementation was associated with significant increases in serologic indices of muscle injury and inflammation *(69)*. Taken together, these reports suggest that high-dose VC supplementation may potentiate harmful, as well as protective, inflammatory responses *(63,64,69)*. Clearly, a discerning approach is essential to identify who is most likely to benefit from increased VC intake.

In addition to apparent modulation of the release of cortisol from the adrenals, VC has also been reported to interfere with the immunosuppressive interactions of the hormone with T lymphocytes. Campbell et al. reported that VC antagonizes corticosteroid-induced apoptosis, as well as spontaneous apoptosis and apoptosis caused by withdrawal of growth factors in murine T lymphocytes, an activity that they suggest may contribute to VC's immunopotentiating activities *(41)*. These observations support the findings of an earlier study in poultry in which VC antagonized the immunosuppressive actions of corticosteroids *(55)*.

3.4. Protection of Vascular Endothelium

Specialized vascular endothelium orchestrates the homeostatic trafficking of lymphocytes between the circulation and secondary lymphoid organs, whereas the movement of leukocytes out of the circulation during inflammatory responses is directed by localized changes in the adhesiveness of vascular endothelium. Clearly, functionally intact vascular endothelium is critically important not only in promoting protective immune and inflammatory responses but also in ensuring that these are stringently regulated.

Recently, it has become increasingly evident that VC is involved crucially in preserving endothelial function. Although this activity of VC is particularly important in preventing or reversing the endothelial dysfunction that leads to the development of cardiovascular disorders, such as hypertension, diabetes, atherosclerosis, idiopathic dilated cardiomyopathy, and congestive heart failure (70–73), maintenance of endothelial integrity would also be expected to favor optimum regulation of the transendothelial migration of leukocytes. There are several, probably related, mechanisms by which VC maintains endothelial function. These include suppression of induction of endothelial cell apoptosis (72); protection of nitric oxide, an important regulator of vasomotor tone, against oxidative inactivation (73); potentiation of nitric oxide synthesis (74,75); maintenance of intracellular glutathione in the reduced state (75); antagonism of homocysteine (76); inhibition of the formation of proatherogenic phospholipids (77,78); and attenuation of ischemia/reperfusion-associated oxidative injury (79,80). In addition to these, antagonism of the prooxidative and proapoptotic effects of hyperglycemia, as described in Section 3.6., may also contribute to VC-mediated preservation of endothelial integrity and function.

3.5. Antiapoptotic Actions

As mentioned, VC prolongs the lifespan of both T lymphocytes and endothelial cells in vitro by mechanisms that remain to be fully characterized (40,72,81) but that may involve prevention of hydrogen peroxide-mediated denaturation and release of cytochrome c, alterations in mitochondrial membrane potential, and caspase activation (82–84). If operative in vivo, as is the case with endothelial cells (72), these antiapoptotic actions of VC may contribute to the maintenance of optimum immune functions.

3.6. Antagonism of the Prooxidative Actions of Glucose

VC in the charged form (ascorbic acid) enters cells by sodium-dependent facilitated transport, whereas the uncharged form, dehydroascorbic acid, is taken up via glucose transporters and is converted to the reduced form of the vitamin (71,85,86). Conversion of dehydroascorbate to ascorbate intracellularly is believed to be an important mechanism of prevention of intracellular oxidative stress that may be compromised by hyperglycemia (71,85). Such a prooxidative mechanism may underlie the vascular and immunologic complications in diabetes (71,85), as well as the transient endothelial dysfunction and the increase in reactive oxidant generation by circulating neutrophils, which accompanies acute experimental hyperglycemia in healthy adult human volunteers (87). These adverse prooxidative effects of acute and chronic hyperglycemia on endothelial and immune functions may be counteracted by VC administration (71).

Table 3
Mechanisms by Which Vitamin C Sustains the Functions of Phagocytes and Lymphocytes

Mechanism	Cell type affected	References
Protection of glyceraldehyde-3-phosphate dehydrogenase and glycolytic activity	Neutrophils and lymphocytes	(18)
Regeneration of vitamin E, with an accompanying decrease in the synthesis of immunosuppressive prostaglandins	Lymphocytes	(51,52)
Augmentation of intracellular glutathione levels	Neutrophils and lymphocytes	(29,45)
Interference with cortisol release and/or production, as well as antiapoptotic actions	Lymphocytes and endothelial cells	(31,38,40,54–65)
Protection of vascular endothelium	Endothelial cells(directly), as well as neutrophils and lymphocytes (indirectly)	(72–76)
Antagonism of the prooxidative effects of hyperglycemia	Endothelial cells, neutrophils, and lymphocytes	(71,85–87)

Exercise-induced oxidative stress may also be exacerbated by high intakes of supplementary glucose, particularly in endurance athletes (63,64,68).

These various mechanisms by which VC sustains the functions of phagocytes, lymphocytes, and endothelial cells are summarized in Table 3.

4. ANTI-INFECTIVE PROPERTIES

The anti-infective effects of VC supplementation, presumably as a consequence of augmentation of host defenses, have been convincingly demonstrated in various animal models of experimental infection (reviewed in refs. [19,38]). However, the relevance of these to spontaneous microbial and viral infections in humans remains has not yet been established. Notwithstanding the well-published clinical trials in the prevention of/amelioration of symptoms in the common cold, there are relatively few controlled studies with large numbers of participants on the anti-infective effects of VC in humans.

Peters et al. have reported that VC administration (500 mg/d) significantly reduces the incidence of postrace symptoms of upper respiratory tract infection in ultradistance runners (88,89), whereas in other studies with fewer participants, administration of VC at 1000 and 200 mg/d has led to significant clinical improvement in patients with recurrent furunculosis and in elderly hospitalized patients with acute respiratory infections, respectively (26,90).

Table 4
Content of Ascorbic Acid in Selected Foods

Fruits and meat	Ascorbic acid (mg/100 g)	Vegetables	Ascorbic acid (mg/100 g)
Fruits of *Terminalia fernandiana*	3000	Peppers	125–200
Acerola	1300	Kale	120–180
Rose hips	1000	Parsley	170
Hawthorn berries	160–800	Turnip greens	139
Guava	300	Horseradish	120
Black currant	150–230	Collard greens	100–150
Lemons	50–80	Brussels sprouts	90–150
Strawberries	40–90	Broccoli	70–160
Oranges	40–60	Spinach	50–90
Grapefruit	35–45	Watercress	79
Red currant	40	Cauliflower	60–80
Tangerines	30	Kohlrabi	66
Pineapples	20–40	Cabbage	30–60
Raspberries	18–25	Turnips	15–40
Melons	13–33	Asparagus	15–30
Apples	10–30	Leek	15–30
Cherries	10	Potatoes	10–30
Peaches	7–14	Beans	10–30
Bananas	5–10	Peas	10–30
Liver, kidney	10–40	Onion	10–30
Fish	0–3	Tomatoes	10–30
Meat (beef and pork)	0–2	Squash	8–25
Milk		Corn (sweet)	12
Human	3–6	Rhubarb	10
Cow	1–2	Celery	7–10
		Carrots	5–20
		Oat, rye, and wheat	0
		Rice	0

Source: Moser U, Bendich A. Vitamin C. In: Machlin LJ, ed. Handbook of Vitamins: Second Edition, Revised and Expanded. Marcel Dekker Inc., New York, 1991, pp. 195–232.

5. RECOMMENDED VITAMIN C INTAKES

Optimum daily intakes of VC remain difficult to establish but are clearly in excess of the 30–60 mg/d advocated by national health authorities in the past. Based on the role of the vitamin in the prevention of degenerative diseases, Carr and Frei suggested a daily intake of 90–100 mg for optimum risk reduction *(90)*. However, as reported by Brubacher and colleagues, the members of an expert panel recently concluded that the plasma concentration of VC required for potential primary prevention should be the determinant of intake and, on this basis, recommended an optimal plasma concentration of 50 µmol/l *(91)*. This can be achieved in the general population by ingesting 100 mg/d of the vitamin d, which is the new recommendation of the Austrian, German, and Swiss Nutrition

Societies *(91)*. However, higher intakes of up to 200 mg/d are required to achieve this level in the elderly and in cigarette smokers *(91)*.

In contrast to disease prevention, the therapeutic applications of the vitamin, such as the correction of endothelial dysfunction in patients with cardiovascular disorders, may require the administration of VC doses considerably in excess of 100 mg/d *(71–75)*. In this setting, potential, albeit apparently minor, side effects of the GI and urinary tracts may be evident *(92,93)*, and concerns remain about the more ominous threat of oxidative damage to DNA *(49)*.

The main dietary sources of VC are listed in Table 4.

6. FUTURE RESEARCH

Clearly, accurate scientific evaluations of the anti-infective properties of VC in humans, as well as the daily intakes of the vitamin required to maximize these effects, especially with respect to age, are priority areas for future research.

7. "TAKE-HOME" MESSAGES

1. Vitamin C maintains host defenses.
2. Phagocyte and lymphocyte functions are sustained by vitamin C.
3. Although antioxidative mechanisms contribute, in large measure, to the immuno-protective actions of VC, additional mechanisms are operative.
4. These include the antiapoptotic and corticosteroid-reducing actions of VC, both of which are currently poorly understood.
5. Optimum intakes of VC with respect to its anti-infective properties, are not yet established but are likely to be in excess of current recommended daily allowances (RDAs), which are generally approx 60–100 mg/d.

REFERENCES

1. Chojkier M, Houglum K, Solis-Herruzo J, Brenner DA. Stimulation of collagen gene expression by ascorbic acid in cultured human fibroblasts. A role for lipid peroxidation? J Biol Chem 1989;264:16957–16962.
2. Otsuka M, Matsuzawa M, Ha TY, Arakawa N. Contribution of a high dose of L-ascorbic acid to carnitine synthesis in guinea pigs fed high fat diets. J Nutr Sci Vitaminol 1999;45:163–171.
3. Dhariwal K, Washko P, Hartzell W, Levine M. Ascorbic acid within chromaffin granules. J Biol Chem 1989;264:15404–15409.
4. Levine M. New concepts in the biology and biochemistry of ascorbic acid. N Engl J Med 1986;314: 892–901.
5. Hemilä H, Herman ZS. Vitamin C and the common cold: a retrospective analysis of Chalmers' review. J Am Coll Nutr 1995;14:116–123.
6. Murata A, Morishige F, Yamaguchi H. Prolongation of survival times of terminal cancer patients by administration of large doses of ascorbate. Int J Vit Nutr Res 1982;(Suppl 23):103–112.
7. Corea P, Fontham ETH, Bravo JC, et al. Chemoprevention of gastric dysplasia: randomized trial of anti-oxidant supplements and anti-*Helicobacter pylori* therapy. J Natl Cancer Inst 2000;92:1881–1888.
8. Frei B, England L, Ames BN. Ascorbic acid is an outstanding anti-oxidant in blood plasma. Proc Natl Acad Sci USA 1989;86:6377–6381.
9. Hu GZ, Zhang X, Chen JS, Peto R, Campbell TC, Cassano PA. Dietary vitamin C and lung function in rural China. Am J Epidemiol 1998;148:594–599.
10. Smit HA, Grievink L, Tabak C. Dietary influences on chronic obstructive lung disease and asthma: a review of the epidemiological evidence. Proc Nutr Soc 1999;58:309–319.

11. Chen RL, Tunstall-Pedoe H, Bolton-Smith C, Hannah MK, Morrison C. Association of dietary anti-oxidants and waist circumference with pulmonary function and airway obstruction. Am J Epidemiol 2001;153:157–163.
12. Cadenas S, Rojas C, Barja G. Endotoxin increases oxidative injury to proteins in guinea pig liver: protection by dietary vitamin C. Pharmacol Toxicol 1998;82:11–18.
13. McCloy R. Chronic pancreatitis at Manchester, UK—focus on antioxidant therapy. Digestion 1998;59(Suppl 4):36–48.
14. Sakai N, Yokoyama T, Date C, Yoshiike N, Matsumura Y. An inverse relationship between serum vitamin C and blood pressure in a Japanese community. J Nutr Sci Vitaminol 1998;44:853–867.
15. Bates CJ, Walmsley CM, Prentice A, Finch S. Does vitamin C reduce blood pressure? Results of a large study of people aged 65 or older. J Hypertens 1998;16:925–932.
16. Ellis GR, Anderson RA, Lang D, et al. Neutrophil superoxide anion-generating capacity, endothelial function and oxidative stress in chronic heart failure: effects of short- and long-term vitamin C therapy. J Am Coll Cardiol 2000;36:1474–1482.
17. Morton DJ, Barrett-Connor EL, Schneider DL. Vitamin C supplement use and bone mineral density in postmenopausal women. J Bone Min Res 2001; 16:135–140.
18. Anderson R, Smit MJ, Jooné GK, Van Staden AM. Vitamin C and cellular immune functions: protection against hypochlorous acid-mediated inactivation of glyceraldehyde-3-phosphate dehydrogenase and ATP generation in human leukocytes as a possible mechanism of ascorbate-mediated immuno-stimulation. Ann NY Acad Sci 1990;587:34–48.
19. Anderson R. Mechanisms of vitamin-mediated anti-inflammatory and immunomodulatory activity. Bib Nutrito Dieta 2001;55:135–147.
20. Khaw KT, Bingham S, Welch A, et al. Relation between plasma ascorbic acid and mortality in men and women in EPIC-Norfolk prospective study: a prospective population study. Lancet 2001;357:657–663.
21. Sotirou S, Gispert S, Cheng J, et al. Ascorbic acid transporter S1c23a1 is essential for ascorbic acid into the brain and for perinatal survival. Nature Med 2002;8:514–517.
22. Peters-Futre EM. Exercise, vitamin C and phagocyte function. The missing link. Exerc Immunol Rev 1997;3:32–52.
23. Bendich A. Micronutrients in women's health and immune function. Nutrition 2001;17:858–867.
24. Washko P, Rotrosen D, Levine M. Ascorbic acid transport and accumulation in human neutrophils. J Biol Chem 1989;264:18996–19002.
25. Tintinger GR, Theron AJ, Steel HC, Anderson R. Accelerated calcium influx and hyperactivation of neutrophils in chronic granulomatous disease. Clin Exp Immunol 2001;123:254–263.
26. Levy R, Shriker O, Porath A, Riesenberg K, Schlaeffer F. Vitamin C for the treatment of recurrent furunculosis in patients with impaired neutrophil functions. J Infec Dis 1996;173:1502–1505.
27. Mulero V, Esteban MA, Meseguer J. Effects of in vitro addition of exogenous vitamins C and E on gilthead seabream (Sparus aurata L.) phagocytes. Vet Immunol Immunopathol 1998;66:185–199.
28. Delrio M, Ruedas G, Medina S, Victor VM, Delafuente M. Improvement by several antioxidants of macrophage function in vitro. Life Sci 1998;63:871–881.
29. Lenton KJ, Therriault H, Cantin AM, Fulop T, Payette H, Wagner JR. Direct correlation of glutathione and ascorbate and their dependence on age and season in human lymphocytes. Am J Clin Nutr 2000;71:1194–1200.
30. Jayachandran M, Rani PJA, Arivazhagan P, Panneerselvam C. Neutrophil phagocytic function and humoral immune response with reference to ascorbate supplementation in aging humans. J Anti-Aging Med 2000;3:37–42.
31. De la Fuente M, Fernandez MD, Burgos MS, Soler A, Prieto A, Miquel J. Immune function in aged women is improved by ingestion of vitamins C and E. Can J Physiol Pharmacol 1998;76:373–380.
32. McFadden ER. Inhaled glucocorticoids and acute asthma: therapeutic breakthrough or non-specific effect? Am J Respir Crit Care Med 1998;157:677–678.
33. Cox G. Glucocorticoid treatment inhibits apoptosis in human neutrophils. J Immunol 1995;154:4719–4725.
34. Krause R, Patruta S, Daxbock F, Fladerer P, Biegelmayer C, Wenisch C. Effect of vitamin C on neutrophil function after high-intensity exercise. Eur J Clin Invest 2001;31:258–263.
35. Brites FD, Evelson PA, Christiansen MG, et al. Soccer players under regular training show oxidative stress but an improved plasma antioxidant status. Clin Sci 1999;96:381–385.

36. Schwager J, Schultze J. Modulation of interleukin production by ascorbic acid. Vet Immunol Immunophathol 1998;64:45–57.

37. Puthpongsiriporn U, Scheideler SE, Sell JL, Beck MM. Effects of vitamin E and C supplementation on performance, in vitro lymphocyte proliferation, and antioxidant status of laying hens during heat stress. Poult Sci 2001;80:1190–1200.

38. Amakye-Anim J, Lin TL, Hester PY, Thiagarajan D, Watkins BA, Wu CC. Ascorbic acid supplementation improved antibody response to infectious bursal disease vaccination in chickens. Poult Sci 2000;79:680–688.

39. Mitsuzumi H, Kusamiya M, Kurimoto T, Yamamoto I. Requirement of cytokines for augmentation of the antigen-specific antibody responses by ascorbate in cultured murine T-cell-depleted splenocytes. Jpn J Pharmacol 1998;78:169–179.

40. Campbell JD, Cole M, Bunditrutavorm B, Vella AT. Ascorbic acid is a potent inhibitor of various forms of T cell apoptosis. Cel Immunol 1999;194:1–5.

41. Allard JP, Aghdassi E, Chau J, et al. Effects of vitamin E and C supplementation on oxidative stress and viral load in HIV-infected subjects. AIDS 1998;12:1653–1659.

42. Muller F, Svardal AM, Nordoy I, Berse RK, Aukrist P, Froland SS. Virological and immunological effects of antioxidant treatment in patients with HIV infection. Eur J Clin Invest 2000;30:905–914.

43. Van Antwerpen VL, Theron AJ, Myer MS, et al. Cigarette-smoke-mediated oxidant stress, phagocytes, vitamin C, vitamin E, and tissue injury. Ann NY Acad Sci 1993;686:53–65.

44. Halliwell B, Wasil M, Grootveld M. Biologically significant scavenging of the myeloperoxidase-derived oxidant hypochlorous acid by ascorbic acid. Implications for antioxidant protection in the inflamed rheumatoid joint. FEBS Lett 1987;213:15–17.

45. Guaiquil VH, Vera JC, Golde DW. Mechanism of vitamin C inhibition of cell death induced by oxidative stress in glutathione-depleted HL-60 cells. J Biol Chem 2001;276:40955–40961.

46. Jackson JH, Gajewski E, Schraufstatter IU, et al. Damage to the bases in DNA induced by stimulated neutrophils. J Clin Invest 1989;84:1644–1649.

47. Brennan LA, Morris GM, Wasson GR, Hannigan BM, Barnett YA. The effect of vitamin C or vitamin E supplementation on basal and H_2O_2-induced DNA damage in human lymphocytes. Br J Nutr 2000;84:195–202.

48. Furumoto K, Inoue E, Nagao N, Hiyama E, Miwa N. Age-dependent telomere shortening is slowed down by enrichment of intracellular vitamin C via suppression of oxidative stress. Life Sci 1998;63:935–948.

49. Podmore ID, Griffiths HR, Herbert KE, et al. Pro-oxidant effect of vitamin C. Nature 1998;392:559.

50. Vojdani A, Bazargan M, Vojdani E, Wright J. New evidence for antioxidant properties of vitamin C. Cancer Detect Prev 2000;24:508–523.

51. Noguchi N, Niki E. Dynamics of vitamin E action against LDL oxidation. Free Rad Res 1998;28:561–572.

52. Meydani SN, Wu D, Santos MS, Hayek MG. Antioxidant and immune responses in aged responses: overview of present evidence. Am J Clin Nutr 1995;62(Suppl):1462–1476.

53. Moore AR, Willoughby DA. The role of cAMP regulation in controlling inflammation. Clin Exp Immunol 1995;101:387–389.

54. Pardue SL, Thaxton JP. Evidence for amelioration of steroid-mediated immunosuppression by ascorbic acid. Poult Sci 1984;63:1262–1268.

55. Satterlee DG. Ascorbic acid and physiological stress in poultry. In: Wenk G, Fenster R, Völker L (eds.). Ascorbic Acid in Domestic Animals: Proceedings of the Second Symposium. F. Hoffmann-La Roche Ltd, Basel, Switzerland, 1992, pp. 43–59.

56. Satterlee DG, Jones RB, Ryder FH. Effects of ascorbyl-2-polyphosphate on adrenocortical activation and fear-related behaviour in broiler chickens. Poult Sci 1994;73:194–201.

57. Jones RB, Satterlee DG, Cadd GG. Timidity in Japanese quail: effects of vitamin C and divergent selection for adrenocorticol response. Physiol Behav 1999;67:117–120.

58. Odumosu A. Ascorbic acid and cortisol metabolism in hypovitaminosis C in guinea pigs. Int J Vit Nutr Res 1982;52:176–185.

59. Douglas NL, Constantopoulos A, Litsios B. Effect of ascorbic acid on guinea pig adrenal adenylate cyclase activity and plasma cortisol. J Nutr 1987;117:1108–1114.

60. Enwonwu CO, Sawiris P, Chanaud N. Effect of marginal ascorbic acid deficiency on saliva level of cortisol in the guinea pig. Arch Oral Biol 1995;40:737–742.

61. Dabrowska H, Dabrowski K, Meyer-Burgdorff K, Hanke W, Gunther KD. The effect of large doses of vitamin C and magnesium on stress responses in common carp, *Cyprinus carpio*. Comp Biochem Physiol 1991;99:681–685.

62. Nathan N, Vandoux JC, Feiss P. Role of vitamin C on adrenocortical effects of etomidate. Ann Francaises Anesthesie Reanimation 1991;10:329–332.

63. Peters EM, Anderson R, Theron AJ. Attenuation of the increase in circulating cortisol and enhancement of the acute phase response in vitamin C-supplemented marathon runners. Int J Sports Med 2001;22:120–126.

64. Peters EM, Anderson R, Nieman DC, Fickl H, Jogessar V. Vitamin supplementation attenuates the increases in circulating cortisol, adrenaline and anti-inflammatory polypeptides following ultramarathon running. Int J Sports Med 2001;22:537–543.

65. Liakakos D, Douglas D, Ikkos C, Anoussakis C, Jouramani G. Inhibitory effect of ascorbic acid (vitamin C) on cortisol secretion following adrenal stimulation in children. Clin Chim Acta 1975;65:251–255.

66. Goralczyk R, Moser UK, Matter U, Weiser H. Regulation of steroid hormone metabolism requires L-ascorbic acid. Ann NY Acad Sci 1992;669:349–351.

67. Moser UK. Physiology and metabolism of ascorbic acid. In: Wenk C, Fenster R, Völker L (eds.). Ascorbic Acid in Domestic Animals: Proceedings of the Second Symposium. F. Hoffmann-La Roche Ltd, Basel, Switzerland, 1992, pp. 3–16.

68. Nieman DC, Henson DA, McAnulty SR, et al. Influence of vitamin C supplementation on oxidative and immune changes after an ultramarathon. J Appl Physiol 2002;92:1970–1977.

69. Childs A, Jacobs C, Kaminski T, Halliwell B, Leeuwenburgh C. Supplementation with vitamin C and N-acetyl-cysteine increases oxidative stress in humans after and acute muscle injury induced by eccentric exercise. Free Rad Biol Med 2001;31:745–753.

70. Horio F, Hayashi K, Mishima T, et al. A newly established strain of spontaneously hypertensive rat with a defect of ascorbic acid biosynthesis. Life Sci 2001;69:1879–1890.

71. Price KD, Price CSC, Reynolds RD. Hyperglycemia-induced ascorbic acid deficiency promotes endothelial dysfunction and the development of atherosclerosis. Atherosclerosis 2001;158:1–12.

72. Rossig L, Hoffmann J, Hugel B, Mallat Z, Haase A, Freyssinet JM. Vitamin C inhibits endothelial cell apoptosis in congestive heart failure. Circulation 2001;104:2182–2187.

73. Richartz BM, Werner GS, Ferrari M, Figulla HR. Reversibility of coronary endothelial vasomotor dysfunction in idiopathic dilated cardiomyopathy: acute effects of vitamin C. Am J Cardiol 2001;88:1001–1005.

74. Heller R, Unbehaum A, Schellenberg B, Meyer B, Werner-Felmayer G, Werner ER. L-ascorbic acid potentiates endothelial nitric oxide synthesis via a chemical stabilization of tetrahydrobiopterin. J Biol Chem 2001;276:40–47.

75. Smith AR, Visioli F, Hagen TM. Vitamin C matters: increased oxidative stress in cultured aortic endothelial cells without supplemental ascorbic acid. FASEB J 2002;16:125–144.

76. Nappo F, De Rosa N, Marfella R, et al. Impairment of endothelial functions by acute hyperhomocysteinemia and reversal by antioxidant vitamins. JAMA 1999;281:2113–2118.

77. Lloberas NR, Torras J, Herrero-Fresneda I, et al. Postischemic renal oxidative stress induces an inflammatory response through PAF and oxidized phospholipids: prevention by antioxidant treatment. FASEB J 2002;16:358–377.

78. Carr AC, Frei B. Human neutrophils oxidize low-density liproprotein by a hypochlorous acid-dependent mechanism. The role of vitamin C. Biol Chem 2002;383:627–636.

79. Mak S, Egri Z, Tanna G, Colman R, Newton GE. Vitamin C prevents hyperoxia-mediated vasoconstriction and impairment of endothelium-dependent vasodilatation. Am J Physiol 2002;282:H2414–H2421.

80. Molyneux CA, Glyn MC, Ward BJ. Oxidative stress and cardiac microvascular structure in ischemia and reperfusion. The protective effect of antioxidant vitamins. Microvasc Res 2002;64:265–277.

81. Ho FM, Liu SH, Liau CS, Huang PJ, Shiah SG, Lin-Shiau SY. Nitric oxide prevents apoptosis of human endothelial cells from high glucose exposure during early stage. J Cell Biochem 1999;75:258–263.

82. Gruss-Fischer T, Fabian I. Protection by ascorbic acid from denaturation and release of cytochrome c, alteration of mitochondrial membrane potential and activation of multiple caspases induced by H_2O_2 in human leukemic cells. Biochem Pharmacol 2002;63:1325–1335.

83. Kowluru RA, Koppulu P. Diabetes-induced activation of caspase-3 in retina: effect of antioxidant therapy. Free Rad Res 2002;36:993–999.

84. Rojas M, Rugeles MT, Gil DP, Patino P. Differential modulation of apoptosis and necrosis by antioxidants in immunosuppressed human lymphocytes. Toxicol Appl Pharmacol 2002;180:67–73.

85. Root-Bernstein R, Busik JV, Henry DN. Are diabetic neuropathy, retinopathy and nephropathy caused by hyperglycemic exclusion of dehydroascorbate uptake by glucose transporters. J Theoret Biol 2002;216:345–359.

86. Wilson JX. The physiological role of dehydroascorbic acid. FEBS Lett 2002;527:5–9.

87. Lee IK, Kim HS, Bae JH. Endothelial dysfunction: its relationship to hyperglycemia and hyperlipidemia. Int J Clin Prac 2002;129(Suppl):59–64.

88. Peters EM, Goetzche JM, Joseph LE, Noakes TD. Vitamin C supplementation reduces the incidence of post-race symptoms of upper respiratory tract infection in ultradistance runners. Am J Clin Nutr 1993;57:170–174.

89. Peters EM, Goetzche JM, Joseph LE, Noakes TD. Vitamin C as effective as combinations of anti-oxidant nutrients in reducing symptoms of upper respiratory tract infections in ultramarathon runners. S Afr J Sports Med 1996;4:23–27.

90. Hunt C, Chakravorty NK, Annan G, Habibzadeh N, Schorah CJ. The clinical effects of vitamin C in elderly hospitalised patients with acute respiratory infections. Int J Vit Nutr Res 1994;64:212–219.

91. Carr AC, Frei B. Toward a new recommended dietary allowance for vitamin C based on antioxidant and health effects in human. Am J Clin Nutr 1999;69:1086–1107.

92. Brubacher D, Moser U, Jordan P. Vitamin C concentrations in plasma as a function of intake: a meta-analysis. Int J Vit Nutr Res 2000;70:226–237.

93. Curhan GC, Willett WC, Speizer FE, Stampfer MJ. Intake of vitamins B6 and C and the risk of kidney stones in women. J Am Soc Nephrol 1999;10:840–845.

94. Schwille PO, Schmiedl A, Herrmann U, et al. Ascorbic acid in idiopathic recurrent calcium urolithiasis in humans—does it have an abettor role in oxalate and calcium oxalate crystallization? Urol Res 2000;28:167–177.

95. Moser U, Bendich A. Vitamin C. In: Machlin LJ (ed.). Handbook of Vitamins: Second Edition, Revised and Expanded. Marcel Dekker Inc., New York, 1991, pp. 195–232.

8 Vitamin E

Sung Nim Han
and Simin Nikbin Meydani

1. INTRODUCTION

Vitamin E is a potent chain-breaking antioxidant that protects membranes from free-radical damage. Evidence suggests that there are beneficial effects of supplemental vitamin E on immune functions and several chronic diseases, including Alzheimer's disease *(1)*, cardiovascular disease *(2)*, and prostate cancer *(3)*. Vitamin E is, perhaps, one of the most studied nutrients in relation to its immunoregulatory effects. Results from animal and human studies indicate that vitamin E deficiency impairs both humoral and cell-mediated immune functions *(4,5)*. Vitamin E supplementation above the recommended levels enhances immune functions and is associated with increased resistance against several pathogens *(6,7)*. This chapter summarizes studies related to the role of vitamin E in modulating immune responses in humans and mechanisms by which vitamin E exerts its effect.

2. VITAMIN E: DEFINITION, SOURCES, AND INTAKES

Vitamin E is a generic description for all tocols and tocotrienols that exhibit the biological activity of α-tocopherol. There are eight naturally occurring forms of vitamin E: α-, β-, γ-, and δ-tocopherols and α-, β-, γ-, and δ-tocotrienols. Chemically synthesized α-tocopherol contains eight stereoisomers and is designated all-*rac*-α-tocopherol (historically called *dl*-α-tocopherol), whereas the naturally occurring stereoisomer of α-tocopherol is RRR-α-tocopherol (formerly called *d*-α-tocopherol). It has been generally accepted that biologic activities of different forms of vitamin E correlate with antioxidant activities in the order of $\alpha > \beta > \gamma > \delta$ *(8)*. However, recent studies *(9,10)* suggest that the biological effects of vitamin E may not necessarily correlate with antioxidant activities of different forms of vitamin E.

The various forms of vitamin E occur in foods in different proportions, and the content of vitamin E in food varies depending on storage, processing, and preparation procedures. Vegetable oils and nuts contain high amounts of vitamin E. Major sources of vitamin E that contribute to dietary vitamin E in the US diet are fats and oils, vegetables, poultry and meat, and fish *(11)*. Although wheat-germ oil, sunflower oil, safflower oil, canola oil, and

From: *Diet and Human Immune Function*
Edited by: D. A. Hughes, L. G. Darlington, and A. Bendich © Humana Press Inc., Totowa, NJ

Table 1
Average Intake of Dietary Vitamin E in Different Countries

Average daily intake of vitamin E	Country	Sample size	Age (yr)	Period when data was collected	Method for collecting dietary intake data	Reference
10 mg (mainly from γ-tocopherol)	US	1047	50–79	1994–1996 (Women's Health Initiative)	Semiquantitative food frequency questionnaire	White et al. (47)
9.6 mg (men); 7.0 mg (women)	US	11,658	>19	1976–1980 (NHANES II)	24-h recall	Murphy et al. (11)
7.1–9.4 mg (α-TE)	US	474	65–98	1990	24-h recall	Ryan et al. (14)
8.4 mg	UK	18,855	All ages	1986	Weekly household food supply	Lewis et al. (48)
10.7 mg (α-TE)	Finland	Whole population	All ages	1987	National food balance sheet	Heinonen et al. (49)
6.4 mg (α-tocopherol)	Canada	Whole population	All ages	1968	Daily per-capita consumption of food	Thompson et al. (50)
8.1–12.3 mg	Ireland	1379	18–64	1997–1999 (North/South Ireland Food Consumption Survey)	7-d food diary	O'Brien et al. (51)

Table 2
Vitamin E Supplementation and Immune Responses in Humans

Subjects	Age	Amount and duration of supplementation[a]	Effects on immune function	Reference
Adults and teenagers (n = 18)	25–30, 13–18	300 mg/d for 3 wk	⇓ Lymphocyte proliferation; ⇔ Delayed type hypersensitivity (DTH); ⇓ Bactericidal activity	Prasad et al., 1980 (52)
Adults (n = 31) and premature infants (n = 10)	24–31	600 mg/d for 3 mo[b]; 40 mg/kg body wt for 8–14 d	⇓ Chemiluminescence	Okanno et al., 1990 (53)
Cigarette smoker (n = 60)	33 ± 4	900 IU/d for 6 wk	⇓ Chemiluminescence	Richards et al., 1990 (54)
Sedentary young and elderly	22–29, 55–74	800 IU/d for 48 d	⇓ Interleukin (IL)-6 secretion; ⇓ Exercise-enhanced IL-1β secretion	Cannon et al., 1991 (36)
Adults (n = 26)	25–35	233 mg/d for 28 d[c]	⇑ Lymphocyte proliferation; ⇑ Total T cells, CD4 T cells; ⇓ Plasma malondialdehyde; ⇓ Urinary 8-OHDG	Lee and Wan, 2000 (18)
Institutionalized elderly	63–93	200 mg/d for 4 mo	⇑ Total serum protein; α-2 and β-2 globulin fractions	Ziemlanski et al., 1986 (55)
Institutionalized adults and elderly (n = 103)	24–104	200, 400 mg/d for 6 mo	⇔ Antibody development to influenza virus	Harman and Miller, 1986 (56)
Elderly (n = 74)	≥ 65	100 mg/d for 3 mo	⇔ Lymphocyte proliferation; ⇔ IgG, IgA levels	De Waart et al., 1997 (19)
Elderly (n = 161)	65–80	50, 100 mg/d for 6 mo	⇑ No. of positive DTH responses with 100 mg; ⇑ Diameter of induration of DTH responses in a subgroup with 100 mg; ⇔ IL-2 production	Pallast et al., 1999 (20)

151

(continued)

Table 2
Continued

Subjects	Age	Amount and duration of supplementation[a]	Effects on immune function	Reference
Elderly ($n = 32$)	≥ 60	800 mg/d for 30 d	⇑ Lymphocyte proliferation ⇑DTH ⇑ IL–2 production ⇓ PGE_2 production	Meydani et al., 1990 (6)
Elderly ($n = 88$)	≥ 65	60, 200, 800 mg/d for 235 d	⇑ DTH and antibody titer to hepatitis B with 200 and 800 mg	Meydani et al., 1997 (17)
Hypertriglyceridemic ($n = 12$) and normolipidemic ($n = 8$) adults	49.5 ± 9.6 55.8 ± 12.1	600 IU/d for 6 wk[b]	⇓ Superoxide production ⇓ Tumor necrosis factor (TNF)-α, IL–1β, IL–8 production	Van Tits et al., 2000 (57)

[a] Supplemented with *dl*-α-tocopherol acetate unless indicated.
[b] Supplemented with RRR-α-tocopherol.
[c] Supplemented with *dl*-α-tocopherol.

152

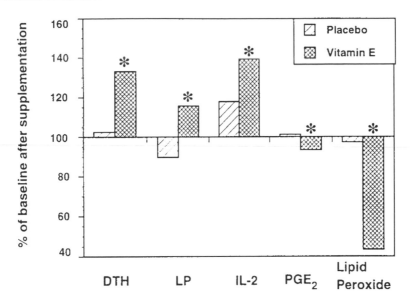

Fig. 1. Effect of vitamin E supplementation (800 mg/d for 30 d) on immune responses of healthy older adults. *Significant changes from baseline at $p < 0.05$. DTH, delayed type hypersensitivity response; LP, lymphocyte proliferation; IL-2, interleukin-2; PGE$_2$, prostaglandin E$_2$. Reproduced from Meydani and Han *(46)*, with permission of ILSI Press, Washington, DC.

olive oil provide vitamin E mostly in the form of α-tocopherol, corn oil, soybean oil, sesame oil, and peanut oil contain mainly γ-tocopherol.

The recommended daily vitamin E intake is currently 15 mg/d of α-tocopherol for adults (ages older than 19 yr) *(12)*, increased from 10 mg recommended in the 10th edition of the recommended dietary allowance (RDA) book *(13)*. Average daily vitamin E intake in the United States and other Western countries is estimated at approx 10 mg (*see* Table 1). Certain groups, such as the elderly, are at greater risk for inadequate dietary vitamin E intake *(14,15)*. Ryan et al. *(14)* reported that more than 40% of the elderly (65–98 yr) had vitamin E intakes that were below two thirds of the 1989 RDA.

3. VITAMIN E AND IMMUNE FUNCTIONS

The beneficial effects of dietary vitamin E supplementation higher than the recommended levels, especially in the aged, have been shown in animal studies and human clinical trials *(6,16,17)*. Table 2 summarizes the studies that have investigated the effects of vitamin E supplementation in humans. Studies in which the immunomodulating effects of vitamin E in combination with other nutrients have been investigated are not included in Table 2, because it would be difficult to attribute any effects to a single nutrient.

Vitamin E supplementation (800 mg/d) in healthy elderly older than 60 yr resulted in an increase in delayed type hypersensitivity (DTH) response, in vitro T-cell proliferation, and interleukin (IL)-2 production and a decrease in plasma lipid peroxide concentration and production of the T cell-suppressive PGE$_2$ *(6)* (*see* Fig. 1). In a subsequent study, Meydani et al. *(17)* investigated the effects of 4.5 mo of vitamin E supplementation on in vivo indices of immune function in healthy elderly aged more than 65 yr; 88 subjects were supplemented with either placebo or 60, 200, or 800 mg *dl*-α-tocopheryl acetate. All three vitamin E-supplemented groups showed a significant increase in DTH response compared with baseline. Subjects in the 200 mg/d group showed a significantly greater increase in median percentage change of DTH response compared with those in the placebo group (65% vs 17%, *p* = 0.04) and a significant increase in antibody titers to hepatitis B and tetanus vaccines. Lee and Wan *(18)* reported a significant increase in proliferative response to phytohemagglutinin (PHA) or lipopolysaccharides (LPS) and a significant decrease in plasma malondialdehyde and urinary DNA adduct 8-hydroxy-2'-deoxyguanosine after short-term vitamin E supplementation (233 mg *dl*-α-tocopherol/d for 28 d) in Chinese adults. De Waart et al. *(19)* observed no significant changes in mitogenic response to concanavalin A (Con A) and PHA or immunoglobulin (Ig)G and A(IgA) levels against *Penicillium* after 3-mo vitamin E supplementation at 100 mg/d. The lower dose of vitamin E, as well as the use of previously frozen lymphocytes for determination of mitogenic response and evaluation of antibody levels without previous specific vaccination, may have contributed to the discrepancy observed between the results from De Waart et al. *(19)* and Meydani et al. *(6,17)*. Pallast et al. *(20)* supplemented healthy elderly subjects (65–80 yr old) with 50 or 100 mg/d of vitamin E for 6 mo. Subjects in the vitamin E-supplemented group showed a significant increase in DTH response (induration diameter and number of positive responses) compared with their own baseline values. Only the change in the number of positive DTH responses tended to be larger in the 100 mg-supplemented group than the placebo group (*p* = 0.06). A significantly greater improvement in cumulative DTH score and the number of positive DTH responses was observed in a subgroup of subjects who received 100 mg vitamin E and had a low baseline DTH reactivity. There was no significant difference in PHA-stimulated IL-2 production in the vitamin E-treated groups compared with the placebo group, and IFN-γ production tended to be lower in the groups receiving vitamin E.

Differences in results among human studies may reflect the differences in vitamin E status at baseline and supplementation dose, resulting in varied levels of changes in plasma vitamin E levels (*see* Table 3) (*see* Fig. 2), as well as differences in methodology. Considering the results from the study by Meydani et al. *(17)*, in which subjects in the upper tertile of serum vitamin E concentration (>48.4 μmol/L) after supplementation had higher antibody response to hepatitis B, as well as higher DTH responses than those in the lower tertile of serum vitamin E (19.9–34.7 μmol/L), the amount of increase in serum vitamin E levels achieved in the studies by others *(19,20)* might not have been adequate to observe a highly significant effect. It is also noteworthy that Lee and Wan *(18)* observed a significant increase in cell-mediated immune response, with a 13.4-μmol/L increase in plasma vitamin E level, a level of increase comparable to those observed by others, e.g., De Waart et al. *(19)* and Pallast et al. *(20)*, with 100 mg supplementation. A difference in vitamin E status at baseline may explain the differences in results, because subjects in the study by Lee and Wan *(18)* had significantly lower plasma vitamin E levels at baseline compared with those in the studies by De Waart et al. *(19)* and Pallast et al. *(20)* (*see* Table 3).

Different forms of vitamin E, other than α-tocopherol, have immunoregulatory functions *(9,10)*. α-Tocopherol is the most common form of vitamin E in plasma and tissues and the most extensively studied for its beneficial effect on immune function, probably because it is the exclusive component in most vitamin E supplements. Wu et al. *(9)*

Table 3
Changes in Plasma Vitamin E Levels Observed in Vitamin E Supplementation Studies

Supplementation dose and duration	Vitamin E level at baseline (μmol/L)	Change in blood vitamin E levels (μmol/L)	Reference
800 mg for 30 d	25.6 ± 1.4	45.3	Meydani et al. *(6)*
60 mg for 235 d	27.2 ± 6.1	11.2	Meydani et al. *(17)*
200 mg for 235 d	25.6 ± 5.7	25.4	
800 mg for 235 d	25.8 ± 6.3	45.7	
233 mg for 28 d	14.25 ± 0.56	13.4	Lee and Wan *(18)*
50 mg for 6 mo	28.8 ± 6.8	10.1	Pallast et al. *(20)*
100 mg for 6 mo	31.3 ± 6.0	15.8	
100 mg for 3 mo	33.0	16.7	De Waart et al. *(19)*

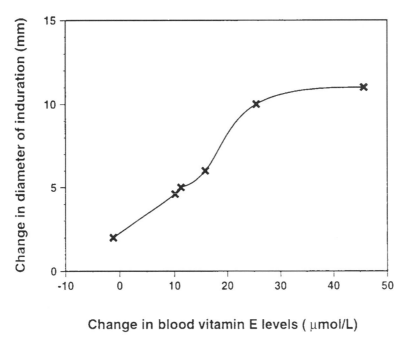

Change in blood vitamin E levels (μmol/L)

Fig. 2. Relationship between changes in delayed type hypersensitivity and changes in blood vitamin E levels after different amounts of vitamin E supplementation. Reproduced from Meydani and Han *(46)*, with permission of ILSI Press, Washington, DC.

investigated the effects of in vitro exposure to different tocopherol homologues on functions of immune cells from old mice. The results showed that all four (α-, β-, γ-, and δ-) tocopherol homologues enhanced lymphocyte proliferation and the magnitude of maximal enhancement was the same. The dose range to produce maximal enhancement varied with different homologues: β- and γ-tocopherols required the lowest dose, and α-tocopherol required the highest dose. All four homologues inhibited cyclooxygenase activity. PGE_2 production by peritoneal macrophages was inhibited by α-, γ-, and δ-tocopherols. Jiang et al. *(10)* also showed that γ-tocopherol reduced PGE_2 synthesis in

LPS-stimulated RAW264.7 cells, a macrophage-like cell line, and in an IL-1β-treated A549 human epithelial cell line.

4. VITAMIN E AND INFECTIOUS DISEASES

The immunostimulatory effect of vitamin E is associated with resistance to infections. Most of the animal studies that investigated the effect of vitamin E on infectious diseases reported a protective effect, despite the variations in the dose and duration of the supplementation, infectious organisms involved, and administration route. Tengerdy and Nockels (21) observed lower mortality after *Escherichia coli* infection in chicks, and Stephens et al. (22) reported a faster recovery, higher food intake and weight gains in lambs infected with *Chlamydia* when given vitamin E supplements. Vitamin E supplementation in old mice resulted in significantly lower viral titer and preserved antioxidant nutrient status after influenza virus infection (23). Vitamin E's protective effect against influenza infection partly results from enhancement of the Th1 response, an increased IL-2 and IFN-γ production (24). Dysregulation of T helper type-1 (Th1) and Th type-2 (Th2) functions are observed with aging, and these changes in Th1/Th2 balance can con-tribute to the delayed clearance and recovery from influenza infection, because Th1 clones are cytolytic in vitro and protective against lethal challenges in vivo, whereas Th2 clones are noncytolytic and not protective (25).

Only a limited number of studies have investigated the effect of vitamin E on resistance against infections in humans. Chavance et al. (26) investigated the relationship between vitamin status and number of infections in healthy individuals aged 60 yr and older. Vitamin E status was negatively associated with the number of infections during the preceding 3 yr. However, it is hard to prove a causal relationship between vitamin E status and incidence of infections from these data, because it is possible that the high incidence of infections in individuals with low vitamin E status may reflect decreased vitamin E levels owing to frequent infections. Chandra (27), Chavance et al. (28), and Girodon et al. (29,30) investigated the effects of vitamin E supplementation in mixture with other nutrients on infections in elderly subjects. Girodon et al. (29,30), investigated the effect of a multitrace element supplement (20 mg of zinc and 100 μg of selenium), multivitamin supplement (120 mg of vitamin C, 6 mg of β-carotene, and 15 mg α-tocopherol), or a combination of these supplements on infectious morbidity and mortality during a 2-yr period in 81 institutionalized elderly (average age of 84 yr), then subsequently among 725 subjects. Subjects who received trace elements alone or in combination with vitamins had significantly less infectious events. Vitamin supplementation alone did not have a significant effect on incidence of infections. Serum vitamin E levels increased from 29.04 μmol/L to 32.2 μmol/L after 1 yr of supplementation. Chavance et al. (28) studied the efficacy of a multivitamin supplement for prevention of common infections in 238 healthy elderly subjects aged 60 yr and older for 4 mo. The supplement contained vitamin A (5000 IU), vitamin D_2 (400 IU), vitamin E (30 IU), ascorbic acid (90 mg), thiamin (2.25 mg), riboflavin (2.6 mg), pyridoxine (3 mg), cyanocobalamin (9 μg), folic acid (0.4 mg), nicotinamide (20 mg), biotin (45 μg), pantothenic acid (10 mg), calcium (162 mg), phosphorus (125 mg), iodine (150 μg), iron (27 mg), magnesium (100 mg), copper (3 mg), manganese (7.5 mg), potassium (7.5 mg), and zinc (22.5 mg). There was no significant difference between the supplemented and the placebo groups in the incidence of infections. No difference in vitamin A status, a slight increase in plasma vitamin C level (3.69 mg/L), and a modest increase in α-tocopherol level (5.81 μmol/L) were observed in the supplemented group. The lack of protective effects of the vitamin mixtures in the previous studies could result from low levels of vitamins used in the mixtures. This is supported by a modest increase in vitamin E levels in the blood. On the other hand, Chandra *(27)* reported a significantly lower number of days of illness due to infections in the group supplemented with nutrient mixtures for 12 mo compared with the placebo group (23 vs 48 d/yr). In this study, 96 healthy elderly aged 65 yr and order were supplemented with either placebo or a multinutrient supplement containing vitamin A (400 RE), β-carotene (16 mg), thiamin (2.2 mg), riboflavin (1.5 mg), niacin (16 mg), vitamin B_6 (3.0 mg), folate (400 μg), vitamin B_{12} (4.0 μg), vitamin C (80 mg), vitamin D (4 μg), vitamin E (44 mg), iron (16 mg), zinc (14 mg), copper (1.4 mg), selenium (20 μg), iodine (0.2 mg), calcium (200 mg), and magnesium (100 mg). The percentage of individuals defined as deficient in vitamin E (serum level <12 μmol/L) was 12.2% (5 of 41) in the placebo group and 2.2% (1 of 45) in the nutrient-supplemented group at the end of the 12-mo supplementation period. Meydani et al. *(17)* also reported a nonsignificant ($p < .09$) 30% lower incidence of self-reported infections among the groups supplemented with vitamin E (60, 200, or 800 mg/d for 235 d) compared with the placebo group. In this study, infection was not the primary outcome, and the study did not have enough power to detect significant differences in infectious incidence. Hemilia et al. *(31)* evaluated the long-term effects of vitamin E and β-carotene supplementation on the incidence of common cold episodes in a cohort of 21,796 male smokers from the Alpha-Tocopherol Beta-Carotene Cancer Prevention Study. The incidence of common cold episodes was documented 3 times/yr during a 4-yr follow-up period. A supplemental dose of 50 mg of vitamin E supplementation resulted in a slightly lower incidence of colds among subjects 65 yr of age or older (rate ratio = .95); this reduction was greatest among older city dwellers who smoked fewer than 15 cigarettes per day (rate ratio = 0.72).

Recently, Graat et al. *(32)* reported that the effect of vitamin E and a multivitamin-mineral supplementation on the incidence and severity of acute respiratory tract infections in elderly noninstitutionalized individuals. A total of 652 individuals aged 60 yr and older (mean age 73 yr) were supplemented with placebo, 200 mg of vitamin E alone, multivitamin-mineral capsule containing retinol (600 μg), β-carotene (1.2 mg), ascorbic acid (60 mg), vitamin E (10 mg), cholecalciferol (5 μg), vitamin K (30 μg), thiamin mononitrate (1.4 mg), riboflavin (1.6 mg), niacin (18 mg), pantothenic acid (6 mg), pyridoxine (2.0 mg), biotin (150 μg), folic acid (200 μg), cyanocobalamin (1 μg), zinc (10 mg), selenium (25 μg), iron (4.0 mg), magnesium (30 mg), copper (1.0 mg), iodine (100 μg), calcium (74 mg), phosphorous (49 mg), manganese (1.0 mg), chromium (25 μg), molybdenum (25 μg), and silicon (2 μg), or vitamin E in combination with the multivitamin-mineral supplement for 15 mo. Incidence and severity of acute respiratory tract infections were self-reported (1024 reports by 443 subjects) and assessed in subsets of patients by a nurse (telephone contact, 757 out of 763 calls were evaluated as acute respiratory tract infections), home visits, and microbiologic and serologic testing (confirmed in 62 of 107 tested). Mean incidence of infections per year was 1.53, 1.73, 1.48, and 1.63 for placebo, vitamin E alone, mutivitamin-mineral, and vitamin E plus multivitamin-mineral groups, respectively. When effects of multivitamin-mineral or vitamin E supplements were analyzed according to the 2 × 2 factorial design, there was no significant effect of multivitamin-mineral supplementation on the incidence rate ratio

(0.95) and severity of infections. There was no significant difference in incidence rate ratio between vitamin E supplemented groups (1.12) and no vitamin E groups (1.00). However, the authors reported that when compared with no vitamin E supplementation (multivitamin-mineral alone or placebo groups), vitamin E supplementation resulted in more severe illness, indicated by significantly higher total illness duration, number of symptoms, presence of fever, and restriction of activities. There are several problems with the data collection methods and interpretation of the results in this study. First, any data collected based on self-report by elderly is questionable, particularly in this case because there was no evaluation of the cognitive function of the subjects. Because vitamin E has been shown to improve cognitive function, this could bias the data so that any beneficial effect of vitamin E in reducing the incidence of infection will be undermined by the subjects' better reporting capability. The authors indicate that a subset of reported infections were confirmed by laboratory tests. However, a close examination of the data indicates that only 107 out of 1024 episodes, i.e., 10% of all episodes, were checked by laboratory tests. Of the cases tested, only 58% of the reported infection was confirmed by laboratory tests. The small percentage of reports tested by laboratory test, and confirmation of only 58% of these, does not generate a high degree of confidence in reliability of the reported data. Second, the 441-d follow-up is reported as the median, indicating that 84% of the subjects could not have achieved the stated 15 mo follow-up. Because the number of infections is time dependent, it is critical that all subjects be evaluated for the same time period. Third, the baseline characteristics of the subjects showed that although there is no significant difference between groups in many of the risk factors, the combined number of chronic obstructive pulmonary diseases (COPD), asthma, allergy, and smoking status is higher in the vitamin E group compared with that of the placebo group (77 in vitamin E group vs 57 in placebo group). It is well-known that COPD, smoking, and asthma increase susceptibility to respiratory infection. In addition, these conditions could directly affect respiratory function and exacerbate the symptoms associated with respiratory infections. Deterioration of airway functions and slower clinical improvement after infection with influenza has been documented in patients with allergy, asthma, or COPD *(33)*. Furthermore, current smokers had higher rates of both asymptomatic and symptomatic influenza than nonsmokers *(34)*. Fourth, compliance by way of post-intervention plasma determination of the nutrients used or returned capsules is neither reported nor discussed, thus making it difficult to determine effectiveness of the supplementation. Fifth, the criteria used for determining illness severity were not well defined. For example, subjects reported symptoms, but it is not clear if a set of predetermined definitions for each symptom was provided to the subjects or if the ability of subjects to accurately determine the symptoms and their duration was validated. Similarly, details regarding methods to define restriction of activity or collection of body temperature data at the same time of the day were not provided. If, indeed, the vitamin E-supplemented group had more severe respiratory infection, this should have been reflected in a higher number of visits to the doctor and more use of prescribed and nonprescribed medication. This apparently was not the case, because the authors report that the number of episode-related medications was the same for the groups. It is also surprising that the authors have included a rise in body temperature as an adverse effect of vitamin E. It is well-known that the elderly do not develop an effective fever response to infection. Previously, we reported that healthy elderly have lower body temperatures compared with young sub-

jects and that vitamin E supplementation corrected the low body temperature in older subjects to that of the younger subjects *(35,36)*. Thus, the higher body temperature observed in this study could be considered a beneficial effect rather than an adverse effect of vitamin E. Furthermore, the data on restriction of activity, a parameter not defined well, was analyzed using a one-tail *t*-test. The authors indicate that a two-tailed *t*-test is necessary, which was used in analysis of other results in the article. If a two-tailed test is used for assessment of the activity data, the difference between vitamin E and placebo group will no longer be significant. In summary, further studies using more rigorous methodology are needed to determine the effect of vitamin E and multivitamin supplements on incidence and severity of infectious diseases in the elderly.

5. MECHANISMS OF IMMUNOENHANCING EFFECT OF VITAMIN E

Several mechanisms have been proposed to explain immunostimulatory effects of vitamin E, including its effect on membrane integrity, PGE_2 production, and signal transduction pathways that are particularly sensitive to oxidative stress, such as those involving the transcription factors, NF-κB and AP-1. Vitamin E can exert its effect either directly on T cells or indirectly through reducing production of suppressive factors from macrophages.

Several lines of evidence indicate that vitamin E exerts its immunostimulatory effects partly by lowering macrophage PGE_2 production *(37,38)*. Preincubation of macrophages from old mice with vitamin E in vitro increased proliferation of cocultures containing T cells from either young or old mice and increased IL-2 production of cocultures containing T cells from old mice accompanied by decreased production of PGE_2 *(37)*. These data suggest that the immunoenhancing effect of vitamin E is partly mediated through lowering PGE_2 production of old macrophages. Vitamin E supplementation of old mice eliminates the age-associated increase in PGE_2 production and suppresses the age-associated increase in Cox-2 activity. Cox-2 is a key isoenzyme involved in the conversion of arachidonic acid to prostaglandins. The vitamin E-induced suppression of Cox activity did not result from a decrease in expression of protein or mRNA for Cox-1 or Cox-2, indicating that regulation of Cox activity by vitamin E is at the posttranslational level *(38)*.

The results from the study by Beharka et al. *(39)* suggest that peroxynitrite plays an important role in vitamin E-induced inhibition of Cox activity. Peroxynitrite, a product of nitric oxide (NO) and superoxide (O_2^-), increased the Cox activity without affecting its expression levels *(40)*. Macrophages from old mice had significantly higher PGE_2 levels, Cox activity, and NO levels compared with young mice; these levels were significantly reduced by vitamin E supplementation in the old macrophages. When NO and O_2^- inhibitors were added together, Cox activity was significantly reduced in the macrophages from old mice fed 30 ppm vitamin E in the diet. However, adding NO or O_2^- inhibitors alone had no effect on inhibiting Cox activity. When peroxynitrite levels were increased by a continuous source of NO and O_2^-, Cox activity in macrophages from old mice fed 500 ppm vitamin E in the diet increased significantly, whereas there was no change in macrophages from old mice fed 30 ppm vitamin E in the diet. These results strongly suggest that vitamin E reduces Cox activity through reduction in peroxynitrite formation, which, at least in part, results from a decrease in NO production by vitamin E.

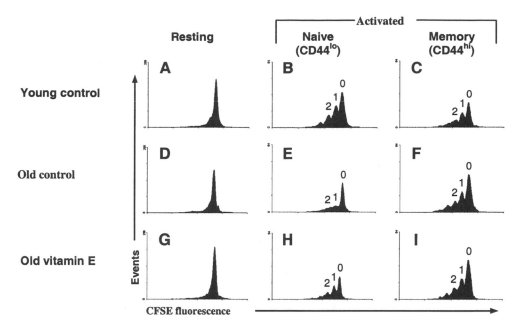

Fig. 3. Effect of age and vitamin E on the progression of T cells through cell cycle division. Purified T cells were preincubated with 46 μm vitamin E for 4 h, labeled with carboxyfluoroscein succinimidyl ester (CFSE) and activated with immobilized anti-CD3 and soluble anti-CD28 MAb for 48 h. Cells were harvested, stained for CD44 expression, and analyzed on a flow cytometer. One representative histogram for each of young control (**A**, **B**, and **C**), old control (**D**, **E**, and **F**), and old preincubated with vitamin E (**G**, **H**, and **I**) are shown. Cell cycle division patterns are shown for unactivated T cells (**A**, **D**, and **G**), activated naive (CD44[lo]) T cells (**B**, **E**, and **D**), and activated memory (CD44[hi]) T cells (**C**, **F**, and **I**). Peaks representing cell division cycles 0, 1, and 2 are also indicated. Reproduced from Adolfsson et al. *(41)* with permission, copyright 2001, The American Association of Immunologists, Inc.

In addition to its effect on reducing PGE_2 production by macrophages, vitamin E has a direct, PGE_2-independent, immunoenhancing effect on T-cell function in the aged. When purified T cells were supplemented with 46 μM vitamin E by an in vitro method, both proliferation and total IL-2 production in response to anti-CD3 and anti-CD28 stimulation by T cells from old mice increased significantly, whereas there was no significant effect on young T cells *(41)*. It is well accepted that aging is accompanied by a phenotypic shift in the peripheral T-cell population, from mostly T cells that have not encountered antigen (naïve) to a much greater proportion of T cells that have (memory). This shift in T-cell phenotype is a major change that influences T cell-mediated immunity in the aged *(42,43)*, because naïve and memory T cells differ in response kinetics to activating stimuli and the requirements for cell activation.

A study by Adolfsson et al. *(41)* demonstrated that vitamin E could enhance the functions of T cells from old mice directly, with preferential effect on naïve but not memory T cells. When young and old T cells supplemented with vitamin E were examined for their ability to go through activation-induced cell division during a 48-h period, vitamin E significantly increased the ability of naïve T cells from old mice to progress through one, as well as two, cell division cycles (*see* Fig. 3). This enhancing effect of

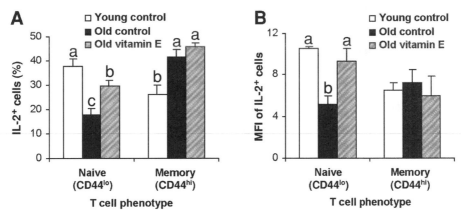

Fig. 4. Effect of age and vitamin E on intracellular interleukin (IL)-2 by naïve and memory T-cell subsets. Purified T cells ($n = 5$) were preincubated with 46 µm vitamin E for 4 h and activated with immobilized anti-CD3 and soluble anti-CD28 MAb for 48 h. Cells were treated with monensin, an IL-2 secretion inhibitor, for the last 10 h of activation. Harvested cells were stained with fluorochrome-conjugated anti-CD44 MAb, permeabilized, and stained with fluorochrome-conjugated anti-IL-2. T cells were divided in to naïve and memory phenotypes based on low or high expression of the CD44 antigen, respectively. Cell fluorescence was measured on a flow cytometer. **(A)** Relative proportion (mean ± SEM) of IL-2$^+$ T cells. **(B)** Linearized mean fluorescence intensity (MFI) of IL-2$^+$ T cells. Bars with different letters within each phenotype are significantly different ($p < 0.05$) by an analysis of variance followed by Tukey's HSD post-hoc procedure. Reproduced from Adolfsson et al. *(41)* with permission, copyright 2001, The American Association of Immunologists, Inc.

vitamin E was not observed for memory T cells from old mice. Furthermore, by performing intracellular staining of IL-2, vitamin E supplementation increased IL-2 production by naïve T cells from old mice, whereas there was no effect on IL-2 production by memory T cells. Both the number of naïve IL-2$^+$ T cells from old mice and the intensity of fluorescence staining, indicating the amount of IL-2 produced per cell, was increased by vitamin E (*see* Fig. 4). The differential effect of vitamin E on naïve and memory T cells may result from an underlying difference in the susceptibility of these cells to oxidative stress-induced damage, because memory T cells from old mice are reported to be more resistant to oxidative injury than naïve T cells *(44)*.

Recently, several tocopherol-binding proteins, α-tocopherol transfer protein (α-TTP) and cellular tocopherol associated proteins (TAPs), have been identified. α-TTP is mainly expressed in the liver, brain, retina, and lymphocytes, and TAPs are present in all cells. These proteins are involved in providing nonantioxidant molecular functions of vitamin E, including regulation of protein kinase C activity at the cellular level *(45)*. Further research will clarify the exact role that these binding proteins play in modulating effects of vitamin E.

6. CONCLUSIONS

Several investigations have demonstrated that vitamin E significantly enhances immune functions in humans, especially in the elderly. Results from cellular and molecular mechanistic studies have shown that immunoregulatory effects of vitamin E are mediated indirectly by reducing the production of suppressive factors, such as PGE$_2$, by macrophages and directly by increasing cell division capacity and IL-2 production by naïve T cells. Animal studies strongly suggest that vitamin E supplementation improves resistance against bacterial and viral infections. However, clinical significances and benefits of vitamin E supplementation in humans have not yet been demonstrated conclusively. Controlled intervention studies in humans are required to establish the clinical significance of vitamin E supplementation. In addition, considering the emerging evidence on differential effects of different forms of vitamin E, more studies investigating the effects of different forms of vitamin E, other than α-tocopherol, on immune functions are needed.

7. "TAKE-HOME" MESSAGES

1. Vitamin E is a chain-breaking antioxidant that protects membrane from free-radical damage. It occurs naturally in eight forms (α-, β-, γ-, and δ-tocopherols and α-, β-, γ-, and δ-tocotrienols) that differ in biological and antioxidant activities.
2. Several intervention studies have shown that vitamin E supplementation higher than recommended levels enhances immune functions in animals and humans, especially the elderly.
3. Differences in results observed in human studies regarding effects of vitamin E on immune functions may reflect the differences in vitamin E status at baseline and supplementation dose, resulting in varied levels of changes in plasma vitamin E levels and methodology.
4. Vitamin E exerts its immunostimulatory effects by lowering macrophage PGE$_2$ production via reduction in cyclooxygenase activity and by directly enhancing T-cell functions in the elderly via increasing naïve T-cell IL-2 production and ability to go through activation-induced cell division.
5. The immunostimulatory effect of vitamin E is associated with increased resistance to infections in animal studies. However, clinical significance and benefits of vitamin E supplementation in humans have not yet been demonstrated, mainly because of a lack of well-controlled intervention studies.
6. Further studies are needed to investigate the effects of different forms of vitamin E, other than α-tocopherol, on immune functions, as well as their clinical significance in humans.

REFERENCES

1. Engelhart MJ, Geerlings MI, Ruitenberg A, et al. Dietary intake of antioxidants and risk of Alzheimer Disease. JAMA 2002;287:3223–3229.
2. Rimm EB, Stampfer MJ, Ascherio A, Giovannucci E, Colditz GA, Willet WC. Vitamin E consumption and the risk of coronary heart disease in men. N Engl J Med 1993;328:1450–1456.
3. Helzlsouer KJ, Huang HY, Alberg AJ, et al. Association between alpha-tocopherol, gamma-tocopherol, selenium, and subsequent prostate cancer. J Natl Cancer Inst 2000;92:2018–2023.
4. Gebremichael A, Levy EM, Corwin LM. Adherent cell requirement for the effect of vitamin E on in vitro antibody synthesis. J Nutr 1984;114:1297–1305.
5. Kowdley KV, Mason JB, Meydani SN, Cornwall S, Grand RJ. Vitamin E deficiency and impaired cellular immunity related to intestinal fat malabsorption. Gastroenterology 1992;102:2139–2142.
6. Meydani SN, Barklund MP, Liu S, et al. Vitamin E supplementation enhances cell-mediated immunity in healthy elderly subjects. Am J Clin Nutr 1990;52:557–563.
7. Han SN, Meydani SN. Vitamin E and infectious diseases in the aged. Proc Nutr Soc 1999;58:1–9.
8. Traber MG. Vitamin E. In: Shils ME, Olson JA, Shike M, Ross AC (eds.). Modern Nutrition in Health and Disease. Williams & Wilkins, Baltimore, 1999, pp. 347–362.

9. Wu D, Meydani M, Beharka AA, Serafini M, Martin KR, Meydani SN. In vitro supplementation with different tocopherol homologues can affect the function of immune cells in old mice. Free Rad Biol Med 2000;28:643–651.
10. Jiang Q, Christen S, Shigenaga MK, Ames BN. γ-Tocopherol, the major form of vitamin E in the US diet, deserves more attention. Am J Clin Nutr 2001;74:714–722.
11. Murphy SP, Subar AF, Block G. Vitamin E intake and sources in the United States. Am J Clin Nutr 1990;52:361–367.
12. Food and Nutrition Board. Dietary Reference Intakes for Vitamin C, Vitamin E, Selenium, Carotenoids. National Academy Press, Washington, DC, 2000.
13. National Research Council. Recommended Dietary Allowances. National Academy Press, Washington, DC, 1989.
14. Ryan AS, Craig LD, Finn SC. Nutrient intakes and dietary patterns of older Americans: a national study. J Gerontol 1992;47:M145–M150.
15. Panemangalore M, Lee CJ. Evaluation of the indices of retinol and α-tocopherol status in free-living elderly. J Gerontol 1992;47:B98–B104.
16. Meydani SN, Meydani M, Verdon CP, Shapiro AA, Blumberg JB, Hayes KC. Vitamin E supplementation suppresses prostaglandin E_2 synthesis and enhances the immune response of aged mice. Mech Ageing Dev 1986;34:191–201.
17. Meydani SN, Meydani M, Blumberg JB, et al. Vitamin E supplementation and in vivo immune response in healthy subjects. JAMA 1997;277:1380–1386.
18. Lee C-YJ, Wan JM-F. Vitamin E supplementation improves cell-mediated immunity and oxidative stress of Asian men and women. J Nutr 2000;130:2932–2937.
19. De Waart F, Portengen L, Doekes G, Verwaal CJ, Kok FJ. Effect of 3 months vitamin E supplementation on indices of the cellular and humoral immune response in elderly subjects. Br J Nutr 1997;78:761–774.
20. Pallast EG, Schouten EG, deWaart FG, et al. Effect of 50- and 100-mg vitamin E supplements on cellular immune function in noninstitutionalized elderly persons. Am J Clin Nutr 1999;69:1273–1281.
21. Tengerdy RP, Nockels CF. Vitamin E or vitamin A protects chickens against *E. coli* infection. Poult Sci 1975;54:1292–1296.
22. Stephens LC, McChesney AE, Nockels CF. Improved recovery of vitamin E-treated lambs that have been experimentally infected with intratracheal cylamydia. Br Vet J 1979;135:291–293.
23. Hayek MG, Taylor SF, Bender BS, et al. Vitamin E supplementation decreases lung virus titers in mice infected with influenza. J Infect Dis 1997;176:273–276.
24. Han SN, Wu D, Ha WK, et al. Vitamin E supplementation increases T helper 1 cytokine production of old mice infected with influenza virus. Immunology 2000;100:487–493.
25. Graham MB, Braciale VL, Braciale TJ. Influenza virus-specific CD4+ T helper type 2 T lymphocytes do not promote recovery from experimental virus infection. J Exp Med 1994;180:1273–1282.
26. Chavance M, Herbeth B, Fournier C, Janot C, Vernhes G. Vitamin status, immunity and infections in an elderly population. Eur J Clin Nutr 1989;43:827–835.
27. Chandra RK. Effect of vitamin and trace-element supplementation on immune responses and infection in elderly subjects. Lancet 1992;340:1124–1127.
28. Chavance M, Herbeth B, Lemoine A, Zhu B-P. Does multivitamin supplementation prevent infections in healthy elderly subjects? A controlled trial. Int J Vit Nutr Res 1993;63:11–16.
29. Girodon F, Lombard M, Galan P, et al. Effect of micronutrient supplementation on infection in institutionalized elderly subjects: a controlled trial. Ann Nutr Metab 1996;41:98–107.
30. Girodon F, Galan P, Monget A-L, et al. Impact of trace elements and vitamin E supplementation on immunity and infections in institutionalized elderly patients. Arch Intern Med 1999;159:748–754.
31. Hemila H, Kaprio J, Albanes D, Heinonen OP, Virtamo J. Vitamin C, vitamin E, and beta-carotene in relation to common cold incidence in male smokers. Epidemiology 2002;13:32–37.
32. Graat JM, Schouten EG, Kok FJ. Effect of daily vitamin E and multivitamin-mineral supplementation on acute respiratory tract infections in elderly persons. JAMA 2002;288:715–721.
33. Nicholson KG. Human influenza. In: Nicholson K, Webster R, Hay AJ (eds.). Textbook of Influenza. Blackwell Sciences Ltd, London, 1998, pp. 219–264.
34. Kark JD, Lebiush M, Rannon L. Cigarette smoking as a risk factor for epidemic A (H1N1) influenza in young men. N Engl J Med 1982;307:1042–1046.

35. Cannon J, Orencole S, Fielding R, et al. Acute phase response in exercise: interaction of age and vitamin E on neutrophils and muscle enzyme release. Am J Physiol 1990;259:R1214–R1219.
36. Cannon JG, Meydani SN, Fielding RA, et al. Acute phase response in exercise. II. Associations between vitamin E, cytokines, and muscle proteolysis. Am J Physiol 1991;260:R1235–R1240.
37. Beharka AA, Wu D, Han SN, Meydani SN. Macrophage prostaglandin production contributes to the age-associated decrease in T cell function which is reversed by the dietary antioxidant vitamin E. Mech Ageing Dev 1997;93:59–77.
38. Wu D, Mura C, Beharka AA, et al. Age-associated increase in PGE_2 synthesis and COX activity in murine macrophages is reversed by vitamin E. Am J Physiol 1998;275:C661–C668.
39. Beharka A, Wu D, Serafini M, Meydani S. Mechanism of vitamin E inhibition of cyclooxygenase activity in macrophages from old mice: role of peroxynitrite. Free Rad Biol Med 2002;32:503–511.
40. Landino LM, Crews BC, Timmons MD, Morrow JD, Marnett LJ. Peroxynitrite, the coupling product of nitric oxide and superoxide, activates prostaglandin biosynthesis. Proc Natl Acad Sci USA 1996;93:15069–15074.
41. Adolfsson O, Huber BT, Meydani SN. Vitamin E-enhanced IL-2 production in old mice: naive but not memory T cells show increased cell division cycling and IL-2-producing capacity. J Immunol 2001;167:3809–3817.
42. Miller RA. The aging immune system: primer and prospectus. Science 1996;273:70–74.
43. Ernst DN, Hobbs MV, Torbett BE, et al. Differences in the expression profiles of CD45RB, Pgp-1, and 3G11 membrane antigens and in the patterns of lymphokine secretion by splenic CD4+ T cells from young and aged mice. J Immunol 1990;145:1295–1302.
44. Lohmiller JJ, Roellich KM, Toledano A, Rabinovitch PS, Wolf NS, Grossmann A. Aged murine T-lymphocytes are more resistant to oxidative damage due to the predominance of the cells possessing the memory phenotype. J Gerontol 1996;51:B132–B140.
45. Azzi A, Ricciarelli R, Zingg J-M. Non-antioxidant molecular functions of α-tocopherol (vitamin E). FEBS Lett 2002;519:8–10.
46. Meydani SN, Han SN. Nutrient regulation of the immune response: the case of vitamin E. In: Bowman BA, Russell RM (eds.). Present Knowledge in Nutrition (8th ed.). ILSI Press, Washington, DC, 2001, pp. 449–462.
47. White E, Kristal AR, Shikany JM, et al. Correlates of serum α- and γ-tocopherol in the women's health initiative. Ann Epidemiol 2001;11:136–144.
48. Lewis J, Buss DH. Minerals and vitamins in the British household food supply. Br J Nutr 1988;60: 413–424.
49. Heinonen M, Piironen V. The tocopherol, tocotrienol, and vitamin E content of the average Finnish diet. Int J Vit Nutr Res 1991;61:27–32.
50. Thompson JN, Beare-Rogers JL, Erdody P, Smith DC. Appraisal of human vitamin E requirement based on examination of individual meals and a composite Canadian diet. Am J Clin Nutr 1973;26:1349–1354.
51. O'Brien MM, Kiely M, Harrington KE, Robson PJ, Strain JJ, Flynn A. The North/South Ireland Food Consumption Survey: vitamin intakes in 18–64-year-old adults. Public Health Nutr 2001;4:1069–1079.
52. Prasad JS. Effect of vitamin E supplementation on leukocyte function. Am J Clin Nutr 1980;33:606–608.
53. Okanno T, Tamai H, Makoto M. Superoxide generation in leukocytes and vitamin E. Int J Vit Nutr Res 1990;61:20–26.
54. Richards G, Theron A, Van Rensburg C, et al. Investigation of the effects of oral administration of vitamin E and beta-carotene on the chemiluminescence responses and the frequency of sister chromatid exchanges in circulating leukocytes from cigarette smokers. Am Rev Respir Dis 1990;142:648–654.
55. Ziemlanski S, Wartanowicz M, Klos A, Raczka A, Klos M. The effects of ascorbic acid and alpha-tocopherol supplementation on serum proteins and immunoglobulin concentration in the elderly. Nutr Int 1986;2:1–5.
56. Harman D, Miller RW. Effect of vitamin E on the immune response to influenza virus vaccine and the incidence of infectious disease in man. Age 1986;9:21–23.
57. van Tits LJ, Demacker PN, de Graaf J, Hak-Lemmers HL, Stalenhoef A. α-Tocopherol supplementation decreases production of superoxide and cytokines by leukocytes ex vivo in both normolipidemic and hypertriglyceridemic individuals. Am J Clin Nutr 2000;71:458–464.

9 Carotenoids

David A. Hughes

1. INTRODUCTION

The consumption of five portions of fruit and vegetables a day is now a common recommendation by many national and international advisory bodies *(1–3)*, which is based on several epidemiologic studies that show a consistent association between a high intake of fruits and vegetables and a reduced incidence of chronic diseases, such as cancer *(4)* and cardiovascular disease *(5)*. However, the active components in fruits and vegetables responsible for these beneficial effects remain uncertain. Recently, considerable attention has been given to the carotenoids found in these foods, mainly their antioxidant properties. After a major review article in *Nature* by Peto and colleagues in 1981 *(6)*, a great deal of attention focused on the potential role of one particular carotenoid, β-carotene, in preventing cancer. Numerous publications have described epidemiologic studies, in vitro experiments, animal studies, and clinical trials that suggest that this carotenoid can protect against not only cancer but also other oxidative damage-associated disorders, as listed in Table 1 (reviewed in *[7]*).

2. SOURCES, BIOAVAILABILTY, AND INTAKES

2.1. Sources

Carotenoids were first isolated from carrots by Wackenroder in 1831. The carotenoids are a group of more than 600 naturally occurring colored pigments that are widespread in plants, of which only approx 20 commonly occur in human foodstuffs. Table 2 details the carotenoid content of commonly eaten vegetables and fruits. More detailed carotenoid databases can be found in the article by O'Neill et al. *(8)* and at the U.S. Department of Agriculture (USDA) Web site at http://www.nal.usda.gov/fnic/foodcomp/Data/Carot/index.html. The most prevalent carotenoids include β-carotene, α-carotene, lycopene, lutein, β-cryptoxanthin, and zeaxanthin. Only three of these (β-carotene, α-carotene, and β-cryptoxanthin) are converted to vitamin A in the body and considered "provitamin" carotenoids. The chemical structures of some carotenoids are shown in Fig. 1.

One of the most potentially beneficial uses of genetically modified foods is the introduction of β-carotene into rice ("Golden rice") *(9)*. Rice is a major staple food for several hundred million people, but the edible part of rice grains consists of the endosperm, filled with starch granules and protein bodies, and it lacks several essential nutrients, such as

From: *Diet and Human Immune Function*
Edited by: D. A. Hughes, L. G. Darlington, and A. Bendich © Humana Press Inc., Totowa, NJ

Table 1
Degenerative Disorders Associated with
Oxidative Damage

Cancer
Cardiovascular disease
Chronic obstruction pulmonary disease
Cataract
Degeneration of the macula region of the retina
Immunosenescence
Aging
Alzheimer's disease
Type 2 diabetes
Stroke
Asthma
HIV infection
Autoimmune disorders

---

carotenoids exhibiting provitamin A activity. Thus, reliance on rice as a primary food staple contributes to vitamin A deficiency, a serious health problem in many parts of Africa and Asia (*see* Chapter 7). It is only now possible to fortify rice with β-carotene by recombinant technologies, because there are no conventional rice cultivars that produce β-carotene in the endosperm. It is hoped that after further improvement and testing this modified rice will contribute to the alleviation of vitamin A deficiency, provided that access to the β-carotene-rich seeds by poor farmers in developing countries is possible at the same cost as current popular cultivars *(9)*.

2.2. Bioavailability

In nature, carotenoids in several plants, animals, and microorganisms are complexed with protein. Therefore, release from the food matrix is an important factor in the absorption process. Studies on the effect of food matrix on carotenoid bioavailability have usually compared the responses of pure, formulated, natural, or synthetic carotenoid preparations with the equivalent carotenoid dose found in a food source. Several investigators have found that pure β-carotene dissolved in oil or aqueous dispersions (i.e., many forms of supplements) is efficiently absorbed (>50%), whereas carotenoids in uncooked vegetables, such as β-carotene in the carrot or lycopene in tomato juice, are poorly absorbed (<3%). Readers interested in a summary of current knowledge of carotenoid bioavailability and bioconversion within the body are referred to a recent review by Yeum and Russell *(10)*.

Because β-carotene is fat soluble, there has been some concern recently regarding the use of vegetable oil spreads enriched with plant sterols or stanols (as their fatty acid esters), which inhibit cholesterol absorption in the small intestine, because the reduced fat absorption might result in low circulating levels of fat-soluble vitamins and carotenoids. However, recent research suggests that this is not a problem, particularly if the spreads are eaten as part of a well-balance diet containing fruits and vegetables *(11)*.

Table 2
The Carotenoid Content of Vegetables and Fruits μg/100 g "Wet Weight" as Eaten (65)

Food		β-Carotene	α-Carotene	Lycopene	Lutein	β-cryptoxanthin	Zeaxanthin
Brussels sprout (frozen)	Raw	553	–	–	610	–	–
Brussels sprout (frozen)	Cooked	555	–	–	621	–	–
Bean, green (frozen)	Raw	376	70	–	494	–	–
Bean, green (frozen)	Cooked	373	26	–	548	–	–
Beans, baked (in tomato sauce)	Canned	30	–	1659	25	–	–
Beans, runner	Raw	343	33	–	555	–	–
Beans, runner	Cooked	538	Trace	–	632	–	–
Broccoli, fresh	Raw	919	–	–	1614	–	–
Broccoli, fresh	Cooked	1381	–	–	1949	–	–
Cabbage, green	Raw	59	–	–	80	–	–
Cabbage, green	Cooked	71	–	–	111	–	–
Carrots	Raw	10,800	3610	–	283	–	–
Carrots	Cooked	12,302	3767	–	313	–	–
Carrots (frozen)	Raw	8538	3268	–	268	–	–
Carrots (frozen)	Cooked	9907	3851	–	300	–	–
Parsley	Raw	4523	–	–	5812	–	–
Peas (frozen)	Raw	438	–	–	1633	–	–
Peas (frozen)	Cooked	670	–	–	1991	–	–
Pepper, green	Raw	298	–	–	660	–	–
Pepper, orange	Raw	416	167	–	503	90	1608
Tomato, fresh	Raw	439	–	2937	78	–	–
Tomato, fresh	Cooked	648	–	3703	120	–	–
Tomatoes, tinned	In sauce	423	–	6205	105	–	–
Watercress	Raw	5912	–	–	10,713	–	–
Apples	Eating	35	Not detectable	–	84	11	13
Apricots	Fresh	1766	37	–	101	231	31
Apricots	Tinned	879	Not detectable	–	59	32	16
Mandarin oranges		285	12	–	50	1774	142
Satsumas		23	Not detectable	–	44	1180	41

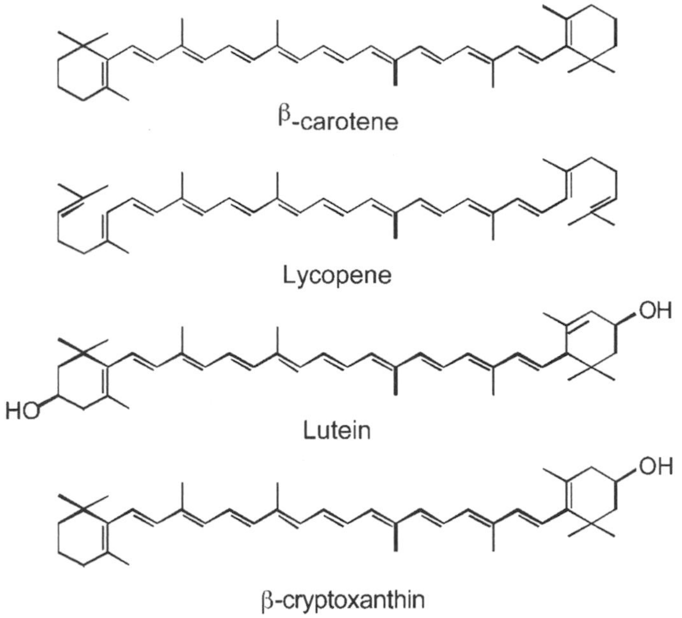

Fig. 1. Chemical structure of some carotenoids found in the diet.

2.3. Intakes

2.3.1. RECOMMENDED INTAKES

Although numerous studies have suggested that high blood concentrations of β-carotene and other carotenoids are associated with low risk of several diseases, the US Institute of Medicine has concluded that this evidence cannot be used to establish a requirement for β-carotene or total carotenoid intake, because these effects may be the result of other compounds present in carotenoid-rich foods or might be related to behaviors correlated with increased fruit and vegetable consumption *(12)*. Therefore, currently there are no Dietary Reference Intakes (DRIs) for carotene intake, because it is believed that the current state of research on these nutrients is not strong and consistent enough to support any recommendations. A 6-mg β-carotene intake is required to meet the vitamin A Recommended Dietary Allowance (RDA) of 1 mg retinol equivalents (RE). (RE is a measurement of vitamin A intake that allows for comparing different forms of the vitamin.) One IU of vitamin A is equivalent to 0.6 μg of β-carotene. Because of insufficient data demonstrating a threshold above which adverse events will occur, no Tolerable Upper Intake Level has been set for any carotenoid *(13)*.

Carotenoids are believed to be safe at fairly high doses. Some areas of skin may become yellow or orange in color (carotenodermia) if high doses of β-carotene (>30 mg/d) are taken for long periods but will return to normal when intake is reduced *(12)*. This effect has been used therapeutically to treat patients with erythropoietic photoporphyria (a photosensitivity disorder). These patients have been treated with doses of approx 180 mg/d without reports of toxic effects *(12)*. However, there is now some concern regarding the use of high levels of synthetic β-carotene supplements in smokers because of the possible association with an increase in lung cancer (*see* section 5).

2.3.2. European and American Estimated Dietary Intakes

It is only recently that the detailed carotenoid composition of foods has been entered in the various food tables used to estimate dietary intakes. Table 3 details a comparison of carotenoid intakes in adults from five European countries (Spain, France, United Kingdom, Republic of Ireland, and the Netherlands) during the winter season, together with data obtained from southern California and Maryland.

The European countries were studied using a newly constructed carotenoid database (8), the Maryland study used a USDA-National Cancer Institute (USDA-NCI) carotenoid food-composition database (14), and the California data were obtained by a modified food-frequency questionnaire (FFQ) collecting additional data on the intake of carotenoid-rich food items (15).

The data for the European countries suggest that the French had a significantly higher median intake of total carotenoids than other participating countries and the Spanish had the lowest (8). No significant differences were observed between men and women in any of the European countries. The same FFQ was also used in the summer in the United Kingdom, Republic of Ireland, and Spain, and there were no seasonal differences in the median total intakes of carotenoids. Analysis of the main foods contributing to the intake of the individual carotenoids showed that carrots are the richest source of β-carotene in the European diet, and, only in Spain, where carrots are not consumed in large amounts, did another food, spinach, make the major contribution to dietary β-carotene. Spinach was also the major contributor to dietary lutein in Spain, as well as the Netherlands and France, whereas peas were the main contributor in the United Kingdom and the Republic of Ireland. The major sources of lycopene in all the European countries were tomatoes, canned tomatoes, tomato soup, and pizza (except Spain). In Spain, pizza consumption was a minor contributor to lycopene intake, and fresh tomatoes and tomato puree in other dishes were the principal food sources. It should be noted that other factors can influence carotenoid intake. Smoking is associated with lower carotenoid intakes in the United Kingdom (16), and Carroll et al. (17) have reported that β-carotene and lycopene intakes were 36% and 58% lower, respectively, in a group of elderly individuals (≥65 yr) compared with a younger age (24–45 yr) group. The US intake data were comparable with the European study, and the only notable difference was that lycopene, rather than β-carotene, is the major source of carotenoids in both US groups.

3. OXIDATIVE STRESS AND THE IMMUNE SYSTEM

In nature, carotenoids serve two essential functions: accessory pigments in photosynthesis and in photoprotection. These two functions are achieved through the chemical structure of carotenoids (*see* Fig. 1), which allows the molecules to absorb light and to quench singlet oxygen and free radicals.

Oxidative stress, resulting from cumulative damage caused by reactive oxygen species (ROS), is present throughout life and is believed to be a major contributor to the aging process (18). The immune system is especially vulnerable to oxidative damage, because many immune cells produce these reactive compounds as part of the body's defense mechanisms to destroy invading pathogens. Higher organisms have evolved several antioxidant defense systems to either prevent ROS generation or intercept any that are generated. Enzymes such as catalase and glutathione peroxidase can safely decompose

Table 3
Comparison of Carotenoid Intakes (mg/d) in Adults in Five European Countries and in Two States in the United States

Sex and age of groups studied	β-Carotene Median Range	α-Carotene Median Range	Lycopene Median Range	Lutein (+ zeaxanthin) Median Range	β-Cryptoxanthin Median Range	Total carotenoids Median Range
Spain (n = 70)[a]	Men and women	2.96 1.58–4.41	0.29 0.15–0.51	1.64 0.50–2.64	3.25 1.75–4.34	1.36 0.74–2.16	9.54 7.16–14.46
France (n = 76)	25–45 yr,	5.84 3.83–8.00	0.74 0.37–1.36	4.75 2.14–8.31	2.50 1.71–3.91	0.45 0.17–0.88	16.06 10.3–22.1
United Kingdom (n = 71)	in all five countries	5.55 3.66–6.56	1.04 0.71–1.66	5.01 3.2–7.28	1.59 1.19–2.37	0.99 0.32–1.64	14.38 11.77–19.1
Republic of Ireland (n = 76)		5.16 3.47–7.42	1.23 0.69–1.78	4.43 2.73–7.13	1.56 1.14–2.1	0.78 0.4–1.44	14.53 10.37–18.9
The Netherlands (n = 75)		4.35 2.93–5.7	0.68 0.30–0.90	4.86 2.79–7.53	2.01 1.42–3.04	0.97 0.50–1.75	13.71 9.98–17.7
Maryland, USA (n = 98)[b]	Women 28.6 ± 5.1[d]	2.70 0.26–11.20	0.55 0.04–3.84	3.01 0.03–15.0	1.87 0.02–9.57	0.03 0.01–0.26	8.54 1.03–24.53
California, USA (n = 215)[c]	Men and women 62.0 ± 6.8[d]	4.80 ± 3.23[d]	0.94 ± 0.79	5.18 ± 3.86	3.23 ± 2.29	0.07 ± 0.07	Not stated

[a]O'Neill et al., 2001. (8).
[b]Yong et al., 1994 (14).
[c]Enger et al., 1995 (15).
[d]Mean ± SD.

170

peroxides, particularly hydrogen peroxide produced during the "respiratory burst" involved in killing invading microorganisms, whereas superoxide dismutase intercepts or "scavenges" free radicals. However, the food we eat provides us with a large amount of our body's total supply of antioxidants in the form of various essential micronutrients and "nonnutrients."

If we imagine oxidative stress in terms of a two-pan balance, with ROS in one pan and antioxidants in the other, tipping the balance in favor of the ROS is believed to be a major contributor to several degenerative disorders, such as cancer and cardiovascular diseases (*see* Table 1), as well as the general aging process. Indeed, it is probably prudent to attempt to keep the balance of ROS to antioxidants as level as possible from as early an age as possible to prolong the onset of, if not prevent, many age-related disorders.

The immune system is particularly sensitive to oxidative stress. Immune cells rely heavily on cell-cell communication, particularly via membrane-bound receptors, to work effectively. Cell membranes are rich in polyunsaturated fatty acids (PUFAs), which, if peroxidized, can lead to a loss of membrane integrity, altered membrane fluidity (19), and alterations in intracellular signaling and cell function. ROS exposure can lead to a reduction in cell membrane receptor expression (20). In addition, the ROS production by phagocytic immune cells can damage the cells themselves if they are not sufficiently protected by antioxidants (21).

4. CAROTENOIDS AND THE HUMAN IMMUNE SYSTEM

The immune system plays a major role in preventing the development of cancer, and it has, therefore, been suggested that β-carotene and possibly other carotenoids present in the diet may enhance the function of immune cells involved in detecting and eliminating tumor cells. In animals, adding carotenoids to the diet prevented stress-related thymic involution, increased the number of circulating lymphocytes, enhanced lymphocyte proliferation and cytotoxic T-cell activity, and increased resistance to infective pathogens (22,23).

4.1. Effects of β-Carotene on Human Immune Function

Repeated exposure to ultraviolet (UV) light markedly suppresses immune function (24). Because carotenoids can provide photoprotection, several studies have assessed the ability of β-carotene to protect the immune system from UV-induced free-radical damage. In one study, a group of young men were placed on a low-carotenoid diet (<1.0 mg/d total carotenoids) and given either placebo or 30 mg β-carotene/d for 28 d before periodic exposure to UV light. Delayed type hypersensitivity (DTH) responses were significantly suppressed in the placebo group after UV treatments, and the suppression was inversely proportional to plasma β-carotene concentrations in this group (25), but no significant suppression of DTH responses was seen in the β-carotene-treated group. In a later study, the same research team studied a group of healthy older men, again given either 30 mg β-carotene or placebo for 28 d before periodic exposure to UV light. They again observed a suppression of DTH response after UV exposure, but in this age group, the extent of protective effect of β-carotene appeared less than had been observed with the younger men (26). The authors suggest that this might have resulted from either a reduced plasma response to supplementation in the older age group and/or to higher plasma vitamin E levels than was observed in the younger men. These workers also observed that stronger

DTH responses were associated with higher plasma β-carotene concentrations in both UV- and non-UV-exposed individuals. β-Carotene's ability to protect against the harmful effects of natural UV sunlight has also been demonstrated by exposing healthy female students to time- and intensity-controlled sunlight exposure: a Berlin-based study involved taking volunteers to the Red Sea and exposing areas of their skin to the sunlight by lifting discretely placed flaps in their specially designed swimsuits *(27)*!

Several studies have examined the effect of β-carotene on immune function by measuring changes in the numbers of lymphocyte subpopulations and on the expression of cell activation markers. However, because of the large variation in intakes of β-carotene and the duration of supplementation, numerous results have been obtained, and it is extremely difficult to make adequate comparisons between the different studies. Indeed, doses ranging from dietary achievable levels of 15 mg/d up to pharmacologic doses of 300 mg/d have been provided for periods of between 14 d and 12 yr (*see* Table 4). What is common to many studies, however, is that more marked changes are observed in those involving older individuals. This might be predicted, because a reduction in the body's ability to mount an immune response is a recognized feature of aging—"immunosenescence" *(28)*. For example, there have been reported increases in the numbers of CD4+ lymphocytes ("helper" T cells that stimulate cell-mediated immune responses) or in the ratio of CD4+ to CD8+ cells ("suppressor" T cells that inhibit responses), and in the percentages of lymphocytes expressing markers of cell activation, such as interleukin (IL)-2 receptors and transferrin receptors *(29,30)*, particularly in older individuals. The potential for increasing the numbers of CD4+ cells led to the suggestion that β-carotene might be useful as an immunoenhancing agent in treating HIV infection. Preliminary studies have shown a slight but insignificant increase in CD4+ numbers in response to β-carotene (60 mg/d for 4 wk) in patients with AIDS *(31)*, but long-term effectiveness in treating HIV infection or AIDS has not been reported.

Other studies have been unable to confirm the increase in T cell-mediated immunity in healthy individuals after β-carotene supplementation. Santos and colleagues *(32)* recently reported the results of two studies in the elderly: a short-term high-dose study (90 mg/d for 21 d) in women and a longer term lower-dose trial (50 mg/alternate days for 10–12 yr) in men. The conclusion of both studies was that there was no significant difference in T-cell function as assessed by DTH response, lymphocyte proliferation, IL-2 production, and lymphocyte subset composition. However, these investigators also examined the effect of β-carotene supplementation on natural killer (NK) cell activity in the longer term trial with male volunteers. Homozygous mice, genetically deficient in NK cell activity, grow tumors and develop leukemia more rapidly than heterozygous littermates with normal NK cell function. Patients with Chediak-Higashi syndrome, a disorder associated with defective NK cell function, show a higher susceptibility to tumor formation. Therefore, the possible effect of β-carotene on NK cell activity is believed to be a link between raised intakes of this nutrient and cancer prevention. In the study by Santos and colleagues *(33)*, β-carotene supplementation resulted in significantly greater NK cell activity compared with subjects of a similar age who were given placebo treatment. This study also highlighted the reduction in NK cell activity that is observed with age, but, interestingly, the increase in NK cell activity observed in older men (65–86 yr) after β-carotene supplementation restored it to the level seen in a group of younger men (51–64 yr). The mechanism for this remains unknown, but it did not result from an

Table 4
Beta-Carotene Supplementation and Immune Responses in Humans

Subjects	Age[a]	Amount and duration of supplementation	Effects on immune function	Reference
Healthy men (n = 17)	20–40	180 mg/d for 14 d	↑% total T cells, ↑% CD4+ cells, ↔ T-cell numbers	(66)
Barrett esophagus, men (n = 9)	35–75 (59)	30 mg/d for 3 mo	↑% interleukin (IL)-2R expression, ↑% natural killer (NK) cells, ↑ NK function, ↔% total T cells, CD4+ and CD8+ cells	(67)
Oral leukoplakia, men (n = 16)	39–79 (62)	30 mg/d for 3 mo	Same effects as above	(67)
Healthy men and women (5 groups of 10 each)	18–54 (34)	0, 15, 45, 180, 300 mg/d + Unicap multivitamin[b]/d for 1 mo	↔ total T cells, CD4+, CD8+, B cells, NK cells, HLA-DR+, IL-2R+, IL-2 production, immunoglobulin (Ig) production	(68)
Healthy men (n = 10) and women (n = 10) (5 groups of 4)	50–65 (56)	0, 15, 30, 45, 60 mg/d for 2 mo	↑% T cells, ↑% NK cells, ↑% IL-2R+, % transferrinR+ (≤30 mg/d), ↔ total T cells and CD8+cells	(29)
Healthy male smokers (n = 45; 21 β-carotene, 24 placebo)	39.1 ± 9.1[c]	0, 20 mg/d for 14 wk	↑ lymphocyte proliferation, ↔ total T cells, CD4+, CD8+, CD16+ NK cells, CD45RA+ T naïve cells, CD45RO+ memory cells	(69)
Healthy men (n = 20; 10 β-carotene, 10 placebo)	20–25 (22)	0 and 60 mg/d for 44 wk	↑ CD4/CD8 ratio (at 9 mo), ↔ % CD4+, CD8+ T cells, B cells, NK cells	(30)
Healthy women (n = 13; 9 treatment, 4 control)	18–42	68 d depletion, repletion of 15 mg/d for 28 d	↔% CD4+, CD8+ T cells, total T cells, B cells, ↔ NK cells, HLA-DR+ cells	(70)
Healthy men (38 middle-aged, 21 β-carotene, 17 placebo; 21 elderly, 8 β-carotene, 13 placebo)	51–64 (57) 65–86 (74)	50 mg/alternate d for 10–12 yr	↔ CD16+ NK cells, IL-2 production, PGE$_2$ production, ↔ NK function in middle-aged subjects, ↑ NK function in elderly subjects	(33)

(continued)

173

Table 4
Continued

Subjects	Age[a]	Amount and duration of supplementation	Effects on immune function	Reference
Healthy women (n = 23; 11 β-carotene, 12 placebo)	60–80 (70)	90 mg/d for 3 wk	↔ delayed type hypersensitivity (DTH) response, lymphocyte proliferation, IL-2 production, PGE$_2$ production, CD3+, CD4+, CD8+, CD19+ B cells, CD16+ NK cells	(32)
Healthy men (n = 54, 27 β-carotene, 27 placebo)	50–86 (63)	50 mg/alternate d for 10–12 yr	Same effects as above, plus ↔% IL-2R+, % transferrinR+ cells	(32)
Healthy men (n = 25)	19–58 (39)	15 mg/d for 26 d	↑% HLA-DR+ cells, % ICAM-1+ cells, % LFA-3+ cells, TNF-α production	(37)
Healthy men (n = 18, 9 β-carotene, 9 placebo) and women (n = 17, 8 β-carotene, 9 placebo)	65–83 (71)	0, 8.2 mg/d for 12 wk	↔ total T or B cells, % CD4+, % CD8+, CD16+ NK cells, MHC class II+ cells, lymphocyte proliferation, IL-2 or IL-4 production	(46)

[a]Mean in parentheses.
[b]Unicap multivitamin capsule, contained no β-carotene (The Upjohn Company, Kalamazoo, MI).
[c]Age range not stated.

174

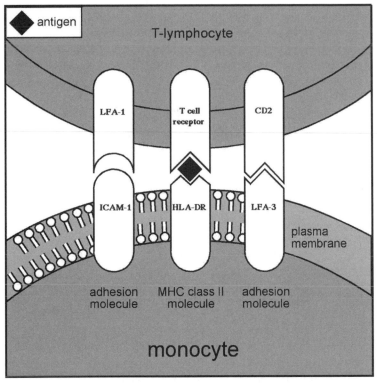

Fig. 2. Cell surface molecules involved in initiating cell-mediated immune responses. LFA, leukocyte function-associated antigen; ICAM-1, intercellular adhesion molecule-1; HLA, human leukocyte-associated antigen; MHC, major histocompatibility complex.

increase in the percentage of NK cells or to an increase in IL-2 production. The authors suggest that β-carotene may act directly on one or more of the lytic stages of NK cell cytotoxicity or on NK cell activity-enhancing cytokines other than IL-2, such as IL-12. This suggestion still awaits confirmation.

Because antigen-presenting cells initiate cell-mediated immune responses, we have investigated whether β-carotene supplementation can influence the function of human blood monocytes, the main antigen-presenting cell type present in the bloodstream. A prerequisite for this function is the expression of major histocompatibility complex (MHC) class II molecules (HLA-DR, HLA-DP, and HLA-DQ) *(34)*, which are present on the majority of human monocytes. The antigenic peptide is presented to the helper T lymphocyte in a groove of the MHC class II molecule (*see* Fig. 2). Because an individual's degree of immune responsiveness is proportional to both the percentage of MHC class II-positive monocytes and the density of these molecules on the cell surface *(35)*, it is possible that one mechanism by which β-carotene may enhance cell-mediated immune responses is by enhancing the cell-surface expression of these molecules. In addition, cell–cell adhesion is critical for the initiation of a primary immune response, and it has been shown that the intercellular adhesion molecule-1 (ICAM-1)-leukocyte function-associated antigen (LFA)-1 ligand-receptor pair is also capable of costimulating an immune response *(36)*, enhancing T-cell proliferation, and cytokine production.

To assess the effect of β-carotene supplementation on the expression of monocyte surface receptors, we undertook a randomized double-blind crossover study of middle-aged nonsmoking men, who participated in two dietary intervention periods of 26 d, during which time they were provided with a daily capsule of either 15 mg β-carotene, a dietary achievable intake (equivalent to 150 g of cooked carrots), or placebo. After dietary supplementation, there were significant increases in β-carotene plasma levels and in the percentages of monocytes expressing the MHC class II molecule, HLA-DR, and the adhesion molecules, ICAM-1 and LFA-3 *(37)*. These results suggest that moderate increases in the dietary intake of β-carotene can enhance cell-mediated immune responses in a relatively short period of time, providing a potential mechanism for the anticarcinogenic properties attributed to this compound. The increase in surface molecule expression could also, in part, account for β-carotene's ability to prevent the reduction in DTH response after exposure to UV radiation, because the latter can inhibit both HLA-DR and ICAM-1 expression on human cell lines. This finding could certainly be relevant to the preventive effect of β-carotene on the formation of skin cancer *(38)*, because immunosuppressed individuals, such as renal transplant patients, are at increased risk of skin cancer.

It has also been suggested that β-carotene can influence immune cell function by modulating the production of prostaglandin (PGE_2). This eicosanoid is the major PG synthesized by monocytes and macrophages and possesses several immunosuppressive properties. It has been suggested that β-carotene might enhance immune responses by altering the activation of the arachidonic acid cascade (from which PGE_2 is derived), because it is capable of suppressing the generation of arachidonic acid products in vitro from nonlymphoid tissues *(39)*.

4.2. Effects of Other Dietary Carotenoids on Human Immune Function

Few studies have examined the influence of other carotenoids on human immune function, even though there is strong epidemiologic evidence to suggest that lycopene (found in tomatoes) and lutein (found in corn, peas, watercress, and other vegetables) can protect against prostate and lung cancer development, respectively. In addition, tomato intake is inversely associated with the risk of diarrheal and respiratory infections in young children in the Sudan *(40)*. To compare the relative ability of different dietary carotenoids to influence the expression of monocyte surface molecules involved in antigen presentation, we undertook comparable studies to the one we had previously conducted with β-carotene, this time providing the same daily intake of either lycopene or lutein (15 mg/ d) to our middle-aged male volunteers. The results suggest that the latter carotenoids have less influence than β-carotene, at least in this particular parameter of immune cell function *(41)*. The less striking effect of either lycopene or lutein supplementation on monocyte surface marker expression that was seen after β-carotene supplementation might be related to the lower plasma levels achieved after supplementation. We previously observed that there might be a threshold effect of plasma β-carotene concentration on the expression of ICAM-1 and LFA-3 *(37)*, and it is possible the lycopene or lutein plasma levels achieved after supplementation were not high enough to cause a significant change in the expression of most of the monocyte surface molecules examined. The reason for the difference in plasma levels of these carotenoids after the same level of supplementation is uncertain but could reflect differences in their uptake, metabolism, and excretion or to selective sequestration of different carotenoids to specific body sites. It is unlikely that lycopene absorption from the supplements is a problem, because it has been shown recently that lycopene bioavailability from tomato juice and dietary supplements is similar *(42)*. However, lycopene is found in higher concentrations in the prostate *(43)* than in serum, and this might contribute to the reduced prostate cancer risk associated with the consumption of tomato-based foods *(44)*. Indeed, one possible factor to explain the different effects seen with different carotenoids might be the preferred location of these compounds within the cell and within the body. Carotenoids are lipid soluble, and, thus, it is believed that most are concentrated in the lipid-rich cell membranes. However, their exact location may influence their effectiveness in modulating specific cellular events. At the whole body level, it is also possible that not all beneficial effects bestowed by carotenoids might be observed systemically, but only at specific locations in the body, suggesting that there might be "hidden" benefits associated with certain dietary components that we have yet to discover. Carotenoid concentrations vary considerably from tissue to tissue, although the mechanism for this remains poorly understood. For instance, the carotenoids, lutein, and zeaxanthin are found in high concentrations in the macular region of the eye, suggesting the presence of a binding protein within this specific eye area *(45)*.

In a further intervention study, we again gave dietary achievable levels of carotenoid supplements, this time to a group of older volunteers (older than 65 yr) living in Ireland. We gave these individuals ($n = 52$) placebo, β-carotene (8.2 mg), or lycopene (13.3 mg) daily for 12 wk and examined changes in various parameters of cell-mediated immunity. We observed no significant changes in T-cell subset numbers, lectin-stimulated lymphocyte proliferation, or surface molecule expression after any of these interventions *(46)*, despite significant increases in carotenoid plasma levels. We concluded that in well-nourished free-living healthy individuals, supplementation with relatively low levels of β-carotene or lycopene is not associated with either beneficial or detrimental effects on cell-mediated immunity. Another group has also shown recently that enriching the diet with lycopene (by drinking 330 mL of tomato juice daily) for 8 wk does not modify cell-mediated immune responses in well-nourished elderly men and women *(47)*. These investigators have also shown an opposing effect of lycopene and lutein, regarding T-lymphocyte proliferation, with lycopene enhancing and lutein inhibiting this activity *(48)*. These results emphasize further that different carotenoids can affect immune cell function differently. Therefore, in a diet containing a good mixture of fruits and vegetables, the influence of the combination of carotenoids they contain on immune function may represent the sum total of these different effects, and, indeed, the potential for synergistic effects must be investigated. The same investigators raised another point of interest: mononuclear cells obtained from volunteers after the lycopene supplementation period had lower endogenous levels of DNA strand breaks, suggesting that tomato juice consumption might induce protective mechanisms in these cells *(49)*. This finding has been also shown by others *(50)* and raises the question of whether enhanced antioxidative DNA protection in immune cells is somehow related to the immunomodulatory effects of carotenoids.

5. CAROTENOID INTAKE AND CANCER RISK

5.1. Epidemiological Studies

In epidemiological studies, the intake of various carotenoids is inversely associated with reduced risk of cancers of the prostate, breast, or head and neck, but the strongest evidence supporting a beneficial association between carotenoids and cancer prevention is β-carotene intake and reductions in the incidence of lung cancer *(51)*. Carotenoid intake has been associated with a reduced lung-cancer risk in 8 of 8 prospective studies and in 18 of 20 retrospective studies *(52)*.

5.2. Prospective Trials

Based on these findings and on earlier studies that found strong beneficial associations between increased β-carotene intake and reduced cancer risk (reviewed by ref. *53*), three major intervention trials were initiated, examining the efficacy of β-carotene in lung cancer prevention *(54–56)*. The now-well-known failure of these trials to show a protective effect, with two of the studies showing a statistically significant increase in lung cancer in smokers receiving β-carotene supplementation, was initially a surprising disappointment to study participants, investigators, supplement manufacturers, and researchers in the area. In addition to affecting the health of smokers involved in these studies, the negative effects have also had an effect on the availability of funds to undertake further studies on the health effects of this compound. The mechanism for the increased lung cancer-risk associated with the supplementation is unclear, but several suggestions have been made. Because the participants in these studies could be classified as "high-risk" for developing lung cancer (long-term smokers or previously exposed to asbestos), it is possible that many of them had undetected tumors before supplementation commencement. The stage (or stages) of carcinogenesis against which β-carotene might be effective is unclear, but if the effect is mediated via the immune system, it is likely to occur during the promotional stages preceding the formation of a malignant tumor. A recent analysis of the Cancer Prevention Study II (CPS-II), a prospective mortality study of more than 1 million US adults, investigated the effects of supplementation with multivitamins and/ or vitamins A, C, and/or E on mortality during a 7-yr follow-up period. The use of a multivitamin plus vitamins A, C, and/or E significantly reduced the risk of lung cancer in former smokers and in never-smokers but increased the risk of lung cancer in male persistent smokers who had used a multivitamin plus vitamins A, C, and/or E, compared with men who had reported no vitamin supplement use. Interestingly, in this study, no association with smoking was seen in women *(57)*.

One of the major unresolved dilemmas of research into β-carotene is what intake is required to help optimize immune function and provide other health benefits. One of the most likely causes of the failure of the prospective studies is the supplementation level provided. Most studies of this compound have been undertaken at levels that are not achievable within a normal healthy diet and that are certainly above the intakes associated with benefits in the epidemiological studies. It is still unclear whether different intakes are associated with different outcomes or, in mechanistic studies, with different effects on various aspects of immune function.

Several authors have suggested that supradietary β-carotene levels may exhibit prooxidant activity, particularly in the presence of high oxygen tensions, as occurs in the lungs (reviewed by *[58]*). In studies of ferrets *(59,60)* (who, like humans, absorb intact β-carotene into their circulation and accumulate it in lung tissue, have a lung architecture similar to humans, and show lung pathology in response to tobacco smoke), the effects of high-dose β-carotene, with or without smoke exposure were examined. Ferrets given β-carotene at a dose equivalent to 30 mg/d in humans and exposed to tobacco smoke had substantially elevated β-carotene oxidation products in their lung tissue. In addition, there was a dramatic decline in the expression of the retinoic acid receptor β (RARβ) in the lungs of ferrets given the high doses of β-carotene, but this was independent of whether they were exposed to cigarette smoke. It has been suggested that this decline in RARβ expression might be a factor regarding the possible promotion of lung carcinogenesis by high intakes of β-carotene, because a decline in the RARβ gene expression has been observed previously in the development of lung cancer *(61)*. However, it should be noted that despite the changes associated with high intakes of β-carotene, no lung tumors were detected in the ferrets, suggesting that the correlation in human populations between smoking, ingestion of high levels of β-carotene, and lung cancer observed in the prospective studies was only partially replicated in the ferrets *(62)*. A further hypothesis, proposed by Bendich *(23)*, is that β-carotene supplementation can enhance lung function in smokers and that this then allows more of the carcinogens and free radicals present in the smoke to reach the smokers' lungs. To support this theory, the Third National Health and Nutrition Examination Survey (NHANES III) associated higher levels of antioxidant nutrients with better lung function in smokers *(63)* and Grievink et al. *(64)* observed that individuals with high β-carotene plasma levels had substantially higher forced vital capacity and higher forced expiratory volume in 1 s than those with low levels, even after adjusting for smoking status and smoking pack years (number of packs smoked per day × number of years smoked). Ongoing clinical trials, such as the Physicians' Health Study II, may provide more insight into the effects of β-carotene supplementation, good or bad.

Of course, the probability remains that the protection of consuming a diet rich in fruits and vegetables is the result of a multifactorial effect of several components of these foods. In support of this, two of the prospective studies mentioned found that higher plasma β-carotene concentrations on entry into the trials, resulting from dietary consumption as opposed to taking supplements, were associated with a lower risk of lung cancer *(13)*. This emphasizes the need for more studies investigating the effects of enriching the diet with carotenoids via real foodstuffs rather than by supplementation.

6. CONCLUSIONS

Because the immune system is critically dependent on accurate cell-cell communication to mount an immune response, immune cell integrity is essential. It is believed that carotenoids might help to maintain this integrity, reducing the damage caused by ROS to cell membranes and their associated receptors, as well as modulating immune cell function by influencing the activity of redox-sensitive transcription factors and cytokine and prostaglandin production. However, the results of the prospective studies with β-carotene in smokers remind us that caution must still be taken in making recommendations regarding taking supplements, which provide a greater intake than can be achieved by eating a diet rich in fruits and vegetables. Furthermore, research must be undertaken to examine the interaction between different carotenoids and, indeed, between combinations of carotenoids and other antioxidant nutrients, such as vitamin E and dietary flavanoids, and to establish the intake levels required to optimize immune responsiveness in different sectors of the population (e.g., the elderly and cigarette smokers). In the next few years, in the postgenomic era, with the new technologies available in genomics, proteomics, and metabolomics, we will hopefully see major advances in our understanding of the influence of carotenoids on human immune function. In addition, further studies must be undertaken to compare the effects observed after enrichment of the diet with antioxidants via real foodstuffs with those seen after dietary supplementation using pills or capsules, because these real foods undoubtedly contain beneficial compounds that we have yet to discover.

7. "TAKE-HOME" MESSAGES

1. Carotenoids evolved to provide protection against UV damage and to act as accessory pigments in photosynthesis.
2. Many epidemiological studies have shown a strong association between diets rich in carotenoids and a reduced incidence of many forms of cancer, particularly lung cancer.
3. Several intervention studies have shown an enhancing effect of β-carotene supplementation on immune function, particularly in the elderly.
4. Carotenoids differ in their modulatory effects on immune function; this may be related to their distribution both within cells and different body tissues.
5. Large prospective studies have failed to show a beneficial effect of β-carotene supplementation in preventing lung cancer, particularly in smokers; this may be related to the levels of intakes used exceeding those showing a beneficial effect in the epidemiologic studies.
6. Further studies are needed to increase our understanding of the molecular mechanisms of action of carotenoids on immune cell function and to define optimal intakes for different sectors of the population. Intervention studies should use dietary achievable levels of carotenoid supplementation in individuals with low baseline levels of carotenoid and/or immune status. Additional studies, comparing supplements with real foodstuffs, are also overdue.

ACKNOWLEDGMENT

This work was supported by the Biotechnology and Biological Sciences Research Council of the United Kingdom.

REFERENCES

1. Committee on Diet and Health, Food and Nutrition Board. Diet and Health. Implications for Reducing Chronic Disease. National Academy Press, Washington, 1989.
2. World Health Organization. Diet, Nutrition and Prevention of Chronic Diseases. WHO Technical Report Series 797. World Health Organization, Geneva, 1990.
3. Department of Health. Nutritional aspects of cardiovascular disease. Report of the Cardiovascular Review Group, Committee on Medical Aspects of Food Policy. Report on Health and Social Subjects 46. HMSO, London, 1994.
4. Block G, Patterson B, Subar A. Fruit, vegetables, and cancer prevention: a review of the epidemiological evidence. Nutr Cancer 1992;18:1–29.
5. Gaziano JM, Manson JE, Branch LG, Colditz GA, Willett WC, Buring JE. A prospective study of consumption of carotenoids in fruits and vegetables and decreased cardiovascular mortality in the elderly. Ann Epidemiol 1995;5:255–260.

6. Peto R, Doll R, Buckley JD, Sporn MB. Can dietary beta-carotene materially reduce human cancer rates? Nature 1981;290:201–208.

7. Mayne SM. Beta-carotene, carotenoids, and disease prevention in humans. FASEB J 1996;10:690–701.

8. O'Neill ME, Carroll Y, Corridan B, et al. A European carotenoid database to assess carotenoid intakes and its use in a five-country comparative study. Br J Nutr 2001;85:499–507.

9. Beyer P, Al Babili S, Ye X, et al. Golden rice: introducing the beta-carotene biosynthesis pathway into rice endosperm by genetic engineering to defeat vitamin A deficiency. J Nutr 2002;132:506S–510S.

10. Yeum KJ, Russell RM. Carotenoid bioavailability and bioconversion. Annu Rev Nutr 2002;22: 483–504.

11. Raeini-Sarjaz M, Ntanios FY, Vanstone CA, Jones PJ. No changes in serum fat-soluble vitamin and carotenoid concentrations with the intake of plant sterol/stanol esters in the context of a controlled diet. Metabolism 2002;51:652–656.

12. Institute of Medicine. Dietary Reference Intakes for Vitamin C, Vitamin E, Selenium, and Carotenoids. National Academy Press, Washington, DC, 2000.

13. McDermott JH. Antioxidant nutrients: current dietary recommendations and research update. J Am Pharm Assoc 2000;40:785–799.

14. Yong LC, Forman MR, Beecher GR, et al. Relationship between dietary intake and plasma concentrations of carotenoids in premenopausal women: application of the USDA-NCI carotenoid food-composition database. Am J Clin Nutr 1994;60:223–230.

15. Enger SM, Longnecker MP, Shikany JM, et al. Questionnaire assessment of intake of specific carotenoids. Cancer Epidemiol Biomarkers Prev 1995;4:201–205.

16. Margetts BM, Jackson AA. The determinants of plasma beta-carotene: interaction between smoking and other lifestyle factors. Eur J Clin Nutr 1996;50:236–238.

17. Carroll YL, Corridan BM, Morrissey PA. Carotenoids in young and elderly healthy humans: dietary intakes, biochemical status and diet-plasma relationships. Eur J Clin Nutr 1999;53:644–653.

18. Drew B, Leeuwenburgh C. Aging and the role of reactive nitrogen species. Ann NY Acad Sci 2002;959:66–81.

19. Baker KR, Meydani M. Beta-carotene in immunity and cancer. J Optim Nutr 1994;3:39–50.

20. Gruner S, Volk HD, Falck P, Baehr RV. The influence of phagocytic stimuli on the expression of HLA-DR antigens; role of reactive oxygen intermediates. Eur J Immunol 1986;16:212–215.

21. Anderson R. Antioxidant nutrients and prevention of oxidant-mediated diseases. In: Bendich A, Deckelbaum RJ (eds.). Preventive Nutrition (2nd ed.). Humana, Totowa, NJ, 2001, pp. 293–306.

22. Roe DA, Fuller CJ. Carotenoids and immune function. In: Klurfeld DM (ed.). Nutrition and Immunology. Plenum, New York, 1993, pp. 229–238.

23. Bendich A. Micronutrients in women's health and immune function. Nutrition 2001;17:858–867.

24. Rivers JK, Norris PG, Murphy GM, et al. UVA sunbeds: tanning, photoprotection, acute adverse effects and immunological changes. Br J Dermatol 1989;120:767–777.

25. Fuller CJ, Faulkner H, Bendich A, Parker RS, Roe DA. Effect of beta-carotene supplementation on photosuppression of delayed-type hypersensitivity in normal young men. Am J Clin Nutr 1992;56: 684–690.

26. Herraiz LA, Hsieh WC, Parker RS, Swanson JE, Bendich A, Roe DA. Effect of UV exposure and beta-carotene supplementation on delayed-type hypersensitivity response in healthy older men. J Am Coll Nutr 1998;17:617–624.

27. Gollnick PM, Hopfenmuller W, Hemmes C, et al. Systemic beta-carotene plus topical UV-sunscreen are an optimal protection against harmful effects of natural UV-sunlight: results of the Berlin-Eilath study. Eur J Dermatol 1996;6:200–205.

28. Lesourd B, Mazari L. Nutrition and immunity in the elderly. Proc Nutr Soc 1999;58:685–695.

29. Watson RR, Prabhala RH, Plezia PM, Alberts DS. Effect of beta-carotene on lymphocyte subpopulations in elderly humans: evidence for a dose-response relationship. Am J Clin Nutr 1991;53:90–94.

30. Murata T, Tamai H, Morinobu T, et al. Effect of long-term administration of beta-carotene on lymphocyte subsets in humans. Am J Clin Nutr 1994;60:597–602.

31. Fryburg DA, Mark RJ, Griffith BP, Askenase PW, Patterson TF. The effect of supplemental beta-carotene on immunological indices in patients with AIDS: a pilot study. Yale J Biol Med 1995;68: 19–23.

32. Santos MS, Leka LS, Ribaya-Mercado JD, et al. Short- and long-term beta-carotene supplementation do not influence T cell-mediated immunity in healthy elderly persons. Am J Clin Nutr 1997;66:917–924.

33. Santos MS, Meydani SN, Leka L, et al. Natural killer cell activity in elderly men is enhanced by beta-carotene supplementation. Am J Clin Nutr 1996;64:772–777.

34. Bach FH. Class II genes and products of the HLA-D region. Immunol Today 1985;6:89–94.

35. Janeway CA, Bottomly K, Babich J, et al. Quantitative variation in Ia antigen expression plays a central role in immune regulation. Immunol Today 1984;5:99–104.

36. Springer TA. Adhesion receptors of the immune system. Nature 1990;346:425–434.

37. Hughes DA, Wright AJA, Finglas PM, et al. The effect of beta-carotene supplementation on the immune function of blood monocytes from healthy male non-smokers. J Lab Clin Med 1997;129:309–317.

38. Mathews-Roth MM. Beta-carotene: clinical aspects. In: Spiller GA, Scala J (eds.). New Protective Roles for Selected Nutrients. Alan R. Liss, Inc., New York, 1989, pp. 17–38.

39. Halevy O, Sklan D. Inhibition of arachidonic acid oxidation by beta-carotene, retinol and alpha-tocopherol. Biochim Biophys Acta 1987;918:304–307.

40. Fawzi W, Herrera MG, Nestel P. Tomato intake in relation to mortality and morbidity among sudanese children. J Nutr 2000;130:2537–2542.

41. Hughes DA, Wright AJ, Finglas PM, et al. Effects of lycopene and lutein supplementation on the expression of functionally associated surface molecules on blood monocytes from healthy male non-smokers. J Infect Dis 2000;182(Suppl 1):S11–S15.

42. Paetau I, Khachik F, Brown ED, et al. Chronic ingestion of lycopene-rich tomato juice or lycopene supplements significantly increases plasma concentrations of lycopene and related tomato carotenoids in humans. Am J Clin Nutr 1998;68:1187–1195.

43. Gerster H. The potential role of lycopene for human health. J Am Coll Nutr 1997;16:109–126.

44. Clinton SK, Emenhiser C, Schwartz SJ, et al. cis-trans lycopene isomers, carotenoids, and retinol in the human prostate. Cancer Epidemiol Biomarkers Prev 1996;5:823–833.

45. Yemelyanov AY, Katz NB, Bernstein PS. Ligand-binding characterization of xanthophyll carotenoids to solubilized membrane proteins derived from human retina. Exp Eye Res 2001;72:381–392.

46. Corridan BM, O'Donoghue M, Hughes DA, Morrissey PA. Low-dose supplementation with lycopene or beta-carotene does not enhance cell-mediated immunity in healthy free-living elderly humans. Eur J Clin Nutr 2001;55:627–635.

47. Watzl B, Bub A, Blockhaus M, et al. Prolonged tomato juice consumption has no effect on cell-mediated immunity of well-nourished elderly men and women. J Nutr 2000;130:1719–1723.

48. Watzl B, Bub A, Rechkemmer G. Modulation of T-lymphocyte functions by the consumption of carotenoid-rich vegetables. Br J Nutr 1999;82:383–389.

49. Pool-Zobel BL, Bub A, Muller H, Wollowski I, Rechkemmer G. Consumption of vegetables reduces genetic damage in humans: first results of a human intervention trial with carotenoid-rich foods. Carcinogenesis 1997;18:1847–1850.

50. Riso P, Pinder A, Santangelo A, Porrini M. Does tomato consumption effectively increase the resistance of lymphocyte DNA to oxidative damage? Am J Clin Nutr 1999;69:712–718.

51. Cooper DA, Eldridge AL, Peters JC. Dietary carotenoids and certain cancers, heart disease, and age-related macular degeneration: a review of recent research. Nutr Rev 1999;57:201–214.

52. Zeigler RG, Mayne ST, Swanson CA. Nutrition and lung cancer. Cancer Causes Controls 1996;7:157–177.

53. Bendich A. Beta-carotene and the immune response. Proc Nutr Soc 1991;50:263–274.

54. The Alpha-tocopherol Beta-carotene Cancer Prevention Study Group. The effect of vitamin E and beta-carotene on the incidence of lung cancer and other cancers in male smokers. N Engl J Med 1994;330:1029–1035.

55. Hennekens CH, Buring JE, Manson JE, Stampfer M. Lack of effect of long term supplementation with beta carotene on the incidence of malignant neoplasms and cardiovascular disease. N Engl J Med 1996;334:1145–1149.

56. Omenn GS, Goodman GE, Thornquist MD. Effects of a combination of beta carotene and vitamin A on lung cancer and cardiovascular disease. N Engl J Med 1996;334:1150–1155.

57. Watkins ML, Erickson JD, Thun MJ, Mulinare J, Heath CW Jr. Multivitamin use and mortality in a large prospective study. Am J Epidemiol 2000;152:149–162.

58. Palozza P. Prooxidant actions of carotenoids in biological systems. Nutr Rev 1998;56:257–265.
59. Wang XD, Liu C, Bronson RT, Smith DE, Krinsky NI, Russell M. Retinoid signaling and activator protein-1 expression in ferrets given beta-carotene supplements and exposed to tobacco smoke. J Natl Cancer Inst 1999;91:60–66.
60. Liu C, Wang XD, Bronson RT, Smith DE, Krinsky NI, Russell RM. Effects of physiological versus pharmacological beta-carotene supplementation on cell proliferation and histopathological changes in the lungs of cigarette smoke-exposed ferrets. Carcinogenesis 2000;21:2245–2253.
61. Zhang XK, Liu Y, Lee MO. Retinoid receptors in human lung cancer and breast cancer. Mutat Res 1996;350:267–277.
62. Wolf G. The effect of low and high doses of beta-carotene and exposure to cigarette smoke on the lungs of ferrets. Nutr Rev 2002;60:88–90.
63. Hu G, Cassano PA. Antioxidant nutrients and pulmonary function: the Third National Health and Nutrition Examination Survey (NHANES III). Am J Epidemiol 2000;151:975–981.
64. Grievink L, Smit HA, Veer P, Brunekreef B, Kromhout D. Plasma concentrations of the antioxidants beta-carotene and alpha-tocopherol in relation to lung function. Eur J Clin Nutr 1999;53:813–817.
65. Hart DJ, Scott KJ. Development and evaluation of an HPLC method for the analysis of carotenoids in foods, and the measurement of the carotenoid content of vegetables and fruits commonly consumed in the UK. Food Chem 1995;54:101–111.
66. Alexander M, Newmark H, Miller G. Oral beta-carotene can increase the number of OKT4 positive cells in human blood. Immunology 1985;9:221–224.
67. Prabhala RH, Garewal HS, Hicks MJ, Sampliner RE, Watson RR. The effects of 13-cis-retinoic acid and beta-carotene on cellular immunity in humans. Cancer 1991;67:1556–1560.
68. Ringer TV, DeLoof MJ, Winterrowd GE, et al. Beta-carotene's effects on serum lipoproteins and immunologic indices in humans. Am J Clin Nutr 1991;53:688–694.
69. van Poppel G, Spanhaak S, Ockhuizen T. Effect of beta-carotene on immunological indexes in healthy male smokers. Am J Clin Nutr 1993;57:402–407.
70. Daudu PA, Kelley DS, Taylor PC, Burri BJ, Wu MM. Effect of a low beta-carotene diet on the immune functions of adult women. Am J Clin Nutr 1994;60:969–972.

10 Multivitamins

Ho-Kyung Kwak
and Jeffrey B. Blumberg

1. INTRODUCTION

Dietary manipulation with vitamins and other nutrients has been used to beneficially affect immunity in patients, and some studies suggest that they may also decrease the risk of infectious disease and chronic conditions associated with impaired immune responsiveness in general populations *(1,2)*. Although many studies have focused on the potential efficacy of interventions with one or two nutrients *(3–10)*, many investigators have suggested the need to explore a more integrated approach that recognizes the dynamic interrelationship between essential nutrients *(11–13)*. The use of a rationally formulated combination of nutrients could take advantage of the associated and independent pathways in immune functions that are dependent on these compounds.

An increased requirement for vitamins and minerals has long been appreciated in patients with infections, cancers, and some types of trauma *(14–16)*. This elevated need for micronutrients is exacerbated by decreased intakes resulting from anorexia, especially in surgical patients, and by increased nutrient losses. Indeed, soon after their discovery, vitamins were recognized to play a role in host resistance against infectious illness and to influence immune responsiveness *(17,18)*, although it has not been until recently that clinical studies were undertaken to exploit this information. Correcting malnutrition and enhancing presumably adequate nutritional status is now effective in some situations to increase immunization responsiveness and opportunistic infection prevention *(2,19)*. It is noteworthy that immunologic tests are being increasingly recognized as a useful complement to traditional methods of nutritional assessment *(10,20,21)*.

Multivitamin supplements are available as over-the-counter commercial products in most countries. Although there are no regulatory definitions of a multivitamin, these products are typically formulated with most or all of the 11 essential vitamins at doses near the recommended dietary allowance (RDA) for each. Many, but not all, are similarly formulated with the essential minerals and other trace elements, although some ingredients, such as calcium, are not included at recommended intake levels. The use of multivitamins to supplement the diet is an increasingly common practice in the United States *(22)*. This situation has presented an opportunity to examine the relationship between vitamin intakes and immune functions and to provide a well-established product category

From: *Diet and Human Immune Function*
Edited by: D. A. Hughes, L. G. Darlington, and A. Bendich © Humana Press Inc., Totowa, NJ

for clinical trials. Importantly, Fletcher and Fairfield *(23)* have recommended that all adults take a multivitamin daily, although they base their suggestion largely on evidence relevant to the prevention of chronic diseases, such as cancer, coronary heart disease, and osteoporosis, rather than on the potential effect of multivitamins on immune functions *per se (24)*. Although Willett and Stampfer *(25)* have provided similar advice concerning the use of multivitamins for the general population, such recommendations have long been proffered as a solution to preventing the micronutrient inadequacies common in institutionalized older adults *(26–28)*.

There are few studies that have directly assessed the effect of multivitamins on health and disease. In prospective studies, the daily use of a multivitamin has been associated with a lower risk of coronary disease *(29)*, colon cancer *(30,31)*, and breast cancer, particularly in regular consumers of alcohol *(32)*. Randomized clinical trials with multivitamins have indicated a beneficial effect on nutrient status *(33–35)*, antioxidant defenses *(36)*, hypertension *(37)*, cerebrovascular disease mortality rates *(37)*, proliferation in esophageal dysplasia *(38)*, fertility *(39)*, age-related macular degeneration *(40)*, stroke *(37)*, and total plasma homocysteine *(41)*.

The number of studies directed to an examination of the effect of multivitamins on immune responses and associated disease outcomes is limited. Although experiments with combinations of vitamins in cell cultures and animal models are useful for screening mixtures and gaining an understanding of the mechanisms of multivitamin prophylaxis and therapies, these studies are not directly relevant to clinical or public health applications. Thus, this review of multivitamins and human immune functions emphasizes results from observational studies and clinical trials in which the effects of combinations of three or more vitamins on immunity have been reported.

2. OBSERVATIONAL STUDIES OF THE RELATIONSHIP BETWEEN COMBINATIONS OF VITAMINS AND IMMUNE FUNCTIONS

Considering the relationships between vitamin intake and status and immune function is useful to assessing the rationale behind the use of multivitamins to affect immunity. Extensive evidence has accumulated that identifies the adverse effect of single vitamin deficiencies, including those of vitamins A, B_6, B_{12}, C, D, and E and folate, on immune functions *(17,42–49)*. Those reports focusing only on one or two vitamins and immunity are not discussed here. Because immune responsiveness declines with age and older adults are more susceptible to infectious disease, it is not surprising the majority of investigations in this area have focused on elderly cohorts *(50,51)*. Several observational studies have assessed an array of vitamin intake and/or status in association with measures of immune functions, partly to determine the degree to which reductions in immune responses are dependent on age vs. nutriture.

Goodwin and Garry *(52)* were among the first to explore the relationship between a range of vitamin supplementation, particularly at doses higher than the RDA, and immunologic function in a healthy elderly population in the United States. Using a cross-sectional design, they investigated 270 independently living men and women over age 65 yr who were free from serious medical diagnoses and daily medication regimens. Subjects consuming vitamin C supplements had increased cell-mediated immune responses assessed in vivo by delayed type hypersensitivity (DTH) skin tests but not by in vitro lymphocyte mitogenic responses to phytohemagglutinin (PHA). Subjects taking high doses of vitamin E or any one or more of several B vitamins (including B_1, B_2, B_6, folate, and/or niacin) presented with lower absolute circulating lymphocyte counts. The group in the highest decile for vitamin A and C intakes had fewer autoimmunity manifestations. The highest decile group for vitamin C and iron intakes had the lowest anergy prevalence. However, none of these statistically significant relationships was considered to be "dramatic," in contrast to the efficacy reported in short-term clinical trials of high doses of single vitamins reported by other investigators. Potentially confounding these results was the strong correlation between supplementation with specific vitamins, i.e., individuals taking "megadoses" supplemented with several products concomitantly, and the absence of data on supplement use duration.

In another cross-sectional study of 230 older free-living and healthy adults, Goodwin and Garry (53) investigated the relationship between subclinical micronutrient deficiencies and immune responsiveness. They found no association between plasma levels of vitamins A, B_{12}, C, and D and folic acid, riboflavin, and immune functions measured by DTH, lymphocyte responses to PHA, absolute lymphocyte and polymorphonuclear leukocyte counts, serum antibodies, and circulating immune complexes. Moreover, no differences were noted in nutritional status between those who were anergic and those who were reactive to the DTH, except for a paradoxic inverse correlation between poor folate status with stronger DTH and higher lymphocyte counts. Although the authors concluded that subclinical vitamin deficiencies did not affect immunologic function, the general good health of the cohort and minor degree of subclinical deficiency may also explain their results.

Chavance et al. (54) characterized the relationship between vitamin status, immunity, and susceptibility to infections in a cohort of 209 healthy free-living subjects aged 60–82 yr in France. Assessment of plasma ascorbic acid, retinol, α-tocopherol, and α-EGOT (aspartate aminotransferase) (for vitamin B_6) revealed few subjects who had levels indicative of risk for deficiency. Vitamin E (but not vitamin A) status was correlated with a reduced frequency of infectious disease episodes during a 3-yr period. A positive correlation was also noted between vitamin B_6 status and the proportion of CD4+ and CD5+ cells. However, these investigators concluded that overall, vitamin status among these healthy elderly was not strongly related to immune functions as assessed by DTH, T-cell subsets, lymphoproliferative responses to PHA, or susceptibility to infections.

In contrast to the studies examining older people with largely adequate nutrient intakes, Ravaglia et al. (55) examined immune functions in a cohort of 62 old (90–106 yr) but noninstitutionalized Italians who presented with a marked prevalence of poor nutritional status. More than 40% of this cohort had low plasma or serum concentrations of vitamin B_6, selenium, zinc, and ubiquinone, and a poor vitamin A status was noted in 27% of women. The percentage of natural killer (NK) cells (CD16+ and CD56+) was associated with selenium and zinc status. In the women, NK cell cytotoxicity at different effector-target cell ratios was positively associated with plasma vitamin E and ubiquinone-10. In contrast, no significant associations were found among the selected nutrients and the percentage of CD2+, CD3+, CD11a+, CD11b+, CD18+, or CD29+ peripheral blood cells. Payette et al. (47), however, were unable to identify any correlation between the activity of NK cells and nutrition in a cross-sectional study of 82 free-living healthy Canadians older than 65 yr. Anthropometry, vitamin intakes assessed by food records, and the status of folate, iron, and zinc (all within normal ranges, except for 19% with suboptimal zinc status) were not related to the cytotoxic action of NK cells or interleukin (IL)-2 activity. Vitamin D and E intakes were inversely correlated with IL-2 activity.

Although they noted lower lymphocyte mitogenic responses to concanavalin A (Con A), PHA, and pokeweed mitogen (PWA) in 61 older adults (70–95 yr) living in a US retirement community compared with 27 younger people (23–38 yr), Gardner et al. *(56)* failed to identify any association in this regard with plasma β-carotene, retinol, α-tocopherol, or zinc or the use of multivitamin supplements (which were consumed by 54% and 33% of the elderly and young volunteers, respectively). Similarly, in France, Mazari and Lesourd *(50)* compared 40 healthy elderly (75–84 yr and screened per the SENIEUR protocol) with 28 younger adults (25–34 yr) and noted an age-related decrease in total T cells, cytotoxic T-cells, and populations of mature T-cell subsets, as well as an increased number of immature T-cell subsets and IL-6 release. The older subjects with low nutritional status, particularly of B vitamins (folate and vitamins B_6 and B_{12}), expressed similar, but more marked, changes in immune response, especially lower CD4+ counts and T-cell functions, whereas nutritional status did not influence the immune response in the young subjects. Mazari and Lesourd *(50)* concluded from their results that nutritional status "seems to exert a great influence on the immune response in aged humans, even in very healthy individuals."

Also employing the SENIEUR protocol, Ahluwalia et al. *(57)* observed no age-related changes in IL-1β, IL-2, and/or IL-6 production from PHA-stimulated monocytes in 35 younger (20–40 yr) vs. older (>60 yr) healthy well-nourished American women. Further, no differences were observed between these groups in the number of circulating monocytes, granulocytes, B cells and T cells, including CD3+ (total T cells), CD4+ (helper T cells), and CD8+ (suppressor/cytotoxic T cells) cells. These results are consistent with an earlier report on the same cohort of no change in monocyte function and few alterations in acquired immunity (lower T-cell proliferation response to PHA) in carefully selected groups of healthy and well-nourished elderly women *(58)*.

Using the National Cancer Institute Health Habits and History Questionnaire, Kemp *(59)* assessed the relationship between immunity and vitamin nutriture in 65 free-living older Americans (53–86 yr) who were not currently taking dietary supplements. The prevalence of folate, vitamin B_6 and E, and zinc intakes below Dietary Reference Intakes (DRIs) was more than 50% in this cohort. Plasma β-carotene and vitamin B_6 concentrations were below reference ranges in 52% and 14% of the subjects, respectively. Serum IL-2 receptor (IL-2R) concentrations were positively associated with serum concentrations of vitamin B_6, homocysteine, and body mass index (BMI) and negatively associated with serum β-carotene and dietary lycopene; together, these five variables explained 52% of the variability in IL-2R. Serum homocysteine was negatively associated with plasma folate and vitamin B_{12} and positively associated with IL-2R. DTH responses were negatively correlated with serum retinol and helper T-cell numbers but not associated with the dietary intake or plasma concentration of β-carotene; vitamins B_6, B_{12}, and C; folate; copper; or zinc. Positive associations were also observed between helper T-cell numbers and serum copper and between NK cell numbers and dietary folate and vitamin B_6.

A more marked relationship between nutritional status and immune function might be anticipated in a group with malnutrition. In England, Dowd et al. *(60)* selected a cohort of 50 malnourished patients and 20 more with largely absent of signs of deficiencies, all hospitalized for several conditions. Leukocyte ascorbate concentrations were positively correlated with NK cell activity, and a poor zinc status was associated with a reduced lymphocyte proliferative response to Con A. However, additional measures of nutritional status, including anthropometry, serum proteins and micronutrients, and a prognostic nutritional index, were not related to antibody-dependent cellular cytotoxicity or lymphocyte transformation responses to PHA or PWM. Of course, pathologic factors beyond nutritional ones in these patients could account for their diminished immunocompetence and might overwhelm the influence of vitamins and other nutrients.

3. CLINICAL TRIALS OF MULTIVITAMINS: EFFECTS ON IMMUNE FUNCTIONS IN FREE-LIVING POPULATIONS

Observational studies can be confounded by known and unknown variables, so clinical trials are often considered the most reliable approach to determining whether an intervention is truly efficacious. Several multivitamin supplement clinical trials have been reported, virtually all with older adults, although the formulations employed and the duration of the studies, as well as the parameters of immune function tested, vary substantially. A summary of clinical trials with multivitamins where a beneficial effect was reported is found in Table 1. A list of the formulas employed in these trials is provided in Table 2.

Bogden et al. *(61)* conducted a 16-mo double-blind partial cross-over trial of 63 healthy and free-living older Americans (60–89 yr) with a supplementary zinc at 15 or 100 mg daily. However, multivitamin supplements (which did not contain zinc) were also provided to all subjects to discourage any self-prescribed use and to prevent other micronutrient deficiencies that could limit the zinc's ability to enhance immune functions. Indeed, dietary intakes of vitamins B_6 and E and folate were consistently below recommended allowances during the course of the trial. A progressive improvement in DTH and lymphocyte responses to PHA and PWM, but not Con A, occurred in all groups, with the greatest increment occurring in the "placebo" group, i.e., among those taking only the multivitamin. Although this immune function enhancement may have resulted from a booster effect of the DTH antigens, changes in subject diets, or other unknown factors, the investigators deduced that the most likely basis for the improvement was the multivitamin treatment. The zinc intervention was associated with a transient increase in NK cell activity. Testing multivitamins directly, Bogden et al. *(62)* examined DTH after 6 and 12 mo in 56 older adults (59–85 yr) in a double-blind clinical trial. The supplement increased ascorbate, β-carotene, folate, and vitamin B_6 and E status at both time points. Significant improvement was found in DTH after 12 mo, with the number of positive skin-test responses highly correlated with increases in serum ascorbate, β-carotene, folate, and α-tocopherol.

Using the same supplement employed by Bogden et al. *(62)*, Boardley and Fahlman *(63)* tested 31 healthy women (65–89 yr) living in a religious residential retirement community in the United States for 10 wk. This group was well nourished, with consumption of only folic acid and zinc falling below recommended intakes. No difference was observed between placebo and treatment groups on any of the immune parameters examined, including CD3+, CD3+/CD4+, CD3+/CD8+, CD3–/CD16+/CD56+ (NK cells),

Table 1

Effects of Multivitamin Supplements[a] on Immune Function of the Healthy Elderly in Clinical Studies

Subjects (n)	Age range (yr)	Supple-mentation (mo)	Effects	Reference
63	60–89	16	(+) Delayed type hypersensitivity (DTH) response	Bogden et al. (61)
			(+) Lymphocyte response to PHA and PWM	
			(=) Lymphocyte response to Con A	
56	59–85	12	(+) DTH response	Bogden et al. (62)
31	65–89	2.5	(=) Lymphocyte subsets and response to Con A	Boardley and Fahlman (63)
96	>65	12	(+) T cell and natural killer (NK) cell numbers, lymphocyte response to PHA, interleukin (IL)-2 production, IL-2 receptor release, NK cell activity, infection-related illness, and antibody response to influenza vaccine	Chandra (19)
44	50–65	12	(+) IL-2 production, CD3+ and CD4+ cell number, antibody response to influenza vaccine, and reduced infection-related illness	Chandra (66)
36	51–78	12	(+) Less days of illness from respiratory infections	Jain (67)
35	61–79	12	(+) NK cell number	Pike and Chandra (65)
			(=) Lymphocyte response to PHA	
80	50–87	2	(=) IL-2, 6, and 10 production and prostaglandin E_2	McKay et al. (34)
204	>60	4	(=) Reduced incidences of infection	Chavance et al. (64)

[a]Vitamin/mineral supplements formulated at 25–400% recommended dietary allowance.

(+), beneficial effect; (=), no significant effect ($p > 0.05$); PHA, phytohemagglutinin; PWM, pokeweed mitogen; Con A, concanavalin A.

CD19+ (B cells), and NK cell-mediated cytotoxicity. Indeed, possibly because of seasonal variations, both groups showed declines in both NK cell activity and percentage of CD3+ cells. Similarly, McKay et al. (34) were unable to detect a change in immune function during an 8-wk trial. They provided 80 healthy and well-nourished older Americans (50–87 yr) with a placebo or multivitamin and found significant increases in plasma concentrations of vitamins B_6, B_{12}, C, D, and E; folate; and riboflavin but no change in vitamin A and thiamin status. Despite a marked decrease in the prevalence of suboptimal plasma levels, particularly in vitamins B_{12}, C, and E, no effect was observed on cytokine production (IL-2, IL-6, or IL-10) or prostaglandin E_2 (PgE_2) production. However, as the authors note, the volunteers possessed a higher nutritional status than found in most other

Table 2

Multivitamin Formulas Associated with Positive Outcomes on Immune Function in Clinical Trials

Nutrient	Bogden (61)	Bogden (62) and Boardley and Fahlman (63)	Chandra (19), Chandra (66), and Jain (67)	Pike and Chandra (65)	Buzina-Suboticanec (70)
Vitamin A (RE)	1100	1000	400	800	
β-carotene (mg)		0.75	16		7.5
Thiamin (mg)	3	3	2.2	2.18	15
Riboflavin (mg)	3.4	3.4	1.5	2.6	15
Niacin (mg)	30	30	16		
Vitamin B_6 (mg)	3	3	3	3.65	10
Folate (μg)	400	400	400	400	
Vitamin B_{12} (μg)	9	9	4	9	10
Nicotinamide (mg)				30	50
Pantothenic acid (mg)	10	10			25
Biotin (μg)	15	30			150
Vitamin C (mg)	120	100	80	90	250
Vitamin D (μg)	10	10	4	5.0	
Vitamin E (mg)	20	20	44	45	200
Iron (mg)	27	27	16	27	
Zinc (mg)	0–100	15	14	22.5	
Copper (mg)	2	2	1.4	1.5	
Selenium (μg)	10	10	20		
Iodine (μg)	150	150	200	225	
Calcium (mg)	40	40	200	162	
Magnesium (mg)	100	100	100	100	
Manganese (mg)	5	5			
Chromium (μg)	15	15			
Molybdenum (μg)	15	15			
Potassium (mg)	7.5	7.5			
Chloride (mg)	7.5	7.5			
Phosphorus (mg)	31	31			

older cohorts, and the duration of the trial was likely too short to have an effect on immune function. In a slightly longer randomized trial conducted in France, Chavance et al. *(64)* tested the effect of a multivitamin formulated according to recommended allowance in 204 people older than 60 yr of age. During a 4-mo treatment period, vitamin B_1, B_2, B_6, and E and folate status were increased markedly by the supplement, but no significant difference between the groups was noted in the number of infections assessed by questionnaires completed at baseline, 2 mo, and the end of the study.

Chandra *(19)* tested a multivitamin containing some ingredients higher than RDA levels in a randomized trial of 96 healthy free-living Canadians older than 65 yr of age. This study employed a placebo containing 100 mg magnesium and 200 mg calcium. The multivitamin significantly reduced the prevalence of poor nutritional status, particularly vitamins A, B$_6$, C, and E; folic acid; and β-carotene. After 1 yr of supplementation, the multivitamin group showed increases in several T-cell subsets (CD3+, CD3+/CD25+ [IL-2R expressing], CD4+), NK cells, and NK cell activity. Significant increases were also seen in PHA-stimulated lymphocyte proliferation, IL-2 production, serum IL-2R concentrations, and antibody responses to influenza vaccine. Importantly, those receiving the multivitamin were 52% less likely to have illness resulting from infections and also used antibiotics for fewer days.

Pike and Chandra (65) conducted a second randomized trial of multivitamin supplementation in a cohort of 35 free-living and healthy older adults (61–79 yr). During the course of the yearlong study, decreases in the number of CD3+ and CD4+ T cells and the CD4/CD8 ratio were found in the placebo but not in the multivitamin group. The supplemented group presented with an increased number of CD57+ NK cells after 6 and 12 mo of treatment. Recently, Chandra (66) extended these observations with a third trial in a slightly younger group (50–65 yr) of 44 healthy Canadians. The multivitamin essentially eliminated the 43% prevalence of poor nutritional status in the cohort, although the level remained unchanged in the placebo group. The supplement also significantly improved the antibody response to influenza virus vaccine (A/Sydney and A/Beijing) and increased the number of T lymphocytes, CD4+ cells, and IL-2 production compared with the placebo. These immune responses were greater among those subjects who presented at baseline with the lowest vitamin status. The multivitamin also reduced by 53% the total number of days of infection as determined by fever, cough, elevated erythrocyte sedimentation rate (ESR) and C-reactive protein, sinus and chest X-rays, and blood, sputum, and urine cultures. Consistent with the observations by Bogden et al. (61,62), the beneficial effect of the supplement was of greater magnitude during the conclusion of the trial (6–12 mo treatment).

Employing the same multivitamin formulation used by Chandra (19,66), Jain (67) conducted a randomized trial of 36 volunteers (51–78 yr) for 1 yr in India. Respiratory illness was self-reported and confirmed by medical examination, total and differential white blood cell counts, sinus and chest X-rays, sputum culture, and ESR. The supplemented group presented with less days of illness (52%) and used antibiotics for fewer days, although, in contrast, the reduction in episodes of respiratory illness (38%) was not statistically significant.

In the Netherlands, Graat et al. (68) conducted a 15-mo randomized trial of 652 free-living old adults (≥60 yr) using a multivitamin alone or with an additional supplement of 200 mg vitamin E. Although the cohort had a low prevalence of poor vitamin C or E status, the multivitamin significantly increased plasma levels of ascorbic acid and α-tocopherol, as well as total carotenoids. No beneficial effect of the multivitamin (with or without the additional vitamin E) supplement was observed on the incidence or severity of respiratory tract infections assessed by the subjects' self-reports and rectal temperature and, in a subset of 97 symptomatic patients, by microbiologic and serologic tests.

Also in the Netherlands, Wouters-Wesseling et al. (69) tested a sample of 19 subjects (≥65 yr) drawn from a larger cohort of residents of a home for the elderly. The subjects, apparently well-nourished but presenting with some chronic condition(s), were included in this substudy, because they consented to both influenza vaccination and blood draw and had adequate compliance with the supplement regimen. The volunteers received a placebo drink or liquid nutritional supplement containing energy (250 kcal), 30–160%

RDA micronutrients, and low supplemental doses of carotenoids, flavonoids, and coenzyme Q10. After 7 mo of treatment, an increase in antibody titer to the influenza vaccine was noted, although it achieved statistical significance only with the A/Sydney strain and not with the A/Beijing or B/Yamanashi strains or in the protective antibody levels (HI titer = 40) after vaccination. The modest effect of the supplement may be accounted for, in part, by the high prevalence of adequate titers before vaccination.

4. CLINICAL TRIALS OF MULTIVITAMINS: EFFECTS ON IMMUNE FUNCTIONS IN INSTITUTIONALIZED POPULATIONS

Although eating-dependent nursing home residents present with poor nutrient intakes, they are rarely provided with micronutrient supplements (28). A few studies have examined the efficacy of micronutrient supplementation on immunity in the elderly people in hospital settings and long-term care facilities (see Table 3).

In a randomized clinical trial conducted in Croatia, Buzina-Suboticanec et al. (70) tested 72 long-term care facility residents (60–89 yr) who were free of acute disease but had a marked prevalence (20–60%) of low plasma levels of vitamins B_2, B_6, and C. After a 10-wk intervention with a multivitamin formulated at several-fold RDA levels, significant increases in DTH and percentage of lymphocytes compared to the placebo group were noted. DTH responses in the supplemented group were greatest in those who presented with the lowest baseline responses. Positive correlations were found between DTH and vitamin A and C status.

Van der Wielen et al. (71) conducted a single-blind randomized supplement trial in three nursing homes in the Netherlands. The supplement, a fruit juice fortified with approx 25% of the Dutch allowances for water-soluble vitamins and minerals or a regular vitamin C-rich fruit juice (as the placebo) were administered for 12 wk to 33 women (≥ 60 yr). Both groups showed improvement in vitamin C status, whereas those subjects receiving the supplement also showed improvements in vitamins B_1 and B_6 status and decreases in plasma homocysteine. However, no differences were noted in immune function, as measured by lymphocyte numbers and C-reactive protein.

Antioxidant nutrients have been shown in several studies to have a beneficial effect on immune functions (72). In England, Penn et al. (73) enrolled 30 patients (mean age >83 yr) in the hospital for more than 3 mo and with a history of stroke in a 28-d randomized trial using a supplement of 8000 IU vitamin A, 100 mg vitamin C, and 50 mg vitamin E. Supplementation was associated with a reduction in the percentage of patients deficient in vitamins A, C, and E and an improvement in the absolute number of CD3+ T cells, CD4+ cells, CD4/CD8 ratio and lymphocyte mitogenic response to PHA, whereas no changes in nutritional status or immune function were observed in the placebo group.

In France, Galan et al. (74) conducted a 12-mo randomized trial of three different supplement regimens in 756 elderly (65–103 yr) residing in 26 nursing homes. The antioxidant supplement group received 120 mg vitamin C, 15 mg vitamin E, and 6 mg β-carotene, and the trace element supplement group received 100 μg selenium and 20 mg zinc; the third group received both supplements, and the placebo group received a supplement containing calcium phosphate. After 6 mo, from a subsample of 134 subjects, those receiving the combination antioxidant supplement showed increases in the status of the vitamins administered and higher levels of mitogen-stimulated IL-1 (but not IL-2) pro-

Table 3
Effect of Multivitamin Supplements on Immune Function of the Institutionalized Elderly in Clinical Studies

Subjects (n)	Age range (yr)	Supplementation (levels)	Mo	Effects	Reference
72	60–89	Multivitamin (5–10 × RDA)	2.5	(+) Delayed type hypersensitivity (DTH) response	(70)
33	>60	Water-soluble vitamins (25% Dutch dietary recommendations) + minerals	3	(=) Lymphocyte count, C-reactive protein	(71)
30	>80 (avg)	Vitamins A (8000 IU), C (100 mg), and E (50 mg)	0.9	(+) CD3+ and CD4+ cell numbers, CD4/CD8 ratio, and lymphocyte response to phytohemagglutinin (PHA)	(73)
134	65–103	β-Carotene (6 mg) and vitamins C (120 mg) and E (15 mg)	6	(+) Interleukin (IL)–1 production (=) Lymphocyte subsets and response to PHA	(74)
81	65–102	β-Carotene (6 mg) and vitamins C (120 mg) and E (15 mg) + trace elements	24	(+) Reduced occurrence of infection events	(36)
505	65–103	β-Carotene (6 mg) and vitamins C (120 mg) and E (15 mg)	24	(=) Incidences of urogenital infection	(75)
140		β-Carotene (6 mg) and vitamins C (120 mg) and E (15 mg) + trace elements	15–24	(+) Antibody response to influenza vaccine	
150			6, 12	(=) DTH response	

(+), beneficial effect; (=), no significant effect ($p > 0.05$).

194

duction but no change in PHA-stimulated lymphocyte proliferation, DTH, percentage of lymphocyte subsets, or thiobarbituric acid reactive substances (a measure of lipid peroxidation). However, the results were confounded by a high variability in immune responsiveness.

Also in France and continuing to use the same supplements employed by Galan et al. *(74)*, these same researchers *(36,75)* extended their randomized trial of institutionalized geriatric patients to a 2-yr investigation. Girodon et al. *(36)* reported that 81 patients (65–102 yr) receiving the trace element supplement alone or in combination with the antioxidant supplement had significantly less infectious events during the trial period, with the benefit attributed principally to the trace elements. Girodon et al. *(75)* later reported their results on 505 patients from this cohort and noted, in a subsample of 140 subjects, a higher antibody titer after influenza vaccination (A/Singapore, A/Beijing, and B/Panama) in those receiving the trace element supplement alone or combined with the antioxidant supplement; however, those receiving only the antioxidant supplement had lower antibody titers. Among a subsample of 150 patients, no effect of treatment was found on DTH. Few respiratory infections were observed in the trace element group, whereas none of the treatments affected the incidence of urogenital infections.

5. CONCLUSIONS

Studies in animal models and observations in the rare patients who present with a single vitamin deficiency have confirmed the crucial role of some vitamins in immunocompetence. It is well established that vitamin A, B_6, C, and E and folic acid deficiencies result in impaired cell-mediated immunity and reduced antibody responses. Although the dynamic interrelationships between these vitamins (as well as essential minerals) and their effect on immune functions is now appreciated, the enormous complexity of addressing questions of optimal combinations and doses (including those higher than the RDA), mechanisms of action, and clinical applications directed to different population groups has yet to be adequately addressed by clinical research studies. Nonetheless, these are the practical questions for which answers must be provided to have an effect on nutrition therapies in patients who are immunocompromised and on prophylaxis in at-risk groups and in general populations.

Drawing conclusions from human studies with multivitamin supplements is difficult because of the usual confounding associated with observational investigations and the many differences between the formulations and outcomes employed in clinical trials. Further, although it is important to examine the potential benefit of multiple vitamin combinations on immune functions in vulnerable groups, such as the elderly, little information is available in other groups, including children; patients with inflammatory disorders such as rheumatoid arthritis; and those at risk for impaired immunocompetence. Multivitamin studies that do indicate some measure of success, i.e., enhancement of some parameters of immune responsiveness and/or decreases in the incidence, duration, or severity of infectious episodes, have generally required at least 1 yr of treatment. Nonetheless, many studies continue to employ much shorter term interventions and focus on parameters of immune physiology that are difficult to extrapolate readily to clinical significance. Clearly, longer term studies with multivitamins are required to observe and define better their benefit. In this work, researchers must apply more careful assessments than self-reports by volunteers and employ new measures to evaluate outcomes, such as infectious diseases.

Recommendations for the use of multivitamin supplements have already been proffered both for the elderly *(26–28,67)* and the general adult population *(24,25)*. Although such recommendations are prudent and some evidence is promising that multivitamins may contribute to promoting immune functions, more research is needed to demonstrate such a benefit.

6. "TAKE-HOME" MESSAGES

1. Multivitamin formulations (including selected minerals) can take advantage of the dynamic interrelationships between essential micronutrients to provide dietary supplements supporting the associated and independent pathways that are critical to functioning of the immune system.
2. An increased requirement for vitamins and minerals has been established in patients with infections, cancers, and some types of trauma. This elevated need is exacerbated by decreased intakes and by increased losses of micronutrients.
3. The interrelationships between vitamins, including vitamins A, B_6, C, and E and folic acid, as well as essential minerals, that affect immune functions is complex. Questions concerning optimal combinations and doses, mechanisms of action, and clinical applications directed to different population groups have not yet been adequately addressed by clinical research studies.
4. Drawing conclusions from human studies with multivitamin supplements is difficult because of the usual confounding variables associated with observational investigations and the many differences between the formulations and outcomes employed in clinical trials.
5. Much of the evidence supporting a beneficial effect of multivitamins is derived from research on older adults. Little information is available for other vulnerable groups.
6. Multivitamin studies that do indicate some measure of success in enhancing immune functions have generally required at least 1 yr of treatment, so translating these results to practical applications suggests a requirement for long-term interventions.
7. Recommendations for the use of multivitamin supplements have been proffered for both the elderly and the general adult population. Although such recommendations are prudent and may contribute to promoting immune functions, more research is needed to demonstrate such a benefit.

REFERENCES

1. Lesourd BM, Mazari L, Ferry M. The role of nutrition in immunity in the aged. Nutr Rev 1998;56:S113–S125.
2. Chandra RK. Nutrition and the immune system from birth to old age. Eur J Clin Nutr 2002;56:S73–S76.
3. Meydani SN, Barklund MP, Liu S, et al. Vitamin E supplementation enhances cell-mediated immunity in healthy elderly subjects. Am J Clin Nutr 1990;52:557–563.
4. Meydani SN, Meydani M, Blumberg JB, et al. Vitamin E supplementation and in vivo immune response in healthy elderly subjects. A randomized controlled trial. JAMA 1997;277:1380–1386.
5. Lee CY, Man-Fan Wan J. Vitamin E supplementation improves cell-mediated immunity and oxidative stress of Asian men and women. J Nutr 2000;130:2932–2937.
6. de la Fuente M, Ferrandez MD, Burgos MS, Soler A, Prieto A, Miquel J. Immune function in aged women is improved by ingestion of vitamins C and E. Can J Physiol Pharmacol 1998;76:373–380.

7. Kennes B, Dumont I, Brohee D, Hubert C, Neve P. Effect of vitamin C supplements on cell-mediated immunity in old people. Gerontology 1983;29:305–310.
8. Anderson R, Oosthuizen R, Maritz R, Theron A, Van Rensburg AJ. The effects of increasing weekly doses of ascorbate on certain cellular and humoral immune functions in normal volunteers. Am J Clin Nutr 1980;33:71–76.
9. Talbott MC, Miller LT, Kerkvliet NI. Pyridoxine supplementation: effect on lymphocyte responses in elderly persons. Am J Clin Nutr 1987;46:659–664.
10. Kwak HK, Hansen CM, Leklem JE, Hardin K, Shultz TD. Improved vitamin B-6 status is positively related to lymphocyte proliferation in young women consuming a controlled diet. J Nutr 2002;132: 3308–3313.
11. Bendich A, Chandra RK (eds.). Micronutrients and immune functions. Ann NY Acad Sci 1990;587: 3–320.
12. Blumberg JB. Nutrient control of the immune system. In: Goldberg I (ed.). Functional Foods: Designer Foods, Pharmafoods, Nutraceuticals. Chapman & Hall, New York, 1994, pp. 87–108.
13. Blumberg JB. Vitamins. In: Forse RA (ed.). Diet, Nutrition, and Immunity. CRC Press, Inc., Boca Raton, FL, 1994, pp. 237–246.
14. Woo J, Ho SC, Mak YT, Law LK, Cheung A. Nutritional status of elderly patients during recovery from chest infection and the role of nutritional supplementation assessed by a prospective randomized single-blind trial. Age Ageing 1994;23:40–48.
15. Linday LA, Dolitsky JN, Shindledecker RD, Pippenger CE. Lemon-flavored cod liver oil and a multi-vitamin-mineral supplement for the secondary prevention of otitis media in young children: pilot research. Ann Otol Rhinol Laryngol 2002;111:642–652.
16. Kurashige S, Akuzawa Y, Fujii N, Kishi S, Takeshita M, Miyamoto Y. Effect of vitamin B complex on the immunodeficiency produced by surgery of gastric cancer patients. Jpn J Exp Med 1988;58:197–202.
17. Beisel WR. Single nutrients and immunity. Am J Clin Nutr 1982;35:417–468.
18. Gross RL, Newberne PM. Role of nutrition in immunologic function. Physiol Rev 1980;60:188–302.
19. Chandra RK. Effect of vitamin and trace-element supplementation on immune responses and infection in elderly subjects. Lancet 1992;340:1124–1127.
20. Cunningham-Rundles S. Analytical methods for evaluation of immune response in nutrient interventions. Nutr Rev 1998;56:S27–S37.
21. Blumberg JB, Hughes DA. Vitamins and immunocompetence. Bibliotheca Nutritio et Dieta 2001;55:200–205.
22. Balluz LS, Kieszak SM, Philen RM, Mulinare J. Vitamin and mineral supplement use in the United States. Results from the third National Health and Nutrition Examination Survey. Arch Fam Med 2000;9:258–262.
23. Fletcher RH, Fairfield KM. Vitamins for chronic disease prevention in adults: clinical applications. JAMA 2002;287:3127–3129.
24. Fairfield KM, Fletcher RH. Vitamins for chronic disease prevention in adults: scientific review. JAMA 2002;287:3116–3126.
25. Willett WC, Stampfer MJ. What vitamins should I be taking, doctor? N Engl J Med 2001;345: 1819–1824.
26. Bales C. Micronutrient deficiencies in nursing homes: should clinical intervention await a research consensus? J Am Coll Nutr 1995;14:563–564.
27. Drinka P, Goodwin J. Prevalence and consequences of vitamin deficiency in the nursing home: a critical review. J Am Geriatr Soc 1991;39:1008–1017.
28. Rudman D, Abbasi A, Isaacson K, Karpiuk E. Observations on the nutrient intakes of eating-dependent nursing home residents: underutilization of micronutrient supplements. J Am Coll Nutr 1995;14: 604–613.
29. Rimm EB, Willett WC, Hu FB, et al. Folate and vitamin B6 from diet and supplements in relation to risk of coronary heart disease among women. JAMA 1998;279:359–364.
30. Giovannucci E, Stampfer MJ, Colditz GA, et al. Multivitamin use, folate, and colon cancer in women in the Nurses' Health Study. Ann Intern Med 1998;129:517–524.
31. White E, Shannon JS, Patterson RE. Relationship between vitamin and calcium supplement use and colon cancer. Cancer Epidemiol Biomarkers Prev 1997;6:769–774.

32. Zhang S, Hunter DJ, Hankinson SE, et al. A prospective study of folate intake and the risk of breast cancer. JAMA 1999;281;1632–1637.
33. Preziosi P, Galan P, Herbeth B, et al. Effects of supplementation with a combination of antioxidant vitamins and trace elements, at nutritional doses, on biochemical indicators and markers of the antioxidant system in adult subjects. J Am Coll Nutr 1998;17:244–249.
34. McKay DL, Perrone G, Rasmussen H, et al. The effects of a multivitamin/mineral supplement on micronutrient status, antioxidant capacity, and cytokine production in healthy older adults consuming a fortified diet. J Am Coll Nutr 2000;19:613–621.
35. Earnest C, Cooper KH, Marks A, Mitchell TL. Efficacy of a complex multivitamin supplement. Nutrition 2002;18:738–742.
36. Girodon F, Blache D, Monget A, et al. Effect of a two-year supplementation with low doses of antioxidant vitamins and/or mineral in elderly subjects on levels of nutrients and antioxidant defense parameters. J Am Coll Nutr 1997:16:357–365.
37. Mark SD, Wang W, Fraumeni JF Jr, et al. Lowered risks of hypertension and cerebrovascular disease after vitamin/mineral supplementation: the Linxian Nutrition Intervention Trial. Am J Epidemiol 1996;143:658–664.
38. Taylor P, Wang G, Dawsey S, et al. Effect of nutrition intervention on intermediate endpoints in esophageal and gastric carcinogenesis. Am J Clin Nutr 1995;62:1420S–1423S.
39. Czeizel A, Metneki J, Dudas I. The effect of preconceptional multivitamin supplementation on fertility. Int J Vitam Nutr Res 1996;66:55–58.
40. AREDS Research Group. A randomized, placebo-controlled, clinical trial of high-dose supplementation with vitamins C and E, beta-carotene, and zinc for age-related macular degeneration and vision loss. Arch Ophthalmol 2001;119:1417–1436.
41. McKay DL, Perrone G, Rasmussen H, et al. The effects of a multivitamin/mineral supplement on B-vitamin status and homocysteine in healthy older adults consuming a folate fortified diet. J Nutr 2000;130:3090–3096.
42. Semba RD, Muhilal, Scott AL, et al. Depressed immune response to tetanus in children with vitamin A deficiency. J Nutr 1992;122:101–107.
43. Meydani SN, Ribaya-Mercado JD, Russell RM, Sahyoun N, Morrow FD, Gershoff SN. Vitamin B-6 deficiency impairs interleukin 2 production and lymphocyte proliferation in elderly adults. Am J Clin Nutr 1991;53:1275–1280.
44. Tamura J, Kubota K, Murakami H, et al. Immunomodulation by vitamin B12: augmentation of CD8+ T lymphocytes and natural killer (NK) cell activity in vitamin B12-deficient patients by methyl-B12 treatment. Clin Exp Immunol 1999;116:28–32.
45. Jacob RA, Kelley DS, Pianalto FS, et al. Immunocompetence and oxidant defense during ascorbate depletion of healthy men. Am J Clin Nutr 1991;54:1302S–1309S.
46. Gross RL, Reid JV, Newberne PM, Burgess B, Marston R, Hift W. Depressed cell-mediated immunity in megaloblastic anemia due to folic acid deficiency. Am J Clin Nutr 1975;28:225–232.
47. Payette H, Rola-Pleszczynski M, Ghadirian P. Nutrition factors in relation to cellular and regulatory immune variables in a free-living elderly population. Am J Clin Nutr 1990;52:927–932.
48. Cantorna MT. Vitamin D and autoimmunity: is vitamin D status an environmental factor affecting autoimmune disease prevalence? Proc Soc Exp Biol Med 2000;223:230–233.
49. Bhaskaram P. Immunobiology of mild micronutrient deficiencies. Br J Nutr 2001;85:S75–S80.
50. Mazari L, Lesourd BM. Nutritional influences on immune response in healthy aged persons. Mech Ageing Dev 1998;104:25–40.
51. High KP. Nutritional strategies to boost immunity and prevent infection in elderly individuals. Clin Infect Dis 2001;33:1892–1900.
52. Goodwin JS, Garry PJ. Relationship between megadose vitamin supplementation and immunological function in a healthy elderly population. Clin Exp Immunol 1983;51:647–653.
53. Goodwin JS, Garry PJ. Lack of correlation between indices of nutritional status and immunologic function in elderly humans. J Gerontol 1988;43:M46–M49.
54. Chavance M, Herbeth B, Fournier C, Janot C, Vernhes G. Vitamin status, immunity and infections in an elderly population. Eur J Clin Nutr 1989;43:827–835.

55. Ravaglia G, Forti P, Maioli F, et al. Effect of micronutrient status on natural killer cell immune function in healthy free-living subjects aged =90 y. Am J Clin Nutr 2000;71:590–598.
56. Gardner EM, Bernstein ED, Dorfman M, Abrutyn E, Murasko DM. The age-associated decline in immune function of healthy individuals is not related to changes in plasma concentrations of beta-carotene, retinol, alpha-tocopherol or zinc. Mech Ageing Dev 1997;94:55–69.
57. Ahluwalia N, Mastro AM, Ball R, Miles MP, Rajendra R, Handte G. Cytokine production by stimulated mononuclear cells did not change with aging in apparently healthy, well-nourished women. Mech Ageing Dev 2001;122:1269–1279.
58. Krause D, Mastro AM, Handte G, Smiciklas-Wright H, Miles MP, Ahluwalia N. Immune function did not decline with aging in apparently healthy, well-nourished women. Mech Ageing Dev 1999;112: 43–57.
59. Kemp FW. Relationships between immunity and dietary and serum antioxidants, trace metals, B vitamins, and homocysteine in elderly men and women. Nutr Res 2002;22:45–53.
60. Dowd PS, Kelleher J, Walker BE, Guillou PJ. Nutrition and cellular immunity in hospital patients. Br J Nutr 1986;55:515–527.
61. Bogden JD, Oleske JM, Lavenhar MA, et al. Effects of one year of supplementation with zinc and other micronutrients on cellular immunity in the elderly. J Am Coll Nutr 1990;9:214–225.
62. Bogden JD, Bendich A, Kemp FW, et al. Daily micronutrient supplements enhance delayed-hypersensitivity skin test responses in older people. Am J Clin Nutr 1994;60:437–447.
63. Boardley D, Fahlman M. Micronutrient supplementation does not attenuate seasonal decline of immune system indexes in well-nourished elderly women: a placebo-controlled study. J Am Diet Assoc 2000;100:356–359.
64. Chavance M, Herbeth B, Lemoine A, Zhu BP. Does multivitamin supplementation prevent infections in healthy elderly subjects? A controlled trial. Int J Vitam Nutr Res 1993;63:11–16.
65. Pike J, Chandra RK. Effect of vitamin and trace element supplementation on immune indices in healthy elderly. Int J Vitam Nutr Res 1995;65:117–121.
66. Chandra RK. Influence of multinutrient supplement on immune response and infection-related illness in 50–65 year old individuals. Nutr Res 2002;22:5–11.
67. Jain A. Influence of vitamins and trace-elements on the incidence of respiratory infection in the elderly. Nutr Res 2002;22:85–87.
68. Graat JM, Schouten EG, Kok FJ. Effect of daily vitamin E and multivitamin-mineral supplementation on acute respiratory tract infections in elderly persons: a randomized controlled trial. JAMA 2002;288:715–721.
69. Wouters-Wesseling W, Rozendaal M, Snijder M, et al. Effect of a complete nutritional supplement on antibody response to influenza vaccine in elderly people. J Gerontol A Biol Sci Med Sci 2002;57: M563–M566.
70. Buzina-Suboticanec K, Buzina R, Stavljenic A, et al. Ageing, nutritional status and immune response. Int J Vitam Nutr Res 1998;68:133–141.
71. van der Wielen RPJ, van Heereveld HAEM, de Groot CPGM, van Staveren WA. Nutritional status of elderly female nursing home residents: the effect of supplementation with a physiological dose of water-soluble vitamins. Eur J Clin Nutr 1995;49:665–674.
72. de la Fuente. Effects of antioxidants on immune system aging. Eur J Clin Nutr 2002;56:S5–S8.
73. Penn ND, Purkins L, Kelleher J, Heatley RV, Mascie-Taylor BH, Belfield PW. The effect of dietary supplementation with vitamins A, C and E on cell-mediated immune function in elderly long-stay patients: a randomized controlled trial. Age Ageing 1991;20:169–174.
74. Galan P, Preziosi P, Monget AL, et al. Effects of trace element and/or vitamin supplementation on vitamin and mineral status, free radical metabolism and immunological markers in elderly long term-hospitalized subjects. Geriatric Network MIN. VIT. AOX. Int J Vitam Nutr Res 1997;67:450–460.
75. Girodon F, Galan P, Monget AL, et al. Impact of trace elements and vitamin supplementation on immunity and infections in institutionalized elderly patients: a randomized controlled trial. MIN. VIT. AOX. geriatric network. Arch Intern Med 1999;159:748–754.

III MINERALS AND IMMUNE RESPONSES

11 Iron

Günter Weiss

1. INTRODUCTION

Iron is the fourth most abundant element in the world; this points to the general importance of this metal for life. Iron is an essential nutrient for cells because of its role as a cofactor for enzymes in the mitochondrial respiration chain and oxidative phosphorylation, in the citric acid cycle (aconitase), and in DNA synthesis (ribonucleotide reductase). Thus, proliferating organisms and cells have an increased need to acquire a sufficient amount of iron. Moreover, because it is a central component of hemoglobin and myoglobin, iron can reversibly bind and transport molecular oxygen, and, thus, its sufficient supply is a prerequisite for human life and growth *(1)*.

A total amount of approx 4 g of iron is stored in the human body, most of this as part of hemoglobin and myoglobin. A balanced European diet contains approx 6 mg of iron per 1000 kcal. Iron is taken up both as molecular iron and heme-bound metal, the latter being found in a high percentage in meat. The need for iron is increased in periods of growth or when iron is lost, mostly by bleeding episodes. It is recommended that infants should receive at least 1 mg iron/kg body weight/day; preterm infants require even more. The same is also true for adolescents. Blood loss by menstruation increases the need of iron by up to 1.0–1.5 mg/kg body weight/d. During pregnancy, the need for iron is increased to 15 mg/d, because of the iron requirements of the growing fetus (250–300 mg) and the placenta (70 mg), for cellular turnover (250 mg), and for erythropoiesis and compensation of blood loss during birth (400–500 mg).

Iron is also important for immunosurveillance because of its opposing functions: a growth-promotion role for immune cells and interference with cell-mediated immune effector pathways and cytokine activities *(2–4)*. Iron deficiency, as well as iron overload, can exert subtle adverse effects on immune status and, thus, on host resistance toward invading pathogens and microorganisms.

2. CELLULAR IRON HOMEOSTASIS

After being taken up from the duodenum, iron is transported in the circulation after binding to the protein, transferrin, with one molecule of transferrin accepting up to two molecules of iron. This iron-transferrin complex binds to specific cell-surface receptors, known as transferrin receptors (TfR), and the resulting TfR-iron complex is then taken

From: *Diet and Human Immune Function*
Edited by: D. A. Hughes, L. G. Darlington, and A. Bendich © Humana Press Inc., Totowa, NJ

up by cells via endocytosis. After acidification of the endosomal vessicle, iron is then released from transferrin and transported by a not fully understood mechanism into the cytoplasm. Iron is then used for either heme biosynthesis or generation of heme/iron enzymes, or the metal is incorporated into the protein, ferritin, which forms a core structure consisting of 24 subunits of H- and L-chain ferritin, where it can be stored mobilized in case of an iron demand. Moreover, a certain percentage of iron (10–20%) is neither ferritin bound nor used and remains in the labile iron pool (1).

Apart from this "classical" pathway, cells can take up molecular-ferrous-iron by a membrane transporter-coupled process. The transmembrane protein divalent metal transporter-1 (DMT-1) has previously been identified in the duodenum, where it is involved in the absorption of ferrous iron by enterocytes. DMT-1 has been identified in most cell types, and evidence has been provided that it can transport ferrous iron into cells and that it may also be involved in the transfer of ferrous iron from endosomes into the cytoplasm (5,6). As a counterpart to DMT-1, enterocytes express a transmembrane protein on their basolateral side, called ferroportin or IREG-1, which is responsible for the transfer of iron from the enterocyte into the circulation. Ferroportin is also expressed in cells and may regulate the release of iron from cells (7–9).

The orchestration of the demands for iron uptake, iron storage, and iron consumption in the cell is well coordinated via regulation of the expression of the major iron proteins at the posttranscriptional/translational level. This is maintained by the interaction of cytoplasmic proteins, called iron regulatory proteins (IRPs) 1 and 2, which serve as major posttranscriptional regulators of cellular iron metabolism. They bind to the iron responsive elements (IREs) of several mRNAs and thereby control their translation or stability. IREs are present within the 5' untranslated regions of the mRNAs coding for the central proteins for iron storage (H-chain and L-chain ferritin) and iron consumption (erythroid-aminolevulinic acid synthase [e-ALAS], the key enzyme in heme-biosynthesis), whereas the mRNA coding for TfR bears five IREs within its 3' untranslated region (for review see 10,11). Iron deficiency in cells stimulates the increase in binding affinity of IRPs to IREs, thus blocking ferritin and e-ALAS expression by affecting the formation of the translation initiation complex. Conversely, binding of IRPs to the IREs within the 3' untranslated region of TfR mRNA results in increased expression of this protein by prolonging TfR mRNA half-life. In contrast, iron overload in cells reduces the target affinity of IRPs to IREs, which then causes derepression of ferritin and e-ALAS translation, while TfR mRNA is degraded, which, in turn, results in limited TfR-mediated iron uptake, whereas iron storage (ferritin synthesis) or iron consumption (heme synthesis) is induced (10,11).

IRP binding affinity to IREs is not only regulated by the needs of iron but also by labile free radicals produced by immune cells. Nitric oxide (NO) and hydrogen peroxide (H_2O_2) can increase the binding affinity of IRP-1 but not of IRP-2 to target IREs, resulting in TfR mRNA stabilization and repression of ferritin synthesis (12–15), thus helping to modulate cellular iron homeostasis during inflammation.

Table 1
Effects of Iron on Immune Cell Proliferation and Differentiation

Iron alters the CD4/CD8 T-cell ratio, with relative expansion of CD8+ cells.

Iron modulates differentiation and proliferation of Th1/Th2 cell, with Th1 cells being more
    sensitive to iron restriction.

B cells are not prominently affected by iron homeostasis changes.

NK cells are sensitive to iron homeostasis imbalances (impaired proliferation in iron
    deficiency and overload).

Monocytes' proliferation/differentiation are not greatly affected by iron restriction.

Neutrophils' proliferation is dependent on surface expression of transferrin receptors.

3. IRON AND IMMUNE CELL PROLIFERATION

3.1. Lymphocytes

The proliferation of lymphocytes, like that of many other cell types, depends on their
ability to take up iron via the transferrin/TfR pathway (2,3). Lymphocytes respond to a
proliferative stimulus with increased formation and expression of TfR on their cell surface. The incubation of cells with an anti-TfR antibody results in inhibition of their
proliferation and differentiation (2,16,17), which is in accordance with studies in animal
models where induction of iron deficiency resulted in defective T-cell mitogen responses
(18,19). Lymphocyte subsets differ in the number of TfRs they express in response to
mitogen stimulation and, thus, in their dependence on iron in general and specifically on
transferrin-mediated iron uptake (see Table 1). In a study measuring TfR expression on
both proliferating T and B cells, the authors demonstrate that T cells express higher
amounts of TfR mRNA than B cells (20). This is functionally relevant for immunity,
remembering the reciprocal regulatory interactions between iron metabolism and T cells
(3,4). Accordingly, the induction of experimental iron overload in rats resulted in a shift
in the ratio between T helper (CD4+) and T suppressor/cytotoxic T cells (CD8+), with
a relative expansion of the latter (21).

It is well established that there are three CD4+ T helper cell subsets in man, termed type
1 (Th1), Th2, and Th3, each of which produces a typical set of cytokines that regulate
different immune effector functions and that crossreact with each other (22). Th1- derived
cytokines, such as IFN-γ or tumor necrosis factor (TNF)-β, activate macrophages, thus
contributing to the formation of proinflammatory cytokines, such as TNF-α, IL-1, or
IL-6, and the induction of macrophage-mediated cytotoxic immune effector mechanisms. By contrast, Th2 cells produce IL-4, IL-5, IL-9, and IL-13, which, in part, exert
antiinflammatory actions via inhibition of various macrophage functions and also activate immune cells involved in allergic reactions (e.g., immunoglobulin (Ig) E-secreting
B cells). In addition, Th3 and regulatory $CD25^+CD4^+$ T (T_R) cells exist that produce the
antiinflammatory cytokines, transforming growth factor-β (TGF-β) and IL-10, respectively (22).

Th cell subsets respond differently to iron availability limitation. Although Th1 clones
are sensitive to treatment with anti-TfR antibodies, resulting in inhibition of their DNA
synthesis, Th2 cells are resistant to this procedure. It has been suggested that this may,
in part, result from the fact that Th2 clones exhibit larger chelatable iron storage pools

than Th1 cells *(23)*. Thus, Th1-mediated immune effector pathways may be much more sensitive to changes in iron homeostasis in vivo.

The activation of T cells by mitogens results in stimulation of TfR expression via an IL-2-dependent pathway, whereas when phorbol esters are used for T-cell stimulation, TfR expression occurs earlier and is IL-2 independent. This may be related to posttranscriptional regulation of TfR mRNA via IRPs (for review *see [24,25]*).

In contrast to T cells, B lymphocytes are less sensitive to changes in iron homeostasis *(26)*. This is in accordance with clinical studies indicating that iron overload/deficiency did not significantly affect B-cell mediated immune effector mechanisms *(25)*. Although TfR expression is induced after induction of B-cell proliferation, B lymphocytes rather than T cells may be capable of taking up iron efficiently by non transferrin-mediated uptake systems, possibly via DMT-1. This is supported by the observation of highly efficient iron uptake by B-lymphoblastic cells in transferrin-free media. Limitation of iron availability to these B cells on addition of the iron chelator, desferrioxamine, resulted in growth arrest *(27)*.

3.2. Natural Killer Cells

Natural killer (NK) cells are sensitive to iron homeostasis imbalances. Both iron deficiency *(28)* and iron overload *(29)* result in impaired NK cell activity. This may result from NK cells, like T cells, needing a sufficient amount of iron for differentiation and proliferation, whereas iron overload may diminish the activity of regulatory cytokines, such as IL-2, IFN-γ, and/or IL-12, acting on NK cells *(4,25)*.

In addition, all these lymphocyte subtypes express surface receptors for H-ferritin, which is most prominent during the S-phase, suggesting that ferritin receptor expression may be associated with proliferation *(30,31)*. It is not clear if these receptors are involved in iron acquisition by lymphocytes or if they have distinct functions, because the addition of H-ferritin to stimulated lymphocytes expressing H-ferritin receptors resulted in inhibition of cell proliferation and colony formation and a modulation of immune function *(32)*.

Another molecule of interest is lactoferrin, an iron-binding protein found in milk, the mucosa, and neutrophil granules *(33)*. Lactoferrin receptors are found on CD4+ and CD8+ T cells, B cells, and NK cells. The expression of the lactoferrin receptor is linked to lymphocyte activation but not to proliferation *(34)*. Lactoferrin uptake may be an alternative mechanism for immune cells to acquire iron when TfR expression is low. Lactoferrin may not only modulate iron homeostasis but also several regulatory effector mechanisms of immune cells, such as cytokine formation, antibody and complement production, and NK cell function *(35)*.

3.3. Monocytes/Macrophages and Neutrophils

Monocytes have evoked different pathways by which they can acquire iron, including transferrin-mediated iron uptake, transmembrane uptake of ferrous and possibly ferric iron, iron acquisition via lactoferrin receptors, ferritin receptors, or erythrophagocytosis. Therefore, the proliferation and/or differentiation of monocytes/macrophages is not affected by the limitation of one of these iron sources (for review *see* ref. *24*). Monocytes/macrophages not only acquire iron for their own needs but also act as a major iron storage pool, which can be increased under inflammatory conditions or in secondary iron overload. Moreover, iron alone is directly involved in cytotoxic immune defense mechanisms, because it is a central catalytic compound for the production of highly toxic hydroxyl radicals in neutrophils or macrophages by the so-called "Haber-Weiss" reaction *(36)*.

Macrophages and neutrophils also express a phagolysosomal protein, which is involved in the regulation of both innate immunity and intracellular iron homeostasis. This protein is termed the natural resistance-associated protein (NRAMP-1), because it is associated with resistance toward infections with intracellular pathogens, such as *Leishmania*, *Salmonella*, and/or *Mycobacteria* species *(37,38)*. However, NRAMP-1's function is still poorly understood. NRAMP-1 is expressed in the late phagosome and causes phagolysosmal acidification, thus leading to strengthening of immune defense against intracellular pathogens *(37)*. Moreover, NRAMP-1 can transport Mn^{2+}, Zn^{2+}, and Fe^{2+}, most likely by a proton gradient-dependent mechanism. However, there are questions about whether such transport is from the cytoplasm to the phagosome or vice versa and if such a driving force is pH dependent *(37,38)*. Interestingly, NRAMP-1 expression is regulated by iron perturbations, with increased NRAMP-1 mRNA and protein levels observed in macrophages loaded with iron *(39,40)*, which would suggest that NRAMP-1 and iron metabolism may regulate one another by a feedback loop. This is also supported by the finding that the overexpression of NRAMP-1 alters iron homeostasis in macrophages in vitro and in vivo *(41)*.

TfR expression on primary human monocytes is rather low, but it is enhanced in cultured macrophages, resulting in a progressive endosomal uptake of iron transferrin complexes and rapid incorporation of iron into ferritin. In addition, human macrophages can take up iron-chelates with a greater efficacy than diferric transferrin by a temperature dependent but pH-independent process *(24,25,42,43)*. The acquisition of the metal by these pathways is influenced by the nature of the iron chelate, whereas other divalent metals inhibit this process. This suggests that DMT-1 may play a role in this uptake mechanism, which would fit nicely with the observation that DMT-1 expression is upregulated by cytokines in activated monocytes *(44)*. Thus, blocking TfR-mediated iron uptake does not affect the proliferation of cultured human monocytes *(45)*.

Like lymphocytes, macrophages and neutrophils express lactoferrin surface receptors, and the subsequent acquisition of lactoferrin exerts subtle effects on their function and iron metabolism. Lactoferrin is internalized most likely via an endocytotic process and is then involved in the transfer of iron to ferritin *(46)*. Once taken up, lactoferrin may play a regulatory role within macrophages by modulating, on the one hand, iron-mediated cytotoxic effector mechanisms against intracellular pathogens via the formation of hydroxyl radicals, whereas, on the other hand, apo-lactoferrin may protect macrophages from membrane peroxidation *(42)*. Moreover, monocytes and macrophages can acquire and recirculate iron from erythrocytes. Erythrocytes are taken up by phagocytosis and are then destroyed within monocytes/macrophages *(47)*.

In granulocytes (e.g., neutrophils, eosinophils, and basophils), an increased TfR expression is associated with proliferation, whereas TfR negative cells prominently express markers of differentiation and activation, such as superoxide radicals or formyl-Met-Leu-Phe receptors *(48)*. Moreover, a balanced iron homeostasis important for many granulocyte functions, such as phagocytosis or killing intracellular pathogens via the formation of toxic radicals *(36)*.

Interestingly, activated neutrophils, such as monocytes, contribute to the release of iron from transferrin via formation and release of superoxide or hydrogen peroxide *(14,15)*. By these pathways, neutrophils may deliver metabolically active iron for cyto-toxic effector functions, such as hydroxyl radical formation or lipid peroxidation *(36)*. On the other hand, neutrophils downregulate the binding of diferric transferrin to their specific surface receptors via the release of myeloperoxidase, an enzyme involved in radical formation by the cells *(49)*. This suggests that activated neutrophils reduce iron uptake, which is sensible, given the deactivating effects of iron on neutrophil function.

Iron handling by these cells is significantly changed on activation. Both Th1- and Th2-derived cytokines regulate iron metabolism via transcriptional and posttranscriptional alterations of ferritin and/or TfR expression by IRE/IRP-dependent and independent pathways (for review, *see* refs. *25,50*). These regulatory cytokines induce a diversion of iron traffic, resulting in iron withdrawal from the circulation and iron storage in the cells of the reticuloendothelial system. This pathway is a major pathogenic mechanism, contributing to the development of chronic disease anemia, the most frequent anemia in hospitalized patients, mainly observed in subjects suffering from diseases with activated cell-mediated immunity, such as autoimmune diseases, chronic infections, or tumors *(51,52)*.

4. REGULATION OF IMMUNE EFFECTOR FUNCTION BY IRON

Just as cytokines influence iron homeostasis, so iron interferes with cytokine activities and the cell-mediated immune effector mechanisms of macrophages, thus altering the immune response toward invading pathogens *(24,50)*. One central mechanism responsible for this is a direct inhibitory effect of iron on IFN-γ activity. Macrophages's iron loading results in an inhibition of IFN-γ-mediated pathways in macrophages, such as formation of the proinflammatory cytokine TNF-α, expression of MHC class II antigens, formation of neopterin, or ICAM-1 expression *(53)*. Consequently, iron-loaded macrophages lose their ability to kill intracellular pathogens, such as *Legionella, Listeria,* and *Eshrlichia,* as well as viruses and fungi, by IFN-γ-mediated pathways, both in vitro and in vivo (for reviews, *see* refs. *24, 45*). Part of this effect results from the reduced formation of nitric oxide (NO) in the presence of iron. This is important, because NO is an essential effector molecule produced by macrophages to fight infectious pathogens and tumor cells *(54)*. Iron blocks the transcription of inducible NO-synthase (iNOS or NOSII), the enzyme responsible for cytokine-inducible high-output formation of NO by hepatocytes or macrophages *(55)*. By inhibiting the binding affinity of the transcription factors, NF-IL6 and the hypoxia inducible factor-1 (HIF-1) to the iNOS promoter, iron impairs iNOS transcription and reduces its inducibility by cytokines *(56,57)*. According to the regulatory feedback loop, NO produced by activated macrophages activates the IRE-binding function of IRP-1, leading to ferritin translation inhibition *(12,13)*, thus linking maintenance of iron homeostasis to NO formation for host defense.

The inhibitory effect of iron toward IFN-γ activity also affects the Th1/Th2 balance, with Th1 effector function being weakened, whereas Th2-mediated cytokine production and function, such as IL-4 activity, is increased; a condition that is rather unfavorable during a malignant disease or an acute infection (*see* Fig. 1).

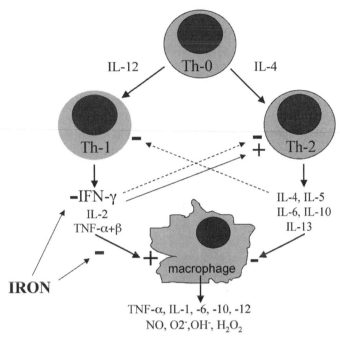

Fig 1. Regulation of Th1/Th2 interaction by iron. By inhibiting IFN-γ activity, iron impairs IFN-γ-induced immune effector pathways in macrophages and also increases Th2 activity, such as IL-4 formation, leading to further deactivation of macrophages, an unfavorable situation for fighting invading pathogens.

Iron overload also has negative effects toward the "first line of cellular host defense," the neutrophil granulocyte. This is supported by the finding that iron therapy used with people on chronic hemodialysis impaired the potential of neutrophils to kill bacteria and reduced their capacity to phagocytoze foreign particles (58), which nicely reflects the observations made by others where iron overload in vitro and in vivo resulted in neutrophil dysfunction (59).

5. CLINICAL EFFECTS OF IRON ON IMMUNE FUNCTION

As shown, both iron overload and iron deficiency may have unfavorable immunologic effects in vivo. This was clearly demonstrated by a study investigating immune function in mice fed with varying amounts of iron. Mice kept on an iron-rich diet had an impaired DTH response and a reduced production of IFN-γ compared with mice fed with a normal diet, whereas animals receiving an iron-deficient diet presented with a decreased T-cell proliferation in response to the mitogen, Con A (60). Moreover, both iron overload and iron deficiency resulted in an increased mortality of mice receiving a lethal dose of lipopolysaccharide (LPS) compared with animals with a balanced iron homeostasis (61). This suggests that changes in iron homeostasis exert subtle effects on cell-mediated immune effector function, which may be clinically relevant in patients with iron deficiency resulting from anemia of chronic disease or iron-deficient anemia, and an opposite effect in patients with primary and secondary iron overload. Thus, it is intriguing to study the net in vivo effects of disturbances in iron homeostasis with respect to the susceptibility towards, and the clinical course of, infections and malignancies.

Iron deficiency is one of the most frequent conditions in the world, with approx 20% of all people being affected and with up to 500 million individuals, mainly children and women, especially in developing countries, suffering from iron deficiency anemia *(62)*. Iron deficiency has been implicated in thymus atrophy, which has been linked to a reduced proliferation of thymocytes when iron availability is low *(63)* and to a diminished terminal differentiation of αβT cell receptor-expressing cells *(17)*.

Several studies were conducted, especially in the tropics, to evaluate the effect of iron deficiency on immune function and susceptibility to infections. These studies were recently summarized in an excellent review *(64)*. Briefly, the major problem in many of these studies arose from the uncertain origin and definition of iron-deficiency anemia, especially in areas where chronic intestinal parasitic infections are a common cause of iron deficiency. Interestingly, results are, therefore, contradictory, because children with iron deficiency had a reduced incidence of infection, whereas others who were not iron deficient had a higher incidence of malaria *(64)*. In a study performed in Malawian children, iron deficiency was associated with a higher percentage of CD8+ cells producing IL-6, a more pronounced expression of T-cell activation markers on lymphocytes, and an increased formation of IFN-γ compared with children with normal iron status *(65)*.

This leads us to question whether iron deficiency is a favorable condition to combat infection. This could also be assumed from studies demonstrating that limitation of iron availability to invading pathogens and tumor cells limits their growth by reducing the amount of this essential nutrient needed for proliferation of these pathogens and malignant cells *(66)* and may strengthen T-cell mediated immune function *(45,65)*.

Accordingly, children suffering from cerebral malaria—resulting from *Plasmodium falciparum* infection—and receiving the iron chelator, desferrioxamine, in addition to a standard antimalarial treatment, had an improved clinical course, which was reflected by a shorter duration of coma and fever and an increased clearance of *Plasmodia* from the circulation *(67)*. Interestingly, the children receiving desferrioxamine had higher levels of Th1 cytokines and NO, whereas serum concentrations of Th2 cytokines (IL-4) were lower *(68)*. This indicates that iron withdrawal also increases Th1-mediated immune function in vivo. This observation has been confirmed by in vitro data showing that desferrioxamine exerted its antiplasmodial activity by stimulating NO formation in neighboring macrophages and not by limiting iron availability to the parasite *(69)*. Nonetheless, desferrioxamine treatment had no effect on mortality, which was traced back to the chemical characteristics of desferrioxamine leading to a poor capacity of the drug to penetrate membranes and to affect intracellular targets *(70)*.

Iron may also play a role in the clinical course of other infections with a worldwide impact, such as hepatitis C. Iron accumulation in the liver may increase tissue damage by catalyzing the formation of toxic radicals, but the metal may also impair the Th1 response directed against the virus *(71)*. Similarly, increased iron concentrations in the liver are associated with impaired patient responses to IFN-α treatment and with faster disease progression *(72)*.

In Africa, an endemic form of secondary iron overload traced back to the consumption of traditional iron-containing beer on an unidentified genetic background, is associated with an increased incidence and mortality from tuberculosis *(73)*. These data are supported by in vitro findings showing that changes in intramacrophage iron availability stimulates mycobacteria proliferation and may weaken macrophages' antimycobacterial defense mechanisms *(74)*. Similar observations were made in patients with HIV infection where the supplementation with iron, a specific haptoglobin polymorphism, or increased iron stores in the bone marrow, are associated with a poor clinical course *(75)*.

Other infectious diseases, ranging from bacterial, viral, and fungal to parasitic disease, where iron overload is associated with an unfavorable course of the infection and/or an impaired immune response, have been well-summarized in a recent review *(66)*. According to in vitro and in vivo evidence, a major mechanism leading to worsening of the disease can be linked to the inhibitory effect of iron toward IFN-γ activity, leading to an impairment of the capacity of macrophages to kill these pathogens.

In addition, iron has been assumed as a risk factor for the occurrence of cancer by impairing immunity, by increasing the supply of the metal to rapidly proliferating cells, or by acting as a carcinogen itself, via catalyzing the formation of radicals, thereby producing tissue damage *(76)*. Such a concept is supported by studies showing that increased iron burden is associated with an increased risk for several tumors, such as colon or hepatocellular carcinoma *(77,78)*.

6. CONCLUSIONS

It is evident that iron has fundamental effects on immune function. Iron is essential for the growth, proliferation, and differentiation of many immune cells, because it is a central component for enzymes involved in oxidative phosphorylation and DNA synthesis. Iron is also involved in immune effector pathways of immune cells, where it catalyzes the formation of toxic radicals involved in host defense. Moreover, iron directly affects cellular immune function. However, later in life, an increased iron burden, leading to iron deposition in immune cells, blocks essential cellular immune effector function and host resistance toward invading pathogens. By impairing the activity of the central T helper cell cytokine, IFN-γ, iron weakens immune effector pathways exerted by this cytokine in macrophages, which is associated with weakening of immune surveillance against microorganisms and tumor cells. Thus, because both iron deficiency and overload have negative effects on immune function, a balanced iron homeostasis is central to determining susceptibility toward, and the fate of, an infection or a malignant disease. Thus, it is essential to gather more knowledge about the optimal level of dietary iron for immune function. Iron availability and the modulation of iron homeostasis by dietary measures or administration of highly active iron chelators may favorably affect immune function and the susceptibility toward and the clinical course of infectious and, possibly, also of malignant diseases.

7. "TAKE-HOME" MESSAGES

1. Iron is a central regulator of immune function.
2. Iron deficiency negatively affects the proliferation of immune cells.
3. During an inflammatory process, iron inhibits T cell-mediated immune-effector pathways and weakens macrophage-mediated immune responses.
4. Control over iron homeostasis is one of the critical determinants deciding the fate of infection and, possibly, tumor development.
5. Because of its negative effects on immune function and its growth-promoting activity toward invading pathogens, iron should never be given to patients with an infectious or a malignant disease.

6. Cytokines lead to iron homeostasis disturbances, resulting in iron storage within immune cells, and, thus, contribute to the development of anemia of inflammation (anemia of chronic disease).
7. The pathophysiologic background underlying a patient's iron deficiency should be carefully explored *before* iron supplementation is started.
8. Sole measurement of serum iron levels is insufficient to gain sufficient information on body iron status and/or possible pathologies underlying an anemia.

ACKNOWLEDGMENT

Support by the Austrian Research Fund, project FWF-15943, is gratefully acknowledged.

REFERENCES

1. Templeton D (ed.). Molecular and Cellular Iron Transport. M. Decker Inc., New York, 2002.
2. Seligman PA, Kovar J, Gelfand EW. Lymphocyte proliferation is controlled both by iron availability and regulation of iron uptake pathways. Pathobiology 1992;60:19–26.
3. De Sousa M. Immune cell functions in iron overload. Clin Exp Immunol 1989;75:1–6.
4. Weiss G, Wachter H, Fuchs D. Linkage of cellular immunity to iron metabolism. Immunol Today 1995;16:495–500.
5. Gunshin H, Mackenzie B, Berger UV, et al. Cloning and characterization of a mammalian proton-coupled metal-ion transporter. Nature 1997; 88:482–488.
6. Andrews NC, Levy JE. Iron is hot: update on the pathophysiology of hemochromatosis. Blood 1998;92:1845–1852.
7. Donovan A, Brownlie A, Zhou Y, et al. Positional cloning of zebrafish ferroportin1 identifies a conserved vertebrate iron exporter. Nature 2000;403:776–781.
8. McKie AT, Marciani P, Rolfs A, et al. A novel duodenal iron-regulated transporter, IREG1, implicated in the basolateral transfer of iron to the circulation. Mol Cell 2000;5:299–309.
9. Abboud S, Haile DJ. A novel mammalian iron-regulated protein involved in intracellular iron metabolism. J Biol Chem 2000;275:19906–19912.
10. Rouault TA, Klausner R. Regulation of iron metabolism in eukaryotes. Curr Top Cell Regul 1997;35:1–6.
11. Hentze MW, Kühn LC. Molecular control of vertebrate iron metabolism: mRNA based regulatory circuits operated by iron, nitric oxide and oxidative stress. Proc Natl Acad Sci USA 1996;93:8175–8180.
12. Weiss G, Goossen B, Doppler W, et al. Translational regulation via iron-responsive elements by the nitric oxide/NO-synthase pathway. EMBO J 1993;12:3651–3657.
13. Drapier JC, Hirling H, Wietzerbin H, Kaldy P, Kühn LC. Biosynthesis of nitric oxide activates iron regulatory factor in macrophages. EMBO J 1993;12:3643–3650.
14. Pantopoulos K, Hentze MW. Rapid responses to oxidative stress mediated by iron regulatory protein. EMBO J 1995;14:2917–2924.
15. Cairo G, Castrusini E, Minotti G, Bernelli-Zazzera A. Superoxide and hydrogen peroxide-dependent inhibition of iron regulatory protein activity: a protective stratagem against oxidative injury. FASEB J 1996;10:1326–1335.
16. Keyna U, Nusslein I, Rohwer P, Kalden JR, Manger B. The role of the transferrin receptor for the activation of human lymphocytes. Cell Immunol 1991;132:411–422.
17. Brekelmans P, van Soest P, Leenen PJ, van Ewijk W. Inhibition of proliferation and differentiation during early T cell development by anti-transferrin receptor antibody. Eur J Immunol 1994;24:2896–2902.
18. Kuvibidila S, Dardenne M, Savino W, Lepault F. Influence of iron deficiency on selected thymus functions in mice: thymulin biological activity, T cells subsets and thymocyte proliferation. Am J Clin Nutr 1990;51:228–232.
19. Mainou-Fowler T, Brock JH. Effect of iron deficiency on the response of mouse lymphocytes to concanavalin A: importance of transferrin bound iron. Immunology 1985;54:325–332.

20. Kumagai N, Benedict SH, Mills GB, Gelfand EW. Comparison of phorbol ester/calicum ionophore and phytohemagglutinin induced signaling in human T lymphocytes. Demonstration of interleukin-2 independent transferrin receptor gene expression. J Immunol 1988;140:37–43.

21. De Sousa M, Reimao R, Porto G, Grady RW, Hilgartner MW, Giardina P. Iron and lymphocytes: reciprocal regulatory interactions. Curr Stud Hematol Blood Transfus 1992;58:171–177.

22. Farrar DJ, Asnagli H, Murphy KM. T helper subset development: roles of instruction, selection, and transcription. J Clin Invest 2002;109:431–435.

23. Thorson JA, Smith KM, Gomez F, Naumann PW, Kemp JD. Role of iron in T cell activation: Th-1 clones differ from Th-2 clones in their sensitivity to inhibition for DNA synthesis caused by IGG MAbs against transferrin receptor and the iron chelator desferrioxamine. Cell Immunol 1991;134:126–127.

24. Weiss G. Iron acquisition by the reticuloendothelial system. In: Templeton D (ed.). Molecular and Cellular Iron Transport. M. Dekker Inc., New York, 2002, pp. 468–487.

25. Brock JH. Iron in infection, immunity, inflammation and neoplasia. In: Brock JH, Halliday JW, Pippard MJ, Powell LW (eds.). Iron Metabolism in Health and Disease. W.B. Saunders, Philadelphia, 1994, pp. 353–391.

26. Brock JH. The effect of iron and transferrin on the response of serum free cultures of mouse lymphocytes to concanavalin A and lipopolysaccharide. Immunology 1981;43:387–392.

27. Seligman PA, Kovar J, Schleicher RB, Gelfand EW. Transferrin-independent iron uptake supports B lymphocyte growth. Blood 1991;78:1526–1531.

28. Rothman-Sherman A, Lockwood JF. Impaired natural killer cell activity in iron deficient rat pups. J Nutr 1987;117:567–571.

29. Kaplan J, Sarnaik S, Gitlin J, Lusher J. Diminished helper/suppressor lymphocyte ratios and natural killer activity in recipients of repeated blood donations. Blood 1984;64:308–310.

30. Anderson GJ, Faulk WP, Arosio P, Moss D, Powell LW, Halliday JW. Identification of H- and L-ferritin subunit binding sites on human T and B lymphoid cells. Br J Haematol 1989;73:260–264.

31. Konijn AM, Meyron-Holtz EG, Levy R, Ben-Bassat H, Matzner Y. Specific binding of placental acidic isoferritins to cells of the T-cell line HD-MAR. FEBS Lett 1990;263:229–234.

32. Gray CP, Arosio P, Hersey P. Heavy chain ferritin activates regulatory T cells by induction of changes in dendritic cells. Blood 2002;99:3326–3334.

33. Brock JH. Lactoferrin. A multifunctional immunoregulatory protein? Immunol Today 1995;16: 417–419.

34. Mincheva-Nilsson L, Hammarstrom S, Hammarstrom ML. Activated human gamma delta T-lymphocytes express functional lactoferrin receptors. Scand J Immunol 1997;46:609–618.

35. Shau H, Kim A, Golub SH. Modulation of natural killer and lymphokine activated killer cell cytotoxiciy by lactoferrin. J Leukoc Biol 1992;51:343–349.

36. Rosen GM, Pou S, Ramos CL, Cohen MS, Britigan BE. Free radicals and phagocytic cells. FASEB J 1995;9:200–205.

37. Forbes JR, Gros P. Divalent metal transport by NRAMP proteins at the interface to host-pathogen interaction. Trends Microbiol 2001;9:397–403.

38. Blackwell JM, Searle S, Goswami T, Miller EN. Understanding the multiple functions of NRAMP1. Microbes Infect 2000;2:317–321.

39. Baker ST, Barton CH, Biggs TE. A negative autoregulatory link between Nramp1 function and expression. J Leukoc Biol 2000;67:501–507.

40. Kuhn DE, Baker BD, Lafuse WP, Zwilling BS. Differential iron transport into phagosomes isolated from the RAW264.7 macrophage cell lines transfected with NRAMP-1^{Gly169} or NRAMP1^{Asp169}. J Leukoc Biol 1999;66:113–119.

41. Biggs TE, Baker ST, Bothman MS, Dhital A, Barton HC, Perry HV. Nramp1 modulates iron homeostasis in vivo and in vitro: evidence for a role in cellular iron release involving de-acidification of intracellular vesicles. Eur J Immunol 2001;31:2060–2070.

42. Oria R, Alvarez-Hernandez X, Licega J, Brock JH. Uptake and handling of iron from transferrin, lactoferrin and immune complexes by a macrophage cell line. Biochem J 1988;252:221–225.

43. Olakamni O, Stokes JB, Britigan BE. Acquisition of iron bound to low molecular weight chelates by human monocyte derived macrophages. J Immunol 1994;153:2691–2703.

44. Wardrop SL, Richardson DR. Interferon-gamma and lipopolysaccharide regulate the expression of Nramp2 and increase the uptake of iron from low relative molecular mass complexes by macrophages. Eur J Biochem 2000;267:6586–6593.

45. Weiss G, Graziadei I, Urbanek M, Grünewald K, Vogel W. Divergent effects of α1-antitrypsin on the regulation of iron metabolism in human erythroleukemic (K562) and myelomonocytic (THP-1) cells. Biochem J 1996;319:897–902.

46. Birgens HS, Kristenesen LO, Borregaard N, Karle H, Hansen NE. Lactoferrin-mediated transfer of iron to intracellular ferritin in human monocytes. Exp Hematol 1988;41:52–57.

47. Moura E, Noordermeer MA, Verhoeven N, Verheul AFM, Marx JJ. Iron release from human monocytes after erythrophagocytosis in vitro: an investigation in normal subjects and hereditary hemochromatosis patients. Blood 1998;92:2511–2519.

48. Kanayasu-Toyoda T, Yamaguchi T, Uchida E, Hayakawa T. Commitment of neutrophilic differentiation and proliferation of HL-60 cells coincides with expression of transferrin receptor. Effect of granulocyte colony stimulating factor on differentiation and proliferation. J Biol Chem 1999;274: 25471–25480.

49. Clark RA, Pearson DW. Inactivation of transferrin iron binding capacity by the neutrophil myeloperoxidase system. J Biol Chem 1989;264:9240–9247.

50. Weiss G. Iron an immunity—a double-edged sword. Eur J Clin Invest 2002;32:S70–S78.

51. Means RT, Krantz SB. Progress in understanding the pathogenesis of the anemia of chronic disease. Blood 1992;80:1639–1647.

52. Weiss G. Iron and the anemia of chronic disease. Kidney Intern 1999;55(Suppl 69):12–17.

53. Weiss G, Fuchs D, Hausen A, et al. Iron modulates interferon-γ effects in the human myelomonocytic cell line THP-1. Exp Hematol 1992;20:605–610.

54. MacMicking J, Xie QW, Nathan C. Nitric oxide and macrophage function. Annu Rev Immunol 1997;15:323–350.

55. Weiss G, Werner-Felmayer G, Werner ER, Grünewald K, Wachter H, Hentze MW. Iron regulates nitric oxide synthase activity by controlling nuclear transcription. J Exp Med 1994;180:969–976.

56. Mellilo G, Taylor LS, Brooks A, Musso T, Cox GW, Varesio L. Functional requirement of the hypoxia responsive element in the activation of the inducible nitric oxide synthase promoter by the iron chelator desferrioxamine. J Biol Chem 1997;272:12236–12242.

57. Dlaska M, Weiss G. Central role of transcription factor NF-IL6 for cytokine and iron-mediated regulation of murine inducible nitric oxide synthase expression. J Immunol 1999;162:6171–6177.

58. Patruta SI, Edlinger R, Sunder-Plassmann G, Horl WH. Neutrophil impairment associated with iron therapy in hemodialysis patients with functional iron deficiency. J Am Soc Nephrol 1998;9:655–663.

59. VanAsbeck BS, Marx JJ, Struyvenberg A, vanKats JH, Verhoef J. Deferoxamine enhances phagocytic function of human polymorphonuclear phagocytes. Blood 1984;64:714–720.

60. Omara FO, Blakley BR. The effects of iron deficiency and iron overload on cell mediated immunity in the mouse. Br J Nutr 1994;72:899–909.

61. Omara FO, Blakley BR, Huang HS. Effect of iron status on endotoxin induced mortality, phagocytosis and interleukin-1 alpha and tumor necrosis factor alpha production. Vet Hum Toxicol 1994;36:423–428.

62. DeMaeyer E, Adiels-Tegman M. The prevalence of anaemia in the world. World Health Stat Q 1985;38:302–316.

63. Kuwibila SR, Porretta C, Surenda Baliga B, Leiva LE. Reduced thymocyte proliferation but not increased apoptosis as a possible cause of thymus atrophy in iron deficient mice. Br J Nutr 2001;86:157–162.

64. Oppenheimer SJ. Iron and its relation to immunity and infectious disease. J Nutr 2001;131:S616–S633.

65. Jason J, Archibald LK, Nwanyanwu OC, et al. The effects of iron deficiency on lymphocyte cytokine production and activation: preservation of hepatic iron but not at all cost. Clin Exp Immunol 2001;126:466–473.

66. Weinberg ED. Iron loading and disease surveillance. Emerg Infect Dis 1999;5:346–350.

67. Gordeuk V, Thuma P, Brittenham G, et al. Effect of iron chelation therapy on recovery from deep coma in children with cerebral malaria. N Engl J Med 1992;327:1473–1477.

68. Weiss G, Thuma PE, Mabeza F, et al. Modulatory potential of iron chelation therapy on nitric oxide formation in cerebral malaria. J Infect Dis 1997;175:226–230.

69. Fritsche G, Larcher C, Schennach H, Weiss G. Regulatory interactions between iron and nitric oxide metabolism for immune defense against *Plasmodium falciparum* infection. J Infect Dis 2001;183: 1388–1394.

70. Hershko C, Gordeuk VR, Thuma PE, et al. The antimalarial effect of iron chelators: studies in animal models and in humans with mild falciparum malaria. J Inorg Biochem 1992;47:267–277.

71. Weiss G, Umlauft F, Urbanek M, et al. Associations between cellular immune effector function, iron metabolism, and disease activity in patients with chronic hepatitis C virus infection. J Infect Dis 1999;180:1542–1548.

72. Shedlofsky SI. Role of iron in the natural history and clinical course of hepatitis C disease. Hepatogastroenterology 1998;45:349–355.

73. Gordeuk VR, McLaren CE, MacPhail AP, Deichsel G, Bothwell TH. Associations of iron overload in Africa with hepatocellular carcinoma and tuberculosis: Strachan's 1929 thesis revisited. Blood 1996;87:3470–3476.

74. Gomes MS, Boelaert JR, Appelberg R. Role of iron in experimental *Mycobacterium avium* infection. J Clin Virol 2001;20:117–122.

75. Gordeuk VR, Delanghe JR, Langlois MR, Boelaert JR. Iron status and the outcome of HIV infection: an overview. J Clin Virol 2001;20:111–115.

76. Weinberg ED. The role of iron in cancer. Eur J Cancer Prev 1996;5:19–36.

77. Stevens RG, Jones DY, Micozzi MS, Taylor PR. Body iron stores and the risk of cancer. N Engl J Med 1988;319:1047–1052.

78. Gangaidzo IT, Gordeuk VR. Hepatocellular carcinoma and African iron overload. Gut 1995;37: 727–730.

12 Selenium

Geoffrey J. Beckett, John R. Arthur,
Sue M. Miller, and Roddie C. McKenzie

1. INTRODUCTION

Selenium (Se) is a dietary trace mineral that has attracted much interest recently, in both the popular and the scientific press, because of its potential as both an anticancer and antiinflammatory agent and its ability to modify human immune function. In this chapter, we discuss why Se is an important component of cellular antioxidant defenses and why it is essential for optimum cellular immunity. We also review the possible role of suboptimal Se status in the pathogenesis of inflammation, infection, certain endocrine/cardiovascular disorders, cancer, and aging. We also consider the research that suggests that Se exerts significant protection against many common human malignancies.

Se was discovered in 1817 by Berzelius, who named it after Selene, the Greek goddess of the moon. The element is widely used in the electronics industry and in the stainless steel and glass manufacturing. In high doses, Se is highly toxic, with signs and symptoms (selenosis) occurring in man if the daily intake exceeds approx 0.8 to 1 mg/d. In the 1940s, studies suggested that Se may be a potential carcinogen, but, paradoxically, it is now recognized that Se has powerful anticancer properties *(1)*. Although initially it was the toxic properties of Se that generated scientific interest, in 1957, Schwartz and Foltz found that Se could prevent hepatic necrosis in vitamin E-deficient rats. This observation led to the acceptance of Se as an essential trace element. In 1973, Se was proven to be a constitutive part of cytoplasmic glutathione peroxidase (cyGPx), an important enzymatic antioxidant. This discovery provided a plausible mechanism by which the trace element could exert its biologic actions *(2)*. Subsequently, it has been found that Se is a constituent of several selenoproteins, which have functions other than antioxidants. Research in the late 1960s and throughout the 1970s associated Se with the optimal function of both cellular and humoral immunity *(2–4)*. During the 1980s and 1990s, clinical trials showed that dietary Se supplements provided protection against carcinogenesis in both animals and humans. These effects probably arise from the direct anticancer properties of selected Se compounds and indirectly as a consequence of Se's effects on the immune system. Also during the 1980s and 1990s, Se's involvement in thyroid and other endocrine functions also became apparent.

From: *Diet and Human Immune Function*
Edited by: D. A. Hughes, L. G. Darlington, and A. Bendich © Humana Press Inc., Totowa, NJ

Table 1
Mammalian Selenoproteins and Their Functions

Selenoprotein	Function
Thioredoxin reductases (TR) TR1, TR2, and TRβ	Dithiol disulphide oxoreductase using NADPH as reducing power. Reduces hydrogen peroxides and lipid peroxides, reduces thioredoxin for growth/synthesis reactions. Maintains redox state of transcription factors.
Glutathione peroxidases (GPXs) Cytosolic GPX (GPX-1)	All generally catalyze the breakdown of lipid peroxides and hydrogen peroxides; breakdowns peroxynitrite. Uses reduced glutathione as electron source.
Gastrointestinal GPX (GPX-II)	Gastrointestinal antioxidant
Plasma GPX (GPX-III)	Antioxidant in plasma
Phospholipid GPX (GPX-IV)	Intracellular and membrane antioxidant and spermatid structural protein
Iodothyronine deiodinase Types I and II	Catalyses conversion of thyroxine (T4) to 3,5,3' triiodothyronine
Types I and III	Catalyses conversion of T4 to 3', 3',′5 reverse triiodothyronine
Selenoprotein P	Se Transport protein Antioxidant Protects endothelia from peroxynitrite
Selenoprotein W	Antioxidant
Selenophosphate synthetase	Synthesises selenophosphate for selenoprotein synthesis
15 kDa selenoprotein	Protects against prostate cancer, tumor suppressor

2. SELENIUM'S MOLECULAR MECHANISMS AND ANTIOXIDATIVE EFFECTS

Selenium is incorporated as selenocysteine—the 21st naturally occurring amino acid—into all mammalian functional selenoproteins (5,6). These include a family of Se-dependent GPxs capable of detoxifying several organic hydroperoxides, hydrogen peroxide, and peroxynitrites produced during oxidative metabolism. Other selenoproteins have been identified that also have important biochemical roles in addition to acting as antioxidants. Such selenoproteins include at least three thioredoxin reductases (TR), which may be involved in modifying cell growth, and three iodothyronine deiodinases, which are essential to maintain thyroid homeostasis (7). Some of the characterized selenoproteins and their functions are listed in Table 1. To date, there are at least 30 selenoproteins that have been identified in mammalian cells by ^{75}Se labeling, but the functions of only approx 22 are partially or fully characterized.

Many selenoproteins have evolved to prevent oxidative damage to DNA, proteins, and cellular membranes by free-radical mechanisms. These antioxidant effects of Se underpin some of the mechanisms by which Se fortifies immune function.

Table 2
Selenium Intake and Dietary Details[a]

Selenium intake around the world	
Country	Intake (µg/d)
Europe	
United Kingdom	29–39
Germany	35
France	29–43
The Netherlands	67
Turkey	30
Sweden	38
Finland	(pre-1984 = 25)
	67–110
Venezuela	300–724
New Zealand	19–80
China	
Keshan disease area	7–11
Selenosis area	750–4990
United States	120–134

Principal forms of selenium	
Inorganic	Organic
Sodium selenite—used in supplementation studies, readily absorbed	Selenomethionine—most common form, readily absorbed used in supplementation studies
Sodium selenate—used in supplementation studies	Selenocysteine—bioactive form that occurs in selenoproteins

Dietary sources of selenium	
Source	(µg of Se/100 g)
Kidney	146
Brazil nuts	124
Crab meat	84
Dairy foods	2

[a]Dietary Reference Intakes, or recommended daily intakes (WHO, 2000), *see* ref. *10* for details. Adult men and women, 55 µg/d; adult women 60 µg/d; safe upper intake limits, 400 µg/d.

3. DIETARY INTAKE

Se comes almost exclusively from food that is consumed in the diet. Because the Se content of food reflects the Se content of the soil in which it was grown, Se deficiencies can arise particularly in areas where the main food staples are grown locally and there is little importation of diet. Selenomethionine and selenocysteine residues are more abundant in protein-rich foods; therefore, grains, nuts, and meat have higher levels of Se than vegetables and dairy foods *(8)*. Specific details of Se dietary requirements and sources are listed in Table 2. Daily human Se intakes vary throughout the world, from fewer than 5 µg/d up to 5000 µg/d, depending on local Se soil content. However, these intakes represent extremes; in most cases, Se intakes are between 30 µg and 200 µg/d. Selenate can be added to fertilizers to increase the Se content of crops and the food chain *(8)*, as

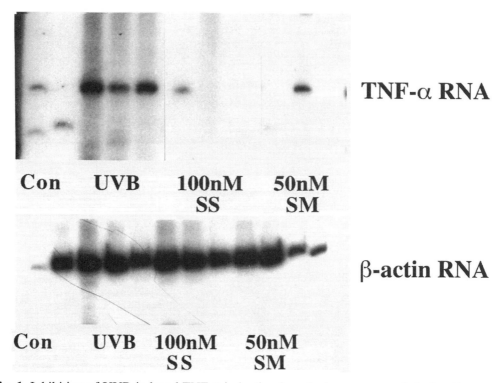

Fig. 1. Inhibition of UVB-induced TNF-α induction by selenium compounds in keratinocytes. Pam 212 cells were supplemented with either sodium selenite (SS) or selenomethionine (SM) for 24 h before cells being exposed to UVB (200 J/m²). Fresh media was returned to the cells, and they were incubated for 6 h before being harvested. The RNA was extracted, and RT-polymerase chain reaction (PCR) analysis was carried out on the samples using ³²P-labeled primers. The PCR products were resolved on SDS-PAGE gels and visualized by exposure to XAR-5 film. The mRNA expression for the housekeeping gene β-actin is shown for comparison in the lower panel. Control cells had no Se added and were mock irradiated. (From Rafferty TS. The Effect of Selenium on Ultraviolet-B Radiation Damage to the Skin [doctoral thesis]. University of Edinburgh, Edinburgh, 2000.)

was done in Finland in 1984 (*see* Table 2). In humans, dietary intake can be monitored by measuring plasma Se or by measuring red cell or plasma GPx activity (8). Recommended daily intakes are calculated as those needed to maximize GPx activity expression in plasma and approx to 1 µg/kg body weight. Excess Se intakes are predominantly excreted as methylated compounds in urine (8).

4. SELENIUM'S EFFECTS ON THE IMMUNE SYSTEM

Proposed mechanisms by which Se influences immunologic events are summarized as follows:

1. Removal of excess hydrogen peroxide and organic hydroperoxides, which also decreases cytokine and adhesion molecule production (*see* Fig. 1 and Table 3).
2. Modulation of eicosanoid synthesis pathways, leading to preferential production of thromboxanes and prostaglandins over leukotrienes and prostacyclins in Se deficiency (*see* Fig. 2).

Table 3
Effect of Selenium on Immune Cell Activity

Cell type	Effect of selenium deficiency	Effect of selenium supplementation
Lymphocytes	Decrease in proliferation to mitogens and leukotriene LTB$_4$ synthesis (cow); restored by Selenium (Se) supplements	Decrease in T- and B-cell responsiveness to mitogens in aged mice restored by supplementation
Cytotoxic T cell	—	Increase in delayed type hypersensitivity (DTH) reaction to phytohemagluttinin in patients who are uremic Increase in T-cell activity by increase in interleukin (IL)-2 receptor expression (mice and humans)
B cell	Immunoglobulin (Ig)M, IgG, and IgA titers decreased in rats. Decrease in IgG and IgM titers in humans.	Improved antibody titers to diphtheria vaccine (humans) Increase in titer response to influenza vaccine in elderly humans Antibody response to *Chlamydia psittaci* increased in poultry
Monocyte/ macrophage	—	Increased survival of mice to *Trypanosoma cruzi* infection, with increase in macrophage chemotaxis
Dendritic cell	Decrease in skin Langerhans cells in mice	Increase in Langerhans cell numbers in diet with 0.1–2 ppm of Se in mice
Neutrophil	Decrease in chemotaxis (Goat), resulting from loss of LTB$_4$ Decrease in candidacidal activity (rat) Increase in thromboxane synthesis (rat)	—
Lymphokine-activated killer cell	—	Increase in cytotoxicity with dietary supplementation (humans)
Endothelial cell	Increase in expression of cellular adhesion molecules in endothelial cells from patients with asthma Greater adhesion of neutrophils	Protection from cell death owing to oxidative stress (human HUVEC cells)
Platelet	Increase in aggregation in atopic humans showing low GPx activity	Decreased aggregation and leukotriene synthesis in humans
Natural killer (NK) cell	—	Restoration of NK-cell activity in aged humans Increase in NK-cell activity in mice and humans

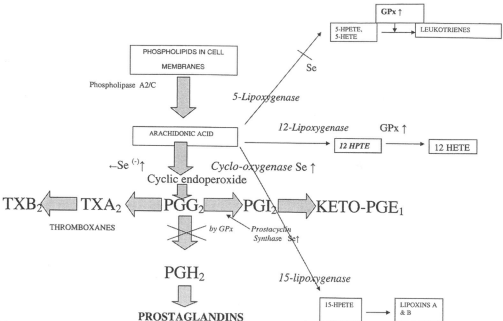

Fig. 2. Effects of selenium on eicosanoid synthesis. Se$^{(-)}\uparrow$, selenium (Se) deficiency stimulates; Se$\uparrow$, Se stimulates; GPx$\uparrow$, stimulated by GPx; $\nrightarrow$, inhibited by Se. The enzymes catalyzing the reactions are in italics. HPETE, hydroperoxyeicosatetraenoic acids; HETE, hydroxyeicosatetraenoic acids.

3. Upregulation of interleukin (IL)-2 receptor expression, enhancing the responsiveness of various immune cells and particularly lymphocytes *(9)*.
4. Protection from DNA damage-mediated release of inflammatory and immunosuppressive cytokines.
5. Regulation of cell redox state, leading to growth inhibition, p53 expression, and apoptotic death of tumor cells *(4,6)* (*see* Tables 3 and 4).

Thus, Se has the potential to influence immunity through several processes. Oxidative stress can initiate the release of inflammatory lipid mediators and cytokines (*see* Fig. 1) and upregulate adhesion molecule synthesis, which, in turn, recruits leucocytes to damaged tissue. Selenoproteins' antioxidant properties can inhibit these and other peroxidation events driven by oxidative damage *(11)*. Many lipid mediators, derived from arachidonic acid metabolism (eicosanoids) *(12)*, require GPx-like activity for several of their synthetic steps (*see* Fig. 2); therefore, Se deficiency impairs their synthesis. Additionally, lack of peroxidase activity can result in spontaneous decomposition of eicosanoid peroxides to more inflammatory intermediates. Mononuclear phagocytes and neutrophils release superoxide anions and other free radicals to destroy microbes. The host cells must have a strong antioxidant enzyme system to prevent being damaged by the release of these radicals *(13)*.

Lipid peroxides produced during oxidative stress induced by agents, such as chemicals or ultraviolet radiation (*see* Fig. 3A), are destructive and lead to free radical-mediated chain reactions, producing more damaging species. These peroxides also impair lymphocytes' ability to proliferate in response to activation *(14)* and inhibit the killing of tumor cell targets by natural killer (NK) cells *(15)*. Selenomethionine or selenite supplementa-

Table 4
Effect of Selenium on Immunologically Important Molecules and Processes

Biological activity/process	Effect of selenium deficiency	Effect of selenium supplementation
Cytokines	—	Inhibition of Ultraviolet B (UVB) induction and constitutive induction of interleukin (IL)-10 and TNF-α in skin cells Downregulation of high IL-8 and TNF-α levels seen in HIV infection
Adhesion molecules	Higher constitutive expression of P- and E-selectins, VCAM-1, and ICAM-1, on endothelial cells of people with asthma	CAM expression returned to normal levels after dietary supplementation with Selenium (Se)
Transcription factors	Loss of activity (AP-1), low levels necessary to keep cysteines in a reduced state	Inhibition of NF-κB and AP-1 activation (dose dependent) in cultured cells Increased expression of MAZ tumor suppressor in adenocarcinoma cells Increase in p53 expression in tumor cells
Virus infectivity/ virulence	Mutation of coxsackievirus to more virulent forms in Se-deficient mice	Decrease in hepatitis B- and HIV-induced mortality in humans
Eicosanoid synthesis	Leukotriene LTB_4 synthesis inhibited—impaired neutrophil chemotaxis Inhibition of prostacyclin synthesis = increase in thromboxane/prostacyclin ratios Inhibition of prostacyclin I_2 synthase	Decrease in prostaglandin $(PG)E_2$ synthesis in selenite-fed rats
Caspase-3 activity	—	Inhibited by selenite
Apoptosis	—	UVB-induced apoptosis inhibited by selenite and selenomethionine in keratinocytes Enhanced apoptosis of tumor cells by selenodiglutathione
Inflammation	Low plasma Se correlated with many inflammatory diseases, but, alone, does not imply a causal relationship Increased synthesis of platelet activating factor	Prevention of *Staphylococcus aureus* induced erysipelas in human skin

TNF, tumor necrosis factor; VCAM, vascular cell adhesion molecule; ICAM, intercellular adhesion molecule; CAM, cell adhesion molecule.

tion of HaCat cells can greatly inhibit lipid peroxide production (*see* Fig. 3B) *(11)*. These compounds inhibit lipid peroxidation in response to hydrogen peroxide in mouse lymphocytes and inhibit lipid peroxidation in mice irradiated with gamma rays *(16)* and in response to ultraviolet radiation (UVR).

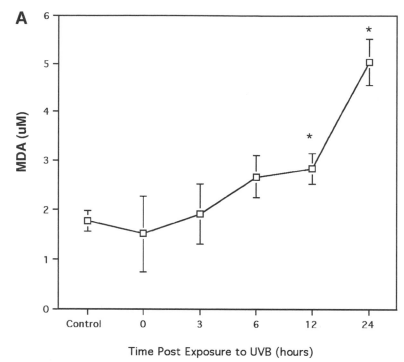

Fig. 3. Effects of selenium on ultraviolet (UV) B-induced lipid peroxidation in keratinocytes. **(A)** Effect of UVB on the formation of malondialdehyde (MDA). HaCaT cells were grown in Petri dishes until they were 70% confluent (1×10^7/dish) and the media was replaced with PBS and cells were irradiated with 1000 J/m^2 UVB. The original media were returned to the cells, and they were incubated 24 h after UVB exposure. The cells were then harvested, and the MDA levels were measured using a commercial assay (Calbiochem, Nottingham, UK). MDA increases time dependently. Control cells were not irradiated. **(A)** *, significantly different ($p < 0.05$) from control.

The induction of transcription factors for cytokine synthesis and the binding of these factors to gene promoters and ligands to receptors are sensitive to cellular redox state. This state is regulated by selenoenzymes' reactive oxygen species (ROS)-scavenging activities *(6)*. Therefore, inadequate selenium levels would be expected to have profoundly deleterious effects on immunity, but high Se intakes in animals also lead to a decrease in immunity *(2,4)*.

Se supplementation augments host antibody and complement responses to both natural and experimental immunogens and increases antibody titers to bacterial and mycotic antigens, as well as increasing B-cell numbers in animals *(2)*. In humans, 297 µg of Se/ d for 99 d raised the antibody titers to diphtheria vaccination by 2.5-fold and stimulated T- and B-lymphocyte proliferation to mitogens *(17)*. Se's protective effects also occur in the cell-mediated arm of the immune system. In animal experiments, increases in neutrophils and lymphocyte GPx activities and concentration of Se in neutrophils also occur with Se supplements *(2)*.

Both T- and B-lymphocyte activities in animals and humans are stimulated by Se supplementation *(2,4,18)*, which may result from increased synthesis of the α and β subunits of the IL-2 receptor *(9)*, leading to the observed increased responsiveness to mitogens *(18)*. In humans, daily supplements of 200 µg/d were given for 8 wk. This

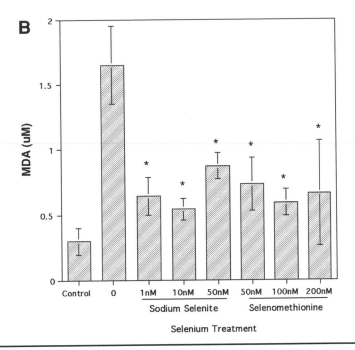

Fig. 3. *(Continued)* **(B)** Effect of selenium (Se) on thiobarbuturic reactive substances (TBAR) formation after UVB. HaCaT cells were treated with either sodium selenite or selenomethionine for 24 h, the media were replaced with phosphate-buffered saline (PBS), and the cells were exposed to 1000 J/m² UVB. The original Se-containing media were returned to the cells, and they were incubated 24 h after UVB exposure. The cells were then harvested, and the malondialdehyde (MDA) levels were measured using a commercial assay (Calbiochem, Nottingham, UK). The experiments were reproducible and were carried out with duplicate samples twice and with triplicate samples once, with similar results. Se decreased MDA formation. Sodium selenite decreased MDA formation at concentrations in the range of 1 to 50 nM and selenomethionine at concentrations between 50 and 200 nM. **(B)** *, significantly different ($p < 0.05$) from UV, O, selenium. (From Rafferty TS. The Effect of Selenium on Ultraviolet-B Radiation Damage to the Skin. University of Edinburgh, 2000.)

created more high affinity IL-2 receptors and enhanced proliferation and differentiation of cytotoxic effector cells *(19)*. The cytotoxicity of both natural and lymphokine-activated killer cells in mice and men is also enhanced by dietary Se supplements *(4,20,21)*. Moreover, these effects were not related to GPx activity, because they occurred at plasma Se levels well above those needed to saturate GPx. In vitro, in mixed lymphocyte-tumor cocultures, Se enhances proliferation and differentiation of cytotoxic effector cells but inhibits suppressor T-cell proliferation *(4,20)*. The in vitro cytotoxicity of human NK cells and the proliferation of human T lymphocytes in vitro is inhibited by doses of 0.5–1.0 μg/mL of selenite *(21)*. This is a high dose but emphasizes the importance of dose in determining whether Se augments or inhibits immune responses. At low levels, immunity is enhanced, but it is inhibited at high doses of Se *(4,6)*.

Se's most striking effects on immunity are noted in patients with subnormal plasma selenium levels. Patients with uremia have lower Se plasma concentration than controls. Se supplementation at 500 μg/d three times a week for 3 mo increased delayed type hypersensitivity (DTH) responses—an index of cell-mediated immunity—compared with preexperimental levels and to the placebo group. The augmented responses dropped to presupplementation values 3 mo after Se supplementation was stopped (22).

Selenium-deficient animals have several impaired immune responses, including defective neutrophil function, abnormal H_2O_2 production during neutrophil phagocytosis, decreased neutrophil numbers, antibody titers to sheep red blood cells (RBCs), and neutrophil fungicidal activity. When Se is unavailable, inactivation of nicotinamide adenine dinucleotide phosphate (NADPH)-dependent generation of superoxide by granulocytes, diminished NK cell activity, and increased mortality resulting from impaired candicidal activity also occurs (2,4). After supplementation, Se accumulates in lymph nodes and immune tissue. However, Se's stimulatory effects on immunity have not been recorded by all investigators, and, in some cases, high (probably toxic) levels of Se supplements decrease immune responsiveness (2). This emphasizes the importance of optimal forms and levels of Se intake to enhance immune processes.

4.1. Selenium and Eicosanoid Metabolism

Eicosanoids are metabolites of arachidonic acid that include the leukotrienes, the thromboxanes, the prostaglandins, and the lipoxins. These lipids have, predominantly, proinflammatory and coagulatory effects, causing platelet degranulation, aggregation, and thrombosis (12). The leukotrienes (LTB_4) and prostaglandins also induce vasodilation and attract leucocytes.

Se acting through GPx-I and GPx-IV, have antiinflammatory effects, preventing the release of inflammatory mediators and blood clotting. Se deficiency has profound effects on eicosanoid production. Chemical reduction of long-chain fatty acid peroxides by peroxidase is necessary to synthesize the mediators (see Fig. 2).

Cyclooxygenases catalyze the conversion of arachidonic acid to the cyclic endoperoxide precursor of prostaglandin (PG) PGG_2. This reaction requires a minimal level of peroxide to stimulate the enzyme, but, if peroxide levels in the cell are excessive, cyclooxygenase activity is inactivated. Thus, Se deficiency results in a decrease in GPx activity, which will inhibit further conversion of arachidonic acid and deplete PGH_2— the pool of substrate for prostacyclin synthase. However, despite that reduction of the hydroperoxieicosatetrenoic acids (HPETEs) to hydroxieicosatetrenoic acids (HETEs) requires the reducing power of the peroxidases; the resultant products are generally proinflammatory. Se's antiinflammatory activity may be explained by the ability of selenoenzymes to inhibit the 5-lipoxygenase enzyme, which converts arachidonic acid to the 5-HPETE precursor of the leukotrienes (23).

A major effect of Se deficiency in rats is a disturbance in the balance of production of the procoagulant thromboxanes and the anticlotting prostacyclin family of metabolites (see Fig. 2). Preferential production of thromboxanes over prostacyclins in Se deficiency would favor the occurrence of atherosclerosis in populations that have low dietary Se intake (7,23,24). Apart from the promotion of blood clotting when Se is suboptimal, the promotion of inflammatory events will occur more readily in a low Se environment. Platelet GPx activity is relatively higher than in other blood cells in humans, and it is, thus, extremely sensitive to the effects of Se deficiency. The platelets of Se-deficient subjects show increased aggregation, thromboxane B_2 production, and the synthesis of lipoxygenase-derived products. In patients with low Se status, Se supplementation increases platelet GPx activity and concomitantly decreases hyperaggregation and leukotriene synthesis *(23)*. Chemical reduction of the HPETEs requires GPx. In aortic endothelial cells cultured in Se-deficient conditions and stimulated with tumor necrosis factor-α (TNF-α), Prostacyclin I_2 accumulation is decreased, and 15-HPETEs and thromboxanes accumulate to higher levels than in Se-replete cells, because HPETE accumulation then inhibits PGI_2 synthase activity *(25)*. Thus, Se-deficiency also alters eicosanoid metabolism by interfering with the activity of key enzymes.

4.2. Oxidative Stress and the Effects of Different Forms of Selenium on Cytokine Induction

Oxidative stress generated by inflammation, chemical insult, or UVR induces cytokines, probably by reactive oxygen species (ROS)-mediated activation of the transcription factors AP-1 and NFκB's binding sites. These sites are present in the promoters of several proinflammatory cytokine genes, including IL-1, IL-6, IL-8, and TNF-α. Cytokine induction is counteracted presumably by selenoproteins breaking down ROS and interrupting ROS-mediated intracellular signaling but also through effects on the redox state of vital cysteine residues in AP-1 and NFκB *(6)*. Preincubation of keratinocytes with selenite or selenomethionine abrogated upregulation of the mRNAs for IL-6, IL-8, IL-10, and TNF-α in response to UVR (*see* Fig. 1) *(6,11,26)*.

Selenite reacts directly with reduced glutathione (GSH) and, at high concentrations, can deplete cellular GSH pools, increasing oxidative stress. Low GSH levels exacerbate redox imbalance, leading to selenite-induced stress *(27)*. In support of this, 9ppm selenite in the diet of Balb/c mice increased the release of IL-1 and TNF-α from splenic macrophages stimulated in vitro with phytohemagluttinin-P, but selenomethionine did not stimulate cytokine release *(28)*. High doses of selenite led to increased H_2O_2 release *(6)*, resulting in oxidative damage to DNA. Damage to DNA induces the release of IL-10 and TNF-α from keratinocytes *(11)*. Supplementation of keratinocytes with selenomethionine was more effective than selenite in inhibiting IL-10 release by Ultraviolet radiation B (UVB) *(26)*. Selenite and selenocystamine, but not selenomethionine, increased oxidative stress, oxidative DNA damage, and apoptosis in keratinocytes *(29)*. Thus, in general, concentrations of Se compounds higher than those encountered in normal diets cause prooxidant toxicity *(30)*.

4.3. Selenium and Protection of Skin Cells from Ultraviolet Radiation Damage

The skin is the largest organ in the body and provides a defensive perimeter against the environment. Skin is continually exposed to oxidative stress because of the products of commensal organisms on the surface and UVR exposure. Some of the studies conducted on skin cells usefully illustrate some of the mechanisms by which Se protects cells and shed light on more global Se effects on immunity and antioxidant defense. They are also important because they help to explain the ability of dietary Se supplements to prevent UVB-induced skin cancer in mice that has implications for human skin cancer *(11)*.

UVR in sunlight is the most common environmental carcinogen and can be divided into two principal wavebands—UVB (290–320 nm) and Ultraviolet radiation A (UVA) (320–400 nm), the latter, by far, the most abundant waveband affecting the skin. UVA and UVB have qualitatively different effects; UVB damages cells directly by energy deposition (DNA-strand breaks and pyrimidine dimer and other photoproduct formation); it also causes damage by decreasing catalase and superoxide dismutase activities *(31)*. UVB exposure causes erythema (sunburn), whereas UVA principally causes tanning and oxidative damage; the latter to DNA, including formation of 8-hydroxy-2-deoxy-guanosine, lipid peroxides, and protein carbonyls *(11)*.

UVR is a complete carcinogen because it both initiates and promotes neoplastic growth. Normal cytotoxic cells are needed to destroy nascent tumors. Thus, promotion is assisted by the UVB-induced suppression of cellular immunity. This occurs, in part, by the release of several soluble mediators that suppress immunity or that generate inflammation and cell damage, which is manifested as erythema *(11,31)*. Among these mediators are cytokines, which are released by UVB irradiation as a result of DNA damage *(11)*.

TNF-α and IL-10 suppress antigen presentation, release of inflammatory mediators, and cell-mediated immunity *(31)*. Se protects the skin from damage caused by inflammatory cytokines by inhibiting their release *(4,11)*, as well as protecting the immune system from UVB-induced suppression by preventing TNF-α release *(see* Fig. 1) and IL-10 *(26)*.

Nanomolar concentrations of selenomethionine and selenite protect keratinocytes, melanocytes, and fibroblasts in culture from UV-induced cell death by a mechanism that implicates selenoproteins. The UVB-induced accumulation of lipid peroxides in keratinocytes *(see* Fig. 3) and fibroblasts is inhibited by preincubation with Se. In addition, selenite and selenomethionine protect keratinocytes from oxidative DNA damage, which possibly abrogates UVB-induced cytokine induction and apoptosis *(11)*. The mechanism by which Se prevents apoptosis is unknown but may reflect the increase in cell viability afforded by inhibition of oxidative damage. Finally, selenite inhibits caspase 3, a key enzyme in the apoptosis pathway, during UVB-induced apoptosis *(32)*. In contrast to these protective effects in normal cells, the anticarcinogenic compound S-methylselenocysteine activates caspase-3 and poly-adenosine 5'-diphospate (ADP) ribose cleavage, both are early events in apoptosis, in the neoplastic HL60 cell line *(33)*.

5. SELENIUM AND INFLAMMATORY DISEASE IN HUMANS

5.1. Subnormal Selenium Levels in Patients—A Caveat

Clinical trials on patients with sepsis and systemic inflammatory response syndrome show that they have relatively low plasma Se concentrations and GPx activity. Two independent prospective studies showed a beneficial therapeutic response in patients given Se supplements *(34)*. The loss of Se in inflammatory conditions may suggest a poor prognosis. However, Se will, like many other trace nutrients (e.g., zinc and iron) decline during acute phase reactions *(35)*. Therefore, it is important to realize that, although correlations may be found between low plasma Se concentrations and diseases *(35)*, this does not necessarily indicate causality. Furthermore, studies on 66 healthy men exposed to physical and psychological stress for 5 d ("Hell week") demonstrated decreases in blood selenium, zinc, and iron and a 266% increase in ceroplasmin, which is characteristic of an acute phase response. This was transitory and returned to normal 7 d after Hell week *(36)*. More work using well-controlled intervention trials are needed in this area before clear conclusions can be drawn.

5.2. Rheumatoid Arthritis

Because of its effects on the immune system, Se could have therapeutic effects on inflammatory, particularly chronic, inflammatory conditions, such as rheumatoid arthritis. However, there are surprisingly few studies of this potential activity reported in the literature. Epidemiologic studies have correlated serum Se levels with disease, but there are few reports of intervention studies. Such work does not report consistent values as to whether GPx activity is normal or abnormal in patients with rheumatoid arthritis. However, this could be because subforms of the disease were not separated in some studies. Moreover, in some forms of the disease, there is an inability of the neutrophil to increase GPx activity with dietary supplementation. This is consistent with lack of effect of Se in alleviating arthritic symptoms *(24,37)*. However, some studies have shown that low Se status may be a risk factor for patients with rheumatoid-factor negative (but not rheumatoid-factor positive) arthritis *(38)*.

5.3. Crohn's Disease

In Crohn's disease, a condition in which immune activation is mediated by ROS, there is a negative correlation between plasma Se and soluble IL-2 receptor (IL-2R) and erythrocyte sedimentation rate *(39)*. The soluble IL-2R concentration is considered a marker for lymphocyte activation.

5.4. Asthma

Oxidative stress and micronutrient deficiencies have been identified, along with Se deficiency and decreased red cell GPx activity, as risk factors for the development of asthma *(40)*. However, some carefully controlled studies show higher GPx activity in the blood of younger patients with asthma *(41)*. Protection against asthmatic wheeze occurred in adult patients with asthma given Se, and the clinical symptoms of children with intrinsic asthma improved when they were given 100 μg/d selenite *(24)*. People with atopic asthma have low platelet and RBC GPx activities that may prolong the inflammatory process *(42)*. More studies into the usefulness of Se supplements in people with asthma are required.

5.5. Selenium and Inflammatory Skin Disease

In 1982, the first study indicating that defective Se metabolism could play a role in certain skin diseases was published *(43)*. This study by Juhlin et al. showed that blood GPx activities were decreased in psoriasis, atopic dermatitis, vasculitis, acne, and *Dermatitis herpetiformis*. These diseases are all inflammatory diseases. Thus, impaired Se metabolism could be a factor in inflammatory dermatoses development. Low serum and platelet GPx activity and low serum Se have been found in both atopic dermatitis and psoriasis patients; because these are inflammatory conditions prompted some investigators to determine whether dietary Se supplements could be therapeutic. However, dietary Se supplements did not improve the clinical score in patients with atopic dermatitis who had been given 600 μg/d of Se as selenomethionine for 12 wk *(44)*. Additional supplementation with 600 μg/d Se or Se and vitamin E together given as a yeast supplement had no effect on the clinical scores of patients with psoriasis *(45)*, despite that the treatments raised the patients' previously relatively low serum Se concentrations. An interesting observation was that there was no correlation between serum Se levels and the skin Se content of these patients. This raises the question of whether dietary Se supplements can influence skin Se levels. A failure to change skin Se levels with dietary Se intake in patients with psoriasis was also noted by other investigators *(46)*.

The availability of dietary Se to the skin is a crucial topic for investigation. Topical application of Se decreases erythema in human skin exposed to UVB *(47)* and diminished disease severity in 92 patients with psoriasis given a combination of Se-enriched water and daily showers in Se-enriched water (balneotherapy) *(48)*. Under this regimen, 86% saw improvement in their clinical (PASI) score, with 7 experiencing complete clearing. Unfortunately, no placebo control group was included in this trial. Erysipelas are a form of skin inflammation associated with streptococcal infection. Injection of a single high dose of selenite completely prevented the erysipelas development *(49)*.

In Behcet's disease, serum Se levels were almost half of the healthy control group and IgM and IgG levels in serum were significantly lower in the disease group, suggesting that the Se deficiency is associated with defective humoral immunity *(50)*. However, there is, as of yet, little hard evidence that Se supplements improve inflammatory skin diseases.

6. SELENIUM'S EFFECTS ON VIRUSES AND MICROBIAL INFECTION

There is accumulating evidence that Se deficiency is associated with increased susceptibility to viral infections and predisposes to a more clinically severe response when infection occurs *(51)*. The first indication that "normal" Se intakes had protective effects against viral infection was the demonstration that the coxsackievirus B mutated and became more cardiotoxic when it passed through an Se-deficient host *(52)*. This is discussed in Section 7.1., Keshan Disease.

RNA viruses are more prone to mutation, in general, in an oxidative environment *(53)* and in GPx-knockout mice *(54)*. In this respect, influenza virus (an RNA virus) epidemics often originate in China, which has low Se intake areas *(55)*. Additionally, when Se-deficient mice are infected with a mild form of influenza virus, they are more susceptible to the infection than Se-adequate animals *(56)*. In people who are hepatitis B positive, Se supplementation protects against hepatitis B-induced hepatocellular carcinoma *(57)*.

Certain viruses have evolved the ability to use host cell oxidant production as a replication signal. Others have acquired, through transduction, GPx-like genes, which are believed to protect the virus from the respiratory burst products of host neutrophils and macrophages. HIV is a particularly good example of a virus that employs this strategy. Selenium has a multifactorial role in HIV infection, and low Se status in HIV-infected patients may be associated with an increased prevalence and progression to AIDS and subsequent mortality. The precise mechanisms behind these relationships remain unclear *(58)*.

7. SELENIUM DEFICIENCY AND CARDIOVASCULAR DISEASE

7.1. Keshan Disease

Keshan disease is an endemic cardiomyopathy affecting mainly children and young peasant women living in areas of China where there is low soil Se. The pathologic features of this disease are distinct, differentiating it from other myocardial diseases and the cardiomyopathy found in patients given inadequate Se supplementation during parenteral nutrition *(59)*. There is strong evidence to suggest that an infective agent, such as coxsackievirus B3, may be a trigger factor for Keshan disease *(52)*. In mice, coxsackievirus B3, which is normally amyocarditic, mutates and becomes cardiotoxic when passed through Se-deficient animals. The same effect occurred in vitamin E-deficient mice and GPx-knockout mice, suggesting that oxidative stress may be involved in the mechanism that causes the mutations *(52–54)*.

7.2. Selenium and Coronary Heart Disease

The risk of developing atherosclerosis and heart disease may be higher in people who have a low dietary Se intake, and animal studies support this view *(59–61)*. The contribution of Se deficiency to the pathogenesis of cardiovascular disease in man is suggested from epidemiologic studies that correlate low Se intake with increased mortality rates from cardiovascular disease *(61)*. A threshold hypothesis suggests that in populations with low Se status, a correlation between serum Se and cardiovascular risk is observed, whereas populations with a high Se intake (serum Se levels >45 µg/L) show no such correlation *(61)*.

7.3. Selenium and Endothelial Dysfunction

Endothelial dysfunction is a primary factor in atherosclerosis pathogenesis, and the ability of certain selenoproteins to protect the endothelium from damage by ROS may explain the inverse association of Se intake and the prevalence of atherosclerosis. For example, Se supplementation (40 nM) of human aortic endothelial cells protects against oxidative damage resulting from tert-butylhydroperoxide. This protection is accompanied by maximal induction of the GPxs and TR *(62)*. Furthermore, Se-deficient bovine endothelial cells also have enhanced levels of 8-isoprostane, a prostaglandin-like peroxidation product, which has been implicated in atherosclerotic disease *(63)*. Human endothelial cells express high concentrations of TR, suggesting that this selenoprotein may have important functions in these cells *(64)*. The TR/thioredoxin (Trx) may be involved in maintaining NOS in a reduced configuration, potentially overcoming the oxidative deactivation of NOS *(65)*. Peroxynitrite formation is believed to contribute to endothelial dysfunction. The glutathione peroxidases, selenoprotein P, and TR/Trx have the potential to detoxify peroxynitrite *(66)*.

Selenium has other beneficial effects on endothelial function. For example, Se supplementation enhances endothelium-dependent relaxation in response to acetylcholine in rat aortic rings *(67)*. In patients with HIV infection, Se supplementation prevents increases in serum soluble thrombomodulin and von Willebrand factor concentrations. These agents are associated with endothelial dysfunction. In culture, Se deficiency promotes prostacyclin and platelet activating factor (PAF) production, giving rise to diminished PGI$_2$ release by the endothelium and increased PAF release *(68)*. In vivo, these effects may alter platelet function, thus contributing to atherosclerosis pathogenesis.

The transmigration of leukocytes into the subendothelial space promotes a proinflammatory response, which is a key feature of endothelial dysfunction observed in early atherogenesis. Neutrophil adherence to bovine mammary artery endothelial cells in response to TNF-α is increased in cells cultured in Se-deficient media compared with culture in Se-sufficient media *(69)*. The Se-deficient cultures also expressed higher levels of the following adhesion molecules: E-selectin, P-selectin, and intercellular adhesion molecule-1 (ICAM-1). A mechanism by which antioxidant selenoproteins may protect the endothelium from the proinflammatory effect of TNF-α and IL-1 by downregulating cytokine signaling has been proposed *(70)*.

Proinflammatory cytokines, such as TNF-α and IL-1, induce many of the adhesion molecules upregulated in inflammation. Existing evidence suggests that Se's effects on adhesion molecule expression are mediated through cytokine release. In general, Se-deficient cells or endothelia from Se-deficient individuals have higher constitutive expression of adhesion molecules, and Se supplementation decreases expression of adhesion molecules. Thus, the Se-induced downregulation of adhesion molecule expression is a mechanism to inhibit inflammation. For example, in endothelial cells obtained from patients with asthma, the constitutive expression of P-selectin, vascular cellular adhesion molecule-1 (VCAM-1), E-selectin, and ICAM-1 is significantly higher than in cells from normal subjects. However, after 3 mo of Se supplementation in vivo, there was a significant decrease in VCAM-1 and E-selectin expression in vitro *(71)*. More direct evidence that the downregulation of adhesion molecules on endothelial cells by Se supplementation results from effects on selenoproteins was provided by the observation that a GPx mimic (ebselen) inhibited ICAM-1 and VCAM-1 expression *(72)*. Furthermore, GPx analogs prevented TNF-α-stimulated expression of P-selectin and E-selectin, as well as TNF-α and IL-1-stimulated IL-8 release in human endothelial cells *(73)*.

8. SELENIUM AND AGING

Aging cells accumulate oxidative damage to both mitochondrial and nuclear DNA *(74)*. Reactive oxygen and nitrogen species also cause an accumulation of carbonyl moieties on protein and thiobarbituric reactive substances (TBARS) from lipid peroxidation. In addition, activated oxygen species may also regulate senescence; the treatment of fibroblasts with nonlethal doses of hydrogen peroxide activates a senescence program, which leads to growth cessation *(75)*. Because the free-radical theory of aging *(74)* suggests that much of the cellular damage that leads to aging is a result of ROS, then the ability of selenoproteins to "mop up" these species suggests that selenoproteins may be important in preventing the damage that leads to cellular aging. Telomere length decreases with age and is accelerated by oxidative stress in fibroblasts *(76)*. The rate of telomere shortening and carbonyl group accumulation was inversely correlated with GPx activity in fibroblasts *(77)*.

The immune system's efficiency declines with age, and the elderly are more prone to infections than young or middle-aged adults. Compared with controls, lymphocyte proliferation in response to mitogens was enhanced by 138% in institutionalized elderly patients who had been taking Se at 100 µg/d as Se-enriched yeast for 6 mo *(78)*. Cancer is a disease often associated with old age and an age-dependent decrease in the immune system's ability to detect and destroy tumors. This may result from a decrease in the effectiveness of NK cells and brought on by inadequate nutrition. In a study of free-living elderly Italians (ages 90–106 yr), the percentage of NK cells in the bloodstream of women was related to the serum Se content *(79)*. In "old" mice, Se supplementation restores lymphocyte responsiveness by upregulating the high-affinity IL-2 receptor *(80)*.

Increased longevity has been reported in areas that have Se-rich soil *(81)*. Relatively fewer people over 80 yr of age were found in areas where the Kashin-Beck and Keshan disease were endemic. An adequate Se intake may also be important in maintaining GPx activity and minimizing oxidative damage in aging cells.

9. SELENIUM AND CANCER

There are many studies that address the role of Se in cancer prevention or incidence; most suggest that Se deficiency may increase the risk of developing cancer in both humans and animals. More importantly, from a mechanistic viewpoint, these studies indicate that optimal protection from malignancy is achieved at Se intakes that are at least three times greater than those currently recommended as adequate (82).

Epidemiologic studies reveal an inverse relationship between Se intake and cancer mortality in several countries (83). Many other trials within countries have shown that low Se status is associated with an increased cancer risk. However, in several studies, average blood Se concentration in cancer cases was only 5–10% less than in controls. Another problem with these associations is that the malignancy may have resulted in a change in Se status, as determined from blood markers. In addition, it is unwise to relate plasma Se concentration to Se concentrations in diseased organs.

More convincing evidence of Se's effect in preventing cancer has come from supplementation trials. A double-blind placebo-control study, conducted for several years, showed that Se supplementation decreased cancer incidence and mortality (84). The incidences of colon, prostate, and lung cancers were decreased by approx 50% when subjects were supplemented with 200 µg of Se/d. The greatest protection was afforded to those subjects with the lowest initial plasma Se concentrations. In the context of Se supplementation acting through an increased selenoprotein activity, this trial raises numerous questions. The American population receiving the supplements already had an Se intake that was considered to saturate selenoprotein activities (84). Thus, Se supplementation was likely to exert its anticancer activity through a mechanism that was unrelated to recognized selenproteins. Several hypotheses could be advanced to explain this, including immune system enhancement, apoptosis, or production of Se metabolites, such as hydrogen selenide, methylated Se compounds, and selenodiglutathione, that are toxic to cancer cells (85,86). The ability to modulate cellular redox status and cellular immune status may account for the chemopreventative properties of 1,4-phenylenebis (methylene) selenocyanate and selenodiglutathione. These compounds can induce the Fas ligand, which activates apoptotic pathways in tumors, as well as activating stress kinase pathways (87).

10. SELENIUM AND ENDOCRINE FUNCTION

10.1. Selenium and the Thyroid

10.1.1. Thyroid Hormone Synthesis

All thyroxine (T4) is synthesized on thyroglobulin within the lumen of the thyroid follicle, a structure composed of thyrocytes clusters. Synthesis of T4 and the bioactive form triiodothyronine (T3) requires iodination of tyrosyl residues on thyroglobulin, followed by coupling of these iodinated derivatives. These reactions take place within the follicular lumen at the surface of the apical membrane. All steps of thyroid hormone synthesis are promoted by thyrotropin (thyroid-stimulating hormone [TSH]) released from the anterior pituitary. Iodination of tyrosyl residues on thyroglobulin requires H_2O_2

generation in high concentrations and also the action of thyroid peroxidase, an enzyme located on the luminal side of the apical membrane. H_2O_2 generation is the rate-limiting step in thyroid hormone synthesis and is regulated by a complex network of interacting second-messenger systems *(88)*. Iodine is essential for thyroid hormone synthesis and is concentrated by the thyroid gland. The thyroid also contains more Se per gram of tissue than any other organ, and Se-like iodine is essential for normal thyroid function and thyroid hormone homeostasis.

10.1.2. SELENIUM AS AN ANTIOXIDANT IN THE THYROID

Although H_2O_2 is essential for thyroid hormone synthesis, it is extremely toxic. The thyrocyte is exposed to high H_2O_2 concentrations and toxic lipid hydroperoxides, but, under normal circumstances, the gland is protected from the products of oxidative stress by antioxidant systems that include selenoenzymes, such as the GPxs and TR. The importance of the peroxide-metabolizing enzymes is further increased in iodine deficiency, where high TSH levels hyperstimulate the thyroid gland to increase H_2O_2 and lipid hydroperoxide production. When Se is available, selenoenzymes are induced and protect against potential oxidative damage *(89)*.

In humans, attention has focused on how Se deficiency may alter the effects of iodine deficiency, particularly, how the deficiencies relate to endemic cretinism pathogenesis *(89,90)*. Two forms of the disorder occur, and, in both, the abnormalities are irreversible once present *(89,90)*. *Myxoedematous cretinism* is associated with severe hypothyroidism, thyroid involution, and stunted growth. In *Neurological cretinism* mental deficiency may be accompanied by neurologic problems, including hearing and speech defects, whereas growth and thyroid functions may be normal. Iodine deficiency plays an important role in both types of cretinism, because both diseases may be prevented by iodine supplementation, but it has been suggested that Se supply may influence the prevalence and type of disease. Some epidemiologic studies imply that increased H_2O_2 generation, produced by iodine deficiency, with an accompanying loss of selenoperoxidase activity caused by Se deficiency, leads to thyroid atrophy and myxedematous cretinism. In contrast, if Se supply is adequate, thyroid destruction may be prevented. More recent reports have failed to provide convincing support for this hypothesis, and the possible role of other additional factors such as thiocyanates must again be considered *(89)*.

10.1.3. SELENIUM AS A REGULATOR OF THYROID HORMONE PRODUCTION

Se may affect thyroid hormone production through regulation of H_2O_2 concentration in the follicular lumen of the thyroid by modulating secretion of extracellular GPx *(89)*. However, Se status also influences iodothyronine deiodinases expression in most tissues, and these enzymes are crucial in regulating the supply of the biologically active thyroid hormone 3,3',5 triiodothyronine (T_3), which is produced by 5'-monodeiodination of T4. The effects of Se deficiency in animals are complex and depend on iodine supply and deficiency duration *(89,91)*.

10.2. Selenium and Diabetes

There are several studies in rats that suggest that Se may influence the consequences of insulin deficiency and diabetes *(91)*. The trace element exerts insulin-like action in cultured adipocytes and rats made diabetic with streptozotocin. For example, when selenate was administered through the intraperitoneal route to diabetic rats for 2 wk, plasma glucose was essentially normalized.

Selenium can prevent or alleviate diabetes' adverse effects on the heart and kidney *(91)*. Unfortunately, there are no reports of Se supplementation trials in humans who are diabetic.

10.3. Selenium and Fertility in Males

One of the first deleterious effects of Se deficiency to be demonstrated in farm livestock was fetal resorption in sheep. Se supplementation prevented these problems. Many subsequent trials with farm animals showed that Se supplementation improved overall reproductive performance *(92)*. Sperm abnormalities have been a consistent feature recognized in Se-deficient animals *(93,94)*. Only recently has the explanation of this phenomenon been fully recognized. Characterization of the selenoprotein that forms a major component of the midpiece of sperm showed that it was a polymeric form of phGPx. This forms up to 50% of the capsule material and is likely to be formed by oxidation of phGPx monomers *(95)*. Further research is required to determine whether male fertility in humans can be associated with the range of Se intakes that are seen throughout the world *(50,95)*. However, one study performed in Scotland (where Se intakes are only 30–40 µg/d) has shown that sperm quality and fertility in humans can be improved by Se supplementation *(96)*.

11. CONCLUSIONS

An adequate dietary Se intake is essential for human and animal health, for optimal immunity and for protection from some types of cancers. Selenium exerts its biologic effects principally through modification of selenoprotein expression. Some of these are selenoenzymes that are essential for the metabolism of harmful products of oxidative metabolism, such as hydrogen peroxide and lipid hydroperoxides. Selenoproteins are, thus, critical to maintaining optimal redox balance and cellular and humoral immunity. Certain selenoproteins, however, have actions that are unrelated to antioxidant effects; for example, Se-containing iodothyronine deiodinases are crucial to maintain thyroid hormone homeostasis. The anticancer action of Se found using high intakes are intriguing because current evidence suggests that such actions must be operating through a mechanism that is independent of selenoprotein synthesis. However, there is some evidence to suggest that with high Se intakes, the enzyme action of some selenoproteins may be impaired and protection from harmful agents, such as UVB, lost. Increasing evidence suggests that Se deficiency may be important in the pathogenesis of several inflammatory diseases, such as asthma, sepsis, arthritis, and in infections and heart and vascular disease. Selenium supplements may have a therapeutic potential in these diseases and in protecting against certain cancers. Furthermore, numerous intervention studies in patients with severe sepsis, burns, and pancreatitis suggest that Se supplementation provides significant clinical beneficial outcome *(97)*.

12. THE VITAL QUESTIONS: TOPICS FOR FUTURE RESEARCH

Despite an explosion in Se research, there are still important questions that are unresolved. Better controlled studies are necessary to answer the following questions:

- Do selenocompounds prevent skin cancer in humans like they do in mice?
- What types of cancers does Se supplementation help to prevent? What Se forms and doses are optimal to give protection?
- Should selenocompounds be used in conjunction with conventional chemotherapy, radiotherapy, or UV therapy?
- Are Se compounds therapeutically useful against chronic inflammatory diseases?
- Does Se deficiency predispose to coronary and vascular disease?
- Is there a case for increasing the Se intake of the population of countries (such as the United Kingdom and other Northern European countries) in which intake does not meet the recommended daily intake? What form of Se should be taken?
- If Se does have an influence on disease, the precise mechanism by which it exerts these effects must be elucidated. Such mechanisms may involve the many selenoproteins for which a biologic role is still unknown.
- Do selenoprotein gene polymorphisms contribute to disease?

13. "TAKE-HOME" MESSAGES

1. Selenium is an essential dietary trace element that has important antioxidant, growth, and anticancer actions. Is also essential for normal thyroid hormone metabolism.
2. Selenium exerts many of its actions by modifying the expression of selenoproteins that have selenocysteine residues incorporated into their active site. Such selenoproteins include the GPx, thioredoxin reductases, and iodothyronine deiodinases.
3. The recommended intake of Se is approx 70 μg/d, an intake that leads to maximum expression of GPx and other characterized selenoproteins. However, in many countries, the dietary Se intake is below this recommended intake, which may leave the population vulnerable to cancer and heart disease.
4. Selenium can improve the immune system's efficiency by modifying peroxide, cytokine, eicosanoid, IL2-receptor, and adhesion molecule production. The trace element can also influence cell redox state, which, in turn, can influence cell growth, p53 expression, and apoptotic death of tumor cells.
5. Se deficiency in the host may encourage viral mutation to produce pathogenic strains. It has been suggested that Keshan disease, HIV, and the influenza virus may have evolved through this mechanism.
6. Increasing evidence suggests that Se deficiency may be important in the pathogenesis of several inflammatory diseases, such as asthma, sepsis, and arthritis.
7. Se's anticancer effects are most potent at intakes that are well above those required to maximize expression of the known selenoproteins. This suggests that Se may exert important biologic effects that are not mediated through selenoproteins.

ACKNOWLEDGMENTS

Our research has been supported by the Foundation for Skin Research, The British Skin Foundation, The Sir Stanley and Lady Davidson Trust, The British Heart Foundation, The Moray Trust, The Agnes Hunter Trust, and the Medical Research Council of the UK. SM was a recipient of a postgraduate studentship from the Faculty of Medicine, University of Edinburgh. JRA's laboratory is funded by the Scottish Executive Environment and Rural Affairs Department (SEERAD).

REFERENCES

1. Vernie LN. Selenium in carcinogenesis. Biochem Biophys Acta 1984;738:203–217.
2. Spallholz JE, Boylan LM, Larsen HS. Advances in understanding Selenium's role in the immune system. Ann NY Acad Sci 1990;587:123–139.
3. McKenzie RC, Rafferty, TS, Beckett GJ. Selenium: an essential element for immune function. Immunol Today 1998;19:342–345.
4. McKenzie RC, Rafferty TS, Arthur JR, Beckett GJ. Effects of selenium on immunity and ageing. In: Hatfield DL (ed.). Selenium: Its Molecular Biology and Role in Human Health. Kluwer Academic Publishers, Boston, 2001, pp. 257–272.
5. Allan CB, Lacourciere GM, Stadtman TC. Responsiveness of selenoproteins to dietary selenium. Ann Rev Nutr 1999;19:1–16.
6. McKenzie RC, Arthur JR, Beckett GJ. Selenium and the regulation of cell signaling, growth and survival: molecular and mechanistic aspects. Antioxid Redox Signal 2002;4:339–351.
7. Rayman MP. The importance of selenium to human health. Lancet 2000;356:233–241.
8. Foster DJ, Sumar S. Selenium in health and disease. Crit Rev Food Sci Nutr 1997;37:211–228.
9. Roy M, Kiremidjian-Schumacher L, Wishe HI, Cohen MW, Stotzky G. Effect of selenium on the expression of high affinity. Interleukin-2 receptors. Proc Royal Soc Exp Biol Med 1992;200:36–43.
10. Levander OA. Evolution of human dietary standards for selenium. In: Hatfield DL (ed.). Selenium: Its Molecular Biology and Role in Human Health. Klewer Academic Publishers, Boston, 2001, pp. 99–311.
11. McKenzie RC. Selenium, ultraviolet radiation and the skin. Clin Exp Dermatol 2000;25:631–636.
12. Funk CD. Prostaglandins and leukotrienes: advances in eicosanoid biology. Science 2001;294:1871–1875.
13. Ebert-Dumig R, Seufert J, Schneider D, Kohrle J, Schutze N, Jakob F. Expression of selenoproteins in monocytes and macrophages—implications for the immune system. Med Klin 1999;94:29–33.
14. Sun EJ, Xu HB, Liu Q, Zhou JY, Zuo P, Wang JJ. The mechanism for the effect of selenium supplementation in immunity. Biol Trace Element Res 1995;48:231–238.
15. Tricarico M, Rinaldi M, Bonmassar E, Fuggetta MP, Barrera G, Fazio VM. Effect of 4-hydroxynonenal, a product of lipid peroxidation, on natural cell mediated cytotoxicity. Anticancer Res 1999;19:5149–5154.
16. Sun EJ, Xu HB, Wen DJ, Zuo P, Zhuo JY, Wang JJ. Inhibition of lipid peroxidation. Biol Trace Element Res 1997;59:87–92.
17. Hawkes WC, Kelley DS, Taylor PC. The effects of dietary selenium on the immune system in healthy men. Biol Trace Element Res 2001;81:189–213.
18. Kiremidjian-Schumacher L, Roy M, Wishe HI, Cohen MW, Stotzky G. Selenium and immune cell functions. I. Effect on lymphocyte proliferation and production of interleukin 1 and interleukin 2. Proc Soc Royal Exp Biol Med 1990;193:136–142.
19. Kiremidjian-Schumacher L, Roy M, Wishe HI, Cohen MW, Stotsky G. Supplementation with selenium and human immune cell functions. II. Effect on cytotoxic lymphocytes and natural killer cells. Biol Trace Element Res 1994;41:115–127.
20. Petrie H, Klassen LW, Kay HD. Selenium and the immune response: 1. Modulation of alloreactive human lymphocyte functions in vitro. J Leukoc Biol 1989;5:207–214.
21. Nair MP, Schwartz SA. Immunoregulation of natural and lymphokine-activated killer cells by selenium. Immunopharmacology 1990;19:177–183.
22. Bonomini M, Forster S, De Risio F, et al. Effects of selenium supplementation on immune parameters in chronic uraemic patients on haemodialysis. Nephrol Dial Transplant 1995;10:1654–1661.
23. Vitoux D, Chappuis P, Arnaud J, Bost M, Accominotti M, Roussel AM. Selenium, glutathione peroxidase, peroxides and platelet functions. Ann Biol Clin 1996;54:181–187.
24. Rayman MP. Dietary selenium: time to act—low bioavailability in Britain and Europe could be contributing to cancers, cardiovascular disease, and subfertility. BMJ 1997;314:387–388.
25. Weaver JA, Maddox JF, Cao YZ, Mullarky IK, Sordillo LM. Increased 15-HPETE production decreases prostacyclin synthase activity during oxidant stress in aortic endothelial cells. Free Rad Biol Med 2001;30:299–308.

26. Rafferty TS, Walker C, Hunter JAA, Beckett GJ, McKenzie RC. Inhibition of ultraviolet radiation B (UVB)-induced IL-10 expression in murine keratinocytes by selenium compounds. Br J Dermatol 2002;146:485–489.

27. Shen HM, Yang CF, Liu J, Ong CN. Dual role of glutathione I selenite-induced oxidative stress and apoptosis in human hepatoma cell. Free Radical Biol Med 2000;28:115–112.

28. Johnson VJ, Tsunoda M, Sharma RP. Increased production of proinflammatory cytokines by murine macrophages following oral exposure to sodium selenite but not to seleno-L-methionine. Arch Environ Contam Toxicol 2000;39:243–250.

29. Stewart MS, Spallholz JE, Neldner KH, Pence BC. Selenium compounds have disparate abilities to impose oxidative stress and induce apoptosis. Free Radical Biol Med 1998;26:42–48.

30. Spallholz JE. Free radical generation by selenium compounds and their pro-oxidant toxicity. Biomed Environ Sci 1997;10:260–270.

31. Duthie MS, Kimber I, Norval M. The effects of ultraviolet radiation on the human immune system. Br J Dermatol 1999;140:995–1009.

32. Park HS, Huh SH, Kim YH, et al. Selenite negatively regulates caspase-3 through a redox mechanism. J Biol Chem 2000;275:8487–8491.

33. Kim T, Jung U, Cho DY, Chung AS. Se-methylselenocysteine induces apoptosis through caspase activation in HL-60 cells. Carcinogenesis 2001;22:559–565.

34. Gartner R, Angstwurm M. Selenium and intensive care medicine. Clinical trials in SIRS and sepsis. Med Klin 1999;94(Suppl 3):54–57.

35. Sattar N, Scott HR, McMillan DC, Talwar D, O'Reilly DSJ, Fell GS. Acute-phase reactants and plasma trace element concentrations in non-small cell lung cancer patients and controls. Nutr Cancer 1997;28:308–312.

36. Singh A, Smoak BL, Patterson KY, LeMay LG, Veillon C, Deuster PA. Biochemical indices of selected trace minerals in men: effect of stress. Am J Clin Nutr 1991;53:126–131.

37. Tarp U. Selenium in rheumatoid-arthritis—a review. Analyst 1995;120:877–881.

38. Knekt P, Heliovaara M, Aho K, Alfthan G, Marniemi J, Aromaa A. Serum selenium, serum alpha-tocopherol, and the risk of rheumatoid arthritis. Epidemiology 2000;11:402–405.

39. Reimund JM, Hirth C, Koehl C, Baumann R, Duclos B. Antioxidant and immune status in active Crohn's disease. A possible relationship. Clin Nutr 2000;19:43–48.

40. Greene LS. Asthma and oxidant stress—nutritional, environmental, and genetic risk-factors. J Am Coll Nutr 1995;14:317–324.

41. Ward KP, Arthur JR, Russell G, Aggett PJ. Blood selenium content and glutathione peroxidase activity in children with cystic fibrosis, coeliac disease, asthma, and epilepsy. Eur J Pediatr 1984;142:21–24.

42. Misso NLA, Powers KA, Gillon RL. Reduced platelet glutathione peroxidase activity and serum selenium concentration in atopic asthmatic patients. Clin Exp Allergy 1996;26:838–847.

43. Juhlin L, Edqvist LE, Ekman LG, Ljunghall K, Olsson M. Blood glutathione-peroxidase levels in skin diseases-effect of selenium and vitamin-E treatment Acta Derm Venereol 1982;62:211–214.

44. Fairris GM, Perkins PJ, Lloyd B, Hinks L, Clayton BE. The effect on atopic dermatitis of supplementation with selenium and vitamin E. Acta Derm Venereol 1989;69:359–362.

45. Fairris GM, Lloyd B, Hinks L, Perkins PJ, Clayton BE. The effect of supplementation with selenium and vitamin E in psoriasis. Ann Clin Biochem 1989;26:83–88.

46. Harvima RJ, Jagerroos H, Kajander EO, et al. Screening of effects of selenomethionine-enriched yeast supplementation on various immunological and chemical parameters of skin and blood in psoriatic patients. Acta Derm Venereol 1993;73:88–91.

47. Burke KE, Burford RG, Combs G, French IW, Skeffington DR. The effect of topical l-selenomethionine on minimal erythema dose of ultraviolet-irradiation in humans. Photodermatol Photoimmunol Photomed 1992;9:52–57.

48. Pinton J, Friden H, Kettaneh-Wold N, et al. Clinical and biological effects of balneotherapy with selenium-rich spa water in patients with psoriasis vulgaris. Br J Dermatol 1995;133:344–347.

49. Kasseroller R. Sodium selenite as prophylaxis against erysipelas in secondary lymphedema. Anticancer Res 1998;18:2227–2230.

50. Delilbasi E, Turan B, Yucel E, Sasmaz R, Isimer A, Sayal A. Selenium and Behcet's disease. Biol Trace Element Res 1991;28:21–25.

51. Beck M. Selenium as an antiviral agent. In: Hatfield DL (ed.). Selenium: Its Molecular Biology and Role in Health. Kluwer Academic Publishers, Boston, 2001, pp. 235–245.
52. Beck AM, Shi Q, Morris VC, Levander OA. Rapid genomic evolution of nonvirulent Coxsackirvirus B3 in selenium deficient mice results in selection of identical virulent isolates. Nature Med 1995;1:433–436.
53. Beck MA. Rapid genomic evolution of a non-virulent coxsackievirus B3 in selenium-deficient mice. Biomed Environ Sci 1997;10:307–315.
54. Beck MA, Esworthy RS, Ho YS, Chu FF. Glutathione peroxidase protects mice from viral-induced myocarditis. FASEB J 1998;12:1143–1149.
55. Combs GF. Selenium and global food systems. Br J Nutr 2001;85:517–547.
56. Beck MA, Levander OA. Dietary oxidative stress and the potentiation of viral infection. Annu Rev Nutr 1998; 18:93–116.
57. Yu SY, Zhu YJ, Li WG. Protective role of selenium against hepatitis B virus and primary liver cancer in Qidong. Biol Trace Element Res 1997;56:117–124.
58. Baum MK, Campa A, Miguez-Burbano MJ, Burbano X, Shor-Posner G. Role of selenium in HIV/AIDS. In: Hatfield DL (ed.). Selenium: Its Molecular Biology and Role in Health. Kluwer Academic Publishers, Boston, 2001, pp. 235–245.
59. Coppinger RJ, Diamond AM. Selenium deficiency and human disease. In: Hatfield DL (ed.). Selenium: Its Molecular Biology and Role in Health. Kluwer Academic Publishers, Boston, 2001, pp. 219–233.
60. Huttunen JK. Selenium and cardiovascular disease—an update. Biomed Environ Sci 1999;10:171–189.
61. Schamberge RJ, Willis CC, McCormack LJ. Selenium and heart disease: blood selenium and heart mortality in 19 states. In: Hemphill DD (ed.). Trace Substance in Environmental Health XIII. University of Missouri Press, Columbia, 1979, pp. 59–63.
62. Miller S, Walker SW, Arthur JR, et al. Selenite protects human endothelial cells from oxidative damage and induces thioredoxin reductase. Clin Sci 2001;100:543–550.
63. Hara S. Effect of selenium deficiency on oxidative stress-induced isoprostane formation by bovine aortic endothelial cells. Toxicol Lett 1998;95:57.
64. Anema SM, Anema SM, Walker SW, Howie AF, Nicol F, Beckett GJ. Thioredoxin reductase is the major selenoprotein expressed in human umbilical-vein endothelial cells and is regulated by protein kinase C. Biochem J 1999;342:111–117.
65. Arteel GE, Mostert V, Oubrahim H, Briviba K, Abel J, Sies H. Protection by selenoprotein P in human plasma against peroxynitrite-mediated oxidation and nitration. Biol Chem 1998;379:1201–1205.
66. Arteel GE, Briviba K, Sies H. Function of thioredoxin reductase as a peroxynitrite reductase using selenocystine or ebselen. Chem Res Toxicol 1999;12:264–269.
67. Lu X, Liu S, Man RYK. Enhancement of endothelium dependent relaxation in the rat aortic ring by selenium supplement. Cardiovasc Res 1994;28:345–348.
68. Hampel G, Watanabe K, Weksler BB, Jaffe EA. Selenium deficiency inhibits prostacyclin release and enhances production of platelet activating factor by human endothelial cells. Biochim Biophys Acta 1989;1006:151–158.
69. Maddox JF, Aherne KM, Reddy CC, Sordillo LM. Increased neutrophil adherence and adhesion molecule mRNA expression in endothelial cells during selenium deficiency. J Leukoc Biol 1999;65: 658–664.
70. McCarty MF. Oxidants downstream from superoxide inhibit nitric oxide production by vascular endothelium—a key role for selenium-dependent enzymes in vascular health. Med Hypoth 1999;53:315–325.
71. Horvathova M, Jahnova E, Gazdik F. Effect of selenium supplementation in asthmatic subjects on the expression of endothelial cell adhesion molecules in culture. Biol Trace Element Res 1999;69:15–26.
72. D'Alessio P, Moutet M, Coudrier E, Darquenne S, Chaudiere J. ICAM-1 and VCAM-1 expression induced by TNF-alpha are inhibited by a glutathione peroxidase mimic. Free Rad Biol Med 1998;24: 979–987.
73. Moutet M, d'Alessio P, Malette P, Devaux V, Chaudiere J. Glutathione peroxidase mimics prevent TNF alpha-and neutrophil-induced endothelial alterations. Free Rad Biol Med 1998;25:270–281.
74. Beckman KB, Ames BN. The free radical theory of aging matures. Physiol Rev 1998;78:547–581.
75. Chen Q, Ames BN. Senescence-like growth arrest induced by hydrogen peroxide in human diploid fibroblast F65 cells. Proc Natl Acad Sci USA 1994;91:4130–4134.

76. von Zglinicki T, Saretzki G, Docke W, Lotze C. Mild hyperoxia shortens telomeres and inhibits prolif-eration of fibroblasts: a model for senescence? Exp Cell Res 1995;220:186–193.

77. Serra V, Grune T, Sitte N, Saretzki G, Von Zglinicki T. Telomere length as a marker of oxidative stress in primary human fibroblast cultures. Ann NY Acad Sci 2000;908:327–330.

78. Peretz A, Neve J, Desmedt J, Duchateau J, Dramaix M, Famaey JP. Lymphocyte-response is enhanced by supplementation of elderly subjects with selenium-enriched yeast. Am J Clin Nutr 1991;53: 1323–1328.

79. Ravaglia G, Forti P, Maioli F, et al. Effect of micronutrient status on natural killer cell immune function in healthy free-living subjects aged ≥ 90 y. Am J Clin Nutr 2000;71:590–598.

80. Roy M, Kiremidjian-Schumacher L, Wishe HI, Cohen MW, Stotzky G. Supplementation with selenium restores age-related decline in immune cell function. Proc Soc Exp Biol Med 1995;209:369–375.

81. Foster HD, Zhang LP. Longevity and selenium deficiency—evidence from the Peoples Republic of China. Sci Total Environ 1995;170:133–113.

82. Combs GF Jr. Selenium as an anticancer agent. In: Hatfield DL (ed.). Selenium: Its Molecular Biology and Role in Health. Kluwer Academic Publishers, Boston, 2000, pp. 205–217.

83. Ip C. Lessons from basic research in selenium and cancer prevention. J Nutr 1998;28:1845–1854.

84. Clark LC, Combs GF Jr, Turnbull BW, et al. Effects of selenium supplementation for cancer prevention in patients with carcinoma of the skin. A randomized controlled trial. JAMA 1996;276:1957–1963.

85. Ip C, Hayes C, Budnick RM, Ganther HE. Chemical form of selenium, critical metabolites, and cancer prevention. Cancer Res 1991;51:595–600.

86. Ip C, Lisk DJ. Characterization of tissue selenium profiles and anticarcinogenic responses in rats fed natural sources of selenium-rich products. Carcinogenesis 1994;15:573–576.

87. Fleming J, Ghose A, Harrison PR. Molecular mechanisms of cancer prevention by selenium compounds. Nutr Cancer 2001;40:42–49.

88. Taurog A. Hormone synthesis and secretion. In: Braverman LE, Utiger RW Werner (eds.). Ingbar's The Thyroid (7th ed.). Lippincott-Raven, Philadelphia, 1996, pp. 47–81.

89. Arthur JR, Beckett GJ, Mitchell JH. The interactions between selenium and iodine deficiencies in man and animals. Nutr Res Rev 1999;12:55–73.

90. Delange FM, Ermans AM. Iodine deficiency. In: Braverman LE, Utiger RD Werner (eds). Ingbar's The Thyroid (7th ed.). Lippincott-Raven, Philadelphia, 1996, pp. 296–316.

91. St. Germain DL. Selenium, deiodinases and endocrine function. In: Hatfield DL (ed.). Selenium. Its Molecular Biology and Role in Health. Kluwer Academic Publishers, Boston, 2000, pp. 189–205.

92. Hansen JC, Deguchi Y. Selenium and fertility in animals and man—a review. Acta Vet Scand 1996;37:19–30.

93. Watanabe T, Endo A. Effects of selenium deficiency on sperm morphology and spermatocyte chromo-somes in mice. Mut Res 1991;262:93–99.

94. Behne D, Weiler H, Kyriakopoulos A. Effects of selenium deficiency on testicular morphology and function in rats. J Reprod Fertil 1996;106:291–297.

95. Flohe L, Flohe RB, Maiorino M, Roveri A, Wissing J, Ursini F. Selenium and male reproduction. In: Hatfield DL (ed.). Selenium: Its Molecular Biology and Role in Health. Kluwer Academic Publishers, Boston, 2001, pp. 273–283.

96. MacPherson SR, Yates RW, Hussain B, Dixon J. The effect of oral selenium supplementation on human sperm motility. Br J Urol 1998;82:76–80.

97. Yamin-Ali R, Khalil N, McCarthy G. Selenium in intensive care: an update. Br J Intensive Care 2001;10:88–94.

13 Zinc

Klaus-Helge Ibs and Lothar Rink

1. INTRODUCTION

Zinc is essential for the growth and development of all organisms. The first observations were made by Raulin in 1869 *(1)*, who described the need for zinc in cultivating *Aspergillus niger*. In 1934, Todd et al. showed the importance of zinc in mammals by establishing a rat model *(2)*. Later, a zinc deficiency syndrome in children was described by Prasad et al. in 1963 *(3)*. These children suffered from anemia, hypogonadism, hepatosplenomegaly, skin alterations, growth, and mental retardation. Then, it was shown that these symptoms occurred because of zinc deficiency resulting from a zinc-specific malabsorption syndrome called *Acrodermatitis enteropathica* (a rare autosomal recessive inheritable disease), which was discovered by Neldner and Hambidge in 1975 *(4)*. *Acrodermatitis enteropathica* leads to death within a few years when it is untreated, because it shows several immunologic alterations and a high frequency of bacterial, viral, and fungal infections. However, pharmacologic zinc supplementation can reverse all of the disease's symptoms *(4)*.

The human body contains 2–4 g zinc total, but only a small amount occurs in the plasma (10–18 μM) and this is influenced by different factors, e.g., age and gender, so the plasma concentration ranges from 10.1 to 16.8 μM in women and 10.6–17.9 μM in men. Although the plasma pool is the smallest zinc pool in the body, it is highly mobile and immunologically important *(5,6)*. In the serum, zinc is predominantly bound to albumin (60%, low affinity), α_2-macroglobulin (30%, high affinity), and transferrin (10%) *(7)*.

Because there is no specialized storage system in the body, a steady state of zinc intake and excretion is necessary. However, the influence of different factors on bioavailability leads to contradictory recommendations regarding daily zinc intake. The recommended intakes in the United States and Germany are shown in Table 1, the results of some intake studies from different countries are summarized in Table 2, and the zinc content of some foods is detailed in Table 3.

These different factors' influences on zinc metabolism, as well as on homeostasis, were recently reviewed by Krebs and Hambidge *(8)*. Intracellular zinc was believed to be available in a cytosolic pool of free or loosely bound Zinc (II) ions in the μM to pM range, but recent data indicate that free zinc concentrations are in the fM range, which suggests a high intracellular zinc-binding capacity *(9)*.

From: *Diet and Human Immune Function*
Edited by: D. A. Hughes, L. G. Darlington, and A. Bendich © Humana Press Inc., Totowa, NJ

Table 1
Actual Recommended Daily Zinc Intake in mg/d

| | Intake | | | |
| Age | Germany (German Society of Nutrition, 2000) | | United States (Food and Nutrition Board, 2001) | |
	Women	Men	Women	Men
Infants				
0–3 mo	1.0	1.0	2.0	2.0
4–6 mo	2.0	2.0	2.0	2.0
7–12 mo	2.0	2.0	3.0	3.0
Children				
1–3 yr	3.0	3.0	3.0	3.0
4–6 yr	5.0	5.0	5.0	5.0
7–9 yr	7.0	7.0	5.0	5.0
10–12 yr	7.0	9.0	8.0	8.0
13–14 yr	7.0	9.5	8.0	8.0
Adolescents/ adults				
15–18 yr	7.0	10.0	9.0	11.0
19–70 yr	7.0	10.0	8.0	11.0
>70 yr	7.0	10.0	8.0	11.0
Pregnancy				
≤18 yr	10.0	12.0		
>18 yr	10.0	11.0		
Lactation				
≤18 yr	11.0	–	13.0	–
>18 yr	11.0	–	12.0	–

Zinc is necessary to maintain normal functioning of the immune system. Even mild zinc deficiency, which is widespread in contrast to severe zinc deficiency, depresses humans' immunity. Individuals with marginal zinc deficiency suffer from impaired taste and smell, onset of night blindness, memory impairment, and decreased spermatogenesis in men (10). Patients with severe zinc deficiency show severely depressed immune function, frequent infections, skin lesions, diarrhea, alopecia, and mental disturbances (10). Some high-risk groups and reasons for zinc deficiency are summarized in Table 4.

2. ZINC SENSORS

As mentioned, free zinc concentrations in the blood are low and they are not easy to assess. A promising technique for precise zinc measurements in vivo is the use of biosensors, which can transduce the presence or concentration of a given chemical analyte into an electronic or optical signal (11). This system is called a biosensor, because the transducer is biological in origin. Using carbonic anhydrase II (CA II) as a transducer, a sensitive and selective system was developed that makes it possible to measure zinc concentrations accurately in the range of 0.1–10 pM. CA II variants, which were obtained from structure-based and random mutagenesis, showed an altered zinc affinity. These

Table 2
Zinc Intake Studies

Country	Year	Participants	Outcome	References
United States	1988–1994	All ages	44.4% with low intake; children, adolescent girls, and aged persons over 71 yr at high risk of inadequate intake	(139)
Australia	1995	Aged persons	43% women with low intake	(140)
China	1992	All ages	Intake between 80% and 90% of RDA	(141)
Spain	2002	Aged persons	No statistically significant difference between intake and RDA	(142)
Pakistan	2002	All ages	No statistically significant difference between intake and RDA	(143)
Italy	2002	Adolescent females	Lower intake than RDA	(144)
Philippines	1993	All ages	Lower intake than RDA	(145)
United Kingdom	2000	Preschool children	20% with low intake	(146)

RDA, recommended dietary allowance.

Table 3
Zinc Content of Some Foods (mg/100 g)

Products from plants		Products from animals	
Wholemeal flour	3.0	Oysters	20–150
Rice	1.3	Liver	4–6
Sweetcorn	1.2	Cheese	1–5
Wheat (white) flour	0.9	Calf fillet	4.3
Carrot	0.64	Pork fillet	3.6
Coconut	0.5	Beef fillet	3.6
Sauerkraut	0.32	Pork shoulder	3.5
Potato	0.2–0.3	Poultry	2–3
Fruit	0.1–0.3	Roast beef	2.5
Cauliflower	0.23	Fish	1–2
Vegetable oil	0.1–0.2	Pork cutlet	1.3
Salad	0.22	Eggs	0.3–0.5
Red cabbage	0.22	Milk	0.2–0.4
Radish	0.16	Butter	0.15
Sugar	0.1		

mutants could potentially allow quantitation of free zinc in a range from 2 fM to 10 μM, when used in an array system (12).

On the cellular level, metal-response element-binding transcription factor-1 (MTF-1) is an important zinc sensor that coordinates the expression of genes involved in zinc homeostasis, protecting against metal toxicity and oxidative stresses (13). In mice, metallothionein (MT), zinc-transporter-1 (ZnT-1), and γ-glutamylcysteine synthetase heavy chain (γ-GCS$_{hc}$) are included in these processes. MTs are widely present in cells

Table 4
Some High-Risk Groups for Zinc Deficiency

Group	Reason
Vegetarians	Decreased absorption
Elderly	Insufficient intake
Children/adolescents	Increased requirements
Pregnant women	Increased requirements
Nursing	Increased requirements
Patients with diabetes	Increased elimination
Persons with allergies	Increased requirements
Renal insufficient patients	Increased elimination
Patients with infectious or inflammatory diseases	Increased requirements
Patients with chronic intestinal diseases (Crohn's disease, celiac disease)	Decreased absorption
Interactions with glucocorticoids, antacids, hormonal contraceptives, diuretics, and other pharmaceuticals	Increased elimination
Alcoholics	Insufficient intake; increased elimination

(14) and bind 5–20% of the total intracellular zinc under physiologic conditions. MTs' functions in protecting against metal toxicity, zinc deficiency, and oxidative stress have been demonstrated (13). ZnT-1 is a member of a mammalian zinc-transporter family, and its main function is regulating zinc efflux from cells. ZnT-1 is localized in the plasma membrane and is expressed in most cell and tissue types (15). γ-GCS is a key regulatory enzyme in the synthesis of GSH (glutathione) (16) that has multiple functions ranging from antioxidant defense to cell proliferation (17). GSH also chelates metal ions with relatively high affinity (18). The actual mechanism discussed is that the zinc-finger domain of MTF-1 binds zinc directly and reversibly (19), then adopts a DNA-binding conformation, and translocates from the cytoplasm to the nucleus (20). There, zinc binds to metal-response elements of the proteins' gene promoters, leading to increased transcription (13). However, the precise mechanism of this process is not yet determined.

3. ZINC TRANSPORT

Within the last decade, great progress has been made in understanding zinc's enterance into the cell. Two families of zinc transporters have been characterized, the zinc-regulated-transporter-(Zrt-), iron-regulated-transporter-(Irt)-like protein (ZIP) and the cation diffusion facilitator (CDF) family (21). One member of the second group, ZnT-1, and its function was mentioned. There are three other members whose functions have been elucidated, ZnT-2, ZnT-3, and ZnT-4. ZnT-2 might play a role in intracellular zinc sequestration and storage (21). The protein is located in the late endosome's membrane (22) that accumulates zinc when cells are grown under high zinc conditions (23). ZnT-3 was detected in synaptic vesicles' membranes in the neurons of the hippocampus and the cerebral cortex *(24)*, and it was suggested that these transport zinc into these compartments. ZnT-4 was found in the mammary gland and is responsible for transporting zinc from serum to milk *(25)*. Moreover, ZnT-4 plays a role in the intestine, because it is expressed in the intestinal enterocytes, where it is localized in the endosomal vesicles *(26)*.

In contrast to members of the CDF family, which are important for zinc efflux and intracellular sequestration, members of the ZIP family regulate zinc uptake into cells. These were named after two of the first members of the family to be identified, Zrt1 from *Saccharomyces cerevisiae* and Irt1 from *Arabidopsis thaliana (27,28)*. Although approx 80 members of the family were already found, only three proteins were detected in humans and only two of them have their function characterized, hZip1 (Zrt-*Irt*-like protein) and hZip2. By screening cDNA libraries, the first member was found to be expressed in several different cell types, whereas hZip2 was only found in prostate and uterine tissues *(21)*. Recently, hZip2 was detected in THP-1 cells, a monocyte cell type *(29)*. Experiments with K562 erythroleukemia cells revealed that hZip1, as well as hZip2, is located in the plasma membrane *(30,31)*. When one of the proteins was overexpressed in these cells, zinc uptake activity increased *(30,31)*. Moreover, there is evidence that hZip1 is the endogenous zinc uptake system in these cells *(31)*. The distribution of hZip3 and its functional characterization must be investigated.

Some researchers have suggested that the transferrin receptor (CD 71) and calcium ion channels can serve as an unspecific transport system for zinc, in addition to facilitated diffusion through amino acids and anionic exchange *(32,33)*. Others could not confirm these mechanisms *(34)*. Intracellular zinc is mostly bound to proteins and only a small amount is freely available. Experiments with immune cells showed that exogenously added zinc enters the cells within minutes and increases the free intracellular zinc pool by approx 70% *(34)*, whereas the total intracellular zinc amount, including the protein-bound zinc, increases by approx 300–600%, indicating that there must be a fast binding process to intracellular proteins *(35)*. Furthermore, the zinc-binding capacity by intracellular proteins, such as MT, is high. The zinc uptake process starts within the first few minutes and is saturated after 30 to 60 min *(34)*. Whether the ZIP family transporter plays a role in these processes has not been investigated.

4. ZINC'S INTRACELLULAR FUNCTIONS

There are more then 300 enzymes that carry zinc as a cofactor *(36,37)*, and nearly 200 three-dimensional structures of these proteins have been identified *(38)*. There are three primary sites of zinc: it is used for structural stability, catalytic activity as the central ion, or as a cocatalytic factor. Amino acids, such as histidine, glutamic acid, aspartic acid, and cysteine, are the main binding partners at these zinc-binding sites. Moreover, zinc influences quaternary protein structures and the protein interface has been identified as the fourth type of zinc-binding. These zinc sites are built by ligands from amino acid residues from two proteins *(38)*. Zinc can also mediate receptor binding that was first observed by investigating binding of superantigens to the major histocompatibility complex class II (MHC II) β-chain. The binding forms a zinc cluster involving histidine-81 of the MHC II β-chain and three amino acids from the superantigen *(39,40)*. In many enzymes, zinc fulfills more than one function. It plays an important role in cell proliferation, because zinc-finger motifs were detected in several replication and transcription factors. Therefore, cell proliferation is impaired when zinc is depleted *(35)*. Thus, highly proliferating cell systems, such as the immune system or the skin, are sensitive zinc deficiency markers, as mentioned.

Apoptosis is a physiologic method of cell death. It is an active and tightly regulated process involving a series of cytoskeletal, membrane, nuclear, and cytoplasmatic changes, leading to nucleus condensation and subsequent fragmentation of the cell into apoptotic bodies *(41)*. Apoptosis ensures the destruction of autoimmune T cells and B cells and amplifies the killing activity of cytotoxic T cells and natural killer (NK) cells *(35)*. On the one hand, zinc deficiency leads to increased occurrence of apoptotic cells in animals in vivo *(42)* and many different in vitro studies showed that culturing cells with zinc-depleted medium or treating them with *N,N,N´,N´*-tetrakis-2-pyridylmethyl-ethylendiamine (TPEN), a zinc chelator, results in apoptosis *(43–45)*. Zinc depletion-induced apoptosis shows all the typical morphologic alterations *(46)* and is dependent on caspase-3 activation *(47)*. Moreover, zinc depletion works synergistically with other apoptotic inducers *(44,48)*; consequently, zinc deficiency makes cells more susceptible to toxin-induced apoptosis.

On the other hand, zinc can protect cells against undergoing apoptosis. Publications by different groups point out an elevated resistance of animals to toxins when they were supplemented with zinc *(49,50)*, and, recently, it was shown that zinc suppresses caspase-3 activity and apoptosis in vivo *(51)*. Three mechanisms are believed to be involved in zinc's antiapoptotic actions. The first is that zinc blocks oxidative damage by protecting cellular membranes directly *(52,53)* or, second, by interacting with glutathione, the main intracellular antioxidant *(54,55)*. Third, zinc interacts with proteins directly involved in apoptotic processes. Many studies show that zinc inhibits caspase-3 *(56)*, caspase-6 *(57,58)*, and caspase-9 *(59,60)*. Moreover, it was observed that zinc supplementation in a monocyte cell line leads to an increased Bcl2/Bax ratio and increased cell resistance to apoptosis *(61)*. Furthermore, there is another antiapoptotic mechanism of zinc. In this case, zinc is described as an inhibitor of tumor necrosis factor-α (TNF-α)-mediated DNA fragmentation and cytolysis *(62)*. These mechanisms show that zinc can protect cells from undergoing apoptosis, which might be interesting in diseases such as diabetes mellitus or Alzheimer's disease. Enhanced apoptosis increases vulnerability to these diseases, and there is often an underlying subclinical or overt state of zinc deficiency recognized *(41)*. Furthermore, a protective function has been reported for many apoptosis-inducing factors, such as dexamethasone, γ-irradiation, cold shock, and hyperthermia *(42)*.

Zinc is also involved in cellular signaling mechanisms. Zinc interacts with calcium signaling as well as receptor tyrosine kinases and mitogen-activated protein kinases *(64)*. Moreover, zinc inhibits phosphodiesterases (PDEs), which are responsible for the degradation of cyclic adenosine monophosphate (cAMP) and cyclic guanosine monophosphate (cGMP) *(64–66)*. cAMP and cGMP, as well as tyrosine kinases, are involved in the direct activation of monocytes by zinc *(34)* (*see* Section 5.4.), but detailed mechanisms are not yet elucidated. Two recent studies detected a direct link between cGMP and zinc. Waetjen et al. revealed a zinc-mediated inhibition of cGMP hydrolysis, leading to increased cGMP in the cells *(67)*, and Haase et al. showed that cGMP modulates zinc uptake *(68)*. Futhermore, zinc has a regulatory function for protein kinase C (PKC), because nm concentrations of zinc can activate PKC, which translocates to the plasma membrane, a central event in PKC activation *(69)*. Zinc also modulates PKC translocation to the cytoskeleton *(70)* and the PKC's autonomous activity *(71)*.

5. ZINC'S ROLE IN THE IMMUNE SYSTEM

5.1. Innate Immunity

The immune system contains highly proliferating cells; consequently, it is strongly influenced by zinc. Innate immunity represents the first steps of the immune response. Altered zinc levels can disturb these processes. In vivo, NK cell activity, phagocytosis of macrophages and neutrophils, and generation of the oxidative burst are impaired by decreased zinc levels *(72,73)*. In neutrophils, not only is cellular recruitment to a site of inflammation affected *(74)*, but also is the chemotactic response, because zinc concentrations of approx 500 μM induce chemotactic activity in polymorphonuclear leukocytes (PMN) directly in vitro *(75)*. The number of neutrophils decreases during zinc deficiency *(76)*. This is easily explained, because 60×10^6 newly derived neutrophils are released from the bone marrow per minute. Zinc is also required by pathogens, such as bacteria and fungi, for proliferation. The human body decreases zinc plasma levels during an acute phase in infection as a defense mechanism. Zinc is chelated by the S-100 Ca^{2+} binding protein, calprotectin, which is released by dying or degranulating neutrophils, e.g., in abscesses and, consequently, reproduction of bacteria and *Candida albicans* is inhibited by zinc depletion *(77–79)*.

NK cells play a role in immunity against infections and tumors, and their activity and number are dependent on serum zinc level *(80)*. Zinc is needed by NK cells for the recognition, via their p58 killer cell inhibitory receptors, of MHC class I molecules on cells *(81)* to inhibit the killing activity. Interestingly, only the inhibitory signals are zinc dependent and not the positive ones. Thus, zinc deficiency might evoke nonspecific killing. However, zinc deficiency decreases NK cell activity and the relative number of precursors of cytolytic cells *(82)*. In healthy elderly, who often show decreased serum zinc levels, the number of NK cells is elevated, but the killing activity is reduced *(83–85)*. It is possible that the immune system might be trying to compensate the loss in killing activity by increasing the number of cells.

The effects of zinc deficiency on cells of the innate immune system are summarized in Table 5. The relationship between serum zinc concentration and cellular function is shown in Table 6.

5.2. T Cells

Zinc not only influences NK cell-mediated killing but also modulates cytolytic T-cell activity *(86)*. Zinc is involved in T-cell development, and zinc deficiency is responsible for thymic atrophy, which can be reversed by zinc supplementation *(87)*. The thymus produces a hormone called thymulin, which is released by thymic epithelial cells *(88,89)* and for which zinc is an essential cofactor. Thymulin regulates the differentiation of immature T cells in the thymus and the function of mature T cells in the periphery, but, moreover, this hormone also modulates cytokine release by peripheral blood mononuclear cells (PBMC), induces CD8+ T cell proliferation, in combination with interleukin (IL)-2 *(90,91)*, and ensures the expression of the high-affinity receptor for IL-2 on mature T cells *(92)*. This is consistent with study results that observed a decreased T-cell proliferation after mitogen stimulation resulting from zinc deficiency *(93,94)*.

Table 5
Effects of Zinc Deficiency on Cells of the Innate Immune System

Subpopulation	Effect		References
Monocytes	Cells	*	
	Phagocytosis	↓	(73)
Neutrophils	Cells	↓	(76)
	Oxidative burst	↓	(73)
Eosinophils	Cells	↓	(76)
	Oxidative burst	↓	(73)
Basophils	Cells	↓	(76)
	Oxidative burst	↓	(73)
Natural killer cells	CD16 (%)	↓	(80)
	CD56 (%)	↓	(80)
	Lytic activity	↓	(72,80,82)

↓ Significantly decreased.
* No data available.

Table 6
Relationship Between Serum Zinc Concentration and Cells Involved in the Innate Immune System

Serum zinc concentrations	Neutrophil granulocytes	Natural killer cells	Monocytes/ macrophages	Effects
Deficiency	Decreased phagocytosis	Decreased cytotoxicity	Decreased functions	Increased number of infections
Physiologic normal	Normal	Normal	Normal	No effects
High dosages	>100 μM: normal	Suppressed killing	>30 μM: normal	
	>500 μM: direct chemotactic activity		>100 μM: direct activation	Positive effects in skin creams

Furthermore, T helper (Th) cells are influenced by zinc, because zinc deficiency causes an imbalance between Th1 and Th2 functions. This can be observed in altered secretion of the typical Th1 and Th2 cytokines during zinc deficiency. The Th1 cell products, interferon (IFN)-γ and IL-2, are decreased in zinc deficiency, whereas Th2 products IL-4, IL-6, and IL-10 remain unchanged (82). Effects of zinc deficiency on T cells are summarized in Table 7, and the relationship between serum zinc levels and T cell function is reviewed in Table 8.

5.3. B Cells

B-cell development is also influenced during zinc deficiency but not as much as those of T cells (95–97), because B cells are less dependent on zinc for proliferation (98,99). These and the following findings have been made by the means of the mouse model. The mouse has an immune system analogous to that of humans, and the effects of zinc deficiency on immune function have been well characterized using it (100). B lympho-

Table 7
Effects of Zinc Deficiency on T Cells

Subpopulation	Effect	References
T cells (total)	↓	(76)
CD8 CD73 (%) (cytotoxic T-cell precursors)	↓	(147,148)
CD4/CD8-ratio	↓	(147)
(CD4: T-helper [Th] cells, CD8: cytotoxic T cells)		
CD4 CD45RA/CD4 CD45RO ratio	↓	(147,148)
(CD45RA: naive T cells, CD45RO: memory T cells)		
Th1/Th2 ratio (imbalance of Th1 and Th2)	↓	(82,147,148)
Interleukin-2 and interferon-γ production	↓	(76,82,148)

↓ Significantly decreased.

Table 8
Relationship Between Serum Zinc Concentration and Cells Involved in Specific Immune Responses

Serum zinc concentrations	T cells	B cells	Effects
Deficiency	Increased autoreactivity and alloreactivity	Apoptosis	Decreased reaction to antigens, increased number of infections, and autoimmunity
Physiologic normal	Normal	Normal	No effects
High dosages	>30 μM: functions decreased >100 μM: functions suppressed	Apoptosis	Suppression of alloreactivity after transplantations Increased number of infections

cytes and their precursors are reduced in absolute number during zinc deficiency, and pre-B and immature B cells are particularly sensitive, whereas changes in mature B lymphocytes are less pronounced. However, low zinc levels have no influence on the cell cycle status of precursor B cells and only modest influences on cycling pro-B cells, in contrast to the cycling status of myeloid cells, which change significantly (101). Moreover, B-lymphocyte antibody production is inhibited during periods of zinc deficiency (102–104). Studies have shown that antibody production in response to T-cell dependent antigens is more sensitive to zinc deficiency than antibody production in response to T-cell independent antigens (102,105). Immunologic memory is also influenced by zinc, because zinc-deficient mice showed reduced antibody recall responses to antigens for which they had been immunized (100,103,104,106). This effect was observed in T-cell independent, as well as T-cell dependent, systems. The relationship between serum zinc level and B-cell function is shown in Table 6, and the effects of zinc deficiency are detailed in Table 9.

5.4. Immunoregulation

Cytokines are modulators within the immune system, and zinc can influence this complicated network. IL-1, IL-6, TNF-α, soluble IL-2 receptor (sIL-2), and IFN-γ were

Table 9
Effects of Zinc Deficiency on B Cells

Subpopulation	Effect	References
B cells (total)	↓	(96)
CD45 Ig-	↓	(96)
CD45 IgM+	↓	(96)
CD45 IgM+ IgD+	↓	(96)
Antibody production	↓	(101–103)
(IgM, IgA, IgG levels)	↑ in elderly	(84)

Ig, immunoglobulin.

released when human PBMCs were stimulated with zinc in vitro *(107–109)*. IL-1, IL-6, and TNF-α are directly induced in monocytes by zinc in the absence of lymphocytes *(109)*. It was shown that TNF-α release after PBMC stimulation by zinc is caused by the induction of mRNA transcription and is not the result of the enhanced translation of already expressed mRNA *(110)*. In vitro supplementation of purified T cells with zinc showed no activation. This suggests that T-cell stimulation depends on monocyte presence *(109,111,112)*. The monocyte-derived cytokines (monokines), IL-1 and IL-6, together with cell-cell contact between monocytes and T cells, are necessary for T-cell stimulation and release IFN-γ and sIL-2 *(109,112)*. Zinc cannot induce cytokine production in isolated and monocyte-depleted T cells *(112,113)*, B cells *(94)*, NK cells *(94)*, or neutrophils (unpublished results). Moreover, activation of T cells and monocytes is dependent on the amount of free zinc ions and protein composition in the culture medium, because transferrin and insulin specifically enhance zinc-induced monocyte stimulation by means of a nonreceptor-dependent mechanism *(94,110,114,115)*. However, high levels of serum proteins in the culture medium inhibit monocyte activation because free zinc is bound by the proteins, and this lowers the available free zinc. In serum-free culture medium, zinc concentrations >100 μM stimulate monocytes but prevent T-cell activation, because T cells have a lower intracellular zinc concentration and are more susceptible to increasing zinc levels than monocytes *(112,116,117)*. This may result from the inhibition of the IRAK (IL-1 type I receptor-associated kinase) by zinc, because T-cell activation is an indirect IL-1-mediated process, the IL-1 being secreted by monocytes *(109,110,112)*. In conclusion, T-cell activation by zinc occurs when zinc concentrations are high enough for monokine induction but do not exceed the critical concentrations for T-cell suppression.

6. ZINC SUPPLEMENTATION AND THERAPY

Although in humans severe zinc deficiency is rare, marginal zinc deficiency is widespread, even in well-nourished industrial societies *(118)*. Studies highlight that zinc supplementation and optimal zinc intake restore impaired immune responses and decrease infection incidence *(119)*. This was shown in the elderly, a group that often suffers from zinc deficiency. Zinc supplementation in physiological amounts for 12 mo resulted in increased numbers of T cells and NK cells and elevated IL-2 and sIL-2R production. Futhermore, lymphocyte response to phytohemagglutinin (PHA) stimulation, as well as NK cell activity, was improved significantly compared with a placebo treated group

(119). CD4+ T cells and cytotoxic T lymphocytes increased significantly after zinc supplementation of 25 mg/d for 3 mo and cell-mediated immune responses also improved *(120)*.

However, the optimal therapeutic dosage to reverse zinc deficiency symptoms is unclear, and pharmacological doses of zinc should be adapted to the actual requirements to avoid zinc's negative side effects on the immune system. Therefore, the zinc plasma level should not exceed 30 μM. On the other hand, zinc is almost nontoxic, even in dosages exceeding the recommended daily intake *(121)*. Zinc concentrations at three to four times the physiological level did not decrease T-cell proliferation in vitro or induce immunosuppressive effects in vivo but did suppress alloreactivity in the MLC (mixed lymphocyte culture) *(122)*, a common in vitro model in transplantation medicine. Thus, this could be a new pathway for the selective suppression of lymphocyte functions, because conventional immunosuppressive drugs currently used to suppress immune responses in transplant patients have several severe side effects. These observations indicate that zinc might be used for the therapeutic treatment of T cell-mediated reactions, such as rheumatoid arthritis or graft rejection, or in transplantation medicine. Furthermore, in elderly persons, high-dose zinc supplementation, representing seven to eight times the physiological zinc level, blocked IFN-α induction *(123)*. Different groups reported a suppression of immune functions at a zinc intake of 100 mg/d *(124–127)*.

Response to vaccination is rather low in zinc-deficient individuals, such as the elderly or patients undergoing hemodialysis *(100,123,129)*. In patients undergoing hemodialysis, it was possible to elucidate a relationship between serum zinc concentrations and the vaccination response. There was a significantly decreased serum zinc level detected in nonresponders, whereas the responders had similar serum zinc levels to the age-matched controls *(130)*. However, there were three trials with either elderly persons or patients undergoing hemodialysis that showed contradictory results in vaccination response when zinc was provided as an adjuvant in concentrations between 3×60 mg/wk and 400 mg/d *(124,131,132)*. Two trials showed that there was no increase in the antibody titer against the vaccine *(124,132)*. The different outcomes of these studies might result from the different zinc dosages used. As mentioned, a 100 mg/d zinc intake is often enough to suppress immune responses. Thus, low-dose zinc supplementation showed an improvement in the humoral response after vaccination in the elderly *(133)*, whereas supplementation with high dosages did not improve the antibody response *(124)*. Improvements might result from restored antibody production of B cells after zinc supplementation, because these were reduced during zinc deficiency *(101–103)*. Other mechanisms might be the increase of IFN-α production by zinc *(123)* or the restoration of impaired T-cell help *(128,134)*. On the other hand, both explanations could explain the negative effects of high zinc dosages in these cases, because IFN-α production and T-cell functions are inhibited by high dosages *(112,123)*.

There are several diseases that are accompanied by altered zinc serum levels. Table 10 details some zinc-therapy trails and summarizes zinc's possible beneficial effects.

7. CONCLUSIONS

It has been known for some time that zinc is an important factor for an intact immune system, but there are many questions without answers, especially concerning the mechanisms by which zinc acts at the molecular level. Zinc is involved in intracellular pro-

Table 10
Zinc Therapy Studies

Disease/ disorder	Study design	Possible positive effects of zinc administration	References
Acrodermatitis enteropathica	100 mg/d zinc sulfate	Reverse of all symptoms by reactivation of enzymes and transcriptions factors, reconstitution of thymocyte functions, increased NK-cell activity, and phagocytosis	(4,149)
Rheumatoid arthritis	45 mg/d for 60 d	Decreased symptoms by impairment of PMN phagocytosis, T-cell suppression, and IL-1 blocking	(150–152)
Herpes simplex virus	Application of zinc oxide/ glycine cream every 2 h	Shortening infection by inhibition of virus functions, increased IFN-α production	(153,154)
Down syndrome	Zinc sulphate supplementation	Symptoms reversed by direct effect on leukocytes and thymus hormones	(155,156)
Crohn's disease	110 mg/d zinc sulphate for 8 wk	Improved intestinal barrier functions, T-cell suppression, and thymus reconstitution	(157–159)
Wilson's disease	5 to 7.5 mg/kg/d zinc salt	Symptoms reduced by inhibited copper resorption, and induced MT synthesis, which prevents copper accumulation	(160–163)
Sickle cell disease	50 to 75 mg/d for 3 yr	Hospitalizations and vasoocclusive pain reduced by reconstitution of thymocyte functions, increase in lymphocyte function, and IL-2 production	(164)
Common cold	13.3 mg zinc every 2 h when cold symptoms are present	Duration of symptoms reduced by zinc gluconate stabilizing the cell membrane against viral penetration and increases IFN-α	(165)
AIDS	200 mg/d zinc sulphate	Frequency of infections reduced by inhibition of T-cell apoptosis and increased thymocytes proliferation	(166–168)

AIDS, acquired immunodeficiency syndrome; IL, interleukin; IFN, interferon; NK, natural killer; PMN, polymorphonuclear leukocytes; MT, metallothionein; AZT, zidovudine.

cesses, such as signaling and apoptosis, but researchers are far from explaining zinc's role in these processes in detail. The recently detected zinc uptake transporter of the ZIP family provides a promising hint of how zinc enters cells. Zinc distribution within the different immune cell types remains to be investigated.

In addition, specific stimulants are needed to investigate the different leukocyte subsets of the immune system. Zinc influences frequently used stimulants, such as lipopolysaccharides (LPS) or superantigens (135–138). LPS is produced by Gramnegative bacteria, and its biologic activity was enhanced by substimulatory zinc concentrations (135,136). This effect depends on a zinc-induced structural alteration of LPS in its biologically more active less fluid form *(137)*. Superantigens are mainly produced by Gram-positive bacteria some of which, such as *Staphylococcus aureus* enterotoxins A, D, and E or the *Mycoplasma arthritidis* superantigen, were able to bind to the MHC II β-chain by forming a zinc cluster. Thus, the interaction between these superantigens and the MHC II β-chain is zinc-dependent, and by adding high zinc concentrations, cytokine induction by superantigens was inhibited *(136)*. These studies indicate that it is important to get zinc-independent stimulants to describe only zinc-dependent effects.

Furthermore, zinc might be used in future therapy, because it has immunosuppressant properties in concentrations where no severe side effects are seen. On the other hand, there are different population groups who are susceptible to low serum zinc concentrations, e.g., elderly individuals who often suffer from high infection rates. Zinc might help to restore their immune system, but still there is no standard therapeutic dosage, and zinc administration must be adjusted to the actual requirements. Thus, zinc is a promising trace element for public health.

8. "TAKE-HOME" MESSAGES

1. Zinc is essential for all highly proliferating systems, especially the immune system.
2. Zinc is involved in regulating apoptosis and intracellular signaling.
3. Proteins of the ZIP and CDF family are zinc transporters.
4. Marginal zinc deficiency is widespread in human populations, and even marginal zinc deficiency results in impaired immune functions.
5. Zinc administration can restore at least some of these immune defects.
6. Serum zinc levels should not exceed 30 μM to avoid negative side effects to the immune system.
7. High dosages of zinc suppress normal immune functions.
8. There is no standard therapeutic dosage; zinc administration must be adapted to the actual requirements.

REFERENCES

1. Raulin J. Etudes Chimique sur al vegetation (chemical studies on plants). Annales des Sciences Naturelles Botanique et Biologie Vegetale 1869;11:293–299.
2. Todd WK, Evelym A, Hart EB. Zinc in the nutrition of the rat. Am J Physiol 1934;107:146–156.
3. Prasad AS, Miaie A Jr, Farid Z, Schulert A, Sandsteadt HH. Zinc metabolism in patients with the syndrome of iron deficiency, hypogonadism and dwarfism. J Lab Clin Med 1963;83:537–549.
4. Neldner KH, Hambidge KM. Zinc therapy in acroderamtitis enteropathica. N Engl J Med 1975;292:879–882.
5. Mills CF. Zinc in human biology. Hum Nutr Rev 1989;4:1–381.
6. Favier A, Favier M. Consequences des deficits en zinc durant la grossesse pour la mere et le nouveau ne. Rev Fr Gynecol Obest 1990;85:13–27.
7. Scott BJ, Bradwell AR. Identification of the serum binding proteins for iron, zinc, cadmium, nickel and calcium. Clin Chem 1983;29:629–633.
8. Krebs NF, Hambidge KM. Zinc metabolism and homeostasis: the application of tracer techniques to human zinc physiology. Biometals 2001;14:397–412.
9. Outten CE, O'Halloran TV. Femtomolar sensitivity of metalloregulatory proteins controlling zinc homeostasis. Science 2001;292:2488–2492.
10. Shankar AH, Prasad AS. Zinc and immune function: the biological basis of altered resistence to infections. Am J Clin Nutr 1998;68:447S–463S.
11. Thompson RB, Walt DR. Emerging strategies for molecular biosensors. Naval Res Rev 1994;46:19–29.

12. Fierke CA, Thompson RB. Fluorescence-based biosensing of zinc using carbonic anhydrase. Biometals 2001;14:205–222.
13. Andrews GK. Cellular zinc sensors: MTF-1 regulation of gene expression. Biometals 2001;14: 223–237.
14. Kägi JHR, Schäffer A. Biochemistry of metallothionein. Biochemistry 1988;27:8509–8515.
15. Palmiter RD, Findley SD. Cloning and functional characterization of mammalian zinc transporter that confers resistence to zinc. EMBO J 1995;14:639–649.
16. Griffith OW, Mulcahy RT. The enzymes of glutathione synthesis: gamma-glutamylcysteine synthtase. Adv Enzymol Relat Areas Mol Biol 1999;73:209–267.
17. Lu SC. Regulation of hepatic glutathione synthesis: current concepts and controversies. FASEB J 1999;13:1169–1183.
18. Ballatori M. Glutathione mercaptides as transport forms of metals. Adv Pharmacol 1994;27:271–298.
19. Bittel D, Daltion T, Samson SL, Gedamu L, Andrews GK. The DNA binding activity of metal resonse element-binding transcription factor-1 is activated in vivo and in vitro by zinc, but not by other transition metals. J Biol Chem 1998;273:7123–7133.
20. Smirnova IV, Bittel, Ravindra R, Jiang H, Andrews GK. Zinc and cadmium can promote rapid response element-binding transcription factor-1. J Biol Chem 2000;275:9377–9384.
21. Gaither LA, Eide DJ. Eukaryotic zinc transporters and their regulation. Biometals 2001;14:251–270.
22. Kobayashi T, Beuchat M, Lindsay M, et al. Late endosomal membranes rich in lysobiphosphatidic acid regulate cholesterol transport. Nature Cell Biol 1999;1:113–118.
23. Palmiter RD, Cole TB, Findley SD. ZnT-2, a mammalian protein that confers resistance to zinc by facilitating vesicular sequestration. EMBO J 1996;15:1784–1791.
24. Palmiter RD, Cole TB, Quiafe CJ, Findley SD. ZnT-3, a putative transporter of zinc into synaptic vesicles. Proc Natl Acad Sci USA 1996;93:14934–14939.
25. Huang L, Gitschier J. A novel gene involved in zinc transport is deficient in the lethal milk mouse. Nature Genet 1997;17:292–297.
26. Murgia C, Vespignani I, Cerase J, Nobili F, Perozzi G. Cloning, expression, and vesicular localization of zinc transporter Dri 27/ZnT4 in intestinal tissue and cells. Am J Physiol 1999;277:G1231–G1239.
27. Eide D, Broderius M, Fett J, Guerinot ML. A novel iron-regulated metal transporter from plants identified by functional expression in yeast. Proc Natl Acad Sci USA 1996;93:5624–5628.
28. Zaoh H, Eide D. The yeast ZRT1 gene encodes the zinc transporter of a high affinity uptake system induced by zinc limitation. Proc Natl Acad Sci USA 1996;93:2454–2458.
29. Cao J, Jeffrey AB, Luzzi JP, Cousins RJ. Effects of intracellular zinc depletion on metallothionein and ZIP2 transporter expression and apoptosis. J Leuk Biol 2001;70:559–566.
30. Gaither LA, Eide DJ. Functional characterization of the human hZIP2 zinc transporter. J Biol Chem 2000;275:5560–5564.
31. Gaither LA, Eide DJ. The human ZIP1 transporter mediates zinc uptake in human K562 erythroleukemia cells. J Biol Chem 2001;276:22258–22264.
32. Bentley PJ. Influx of zinc by channel catfish (*Ictalurus punctatus*): uptake from external environmental solutions. Comp Biochem Physiol C 1992;101:215–217.
33. Hogstrand C, Verbost PM, Bonga SE, Wood CM. Mechanisms of zinc uptake in gills of freshwater rainbow trout interplay with calcium transport. Am J Physiol 1996;270:R1141–R1147.
34. Wellinghausen N, Fischer A, Kirchner H, Rink L. Interaction of zinc ions with human peripheral blood mononuclear cells. Cell Immunol 1996;171:255–261.
35. Rink L, Gabriel P. Zinc and the immune system. Proc Nutr Soc 2000;59:541–552.
36. Coleman JE. Zinc proteins: enzymes, storage proteins, transcription factors and replications proteins. Annu Rev Biochem 1992;16:897–946.
37. Valle BL, Falchuk KH. The biochemical basis of zinc physiology. Physiol Rev 1993;73:79–118.
38. Auld DS. Zinc coordination sphere in biochemial zinc sites. Biometals 2001;14:271–313.
39. Fraser JD, Urban RG, Strominger JL, Robinson H. Zinc regulates the function of two superantigens. Proc Natl Acad Sci USA 1992;89:5507–5511.
40. Bernatchez C, Al-Daccak R, Mayer PE, et al. Functional analysis of *Mycoplasma arthritidis*-derived mitogen interaction with class II molecules. Infect Immunol 1997;65:2000–2005.

41. Trung-Tran AQ, Carter J, Ruffin RE, Zalewski PD. The role of zinc in caspase activation and apoptotic cell death. Biometals 2001;14:315–330.

42. Zalewski PD, Frobes IJ. Intracellular zinc and the regulation of apoptosis. In: Lavin M, Watters D (eds.). Programmed Cell Death: The Cellular and Molecular Biology of Apoptosis. Harwood Academic Publishers, Melbourne, 1993, pp. 73–86.

43. Zalewski PD, Forbes IJ, Giannakis C. Physiological role for zinc in prevention of apoptosis (gene-directed death). Biochem Int 1991;24:1093–1101.

44. Zalewski PD, Forbes IJ, Betts WH. Correlation of apoptosis with change in intracellular labile Zn (II) Zn, using zinquin, a new specific fluorescent probe for Zn (II). Biochem J 1993;296:403–408.

45. Treves S, Trentini PL, Ascanelli M, Bucci G, Di Virgilio F. Apoptosis is dependent on intracellular zinc and independent of intracellular calcium in lymphocytes. Exp Cell Res 1994;211:339–343.

46. Toung-Tran AQ, Ho LH, Chai F, Zalewski PD. Cellular zinc fluxes and the regulation of apoptosis/gene-directed cell death. J Nutr 2000;130(Suppl):1459S–1466S.

47. Chai F, Tuong-Tran AQ, Evdokiou A, Young GP, Zalewski PD. Intracellular zinc depletion induces caspase activation and p21$^{Waf1/Cip1}$ cleavage in human epithelial cell lines. J Infect Dis 2000;182: S85–S92.

48. Meerarani P, Ramadass P, Toborek M, Bauer HC, Bauer H, Hennig B. Zinc protects against apoptosis of endothelial cells induced by linoleic acid and tumor necrosis factor alpha. Am J Clin Nutr 2000;71: 81–87.

49. Matsushita K, Kitagawa K, Matsuyama T, et al. Effect of systemic zinc administration on delayed neuronal death in the gerbil hippocampus. Brain Res 1996;743:362–365.

50. Kuo IC, Seitz B, LaBree L, McDonnell PJ. Can zinc prevent apoptosis of anterior keratocytes after superficial keratectomy? Cornea 1997;16:550–555.

51. Kown MH, Van Der Steenhoven T, Blankenberg FG, et al. Zinc-mediated reduction of apoptosis in cardiac allografts. Circulation 2000;102(Suppl 3):228–232.

52. Bettger WJ, O'Dell BL. A critical physiological role of zinc in the structure and function of biomembranes. Life Sci 1981;28:1425–1438.

53. Powell SR. The antioxidant properties of zinc. J Nutr 2000;130:1447S–1454S.

54. Grutter MG. Caspases: key players in programmed cell death. Curr Opin Struct Biol 2000;10:649–655.

55. Nakatani T, Tawaramoto M, Kennedy D, Kojima A, Matsui-Yuasa I. Apoptosis induced by chelation of intracellular zinc is associated with depletion of cellular reduced glutathione level in rat hepatocytes. Chem Biol Interact 2000;125:151–163.

56. Maret W, Vallee BL, Fischer EH. Inhibitory sites in enzymes: zinc removal and reactivation by thionein. Proc Natl Acad Sci USA 1999;96:1936–1940.

57. Takahashi A, Alnemri ES, Lazebnik YA, et al. Cleavage of lamin A by Mch2 alpha but not CPP32: multiple interleukin 1 beta-converting enzyme-related proteases with distinct substrate recognition properties are active in apoptosis. Proc Natl Acad Sci USA 1996;93:8395–8400.

58. Stennicke HR, Salvesen GS. Biochemical characteristics of caspases-3, -6, -7, and -8. J Biol Chem 1997;272:25719–25723.

59. Mesner PW, Bible KC, Martins LM, et al. Characterization of caspase processing and activation in HL-60 cell cytosol under cell-free conditions. Nucleotide requirement and inhibitor profile. J Biol Chem 1999;274:22635–22645.

60. Wolf CM, Eastman A. The temporal relationship between protein phosphatase, mitochondrial cytochrome c release, and caspase activation in apoptosis. Exp Cell Res 1999;247:505–513.

61. Fukamachi Y, Karasaki Y, Sugiura T, et al. Zinc suppresses apoptosis of U937 cells induced by hydrogen peroxide through an increase of Bcl-2/Bax ratio. Biochem Biophys Res Comm 1998;246:364–369.

62. Flieger D, Riethmuller G, Ziegler-Heitbrock HW. Zn++ inhibits both tumor necrosis factor-mediated DNA fragmentation and cytolysis. Int J Cancer 1989;44:315–319.

63. Beyersmann D, Haase H. Functions of zinc in signaling, proliferation and differentiation of mammalian cells. Biometals 2001;14:331–341.

64. Francis SH, Colbran JL, McAllister-Lucas LM, Corbin JD. Zinc interactions and conserved motifs of the cGMP-binding cGMP specific phosphodiesterase suggest that it is a zinc hydrolase. J Biol Chem 1994;269:22477–22480.

65. Percival MD, Yeh B, Falgueyret JP. Zinc dependent activation of cAMP-specific phosphodiesterase (PDE4A). Biochem Biophys Res Comm 1997;241:175–180.
66. He F, Seryshev AB, Cowan CW, Wensel TG. Multiple zinc binding sites in retinal rod cGMP phosphodiesterase, PDE6ab. J Biol Chem 2000;20752–20577.
67. Waetjen W, Benters J, Haase H, Schwede F, Jastorff B, Beyersmann D. Zn^{2+} and Cd^{2+} increase the cyclic GMP level in PC 12 cells by inhibition of the cyclic nucleotide phosphodiesterase. Toxicology 2001;157:167–175.
68. Haase H. Zinkhomöostase in Säugerzellen: Untersuchungen zur Aufnahme, intrazellulären Verteilung und Toxizität. GCA-Verlag, Herdecke, Germany 2001.
69. Csermely P, Szamel M, Resch K, Somogyi J. Zinc can increase the activity of protein kinase C and contributes to its binding to the plasma membrane in T lymphocytes. J Biol Chem 1988;263:6487–6490.
70. Zalewski PD, Forbes IJ, Giannakis C, Cowled PA, Betts WH. Synergy between zinc and phorbol ester in translocation of protein kinase C to cytoskeleton. FEBS Lett 1990;273:131–134.
71. Knapp LT, Klann E. Superoxide-induced stimulation of protein kinase C via thiol modification and modulation of zinc content. J Biol Chem 2000;275:24136–24145.
72. Allen JL, Perri RT, McClain CJ, Kay NE. Alterations in human natural killer cell activity and monocyte cytotoxicity induced by zinc deficiency. J Lab Clin Med 1983;102:577–589.
73. Keen Cl, Gershwin ME. Zinc deficiency and immune function. Ann Rev Nutr 1990;10:415–431.
74. Chavakis T, May AE, Preissner KT, Kanse SM. Molecular mechanisms of zinc-dependent leukocyte adhesion involving the urokinase receptor and b2-integrins. Blood 1999;93:2976–2983.
75. Hujanen ES, Seppä ST, Virtanen K. Polymorphonuclear leukocyte chemotaxis induced by zinc, copper and nickel *in vitro*. Biochem Biophys Acta 1995;1245:145–152.
76. Prasad AS. Effects of zinc deficiency on immune functions. J Trace Elem Exp Med 2000;13:1–20.
77. Sohnle PG, Collins-Lech C, Wiessner JH. The zinc-reversible antimicrobial activity of neutrophil lysates and abscess fluid supernatants. J Infect Dis 1991;164:137–142.
78. Murthy AR, Lehrer RI, Harwig SSl, Miyasaki KT. *In vitro* candidastic properties of the human neutrophil calprotectin complex. J Immunol 1993;151:6291–6301.
79. Clohessy PA, Golden BE. Calprotectin-mediated zinc chelation as a biostatic mechanism in host defense. Scand J Immunol 1995;42:551–556.
80. Ravaglia G, Forti P, Maioli F, et al. Effect of micronutrient status on natural killer cell immune function in healthy free-living subjects ≥ 90 yr. Am J Clin Nutr 2000;71:590–598.
81. Rajagopalan S, Winter CC, Wagtmann N, Long EO. The Ig-related killer cell inhibitory receptor binds zinc and requires zinc for recognition of HLA-C on target cells. J Immunol 1995;155:4143–4146.
82. Prasad AS. Effects of zinc deficiency on Th1 and Th2 cytokine shifts. Infect Dis 2000;182(Suppl 1):S62–S68.
83. Rink L, Cakman I, Kirchner H. Altered cytokine production in the elderly. Mech Ageing Dev 1998;102:199–210.
84. Rink L, Seyfarth M. Characteristics of immunologic test values in elderly. Z Gerontol Geriatr 1997;30:220–225.
85. Ibs KH, Rink L. The immune system of elderly. Z Gerontol Geriatr 2001;34:480–485.
86. Minigari MC, Moretta A, Moretta L. Regulation of KIR expression in human T cells: a safety mechanism that may impair protective T cell responses. Immunol Today 1998;19:153–157.
87. Mocchegiani E, Santarelli L, Muzzioli M, Fabris N. Reversibility of the thymic involution and age-related peripheral immune dysfunction by zinc supplementation in old mice. Int J Immunopharmacol 1995;17:703–718.
88. Dardenne M, Pléaz JM, Nabarra B, et al. Contribution of zinc and other metals to the biological activity of the serum thymic factors. Proc Natl Acad Sci USA 1982;79:5370–5373.
89. Hadden JW. Thymic endocrinology. Int J Immunopharmacol 1992;14:345–352.
90. Coto JA, Hadden EM, Sauro M, Zorn N, Hadden JW. Interleukin 1 regulates secretion of zinc-thymulin by human thymic epithelial cells and its action on T-lymphocyte proliferation and nuclear protein kinase C. Proc Natl Acad Sci USA 1992;89:7752–7756.
91. Safie-Garabedian B, Ahmed K, Khamashta MA, Taub NA, Hughes GRV. Thymulin modulates cytokine release by peripheral blood mononuclear cells: a comparsion between healthy volunteers and patients with systemic lupus erythrematodes. Int Arch Allergy Immunol 1993;101:126–131.

92. Tanaka Y, Shiozawa S, Morimoto I, Fujita T. Zinc inhibits pokeweed mitogen-induced development of immunglobulin-secreting cells through augmentation of both CD4 and CD8 cells. Int J Immunopharmacol 1989;11:673–679.

93. Dowd PS, Kelleher J, Guillou PJ. T-lymphocyte subsets and interleukin-2 production in zinc-deficient rats. Br J Nutr 1986;55:59–69.

94. Crea A, Guérin V, Ortega F, Hartemann P. Zinc et système immunitaire. Ann Med Intern 1990;141: 447–451.

95. Fraker PJ, King LE, Garvy BA, Medina CA. The immunopathology of zinc deficiency in humans and rodents: a possible role for programmed cell death. In: Klurfeld DM (ed.). Human Nutrition: A Comprehensive Treatise. Plenum, New York, 1993, pp. 267–283.

96. Fraker PJ, Osatiashtiani E, Wagner MA, King LE. Possible roles for glucocorticoides and apoptosis in the suppression of lymphopoiesis during zinc deficiency: a review. J Am Coll Nutr 1995;14:11–17.

97. Fraker PJ, Telford WG. A reappraisal of the role of zinc in life and death decisions of cells. Proc Soc Exp Biol Med 1997;215:229–236.

98. Zazonico R, Fernandes G, Good RA. The differential sensitivity of T cell and B cell mitogenesis to in vitro Zn deficiency. Cell Immunol 1981;60:203–211.

99. Flynn A. Control of in vitro lymphocyte proliferation by copper, magnesium and zinc deficiency. J Nutr 1984;114:2034–2042.

100. Fraker PJ, Jardieu P, Cook J. Zinc deficiency and the immune function. Arch Dermatol Res 1987;123:1699–1701.

101. King LE, Fraker PJ. Variations in the cell cycle status of lymphopoietic and myelopoietic cells created by zinc deficiency. J Infect Dis 2000;182(Suppl 1):S16–S22.

102. Fraker PJ, De Pasquale-Jardieu R, Zwickl CM, Luecke RW. Regeneration of T-cell helper function in zinc-deficient adult mice. Proc Natl Acad Sci USA 1978;75:5660–5664.

103. Fraker PJ. Zinc deficiency: a common state. Surv Immunol Res 1983;2:155–163.

104. Depasquale-Jardieu P, Fraker PJ. Interference in the development of a secondary immune response in mice by zinc deprivation: persistence of effects. J Nutr 1984;114:1762–1769.

105. Moulder K, Steward MW. Experimental zinc deficiency: effects on cellular responses and the affinity of humoral antibody. Clin Exp Immunol 1989;77:269–274.

106. Fraker PJ, Gershwin ME, Good RA, Prasad AS. Interrelationships between zinc and immune function. Fed Proc 1986;45:1474–1479.

107. Salas M, Kirchner H. Induction of interferon-γ in human leukocyte cultures stimulated by Zn^{2+}. Clin Immunol Immunpathol 1987;45:139–142.

108. Scuderi P. Differential effects of copper and zinc on human peripheral blood monocyte cytokine secretion. Cell Immunol 1990;126:391–405.

109. Driessen C, Hirv K, Rink L, Kirchner H. Induction of cytokines by zinc ions in human peripheral blood mononuclear cells and separated monocytes. Lymphokine Cytokine Res 1994;14:15–20.

110. Wellinghausen N, Fischer A, Kirchner H, Rink L. Interaction of zinc ions with human peripheral blood mononuclear cells. Cell Immunol 1996;171:255–261.

111. Rühl H, Kirchner H. Monocyte-dependent stimulation of human T-cells by zinc. Clin Exp Immunol 1978;32:484–488.

112. Wellinghausen N, Martin M, Rink L. Zinc inhibits IL-1 dependent T cell stimulation. Eur J Immunol 1997;27:2529–2535.

113. Hadden JW. The treatment of zinc is an immunotherapy. Int J Immunopharmacol 1995;17:697–701.

114. Phillips JL, Azari P. Zinc transferring: enhancement of nucleic acid in phytohemagglutinin-stimulated human lymphocytes. Cell Immunol 1974;10:31–37.

115. Driessen C, Hirv K, Wellinghausen N, Kirchner H, Rink L. Influence of serum on zinc, toxic shock syndrome toxin-1, and lipopolysaccharide-induced production of IFN-γ and IL-1β by human mononuclear cells. J Leukoc Biol 1995;57:904–908.

116. Bulgarini D, Habetswallner D, Boccoli G, et al. Zinc modulates the mitogenic activation of human peripheral blood lymphocytes. Ann Inst Super Sanita 1989;25:463–470.

117. Goode HF, Kelleher J, Walker BE. Zinc concentrations in pure populations of peripheral blood neutrophils, lymphocytes and monocytes. Ann Clin Biochem 1989;26:85–95.

118. Chandra RK. Nutrition and the immune system: an introduction. Am J Clin Nutr 1997;66:460S–463S.

119. Chandra RK. Effects of vitamin and trace-element supplementation on immune responses and infections in the elderly. Lancet 1992;340:1124–1137.

120. Fortes C, Forastiere F, Agabiti N, et al. The effect of zinc and vitamin A supplementation on immune response in an older population. J Am Geriatr Soc 1998;46:19–26.

121. Fosmire GJ. Zinc toxicity. Am J Clin Nutr 1990;15:225–227.

122. Campo CA, Wellinghausen N, Faber C, Fischer A, Rink L. Zinc inhibits the mixed lymphocyte culture. Biol Trace Elem Res 2001;79:15–22.

123. Cakman I, Kirchner H, Rink L. Reconstitution of interferon-γ production by zinc-supplementation of leukocyte cultures of elderly individuals. J Interferon Cytokine Res 1997;13:15–20.

124. Provinciali M, Montenovo A, Di-Stefano G, et al. Effect of zinc or zinc plus arginine supplementation on antibody titre and lymphocyte subsets after influenza vaccination in elderly subjects: a randomized controlled trial. Age Ageing 1998;27:715–722.

125. Chandra RK. Excessive intake of zinc impairs immune responses. JAMA 1984:252:1443–1446.

126. Reinhold D, Ansorge S, Grüngreiff K. Immunobiology of zinc and zinc therapy. Immunol Today 1999;20:102.

127. Rink L, Kirchner H. Reply to Reinhold et al. Immunol Today 1999;20:102–103.

128. Sandstaed HH, Henriksen LK, Greger JL, Prasad AS, Good RA. Zinc nutriture in the elderly in relation to taste acuity, immune response, and wound healing. Am J Clin Nutr 1982;36:1046–1059.

129. Cakman I, Rohwer J, Schütz RM, Kirchner H, Rink L. Dysregulation between Th1 and Th2 cell subpopulations in the elderly. Mech Ageing Dev 1996;87:197–209.

130. Kreft B, Fischer A, Krüger S, Sack K, Kirchner H, Rink L. The impaired immune response to diphtheria vaccination in elderly chronic hemodialysis patients is related to zinc deficiency. Biogerontology 2000;1:61–66.

131. Brodersen HP, Holtkamp W, Larbig D, et al. Zinc supplementation and hepatitis B vaccination in chronic haemodialysis patients: a multicentre study. Nephrol Dial Transplant 1995;10:1780.

132. Turk S, Bozfakioglu S, Ecder ST, et al. Effects of zinc supplementation on the immune system and on antibody response to multivalent influenza vaccine in hemodialysis patients. Inter J Atif Organs 1998;21:274–278.

133. Girodon F, Galan P, Monget AL, et al. Impact of trace elements and vitamin on immunity and infections in institutionalized elderly patients: a randomized controlled trial. MIN VIT AOX Geriatric network. Arch Intern Med 1999;159:748–754.

134. Mocchegiani E, Santarelli L, Muzzioli M, Fabris N. Reversibility of the thymic involution and of age-related peripheral immune dysfunction by zinc supplementation in old mice. Int J Immunopharmacol 1995;17:703–718.

135. Driessen C, Hirv K, Kirchner H, Rink L. Divergent effects of zinc on different bacterial pathogenic agents. J Infect Dis 1995;171:486–489.

136. Driessen C, Hirv K, Kirchner H, Rink L. Zinc regulates cytokine induction by superantigens and lipopolysaccharide. Immunology 1995;84:272–277.

137. Wellinghausen N, Schromm AB, Seydel U, et al. Zinc enhances lipopolysaccharide-induced monokine secretion by a fluidity change of lipopolysaccharide. J Immunol 1996;157:3139–3145.

138. Wellinghausen N, Rink L. The significance of zinc for leukocyte biology. J Leukoc Biol 1998;571–577.

139. Briefel RR, Bialostoky K, Kennedy-Stephenson J, McDowell MA, Ervin RB, Wright JD. Zinc intake of the U.S. population: findings from the Third National Health and Nutrition Examination Survey, 1988–1994. J Nutr 2000;130:1367–1373.

140. Bannerman E, Magarey AM, Daniels LA. Evaluation of micronutrient intakes of older Australians: The National Nutrition Survey—1995. J Nutr Health Aging 2001;5:234–247.

141. Ge KY, Chang SY. Dietary intake of some essential micronutrients in China. Biomed Environ Sci 2001;14:318–324.

142. Campillo JE, Perez G, Rodriguez A, Torres MD. Vitamins and mineral intake in elderly people from Extremadura. J Nutr Health Aging 2002;6:55–56.

143. Akhter P, Akram M, Orfi SD, Ahmad N. Assessment of dietary zinc ingestion in Pakistan. Nutrition 2002;18:274–278.

144. Cupisti A, D'Alessandro C, Castrogiovanni S, Barale A, Morelli E. Nutrition knowledge and dietary composition in Italian adolescent female athletes and non-athletes. Intl Sport Nutr Exerc Metab 2002;12:207–219.

145. Natera E, Trinidad T, Valdez D, Kawamura H, Palad L, Shiraishi K. Estimation of daily micronutrient intake of Filipinos. Food Nutr Bull 2002;23:222–227.
146. Thane CW, Bates CJ. Dietary intakes and nutrient status of vegetarian preschool children from a British national survey. J Hum Nutr Diet 2000;13:149–162.
147. Beck FW, Prasad AS, Kaplan J, Fitzgerald JT, Brewer GJ. Changes in cytokine production and T cell subpopulations in experimentally induced zinc-deficient humans. Am J Physiol 1997;272:E1002–E1007.
148. Prasad AS. Zinc and immunity. Mol Chem Biochem 1998;188:63–69.
149. Prasad AS. Zinc: an overview. Nutrition 1995;11:93–99.
150. Peretz A, Cantinieaux B, Neve J, Sidoerova V, Fondu P. Effects of zinc suppplementation on the phagocytic functions of polymorphonuclears in patients with inflammatory rheumatic diseases. J Trace Elem Electr Health Dis 1994;8:189–194.
151. Naveh Y, Schapira D, Ravel Y, Geller E, Scharf Y. Zinc metabolism in rheumatoid arthritis: plasma and urinary zinc and relationship to disease activity. J Rheumatol 1997;24:643–646.
152. Simkin PA. Oral zinc sulphate in rheumatoid arthritis. Lancet 1976;2:539–542.
153. Varadinova TL, Bontchev PR, Nachev CK, et al. Mode of action of Zn-complexes on herpes simplex virus type 1 infection in vitro. J Chemother 1993;5:3–9.
154. Godfrey HR, Godfrey NJ, Godfrey JC, Riley D. A randomized clinical trial on the treatment of oral herpes with topical zinc oxide/glycine. Altern Ther Health Med 2001;7:49–56.
155. Trubiani O, Antonucci A, Palka G, Di-Primo R. Programmed cell death of peripheral myeloid precursor cells in Down patients: effect of zinc therapy. Ultrastruct Pathol 1996;20:457–462.
156. Antonucci A, Di-Baldassarre A, Di-Giacomo F, Stuppia L, Palka G. Detection of apoptosis in peripheral blood cells of 31 subjects affected by Down syndrome before and after zinc therapy. Ultrastruct Pathol 1997;21:449–452.
157. Krasovec M, Frenk E. Acrodermatitis enteropathica secondary to Crohn's disease. Dermatology 1996;193:361–363.
158. Myung SJ, Yang SK, Jung HY, et al. Zinc deficiency manifested by dermatitis and visual dysfunction in a patient with Crohn's disease. J Gastroenterol 1998;33:876–879.
159. Struniolo GC, Di Leo V, Ferronato A, D'Odorico A, D'Inca R. Zinc supplementation tightens "leaky gut" in Crohn's disease. Inflamm Bowel Dis 2001;7:94–98.
160. Brewer GJ, Yuzbasiyan-Gurkan V. Wilson disease. Medicine 1992;71:139–164.
161. Brewer GJ, Dick RD, Yuzbasiyan-Gurkan V, Johnson V, Wang Y. Treatment of Wilson's disease with zinc. XIII: therapy with zinc in presymptomatic patients from the time of diagnosis. J Lab Clin Med 1994;123:849–858.
162. Struniolo GC, Mestriner C, Irato P, Albergoni V, Longo G, D'inca R. Zinc therapy increases duodenal concentrations of methallothionein and iron in Wilson's diesease patients. Am J Gastroenterol 1999;94:334–338.
163. Shimizu N, Yamauchi Y, Aoki T. Treatment and management of Wilson's disease. Pediatr Intl 1999;41:419–422.
164. Prasad AS, Beck FW, Kaplan J, et al. Effect of zinc supplementation on incidence of infections and hospital admission in sickle cell disease (SCD). Am J Hematol 1999;61:194–202.
165. Mossad SB, Macknin ML, Medendrop SV, Mason P. Zinc gluconate lozenges for treating the common cold. Ann Intern Med 1996;125:81–88.
166. Mocchegiani E, Veccia S, Ancarani F, Scalise G, Fabris N. Benefit of oral zinc supplementation as an adjust to zidovudine (AZT) therapy against opportunistic infections in AIDS. Int J Immunopharmacol 1995;17:719–727.
167. Wellinghausen N, Kern WV, Jöchle W, Kern P. Zinc serum level in human deficiency virus infected patients in relation to immunological status. Biol Trace Elem Res 2000;73:79–89.
168. Neves I Jr, Bertho AL, Veloso VG, Nascimento DV, Campos-Mello DL, Morgado MG. Improvement of the lymphoproliferative immune response and apoptosis inhibition upon in vitro treatment with zinc of peripheral blood mononuclear cells (PBMC) from HIV+ individuals. Clin Exp Immunol 1998;111:264–268.

IV Nutrition, Immunity, and Disease

14 Rheumatoid Arthritis

L. Gail Darlington

1. INTRODUCTION

Historically and understandably, nutrition and dietary manipulation in the rheumatoid disease field has been highly controversial. Most of the early reports of benefit from dietary changes were anecdotal, and many of the early trials were poorly designed with results of doubtful credibility.

Disorders such as rheumatoid arthritis (RA) have fluctuating disease activity, which makes it all too easy to misinterpret improving fluctuations during dietary treatment as genuine improvements resulting from the changes in the diet. Moreover, because rheumatologic diseases are frequently painful, there is a high potential placebo-response rate that may be increased by any form of treatment that involves frequent visits to a sympathetic physician, particularly if a complex unusual form of treatment, such as dietary manipulation, is involved. In such cases, placebo-response rates may be more than 40%, which makes well-designed and controlled research studies essential if results are to be believed.

Until the 1980s, such well-designed studies were rare and a highly unsatisfactory situation occurred, which has persisted, to some degree, until today, in which those patients suffering from painful chronic diseases of unknown cause and without a cure have desperately sought help outside of the conventional treatment offered to them. They have turned to alternative medicine practitioners who have given advice that has ranged in value from useful to ridiculous. The result of this situation has been, and still remains, a stalemate, in which patients politely refrain from telling their doctors what alternative medical maneuvers they are using, while their doctors assume that any improvements in disease activity result only from the medication they have given patients and ignore any effects that may have resulted from dietary manipulation. Many doctors are also unaware that rates of compliance with conventional drug regimens for different illnesses converge to only approx 50% (1). Such a situation is obviously unacceptable, because much of the damage done to joints in diseases such as RA occurs in the first months or years of the disease (2) and effective drug treatment must not be delayed by ineffective dietary manipulation. Furthermore, patients must be protected from the cost of expensive alternative treatment unless it is of proven benefit.

Unless orthodox researchers investigate unusual forms of therapy, however, patients and practitioners will have no scientific evidence on which to base their treatment choice.

From: *Diet and Human Immune Function*
Edited by: D. A. Hughes, L. G. Darlington, and A. Bendich © Humana Press Inc., Totowa, NJ

The role of nutrition in diseases such as arthritis has been understood more fully by the development of nutritional biochemistry, immunology, and pharmacology and the ever-increasing scientific data on free-radical disease, antioxidants, prostaglandins, flavonoids, etc., have lifted nutrition out of the realm of anecdotal uncertainty into the province of credible science.

The study of nutrition in arthritis may be divided into two areas: *elimination therapy,* in which foods are removed from the diet, and *supplementation therapy*, in which substances are added to the diet.

2. FASTING AND DIETARY ELIMINATION THERAPY

2.1. Fasting

Fasting is an extreme form of elimination dieting. Fasting, for short periods, although undoubtedly helpful to some patients with RA *(3–5)*, is not to be recommended regularly because it may lead to malnutrition. However, when used briefly and occasionally, fasting may give some predictable benefit.

Fasting, either as water only or with fruit and vegetable juices to supply up to 500 cal/d, may exert its beneficial effects by reducing inflammation, altering pain perception and immune function, and reducing gut permeability *(6,7)*. It should only be undertaken with an ample fluid intake and never for more than an absolute 7-d maximum. Fasting is usually ineffective in osteoarthritis and should be avoided in patients with gout, because it causes a rise in lactic acid levels in the blood, which may provoke acute gouty arthritis.

2.2. Dietary Elimination

Our own experience (unpublished work, Darlington and Ramsey) has been that a subgroup of patients with RA remain well, off all medication, and controlled by diet alone for follow-up periods of up to 13 yr. Others relapse, either spontaneously or by failing to comply with the diet. This response to diet is not universal in RA but occurs in a minority of patients (35–40% of RA patients on dietary therapy in our rheumatology unit). The elimination-diet program has three phases: first is an *elimination phase*, in which the patient has only a small number of foods, albeit consumed liberally, and all other foods are excluded. The second phase, usually after 7 d, is the *reintroduction* of foods, one at a time, to determine which foods cause symptoms. The third phase, which is essential for scientific creditability, is *double-blind testing* to confirm that foods identified as culpable in the reintroduction phase are culpable and not just subject to a placebo response or other factors. In 1980, Hicklin et al. *(8)* reported clinical improvement in 24 out of 72 patients with RA on exclusion dieting and, in 1981, Parke and Hughes *(9)* described a patient with RA who responded well to dairy product restriction by objective clinical improvement (grip strength, Ritchie index, visual analog pain score), by a fall in erythrocyte sedimentation rate (ESR), and by disappearance of circulating immune complexes, with reversal of these improvements on rechallenging with dairy produce. (Response to treatment is often difficult to assess in RA because it is a disease associated with pain and stiffness, which are subjective variables. Several tests have, therefore, been agreed internationally to ensure that as much objective evidence as possible is obtained from each research study so that data from studies from different centers can usefully be compared. The ESR was chosen as a simple measurement of inflammation in RA, which is quickly, easily, and

Table 1
Significant Changes in Diet Group After First and Sixth Week on Elimination Diet *(13)*

Parameter	Baseline (mean ± SD)	Week 1 (mean ± SD)	P	Week 6 (mean ± SD)	P
Percentage with severe pain					
By day	44	4	<0.01	14	<0.05
By night	40	4	<0.01	10	<0.01
Pain in 24 h	5.3 ± 2.5	2.9 ± 2.0	<0.001	1.9 ± 1.7	<0.001
Duration of morning stiffness (min)	60	10	<0.01	n.d.	n.d.
No. of painful joints	20.0 ± 9.4	15.6 ± 9.7	<0.005	13.6 ± 10.0	<0.02
Grip strength (mmHg)					
Right	142 ± 83	174 ± 84	<0.01	n.d.	n.d.
Left	142 ± 83	168 ± 84	<0.005		
Fibrinogen (mg/dL)	371 ± 88	421 ± 119	<0.05	n.d.	n.d.
ESR (mm/h)	33.5 ± 18.6	n.d.	n.d.	28.1 ± 15.8	<0.02
Platelets (×10⁹/L)	377 ± 104	n.d.	n.d.	341 ± 108	<0.05
C3 (IU/mL) (C3 is one component of the complement pathway)	151 ± 34	n.d.	n.d.	130 ± 24	<0.001

n.d., not done.

cheaply undertaken in any laboratory. Rheumatoid factors, which are antibodies directed against the patient's own gammaglobulins, are helpful in diagnosing RA but less valuable in following response to treatment.) In 1981, Williams *(10)* described another patient with RA who showed clinical improvement and a significant fall in ESR on corn withdrawal and rapid deterioration on its blind reintroduction.

In 1983, however, Denman et al. *(11)* found no link between food and RA in 18 patients. This study, however, failed to eliminate wheat and other foods that are commonly incriminated in the production of symptoms and also used a diet program from which 13 out of 18 patients defaulted early. In 1983, Panush et al. *(12)* used a commercially popular diet (the Dong diet) in a 10-wk controlled double-blind randomized trial in 26 patients with RA. They obtained a good response in only a small percentage of patients, but that subgroup responded excellently, suggesting that individualized dietary manipulation may be beneficial for certain patients with RA as a subgroup response. In 1986, we published results of a placebo-controlled study of 6 wk of dietary manipulation therapy in 53 patients with RA *(13)*. Significantly greater benefit occurred with diet than with placebo, with significant improvement in pain by day, by night, and in 24 h, duration of morning stiffness, number of painful joints, grip strength, time to walk 18 m, ESR, hemoglobin, fibrinogen, and platelet and C3 levels (Tables 1 and 2). Twenty-five

Table 2
Significant Changes in Control Group in Crossover Stage of Trial After First and Sixth Weeks
on Elimination Diet *(13)*

Parameter	Baseline (mean ± SD)	Week 1 (mean ± SD)	P	Week 6 (mean ± SD)	P
Percentage with severe pain					
By day	27	5	<0.01	n.d.	n.d.
By night	14	9	<0.02		
Pain in 24 h	4.1 ± 2.5	3.0 ± 2.6	<0.01	2.2 ± 2.0	<0.02
Duration of morning stiffness (min)	45	10	<0.01	n.d.	n.d.
No. of painful joints	25.1 ± 13.1	20.3 ± 12.3	<0.005	18.4 ± 12.3	<0.005
Time to walk 18 m (s)	14.3 ± 3.4	13.2 ± 2.7	<0.02	n.d.	n.d.
Hemoglobin (g/dL)	11.7 ± 3.0	13.1 ± 1.0	<0.001	n.d.	n.d.
Platelets (×10⁹/L)	389 ± 102	n.d.	n.d.	337 ± 112	<0.05
C3 (IU/mL)	149 ± 38	n.d.	n.d.	116 ± 17	<0.02

n.d., not done.

percent of patients in both treatment and control groups did not respond to dietary treatment, 40% showed some improvement, but approx 35% responded well and were considered to be a subgroup of good responders.

Energy deprivation is believed to affect immune response *(14)*, and it was believed possible, therefore, that improvement on dietary treatment could be related to weight loss. In 1987, we investigated the mean weight loss of 4.78 kg occurring in 41 patients with RA who underwent dietary therapy for 6 wk *(15)*. Correlations were sought between weight reduction and variables that improved significantly during the diet, but no significant correlations were found, suggesting that weight loss did not play a causal role in the improvement of patients with RA during dietary elimination therapy.

Also in 1987, we investigated 59 patients with RA for evidence of a type 1 (immediate hypersensitivity) reaction that would suggest food allergy *(15)*. A history of atopy was given by 45.8% of patients, but 83% had normal total immunoglobulin (IG) E (IgE) levels (i.e., <300 IU/mL), with median total IgE levels before and after dietary therapy of 62.5 IU/mL and 62.0 IU/mL, respectively. Mean absolute eosinophil counts were normal (i.e., <440/mm³) before and after dietary therapy, and there were no significant correlations to suggest a type 1, immediate hypersensitivity, reaction in patients with RA on dietary treatment.

In 1987, Wojtulewski described a group of 41 patients with RA on a 4-wk elimination diet. The 23 patients who improved were challenged with four different food groups, with positive reactions to challenge in 10 patients. Disodium cromoglycate did not protect against these challenges *(16)*. In 1987, we sought to identify foods to which patients with RA were most often intolerant *(17)*. Forty-eight patients with RA underwent 6 wk of dietary elimination therapy. Forty-one patients identified foods that produced symptoms. Cereal foods were particularly troublesome, with corn and wheat each producing symp-

Table 3
Foods Most Likely to Cause Intolerance
in Patients with Rheumatoid Arthritis *(33)*

Food	Symptomatic patients affected by food (%)
Corn	57
Wheat	54
Bacon/pork	39
Oranges	39
Milk	37
Oats	37
Rye	34
Eggs	32
Beef	32
Coffee	32
Malt	27
Cheese	24
Grapefruit	24
Tomato	22
Peanuts	20
Sugar (cane)	20
Butter	17
Lamb	17
Lemons	17
Soya	17

toms in more than 50% of patients who were symptomatic and, indeed, cereal foods comprised four of the top seven symptom-inducing foods (*see* Table 3).

It has been suggested that the offending element in wheat may be gluten, which is composed of glutenins and gliadins. O'Farrelly et al. *(18)* tested 93 patients with RA for humoral sensitization to gliadin and compared their small intestinal biopsies with those from controls. Of the 93 patients with RA, 44 had raised IgG levels to gliadin and, 38 of whom (86%) were also positive for IgA rheumatoid factor (RF). Patients with raised antibody levels had lower villous surface/volume ratio and lower intestinal lactose concentrations on jejunal biopsy than patients without antibodies or age-matched controls. The authors concluded that the gut may play a more important part in the immuno-pathogenesis of some RA cases than of others and that raised IgA RF levels and wheat protein IgG may identify the former.

Blind challenge studies are needed to confirm symptoms obtained during unblind food challenge. In 1986, Panush et al. *(19)* described prospective placebo-controlled blind challenges with milk in a patient with RA, with exacerbation of arthritis on milk challenge (shown by deterioration in duration of morning stiffness and in numbers of tender and swollen joints). Beri et al., in India, published an uncontrolled dietary treatment study with 71% of good responses *(20)* and, in 1989, we completed a prospective blind challenge study during which 15 patients with RA undertook an exclusion diet followed by reintroduction of foods, after which three symptomatic foods were selected for each patient with which that patient was challenged. Results suggested that, although patients with RA improved significantly on dietary manipulation, 3 wk of food challenge rapidly produced deterioration *(21)*.

In 1990, Panush *(22)* reported food sensitivities, confirmed by double-blind challenges in 3 patients with palindromic arthritic symptoms who were sensitive to milk, shrimp, and nitrate, respectively. In 1991, Kjeldsen-Kragh et al. *(23)* reported good responses to dietary elimination therapy. Their patients (27 in a diet group and 27 controls) were treated for 1 mo on a health farm, where for 7–10 d they consumed only herbal teas and vegetable juices. This was followed by reintroduction of foods: any foods that provoked symptoms were excluded for 7 d, retested and, if they still caused symptoms, were excluded permanently. Milk, eggs, gluten, and citrus fruits continued to be avoided for 3.5 mo, at which stage they were tested individually and reintroduced if they did not produce symptoms. Patients thus treated with diet improved significantly when compared with a placebo group. There was a subset of responders (44% of the total), and 30.6% of the diet group were described as having a high improvement index *(24)*—a percentage similar to our 35% of good responders *(13)*. Benefit was maintained for 1 yr, and most of Kjeldsen-Kragh's good responders showed improvement in laboratory as well as clinical variables *(25)*.

Certain Swedish trials reported similar fasts, followed by a normal diet *(26)*, by a vegan diet *(27,28)*, or by a lactovegetarian diet *(7)* with some benefit. In 1997, Gamlin and Brostoff suggested that an elimination process may be required to give sustained benefit and that a vegetarian or vegan diet alone is insufficient *(29)*. One study that reported a much smaller proportion of patients with symptoms provoked by food was that by Panush, in 1990, who estimated that only 5% of patients with RA were sensitive to food *(22)*. Gamlin and Brostoff *(29)* suggested that this may be an underestimate; they doubted whether patients could be sure that they had food sensitivities or that they could determine culpable foods without going through an elimination diet. They also queried whether the food challenges undertaken by Panush contained sufficient quantities of food in the capsules given to the patients, because patients who were *food-intolerant* (in contrast to patients who were *food-allergic*) are believed to need a reasonable quantity of the food concerned to provoke a response.

In 1992, van de Laar and van der Korst described a double-blind controlled trial of clinical effects of elimination of milk and azo dyes in 94 patients with RA *(30)*. Only subjective improvements were seen on treating patients with two types of artificial elementary food, but a subgroup of patients showed favorable responses, followed by marked disease exacerbation during rechallenge, and the authors felt that food intolerance may influence seropositive RA activity, at least in some patients. The same authors in a further article *(31)* also described 6 patients with seropositive RA who showed a marked improvement after 4 wk of a hypoallergic artificial diet, with placebo-controlled rechallenges showing intolerance for specific foodstuffs in four patients. Improving changes in biopsy material from synovial membrane and proximal small intestine in 3 patients with RA treated with the hypoallergenic diet showed changes suggesting an underlying immunoallergic mechanism.

In 1995, Kavanagh et al. found a significant improvement in grip strength ($p = .008$) and Ritchie articular pain index ($p = .006$) in patients on an *elemental* diet when compared with a control group, i.e., an effective alternative to an elimination diet *(32)* but, unfortunately, one that patients do not like and for which long-term compliance is poor.

Our own experience (unpublished work, Darlington and Ramsey, 1998) has been that a subgroup of patients remain well—off all medication and controlled by diet alone—for follow-up periods of up to 12 yr. Other patients relapsed, either spontaneously or on failing to comply with the diet. As we described in 1993 *(33)*, there are certain practical problems associated with elimination diets: they are not universally effective, they may cause nutritional difficulties, they may cause social disruption, they require considerable commitment from the patient, and they may be taken to extremes by patients if not correctly supervised. *Thus, elimination diets should only be undertaken under medical supervision.*

3. MECHANISMS AFFECTING RESPONSE TO DIETARY MANIPULATION

Patients improvement on dietary therapy may be the result of several different mechanisms, acting singly or in combination.

3.1. Placebo Response

It is important that the placebo response to dietary treatment should be investigated. In our experience, however, the placebo effect detected was insufficient to explain the significant improvement on treatment *(13)*. Furthermore, if benefit resulted only from placebo, one would expect the benefit to fade after a few months on diet, which is not the case, as confirmed by the study by Kjeldsen-Kragh et al. *(23)* that showed persistent benefit for a follow-up of 1 yr.

3.2. Suppression of a Type 1 Reaction

Food sensitivities in patients with RA are not acute allergic (type 1) reactions. We have not shown abnormal IgE levels in patients with RA undergoing dietary therapy *(15)* and neither did Little et al. *(34)*, nor did they show positive skins tests to food extracts.

3.3. Weight Loss

Because energy deprivation is believed to affect the immune response *(14)*, it is possible that weight loss during a diet could cause improvement, but many patients with RA lose weight, without benefit, during disease activity periods. Furthermore, in studies of weight loss during dietary therapy, no correlation was shown between weight loss and the variables that improved significantly *(15,23)*.

3.4. Altered Gastrointestinal Permeability and Bacterial Antigens

In 1968, Olhagen and Mansson *(35)* reported that two thirds of patients with RA have an abnormally abundant faecal flora of atypical *Clostridium perfringens*, and an increase in *C. perfringens* α-antitoxin titer; controls did not. In 1978, Bennett *(36)* suggested that gut bacteria have a role in RA development. Pigs on a diet rich in fish developed abnormal gut flora, with increased numbers of atypical *C. perfringens* type A, and this was followed by arthritis, believed to result from an immunologic reaction to the altered intestinal flora *(37)*. When rabbits were fed cow's milk daily, they developed infiltrative synovial lesions, believed to result from stimulation by antigens absorbed from the gut *(38)*.

Patients with RA who are untreated by nonsteroidal antiinflammatory drugs (NSAIDs) have normal gastrointestinal (GI) permeability, but patients on NSAIDs *(39,40)* and, perhaps, also those on disease-modifying antirheumatic drugs (DMARDs) *(41)* show increased permeability. Such increased permeability may allow food or bacterial antigens to be absorbed in greater quantities than usual, overwhelming normal gut defenses and, possibly, producing RA symptoms. Dietary manipulation could, theoretically, reduce GI permeability, with reduced absorption of food and/or bacterial antigens. In 1985, Ebringer et al. *(42)* proposed that both ankylosing spondylitis and RA are forms of reactive arthritis, to *Klebsiella* spp. and *Proteus* spp., respectively, probably mediated by cross-reactivity to human leucocyte antigens (HLAs). In 1988, Ebringer et al. *(43)* reported raised levels of antibodies against *Proteus mirabilis*—a bacterium found in the gut and urinary tract in patients with RA—and, in 1992, suggested a mechanism involving molecular mimicry between *Proteus* antigen and part of the HLA-DR1/DR4 molecule, which is associated with an increased risk of RA *(44)*.

However, the molecular mimicry hypothesis has not been proven, and a range of hypotheses have been suggested for association of HLA B27 with spondyloarthropathies *(45)*. Nonetheless, in 1995, Kjeldsen-Kragh et al. *(46)* investigated antibodies against *P. mirabilis* and against *Escherichia coli* in patients treated with diet. Patients on the vegetarian diet had a significant reduction in mean anti-*Proteus* titers compared with baseline values *(p < .05)*. No significant change in titer was observed in patients taking an omnivorous diet. Good responders showed greater antibody reduction than nonresponders or omnivores. Antibodies against *E. coli* were almost unchanged in all patient groups during the trial. In view of the various types of bacteria suspected of playing a role in RA pathogenesis *(37,42,47)*, it is theoretically possible that different bacteria could be relevant to different RA subgroups.

Seignalet proposed that RA results, in part, from a food or bacterial peptide crossing the gut wall and proceeding toward the joints *(48)*. In 1991, Hunter *(49)* suggested that a disturbance of normal gut flora may occur, perhaps originating from a severe bout of diarrhea or prolonged antibiotic therapy, which results in beneficial bacteria becoming less abundant and being replaced by more damaging organisms. The gut wall may become irritated by toxins released by the bacteria and become more permeable to undigested food molecules, which could pass through it and promote an immunologic reaction. Alternatively, the more damaging bacteria may feed on particular foods and then produce toxins that produce symptoms. If abnormal bacterial toxins were produced, enzyme defects might also be relevant, and the lack of certain detoxification enzymes could exacerbate the effects of the disturbed gut flora.

Mechanisms for effects of dietary therapy on gut flora are presently hypothetical. The mechanism may be simple, with dietary manipulation removing from the diet certain nutrients needed by the relevant bacteria and reducing their pathogenicity. Alternatively, dietary toxins, e.g., lectins, may affect bacteria or the gut itself directly. Furthermore, when patients underwent dietary therapy with an individually adjusted vegetarian diet, their fecal bacterial fatty acids were shown by Peltonen in 1994 to alter in ways which differed according to whether they responded well *(24)*.

In 1997, Peltonen et al. *(50)* investigated fecal microbial flora and disease activity in RA during a vegan diet and concluded that a vegan diet changes the fecal microbial flora and that these changes are associated with improvement in disease activity. In 1998, Nenonen et al. *(51)* investigated the effects of an uncooked vegan diet, rich in lactobacilli, in patients with RA and found that subjective RA symptoms were reduced. They concluded that large amounts of living lactobacilli consumed daily might have positive effects on objective RA measures (*see* Chapter 17 on Probiotics).

In conclusion, there are still too few data definitely to confirm or refute the suggestion that dietary manipulation may have a beneficial effect on disease activity by affecting gut flora, but the hypothesis is interesting and further investigation is required.

3.6. Secretory IgA Deficiency

Evidence exists that people with food intolerance may have less secretory IgA (SIgA) than healthy people *(52)*, but this is not believed to be sufficient alone to cause food intolerance, because many severely SIgA-deficient patients have no greater evidence of food intolerance than the general population.

3.7. Direct Immunological Response

There may be a direct immunologic response to food. Most patients with food-sensitive RA do not have raised IgE levels *(15)*, although Parke and Hughes' milk-and cheese-sensitive patient was an exception *(9)*. IgG antibodies to relevant foods were described by Panush in two patients with food intolerance *(22)* and by Ratner in 1984 *(53)* in a patient with juvenile RA, but the significance of such antibodies in many patients is arguable, because food antibodies may be present without being pathogenically significant, and further work is necessary to clarify their role. We investigated patients with RA who were undergoing a program of elimination dieting followed by reintroduction of foods, and we could not detect any significant pattern in the immunoglobulin or food antibody results (unpublished work, Darlington and Panush, 1989).

In 1995, Kjeldsen-Kragh, in a comprehensive review of his patients, found only one food-sensitive patient with raised levels of antibody to the food that provoked symptoms *(54)*. Other immunologic changes that have been described include immediate and delayed reactivity of skin and mononuclear cells to the food in question *(19)* and impaired clearance of heat-damaged red cells, which may suggest an abnormally functioning reticuloendothelial system *(19)*. In 1983, Little et al. *(34)* described the release of 5-hydroxytryptamine (5HT) (serotonin) from platelets in response to food challenges. In 1995, Kjeldsen-Kragh et al. *(25)* found that platelet counts and calprotectin levels fell as patients improved on dietary treatment and were lower in responsive than in unresponsive patients. Immune complexes are not raised in food-sensitive patients *(22)*, nor do they fall when patients respond to dietary therapy *(25)*.

3.8. Conclusion

Whatever the mechanism(s) of action, and although dietary elimination therapy only helps a proportion of patients, for those who do respond it can be a safe and useful way to control symptoms in a range of rheumatologic diseases (*see* Table 4), although more work is needed to determine whether its clinically beneficial effects can also control disease progression and prevent erosive change.

4. LITERATURE ON NUTRITION AND ARTHRITIS

In an attempt to see what literature was available to patients about nutrition and arthritis, we investigated 21 books offering dietary advice for patients with arthritis *(55)*. These books were readily available from bookshops and health food shops. Seventeen

Table 4
Application of Elimination Dieting to a Range of Arthritic Diseases *(140)*

Disease	Result
Rheumatoid arthritis	Subgroup achieves benefit
Palindromic arthritis	Frequently helpful
Osteoarthritis	Any benefit is probably by weight reduction
Gout	Drugs are usually required to lower uric acid significantly, but a low purine diet may assist
Enteropathic arthritis	Crohn's disease: dietary change may help but medical supervision is essential
	Celiac disease: gluten-free diets help bowel and joint symptoms
	Ulcerative colitis: no benefit from diet
Psoriatic arthritis	Variable response reported
Systemic lupus erythematosus	Avoid alfalfa products that contain 6-canavanine, because they increase disease activity
Ankylosing spondylitis	Insufficient data to comment
Behçet's syndrome	Insufficient data to comment

books were strongly in favor of dietary manipulation therapy, three stated that diet was of no value in controlling arthritic symptoms, and one was noncommittal.

Dietary advice varied from book to book and was sometimes contradictory; it is hardly surprising, therefore, that patients are confused. However, patients will continue to read the literature available to them in such books, and they must be educated about conflicting and often inappropriate advice from such sources. Thus, healthcare providers should be aware of the current consumer-focused books that their patients may be reading.

5. EPIDEMIOLOGIC DATA ON NUTRITION AND ARTHRITIS

RA has been described as being more prevalent in developed rather than in developing countries *(56)*. This could be explained on the basis of genetic factors, but the need for some environmental factor, such as diet, to trigger the genetic predisposition is enforced by the finding from 1995 by McDaniel et al. *(57)* that African Americans with RA do not have the usually accepted RA genetic markers. Epidemiologic data on nutritional macronutrients and RA have been reviewed recently by Darlington elsewhere *(58)*.

6. SUPPLEMENTATION THERAPY

The best studied supplements are fish oils, evening primrose oil (EPO), New Zealand green-lipped mussels, vitamins, and selenium. Garlic, honey (with or without cider vinegar), herbs, kelp, royal jelly, and ginseng are also popular with patients but have little scientific evidence to support their use in arthritic disease. In the context of this book, this chapter only considers conditions in which foods and their constituent parts are believed to play a part in the development of arthritis and rheumatologic disease, by either their presence or their absence.

6.1. Hypothesis

It is possible that diets poor in certain nutrients may predispose to arthritic disease and that supplementation with the nutrients that are in poor supply could, therefore, reduce arthritic activity.

7. OXIDATIVE STRESS AND ANTIOXIDANTS

Reactive oxygen species (ROS), i.e., highly reactive atoms and molecules with unpaired electrons, are formed continuously in tissues by endogenous and exogenous mechanisms. ROS can damage many macromolecules, including cell membranes, lipoproteins, proteins, and DNA. There is evidence that intraarticular cells, such as chondrocytes, produce ROS *(59)* and that oxidative damage is important in arthritic processes *(60)*. Superoxide anions can adversely affect the structure and integrity of collagen in vitro and may cause depolymerization of hyaluronate in synovial fluid *(61,62)*.

Diseases like RA, systemic lupus erythematosus (SLE), and psoriatic arthritis involve chronic inflammation of joint tissues, with oxidant-associated deterioration of joint structure *(63–66)*. Intraarticular injection of agents that generate hydrogen peroxide (H_2O_2) causes severe joint damage in experimental animals *(67)*, and there is much in vitro evidence suggesting that ROS can damage, or interfere with, joint components, including hyaluronic acid *(62,68)*, glycoproteins *(69)*, collagens *(70)*, and tissue and fluid proteinase inhibitors, such as α-antiproteinase *(71)*. There is also a considerable body of evidence that oxidative stress occurs within the inflamed joint in vivo *(68,72–76)* and that ROS probably damages joints. Inflamed joints are infiltrated by activated neutrophils, and rheumatoid pannus contains many macrophage-like cells. Both of these cell groups produce $O_2^{\cdot-}$ and H_2O_2 *(77,78)* and, perhaps, also nitric oxide (NO) *(79)*. Neutrophils can also make HOCl. $O_2^{\cdot-}$ and H_2O_2 become converted into the highly reactive hydroxyl radical OH· in the presence of free-iron ions, and synovial fluid from RA patients often contains measurable quantities of iron *(80)* capable of catalyzing oxidative damage in vivo *(81)*. The question arises, therefore, whether diets poor in antioxidants may predispose to arthritic disease.

Many raw food materials contain natural antioxidants that affect oxidative processes in living cells. These include enzymes, such as superoxide dismutase, glutathione peroxidase, glucose oxidase, and catalase, which are usually inactivated during food processing and nonenzyme antioxidants, such as fat-soluble carotenoids, especially astaxanthin (e.g., in salmon and certain shellfish), vitamin C (water soluble) tocopherols (in oils), and other phenolic compounds in plants. Nonenzymic antioxidants, such as β-carotene and vitamin E, can remain active after heating and, possibly, after food consumption. Vitamin C acts as a reducing substance that acts synergistically with other antioxidants and, indeed, two or more antioxidants can act synergistically. In the human body, antioxidant enzymes, such as superoxide dismutase, catalases, and peroxidases, provide the major part of the intracellular defense, whereas in the extracellular space, small-molecule antioxidants play an important defensive role *(82)*. These small-molecular antioxidants include α-tocopherol (vitamin E), β-carotene (a vitamin A precursor), other carotenoids, and ascorbate (vitamin C), and their plasma concentrations are largely determined by dietary intake.

Micronutrient antioxidants may protect against tissue injury and, when intracellular enzymes are overwhelmed, can also protect against ROS-mediated damage, which accumulates with age and causes chronic diseases *(83–85)*. More work is required on tissue distributions and bioavailability of antioxidant molecules within joints, because lipophilic antioxidant molecules, such as vitamin E or β-carotene, may not have the same access to tissues as hydrophilic antioxidants, such as vitamin C, although some work has been done on the vitamin E content of fruits *(86,87)*. It is possible that different effects in disease processes may depend on lipophilia or hydrophilia of the antioxidant molecules concerned in different tissue areas.

7.1. Tocopherols and Ascorbic Acid

Tocopherols, of which α-tocopherol (vitamin E) is the most effective, protect cell membranes and other lipids by scavenging free radicals, such as lipid peroxyl radicals, much more quickly than these radicals can react with adjacent fatty-acid side chains or with membrane proteins. Vitamin E is oxidized but may be regenerated by reduced glutathione (GSH) and by ascorbic acid (vitamin C). Because ascorbic acid is a water-soluble vitamin that cannot enter the hydrophobic interior of membranes, this mechanism presupposes that the tocopherol radical can move close to the membrane surface for reduction by ascorbic acid outside the membrane.

In 2001, Niki *(88)* produced an excellent overview of the past work, present problems, and future perspectives of free radicals in life science.

Certain cells contain enzymes that can reduce dehydroascorbate back to ascorbate using either nicotinamide adenine dinucleotide (NADH) or GSH. Any dehydroascorbate that does not enter cells for regeneration may breakdown; hence, ascorbate is lost irretrievably at oxidative damage sites. The role of antioxidant nutrients in preventing oxidant-mediated diseases has been excellently reviewed by Anderson *(89)*.

7.2. α-Tocopherol (Vitamin E)

Benefit from vitamin E treatment has been suggested from rheumatologic studies in humans *(90)*. Because vitamin E blocks arachidonic acid formation from phospholipids and inhibits lipoxygenase activity, although it has little effect on lipoxygenase, vitamin E was believed to have a mild antiinflammatory effect, which could be beneficial in arthritis.

In 1997, Edmonds et al. *(91)* in a double-blind randomized study in 42 patients investigated whether there were additional antiinflammatory or analgesic effects or both when patients with RA who were already receiving antirheumatic drugs were also given orally administered α-tocopherol ($n = 20$) at a dose of 600 mg twice daily. A broad spectrum of clinical and laboratory variables were measured, and all laboratory measures of inflammatory activity and oxidative modification were unchanged. Furthermore, the clinical indices of inflammation were not influenced by treatment. However, pain variables significantly reduced after vitamin E treatment when compared with placebo, suggesting that vitamin E may exert a small but significant analgesic effect, independent of an antiinflammatory effect, to complement standard antirheumatic treatment.

In 2001, Helmy et al. *(92)* undertook a preliminary study with 30 patients with rheumatoid disease divided into three groups. Each group received standard therapy with methotrexate, sulphasalazine, and indomethacin, group I received only this standard therapy, group II also received a combination of antioxidants, and group III received standard treatment with a high dose of vitamin E (400 mg three times daily). By the end of the second month, results of monitoring tests indicated better disease control. Patients on standard treatment alone felt tangible improvement by the end of the second month, but, with adjuvant therapy of either the antioxidant combination or a high dose of vitamin E, arthritic symptoms were better controlled from the first month—suggesting that the use of antioxidants as adjuvant therapy is worth pursuing.

In 2001, we examined plasma levels of the lipid peroxidation products 4-hydroxynonenal and malondialdehyde in a carefully controlled study of age- and gender-matched subjects with RA in whom potentially confounding influences, such as disease modifying antirheumatic drugs, self medication, and vitamin supplements were eliminated (93). We measured plasma concentrations of the antioxidants uric acid and vitamin E. The results revealed a strong consistent inverse correlation between the levels of lipid peroxidation products in the plasma and the erythrocyte sedimentation rate (ESR)—a result suggesting a more complex relationship than had been assumed. There was no indication that either vitamin E or uric acid functions as the major antioxidant in arthritis, as had been suggested in more seriously affected patients.

7.3. Ascorbic Acid (Vitamin C)

In 1996, Jeng et al. showed that supplementation with vitamins C and E enhanced cytokine production by peripheral blood mononuclear cells in healthy adults; combined supplementation was more immunopotentiating than supplementation with either vitamin alone (94).

Vitamin C has nonantioxidant effects, and its deficiency is associated with defective connective tissue, and ascorbate stimulates procollagen secretion (95). Vitamin C is needed by the vitamin C-dependent enzyme lysyl hydroxylase for the posttranslational hydroxylation of specific prolyl and lysyl residues in procollagen—actions necessary to stabilize the mature collagen fibril (96). Vitamin C is also believed to be necessary for glycosaminoglycan synthesis (97). Furthermore, Schwartz and Adamy (97) found decreased levels of arylsulphatase A and B in the presence of ascorbic acid. They also found that sulphated proteoglycan biosythesis, a presumed repair measure, was increased significantly in chondrocyte cultures in the presence of ascorbic acid. Vitamin C is important in the biosynthesis of prostaglandin (PG) E_1, which has been suggested as having a key role in Sjögren's syndrome, which is frequently associated with RA. In 1980, Horrobin and Campbell reported that an attempt to treat patients who had Sjögren's syndrome by raising endogenous PGE_1 production by giving essential fatty-acid PGE_1 precursory of pyridoxine and vitamin C, successfully raised tear and saliva production rates (98).

7.4. Selenium

Abnormalities in the metabolism of the essential trace element selenium (Se) have been described in patients with RA—Se concentrations are relatively low in the serum of patients with RA when compared with healthy controls (99). Se is an essential part of the enzyme glutathione peroxidase (GPx) at the active center of which Se catalyses reduction of hydroperoxides produced from oxidized species (100).

In 1987, Tarp et al. (101) described long-term supplementation of six patients with RA and six controls with selenium as 256 µg of Se in Se-enriched yeast (Selena, Leiras Pharmaceuticals, Turku, Finland). Even after 26 wk of treatment, patients with RA had significantly lower granulocyte GPx activities than those of controls. The low granulocyte GPx activities of patients with RA, regardless of nutritional Se status, may result in maintenance of inflammation from intracellular accumulation of reactive oxygen radicals. The unresponsiveness of granulocyte GPx to Se treatment may explain the predominantly negative effects after treatment with Se in 40 patients with RA *(102)*.

Data are conflicting: some clinical improvement has been reported for patients with RA treated with Se *(103)*, but other evidence suggests that any role of GPx in RA must be indirect because D-penicillamine (a disease modifying drug in RA) is a specific GPx inhibitor *(104)*.

7.5. Vitamin A—Retinol

In 1988, Fairney et al. *(105)* reported a difference in vitamin A metabolism or intake between patients with RA and controls; serum retinol levels were lower in RA than in matched control sera $(p < 0.01)$ and in osteoarthritis (OA) patients $(p < 0.001)$. Serum retinol-binding protein (RBP) values were lower in RA than in matched control sera $(p < 0.001)$, but in OA they were not different from normal $(p < 0.3)$. The mean serum *osteocalcin* was higher than normal in both RA and OA $(p < 0.001$ and < 0.005, respectively—osteocalcin is a vitamin K-dependent calcium-binding protein synthesized by osteoblasts and found primarily in bone. Osteocalcin contains three residues of the amino acid, γ-carboxy glutamic acid, which, in the presence of calcium, promotes binding to hydroxyapatite and subsequent accumulation in the bone matrix.

7.6. β-Carotene

If the diet of healthy volunteers is supplemented with a dietary-achievable level of β-carotene, significant increases occur in the percentage of monocytes expressing the major histocompatibility complex (MHC) class II molecule, HLADR; the intercellular adhesion molecule-1 (ICAM-1); and leukocyte function-associated antigen-3 *(106)*. It is possible that β-carotene also quenches singlet oxygen, which may reduce the free-radical burden and protect membrane lipids from peroxidation in arthritis and other diseases associated with oxidative stress (*see* Chapter 9 on Carotenoids).

A 1994 study in Finland *(107)* measured antioxidant levels in the blood of more than 1400 people and reviewed their health after 20 yr. During that period, 14 people developed RA. Elevated risks of RA were observed at low serum levels of α-tocopherol, β-carotene, and Se. A significant association was observed with a low antioxidant index $(p$ for trend $= 0.03$, the relative risk of RA between the lowest tertile and the higher tertiles of its distribution being 8.3, 95% confidence interval 1.0–71.0). This was particularly interesting work because it measured antioxidant levels *before the onset of disease* and, hence, may well have measured a contributory factor in RA pathogenesis rather than simply measuring the *effects* of the disease, i.e., exhausted antioxidant supplies. In 1997, Mohan and Das *(108)* suggested that measurement of lipid peroxides, NO, and antioxidants can be used as markers to predict progress in patients with SLE.

Also in 1997, Comstock et al. *(109)* undertook a prospective case-controlled study of 21 patients with RA and 6 patients with SLE, which developed 2 to 15 yr after blood donation for a serum bank in 1974. These patients were designated as cases. For each case, four controls were selected from the serum bank donors, matched for race, gender, and age, and stored. Serum samples from cases and controls were assayed for α-tocopherol, β-carotene, and retinol. Cases with both diseases had lower serum concentrations of α-tocopherol, β-carotene, and retinol in 1974 than their matched controls, and, for RA, the difference for β-carotene (–29%) was statistically significant, suggesting that low antioxidant status is a risk factor for RA with, possibly, a similar association for SLE.

7.7. The French Paradox

It has been suggested that the French diet, rich in antioxidants from fruit, vegetables, and red wine, could be the reason for the French paradox, i.e., that cardiovascular disease in France is a lesser problem than would be expected from the fat content of the average French diet *(110)*. The antioxidant-rich diet of the French could also be protective against arthritis.

7.8. Conclusion

Much more work is required to clarify the role of antioxidant supplements in arthritic disease and their possible therapeutic potential.

8. DIETS POOR IN POLYUNSATURATED FATTY ACIDS

8.1. Omega-3 (n–3) Fatty Acids

The suggestion that a diet rich in omega-3 fatty acids found in fish oil may protect against arthritis has a long history. Conversely, a diet poor in fish and fish oil may fail to offer this protection. For many years, both patients and normal healthy people have taken oils to improve their health. In a recent analysis of data from our own patients with RA (unpublished work), two thirds tried fish oil and one third tried an omega-6 fatty-acid-rich product, evening primrose oil (EPO). There is a huge market for such oils, which have a traditional reputation for being good for health and protective against arthritis but long-term safety has not been evaluated and efficacy is uncertain in the small doses taken by many people. The antiinflammatory properties of fish oil and its therapeutic role in RA were reviewed in 1991 by Cleland *(111)*, in 1993 by Darlington *(112)*, and in 2001 by Belluzzi *(113)*. It is well accepted that ingestion of long-chain omega-3 fatty acids, such as eicosapentaenoic acid (EPA) and docosahexaenoic acids (DHA), from fish oil and/or algal sources is likely to have an antiinflammatory effect.

Enthusiasm for fish oils is widespread among patients with arthritis, but doctors are cautious *(114)*. In 1959, Brusch and Johnson *(115)* reported that patients with arthritis on cod liver oil showed biochemical and clinical improvement, and, in 1987, Sperling et al. *(116)*, in an open study, showed a significant decrease in joint pain index and in patients' assessment of disease activity after 6 wk of dietary supplementation with concentrated fish oil (20 g MaxEPA/d). In 1985, Kremer et al. *(117)*, in an open study, gave 10 g MaxEPA/d for 12 wk to patients with RA, in combination with other dietary modifications, and reported modest improvement in morning stiffness and in the number of painful joints—improvements that deteriorated during follow-up after treatment cessation. In 1987, Kremer et al. then completed a well-controlled, crossover study *(118)* using 15 g MaxEPA/d vs 15 g olive oil and reported significantly fewer tender joints and improvement in time to onset of fatigue after 14 wk of fish oil compared with olive oil treatment. In 1988, Belch et al. *(119)* investigated the effect of EPO, alone and in combination with fish oil, on the requirements for NSAIDs in 49 patients with RA and claimed that EPO, both alone and when used with fish oil, produced significant subjective improvement and allowed more than 70% of patients to reduce or even to terminate NSAID therapy, although no significant objective changes in clinical or laboratory measurements were demonstrated.

8.2. Possible Risks Associated with Long-Term Fish Oil Therapy

The concept that fish oil therapy, although of uncertain therapeutic benefit in the doses taken by most people, is at least completely safe is now less certainly correct. A commonly recommended dose would be 1.8 g EPA per day (equivalent to 3 g of total omega-3s in most supplements) but not in whole fish, where a larger intake of total omega-3s would be required to give 1.8 g of EPA. In 1991, Meydani et al. *(120)* in a 3-mo fish oil supplementation study (1.68 g EPA/d and 720 mg DHA/d) in 25 women found significant reductions in plasma triglycerides and a fall in plasma α-tocopherol, with an increase in lipid peroxide. Sanders and Hinds *(121)* found that the α-tocopherol (vitamin E) blood level was decreased to below the normal range during supplementation with fish oil. These results of the Meydani et al. *(120)* and Sanders and Hinds *(121)* studies indicate that the vitamin E content of certain fish oil supplements may not be sufficient to provide adequate antioxidant protection and that increased fish oil may require an increment in vitamin E intake—a fact not appreciated by many doctors and certainly not known by many patients who take fish oil. Such *increased oxidative stress induced by fish oil* varies between species but certainly may be seen in primates other than man *(122)*.

In 1993, Meydani et al. *(123)* described a reduced delayed type hypersensitivity (DTH) response in a measurement of cell-mediated immunity in vivo for several antigens in subjects supplemented with 1.23 g EPA and DHA/d. When fish oil supplements of 1.27 g/d EPA and DHA were given for 24 wk, they found a fall in the percentage of peripheral blood CD4+ cells and an increase in the percentage of CD8+ cells. Fish oil reduces cytokine production, interleukin (IL)-1α, IL-1β, IL-2, IL-6, and tumor necrosis factor (TNF)-α *(120,121,124–126)* from human peripheral blood mononuclear cells ex vivo, in addition to a reduction in proinflammatory leukotrienes *(127)*. In 1996, Hughes et al. *(128)* found that supplementation with n–3 polyunsaturated fatty acids (PUFAs) depressed immune reactivity by suppressing expression of monocyte surface molecules associated with their antigen-presenting function. A combination of all these reasons could explain why fish oil was beneficial in patients with RA. Effects of fish oil administration on lymphocyte functions in vitro, judged by mitogen stimulation, have consistently shown reduced responses in human and nonhuman primate studies *(129)*.

In summary, the long-term consequences of alteration of the n–3/n–6 balance in favor of the n–3 is incompletely understood in man, but it is possible that it could lead to detrimental immunologic and hematologic effects, even in individuals where immunomodulation could have benefits. The lowest possible effective dose should, therefore, be used to relieve pain and stiffness in RA, i.e., for long-term use, a dose of 500–750 mg EPA/d should not be exceeded at this time. More studies are required to investigate the *safety* of long-term supplementation with fish oil in man. Furthermore, studies are needed to determine whether *low-dose* fish oil, as taken by patients without prescription, is effective, because many of the good results reported so far have been in studies using high-dose fish oil concentrates, such as MaxEPA, not available without prescription and fairly expensive to prescribe.

Table 5
Supplements for Rheumatoid Arthritis

Supplement	Result
α-tocopherol (vitamin E)	Analgesic effect
	? Antiinflammatory effect
Ascorbic acid (vitamin C)	In combination increase cytokine production by peripheral
+	blood mononuclear cells
α-tocopherol (vitamin E)	
Ascorbic acid (vitamin C)	Needed for production of:
	Mature collagen
	Glycosaminoglycan
	Sulphated proleoglycan—a presumed measure of repair
	Increased tear and saliva production in Sjögren's
	Syndrome
Selenium	No confirmed benefit
Retinol (vitamin A)	No clear information on supplementation
β-carotene	Low levels predispose to development of rheumatoid
	arthritis and, possibly of systemic lupus erythmatosus
Fish oil (omega-3 fish oils)	Antiinflammatory effect (should not exceed 500–750 mg
	EPA/d)
Evening primrose oil ± fish oil	Subjective improvement
Other oils	No consensus on effectiveness currently available

Other oils have been used to supplement the diet to reduce the disease-associated pain and swelling, and some benefits have been demonstrated from EPO in RA *(119,130,131)*, olive oil in RA *(132,133)*, borage seed oil or starflower oil in RA *(134)*, blackcurrant seed oil in RA *(135)*, and, more controversially, mussel oil in RA and OA *(136–138)*. However, these are small studies of relatively short duration, and a consensus on effectiveness is not currently available.

Current state of knowledge for major supplements in rheumatoid arthritis is shown in Table 5.

9. "TAKE-HOME" MESSAGES

1. We accept the statement by McAlindon and Felson in 1997 *(139)* that research into the effects of nutritional factors in arthritic disease may be made more difficult by many confounding factors.
2. Nutritional immunology, biochemistry, and pharmacology, however, are research areas now recognized as fields of great scientific interest, too long underresearched.
3. Most research into dietary manipulation in arthritis has been undertaken in patients with rheumatoid disease. In other arthritides, its effects have been less well investigated.
4. Dietary treatment may be divided into two areas: elimination therapy, in which foods are removed from the diet, and supplementation therapy, in which substances are added to the diet.
5. Dietary manipulation should be undertaken only under medical supervision, and patients should not delay disease-modifying drug therapy for long if they are at risk of erosive arthritic disease.

6. The time has arrived for nutrition in arthritis to be researched fully to use its full potential benefits and to ensure a dialogue between doctors and patients.

ACKNOWLEDGMENTS

The author gratefully acknowledges untiring help from Ms. L. Gamlin and from Mr. Gordon Smith, Mrs. Marion Morrison, and Mrs. Fiona Rees from the Sally Howell Library at Epsom General Hospital, and also the unfailing support of Mrs. Alison Smith and Mrs. Glenda Primarolo.

REFERENCES

1. Sackett DL, Snow JC. The magnitude of compliance and non-compliance. In: Haynes RB, Taylor WD, Sackett DL (eds.). Compliance in Health Care. The Johns Hopkins University Press, Baltimore, 1979, pp. 11–22.
2. Wolfe F, Cathey MA. The assessment and prediction of functional disability in rheumatoid arthritis. J Rheumatol 1991;18:1298–1306.
3. Hafström I, Ringertz B, Gyllenhammar H, et al. Effects of fasting on disease activity, neutrophil function, fatty acid composition, and leukotriene biosynthesis in patients with rheumatoid arthritis. Arthritis Rheum 1988;3:585–592.
4. Kroker GP, Stroud RM, Marshall RT, et al. Fasting and rheumatoid arthritis. A multi-centre study. Clin Ecol 1984;2:137–144.
5. Sköldstam L, Larsson L, Lindström FD. Effects of fasting and lacto-vegetarian diet on rheumatoid arthritis. Scand J Rheumatol 1979;8:249–255.
6. Palmblad J, Hafström I, Ringertz B. Antirheumatic effects of fasting. Rheum Dis Clin N Am 1991;2:17.
7. Sundqvist T, Lindström F, Magnusson K-E, Skoldstam L, Stjernstrom L, Tagesson C. Influence of fasting on intestinal permeability and disease activity in patients with rheumatoid arthritis. Scand J Rheumatol 1982;11:33–38.
8. Hicklin JA, McEwan LM, Morgan JE. The effect of diet in rheumatoid arthritis. Clin Allergy 1980;10:463.
9. Parke AC, Hughes GRV. Rheumatoid arthritis and food. A case study. BMJ 1981;282:2027–2029.
10. Williams R. Rheumatoid arthritis and food: a case study. BMJ 1981;283:563.
11. Denman AM, Mitchell B, Ansell BM. Joint complaints and food allergic disorders. Ann Allergy 1983;51:260–263.
12. Panush RS, Carter RL, Katz P, Kowsari B, Longley S, Finnie S. Diet therapy for rheumatoid arthritis. Arthritis Rheum 1983;26:462–471.
13. Darlington LG, Ramsey NW, Mansfield JR. Placebo-controlled, blind study of dietary manipulation therapy in rheumatoid arthritis. Lancet 1986;i:236–238.
14. Fernandes G, Yunis EJ, José DG, Good RA. Dietary influence on anti-nuclear antibodies and cell-mediated immunity in NZB mice. Int Arch Allergy Appl Immunol 1973;44:770–782.
15. Darlington LG, Ramsey NW. Weight loss, IgE levels and fish oils in rheumatoid arthritis. In: Machtey I (ed.). Progress in Rheumatology III. Rheumatology Service, Golda Medical Centre, Petah-Tiqva, Israel, 1987, pp. 137–140.
16. Wojtulewski JA. Joints and connective tissue. In: Brostoff J, Challacombe SJ (eds.). Food Allergy and Intolerance. Baillière Tindall, London, 1987, pp. 723–735.
17. Darlington LG, Ramsey NW. Dietary manipulation therapy in rheumatoid arthritis. In: Machtey I (ed.). Progress in Rheumatology III. Rheumatology Service, Golda Medical Center, Petah-Tiqva, Israel, 1987, pp. 128–132.
18. O'Farrelly C, Melcher D, Price R, et al. Association between villous atrophy in rheumatoid arthritis and a rheumatoid factor and gliadin-specific IgG. Lancet 1988;ii:819–822.
19. Panush RS, Stroud RM, Webster EM. Food induced (allergic) arthritis. Inflammatory arthritis exacerbated by milk. Arthritis Rheum 1986;29:220–226.
20. Beri D, Malaviya AN, Shandiya R, Singh RR. Effects of dietary restrictions on disease activity in rheumatoid arthritis. Ann Rheum Dis 1988;47:69–72.

21. Darlington LG, Jump A, Ramsey NW, Spurgeon S, Street P. A prospective study of clinical and serological responses to single or double-blind food challenges in patients with rheumatoid arthritis subject to dietary manipulation. Br J Rheumatol 1989;28(Suppl):116.

22. Panush RS. Food induced ("allergic") arthritis: clinical and serologic studies. J Rheumatol 1990;17:291–294.

23. Kjeldsen-Kragh J, Haugen M, Borchgrevink CF, et al. Controlled trial of fasting and one-year vegetarian diet in rheumatoid arthritis. Lancet 1991;338:899–902.

24. Peltonen R, Kjeldsen-Kragh J, Haugen M, et al. Changes of faecal flora in rheumatoid arthritis during fasting and one-year vegetarian diet. Br J Rheumatol 1994;33:638–643.

25. Kjeldsen-Kragh J, Mellbye OJ, Haugen M, et al. Changes in laboratory variables in rheumatoid arthritis patients during a trial of fasting and one-year vegetarian diet. Scand J Rheumatol 1995;24:85–93.

26. Sköldstam L, Magnusson K-E. Fasting, intestinal permeability, and rheumatoid arthritis. Rheum Dis Clin N Am 1991;17:363–371.

27. Rasmussen GG, Svendsen H. Fasting and vegan diet in rheumatoid arthritis. Scand J Rheumatol 1984;53 (Suppl):88.

28. Sköldstam L. Fasting and vegan diet in rheumatoid arthritis. Scand J Rheumatol 1986;15:219–223.

29. Gamlin L, Brostoff H. Food sensitivity and rheumatoid arthritis. Environ Toxicol Pharmacol 1997;4: 43–49.

30. van de Laar MAFJ, van der Korst JK. Food intolerance in rheumatoid arthritis. I. A double-blind, controlled trial of the clinical effects of elimination of milk allergens and azo dyes. Ann Rheum Dis 1992;51:298–302.

31. van de Laar MAFJ, Aalbers M, Bruins FG, et al. Food intolerance in rheumatoid arthritis. II. Clinical and histological aspects. Ann Rheum Dis 1992;51:303–306.

32. Kavanagh R, Workman E, Nash P, Smith M, Hazleman BL, Hunter JO. The effect of elemental diet and subsequent food reintroduction on rheumatoid arthritis. Br J Rheumatol 1995;34:270–273.

33. Darlington LG, Ramsey NW. Clinical review. Review of dietary therapy for rheumatoid arthritis. Br J Rheumatol 1993;32:507–514.

34. Little CH, Stewart AG, Fennessy MR. Platelet serotonin release in rheumatoid arthritis: a study in food intolerant patients. Lancet 1983;ii:297–299.

35. Olhagen B, Mansson I. Intestinal *Clostridium perfringens* in rheumatoid arthritis and other collagen diseases. Acta Med Scand 1968;184:395–402.

36. Bennett JC. The infectious etiology of rheumatoid arthritis—new considerations. Arthritis Rheum 1978;21:531–538.

37. Mansson I, Norberg R, Olhagen B, Björklund N-E. Arthritis in pigs induced by dietary factors. Microbiologic, clinical and histologic studies. Clin Exp Immunol 1971;9:677–693.

38. Coombs RRA, Oldham G. Early rheumatoid joint lesions in rabbits drinking cow's milk. Int Arch Allergy Appl Immunol 1981;64:287–292.

39. Bjarnason I, Williams P, So A, et al. Intestinal permeability and inflammation in rheumatoid arthritis. Effects of non-steroidal anti-inflammatory drugs. Lancet 1984;ii:1171–1174.

40. Mielants H, de Vos M, Goemaere S, et al. Intestinal mucosal permeability in inflammatory rheumatic diseases. II. Role of disease. J Rheumatol 1991;18:394–400.

41. Behrens R, Devereaux M, Hazleman B, et al. Investigation of auranofin-induced diarrhoea. Gut 1986;27:59–65.

42. Ebringer A, Ptaszynska T, Corbett M, et al. Antibodies to Proteus in rheumatoid arthritis. Lancet 1985;ii:305–307.

43. Ebringer A, Cox NL, Abuliadayel I, et al. Klebsiella antibodies in ankylosing spondylitis and Proteus antibodies in rheumatoid arthritis. Br J Rheumatol 1988;ii:72–85.

44. Ebringer A, Cunningham P, Ahmadi K, Wrigglesworth J, Hosseini R, Wilson C. Sequence similarity between HLA-DR1 and DR4 subtypes associated with rheumatoid arthritis and Proteus serratia membrane haemolysins. Ann Rheum Dis 1992;52:1245–1246.

45. Nuki G. Ankylosing spondylitis, HLAB27, and beyond. Lancet 1998;351:767–769.

46. Kjeldsen-Kragh J, Rashid T, Dybwad A, et al. Decrease in anti-Proteus mirabilis but not anti-Escherichia coli antibody levels in rheumatoid arthritis patients treated with fasting and a one-year vegetarian diet. Ann Rheum Dis 1995;54:221–224.

47. Mansson I, Olhagen B. Intestinal *Clostridium perfringens* in rheumatoid arthritis and other connective tissue disorders. Acta Rheum Scand 1966;12:167–174.
48. Seignalet J. Les associations entre HLA et polyarthrite rhumatoide 11. – Une théorie sur la pathogenie de la polyarthrite rhumatoide. Rev Int Rhumatoide 1989;19:155–170.
49. Hunter JO. Food allergy—or entero metabolic disorder? Lancet 1991;338:495–496.
50. Peltonen R, Nenonen M, Helve T, Hänninen O, Toivanen P, Eerola E. Faecal microbial flora and disease activity in rheumatoid arthritis during a vegan diet. Br J Rheumatol 1997;36:64–68.
51. Nenonen MT, Helve TA, Rauma A-L, Hänninen OO. Uncooked, lactobacilli-rich, vegan food and rheumatoid arthritis. Br J Rheumatol 1998;37:274–281.
52. Brostoff J, Gamlin L. What Causes Food Intolerance? The Complete Guide to Food Allergy and Intolerance. Bloomsbury, London, 1989, pp. 76–77.
53. Ratner D, Eshel E, Vigder K. Juvenile rheumatoid arthritis and milk allergy. J R Soc Med 1984;78: 410–413.
54. Kjeldsen-Kragh J, Hvatum M, Haugen M, Førre Ø, Scott H. Antibodies against dietary antigens in rheumatoid arthritis patients treated with fasting and a one-year vegetarian diet. Clin Exp Rheumatol 1995;13:167–172.
55. Darlington LG, Jump A, Ramsey NW. Literature on dietary treatment of rheumatoid arthritis available to the public. Practitioner 1990;234:456–460.
56. Silman AJ, Hochberg MC. Epidemiology of the Rheumatic Diseases. Oxford University Press, Oxford, 1993.
57. McDaniel DO, Alarcón GD, Pratt PW, Reveille JD. Most African-American patients with rheumatoid arthritis do not have the rheumatoid antigenic determinant (epitope). Ann Intern Med 1995;123: 181–187.
58. Darlington LG. Joints and arthritic disease. In: Brostoff J, Challacombe SJ (eds.). Food Allergy and Intolerance (2nd ed.). Saunders, London, 2002, pp. 747–760.
59. Henrotin Y, Deby-Dupont G, Deby C, Debruiyn M, Lamy M, Franchimont P. Production of active oxygen species by isolated human chondrocytes. Br J Rheumatol 1993;32:562–567.
60. Henrotin Y, Deby-Dupont G, Deby C, Franchimont P, Emerit I. Active oxygen species, articular inflammation and cartilage damage. EXS 1992;62:308–322.
61. Greenwald RA, Moy WW. Inhibition of collagen gelation by action of the superoxide radical. Arthritis Rheum 1979;22:251–259.
62. McCord JM. Free radicals and inflammation: protection of synovial fluid by superoxide dismutase. Science 1974;185:529–531.
63. Chidwick K, Winyard PG, Zhang Z, Farrell AJ, Blake DR. Inactivation of the elastase inhibitory activity of alpha 1 antitrypsin in fresh samples of synovial fluid from patients with rheumatoid arthritis. Ann Rheum Dis 1991;50:915–916.
64. Davies JMS, Horwitz DM, Davies KJA. Inhibition of collagenase activity by N-chlorotaurine, a product of activated neutrophils. Arthritis Rheum 1994;37:424–427.
65. Situnayake RD, Thurnham DI, Kootathep S, et al. Chain-breaking antioxidant status in rheumatoid arthritis: clinical and laboratory correlates. Ann Rheum Dis 1991;50:81–86.
66. Stevens CR, Benboubetra M, Harrison R, Sahinoglu T, Smith EC, Blake DR. Localisation of xanthine oxidase to synovial endothelium. Ann Rheum Dis 1991;50:760–762.
67. Schalkwijk J, van den Berg WB, van de Putte LBA, Joosten LAB. An experimental model for hydrogen peroxide-induced tissue damage. Effects of a single inflammatory mediator on (peri-)articular tissues. Arthritis Rheum 1986;29:532–538.
68. Grootveld M, Henderson EB, Farrell A, Blake DR, Parkes HG, Haycock P. Oxidative damage to hyaluronate and glucose in synovial fluid during exercise of the inflamed rheumatoid joint. Detection of abnormal low-molecular-mass metabolites by proton-n.m.r. spectroscopy. Biochem J 1991;273: 459–467.
69. Cooper B, Creeth JM, Donald ASR. Studies of the limited degradation of mucus glycoproteins—the mechanism of the peroxide reaction. Biochem J 1985;228:615–626.
70. Davies JMS, Horwitz DA, Davies KJA. Potential roles of hypochlorous acid and N-chloroamines in collagen breakdown by phagocyte cells in synovitis. Free Radic Biol Med 1993;15:637–643.

71. Wasil M, Halliwell B, Moorhouse CP, Hutchison DCS, Baum H. Biologically significant scavenging of the myelo peroxidase-derived oxidant hypochlorous acid by some anti-inflammatory drugs. Biochem Pharmacol 1987;36:3847–3850.

72. Blake DR, Hall ND, Treby DA, Halliwell B, Gutteridge JMC. Protection against superoxide and hydrogen peroxide in synovial fluid from rheumatoid patients. Clin Sci 1981;61:483–486.

73. Chapman ML, Rubin BR, Gracy RW. Increased carbonyl content of proteins in synovial patients with rheumatoid arthritis. J Rheumatol 1989;16:15–18.

74. Grootveld M, Halliwell B. Aromatic hydroxylation as a potential measure of hydroxyl-radical formation in vivo. Identification of hydroxylated derivatives of salicylate in human body fluids. Biochem J 1986;237:449–504.

75. Lunec J, Blake DR, McCleary SJ, Brailsford S, Bacon PA. Self-perpetuating mechanisms of immunoglobulin G aggregation in rheumatoid inflammation. J Clin Invest 1985;76:2084–2090.

76. Rowley DA, Gutteridge JMC, Blake DR, Farr M, Halliwell B. Lipid peroxidation in rheumatoid arthritis: thiobarbituric acid—reactive material and catalytic iron salts in synovial fluid from rheumatoid patients. Clin Sci 1984;66:691–695.

77. Nurcombe HL, Bucknall RC, Edwards SW. Neutrophils isolated from the synovial fluid of patients with rheumatoid arthritis: priming and activation in vivo. Ann Rheum Dis 1991;50:147–153.

78. Robinson J, Watson F, Bucknall RC, Edwards SW. Activation of neutrophil reactive-oxidant production by synovial fluid from patients with inflammatory joint disease. Soluble and insoluble immunoglobulin aggregates activate different pathways in primed and unprimed cells. Biochem J 1992;286:345–351.

79. Farrell AJ, Blake DR, Palmer RMJ, Moncada S. Increased concentrations of nitrite in synovial fluid and serum samples suggest increased nitric oxide synthesis in rheumatic diseases. Ann Rheum Dis 1992;51:1219–1222.

80. Gutteridge JMC. Bleomycin-detectable iron in knee-joint synovial fluid from arthritic patients and its relationship to the extra-cellular antioxidant activities of caeruloplasmin, transferrin and lactoferrin. Biochem J 1987;245:415–421.

81. Gutteridge JMC, Rowley DA, Halliwell B. Superoxide-dependent formation of hydroxyl radicals and lipid peroxidation in the presence of iron salts. Detection of "catalytic" iron and anti-oxidant activity in extracellular fluids. Biochem J 1982;206:605–609.

82. Briviba K, Seis H. Nonenzymatic antioxidant defense systems. In: Frei B (ed.). Natural Antioxidants in Human Health and Disease. Academic, San Diego, 1994, pp. 107–128.

83. Hankinson SE, Stampfer MJ, Seddon JM, et al. Nutrient intake and cataract extraction in woman: a prospective study. BMJ 1992;305:335–339.

84. Jacques PF, Chylack LT Jr. Epidemiological evidence of a role for the antioxidant vitamins and carotenoids in cataract prevention. Am J Clin Nutr 1991;53:352S–355S.

85. Rimm EB, Stampfer MJ, Ascherio A, Giovannucci EL, Colditz GA, Willett WC. Vitamin E supplementation and the risk of coronary heart disease in men. N Engl J Med 1993;328:1450–1456.

86. Abushita AA, Hebshi EA, Daood HG, Biacs PA. Determination of antioxidant vitamins in tomatoes. Food Chem 1997;60:207–212.

87. Koch M, Arango Y, Mock H-P, Heise K-P. Factors influencing a-tocopherol synthesis in pepper fruits. J Plant Physiol 2002;159:1015–1019.

88. Niki E. Free radicals in the 1900s: from in vitro to in vivo. Free Rad Res 2001;33:693–704.

89. Anderson R. Antioxidant nutrients and prevention of oxidant-mediated diseases. In: Bendich A, Deckelbaum RJ (eds.). Preventive Nutrition: The Comprehensive Guide for Health Professionals (2nd ed.). Humana, Totowa, NJ, 2001, pp. 293–306.

90. Doumerg C. Etude clinique experimental de l'alpha-tocopheryle-quinone en rheumatologie et an re-education. Therapeutique 1969;43:676–678.

91. Edmonds SE, Winyard PG, Guo R, et al. Putative analgeric activity of repeated oral doses of vitamin E in the treatment of rheumatoid arthritis. Results of a prospective placebo controlled double blind trial. Ann Rheum Dis 1997;56:649–655.

92. Helmy M, Shohayeb M, Helmy MH, el-Bassiouni EA. Antioxidants as adjuvant therapy in rheumatoid disease. A preliminary study. Arzneimittel-Forschung 2001;51:293–298.

93. Deaney CL, Feyi K, Forrest CM, et al. Levels of lipid peroxidation products in a chronic inflammatory disorder. Res Comm Mol Pathol Pharmacol 2001;110:87–95.

94. Jeng K-CG, Yang C-S, Sim W-Y, Tsai Y-S, Liao W-J, Kuo J-S. Supplementation with vitamins C and E enhances cytokine production by peripheral blood mononuclear cells in healthy adults. Am J Clin Nutr 1996;64:960–965.

95. Peterkofsky B. Ascorbate requirement for hydroxylation and secretion of procollagen: relationship to inhibition of collagen synthesis in scurvy. Am J Clin Nutr 1991;54:1135S–1140S.

96. Spanheimer RG, Bird TA, Peterkofsky B. Regulation of collagen synthesis and mRNA levels in articular cartilage of scorbutic guinea pigs. Arch Biochem Biophys 1986;246:33–41.

97. Schwartz ER, Adamy L. Effect of ascorbic acid on arylsulfatase activities and sulfated proteoglycan metabolism in chondrocyte cultures. J Clin Invest 1977;60:96–106.

98. Horrobin DF, Campbell A. Sjögren's syndrome and the sicca syndrome: the role of prostaglandin E_1 deficiency. Treatment with essential fatty acids and vitamin C. Med Hypotheses 1980;6:225–232.

99. Aeseth J, Munthe E, Førre Ø, Steinnes E. Trace elements in serum and urine of patients with rheumatoid arthritis. Scand J Rheumatol 1978;7:237–240.

100. Comb GF Jr, Comb SB. In: The Role of Selenium in Nutrition. Academic, New York, 1986, pp. 205–263.

101. Tarp U, Hansen JC, Overvad K, Thorling EB, Tarp BD, Grandal H. Glutathione peroxidase activity in patients with rheumatoid arthritis and in normal subjects. Effects of long-term selenium supplementation. Arthritis Rheum 1987;30:1162–1166.

102. Tarp U, Overvad K, Thorling EB, Grandal H, Hansen JC. Selenium treatment in rheumatoid arthritis. Scand J Rheumatol 1985;14:364–368.

103. Munthe E, Aeseth J, Jellum E. Trace elements and rheumatoid arthritis (RA)—pathogenic and therapeutic aspects. Acta Pharmacol Toxicol 1986;59(Suppl 1):365–373.

104. Chaudière J, Wilhelmsen EC, Tappel AL. Mechanism of selenium-glutathione peroxidase and its inhibition by mercapto carboxylic acids and other mercapatans. J Biol Chem 1984;259:1043–1050.

105. Fairney A, Patel KV, Fish DE, Seifert MH. Vitamin A in osteo- and rheumatoid arthritis. Br J Rheumatol 1988;27:329–330.

106. Hughes DA, Wright AJ, Finglas PM, et al. The effect of beta-carotene supplementation on the immune function of blood monocytes from healthy male nonsmokers. J Lab Clin Med 1997;129:309–317.

107. Heiövaara M, Knekt P, Aho K, Aaran R-K, Alfthan G, Aromaa A. Serum antioxidants and risk of rheumatoid arthritis. Ann Rheum Dis 1994;53:51–53.

108. Mohan IK, Das UN. Oxidant stress, antioxidants and essential fatty acids in systemic lupus erythematosus. Prostaglandins Leuko Essen Fatty Acids 1997;56:193–198.

109. Comstock GW, Burke AE, Hoffman SC, et al. Serum concentrations of a tocopherol, b carotene and retinol preceding the diagnosis of rheumatoid arthritis and systemic lupus erythematosus. Ann Rheum Dis 1997;56:323–325.

110. Renaud S, De Lorgeril M. Wine, alcohol, platelets, and the French paradox for coronary heart disease. Lancet 1992;339:1523–1526.

111. Cleland LG. Diet and arthritis. Curr Ther 1991;Sept:51–56.

112. Darlington LG. Fish oils: what is the current view on their benefits in various diseases? Med Dialog 1994;429.

113. Belluzi A. Polyunsaturated fatty acids and autoimmune diseases. In: Bendich A, Deckelbaum RJ (eds.). Primary and Secondary Preventive Nutrition. Humana, Totowa, NJ, 2001, pp. 271–287.

114. Fish oils in rheumatoid arthritis [editorial]. Lancet 1987;ii:720–721.

115. Brusch CA, Johnson ET. A new dietary regimen for arthritis. Value of cod liver oil on a fasting stomach. J Nat Med Assoc 1959;51:266–270.

116. Sperling RA, Weinblatt M, Robin JL, et al. Effects of dietary supplementation with marine fish oil on leucocyte lipid mediator generation and function in rheumatoid arthritis. Arthritis Rheum 1987;30:988–997.

117. Kremer JM, Michalek AV, Lininger L, et al. Effects of manipulation of dietary fatty acids on clinical manifestations of rheumatoid arthritis. Lancet 1985;i:184–187.

118. Kremer J, Jubiz W, Michalek A, et al. Fish oil fatty acid supplementation in active rheumatoid arthritis. Ann Intern Med 1987;106:497–503.

119. Belch JJF, Ansell D, Madhok R, O'Dowd A, Sturrock RD. Effects of altering dietary essential fatty acids on requirements for non-steroidal anti-inflammatory drugs in patients with rheumatoid arthritis: a double-blind placebo-controlled study. Ann Rheum Dis 1988;47:96–104.

120. Meydani M, Natiello F, Goldin B, et al. Effect of long-term fish oil supplementation on vitamin E status and lipid peroxidation in women. J Nutr 1991;121:484–491.

121. Sanders TAB, Hinds A. The influence of a fish oil high in docosahexaenoic acid on plasma lipoprotein and vitamin E concentrations and haemostatic function in healthy male volunteers. Br J Nutr 1992;68:163–173.

122. Harbige LS, Ghebremeskel K, Williams G, Summers P. N-3 and N-6 phosphoglyceride fatty acids in relation to in vitro erythrocyte haemolysis induced by hydrogen peroxide in captive common marmosets (*Callithrix jacchus*). Comp Biochem Physiol 1990;97B:167–170.

123. Meydani SN, Lichtenstein SH, Cornwall S, et al. Immunologic effects of national cholesterol education panel step-2 diets with and without fish-derived n-fatty acid enrichment. J Clin Invest 1993;92:105–113.

124. Bonner SA, Rotondo D, Davidson J. Eicosapentaenoic acid supplementation modulates the immune responsiveness of human blood. Prostaglandins Leukot Essent Fatty Acids 1997;57:462–471.

125. Caughey GE, Mantzioris E, Gibson RA, Cleland LG, James MJ. The effect on human tumor necrosis factor-a and interleukin-1b production of diets enriched in n–3 fatty acids from vegetable oil or fish oil. Am J Clin Nutr 1996;63:116–122.

126. Endres S, Meydani SN, Ghorbani R, Schindler R, Dinarello CA. Dietary supplementation with n–3 fatty acids suppresses interleukin-2 production and mononuclear cell proliferation. J Leuk Biol 1993;54:599–603.

127. Schmidt EB, Dyerberg J. N–3 fatty acids and leucocytes. J Intern Med 1989;22:151–158.

128. Hughes DA, Pinder AC, Piper Z, Johnson IT, Lund EK. Fish oil supplementation inhibits the expression of major histocompatibility complex (MHC) class II molecules and adhesion molecules on human monocytes. Am J Clin Nutr 1996;63:267–272.

129. Wu D, Meydani M, Hayek MG, Huth P, Nicolosi RJ. Immunologic effects of marine- and plant-derived n–3 polyunsaturated fatty acids in non-human primates. Am J Clin Nutr 1996;63:273–280.

130. Hansen TM, Lerche A, Kassio V, Lorenzen E, Søndergaard J. Treatment of rheumatoid arthritis with prostaglandin E precursors cis-linoleic acid and gamma-linolenic acid. Scand J Rheumatol 1983;12:85–88.

131. Jantti J, Nikkari T, Solakivi T, Vapaatalo H, Isomäki H. Evening primrose oil in rheumatoid arthritis: changes in serum lipids and fatty acids. Ann Rheum Dis 1989;48:124–127.

132. Brzeski M, Madhok R, Capell HA. Evening primrose oil in patients with rheumatoid arthritis and side effects of non-steroidal antiinflammatory drugs. Br J Rheumatol 1991;30:370–372.

133. Cleland LG, French JK, Betts WH, Murphy GA, Elliott MJ. Clinical and biochemical effects of dietary fish oil supplements in rheumatoid arthritis. J Rheumatol (Canada) 1988;15:1471–1475.

134. Levanthal LJ, Boyce EG, Zurier RB. Treatment of rheumatoid arthritis with gamma-linolenic acid. Ann Intern Med 1993;119:867–873.

135. Watson J, Byars ML, McGill P, Kelman AW. Cytokine and prostaglandin production by monocytes of volunteers and rheumatoid arthritis patients treated with dietary supplements of blackcurrant seed oil. Br J Rheumatol 1993;32:1055–1058.

136. Gibson RG, Gibson SLM, Conway V, Chappell D. Perna canaliculus in the treatment of arthritis. Practitioner 1980;224:955–960.

137. Huskisson EC, Scott J, Bryans R. Seatone is ineffective in rheumatoid arthritis. BMJ 1981;282:1358–1359.

138. Larkin JG, Capell HA, Sturrock RD. Seatone is rheumatoid arthritis: a six month placebo-controlled study. Ann Rheum Dis 1985;44:199–201.

139. McAlindon T, Felson DT. Nutrition risk factors for osteoarthritis. Ann Rheum Dis 1997;56:397–400.

140. Darlington LG, Gamlin L. Diet and Arthritis. Vermilion, London, 1996, pp. 79–251.

15 Osteoporosis, Nutrition, and the Immune System

Marco Di Monaco

1. INTRODUCTION

Osteoporosis is a condition of low bone mass and microarchitectural disruption, resulting in fractures with minimal trauma. A World Health Organization (WHO) panel recommended that an absolute bone mineral density (BMD) standard should be used to make the diagnosis of the disease: a person whose BMD value falls more than 2.5 standard deviations (SD) below the mean value for a large sample of young-adults is defined as having osteoporosis, whereas individuals whose BMD values fall between 1.0 and 2.5 SD below the mean are defined as having osteopenia *(1)*. Severe or established osteoporosis denotes the disease as defined above in the presence of one or more documented fragility fractures (bone fractures resulting from trauma equal to or less than a fall from a standing position). Currently, this is the internationally agreed definition of osteoporosis, although it presents several problems regarding the validity of its use for men, children, and non-Caucasian populations. It also does not consider the pivotal role exerted by qualitative abnormalities of bone, as well as changes in bone size, geometry, and turnover in causing bone fragility. Moreover, the WHO criteria were established largely with dual-energy X-ray absorptiometry (DXA) results in mind. Consequently, the definition should be reserved for BMD assessment by DXA, and uncertainty exists about corresponding thresholds for other techniques employed in BMD measurement and for different body assessment sites. Finally, BMD predicts fracture risk along a continuous, progressive relationship, which is not adequately expressed by one threshold.

The clinical significance of having osteoporosis is realized in fractures resulting from a fragile skeleton. Common sites of fragility-related fractures include vertebrae, the distal forearm, and the proximal femur; however, because the skeletons of patients with osteoporosis are diffusely fragile, many other sites undergo fractures with high frequency. From the etiologic viewpoint, secondary osteoporosis results from specific clinical disorders, such as endocrine diseases, malabsorption syndromes, hematological diseases, rheumatoid arthritis, chronic obstructive airways disease, or treatment with certain drugs, such as corticosteroids, anticonvulsants, cytotoxic drugs, or lithium. Conversely, in primary osteoporosis, no underlying cause can be detected, although several risk factors have been elucidated, leading to the concept of a multifactorial disease.

From: *Diet and Human Immune Function*
Edited by: D. A. Hughes, L. G. Darlington, and A. Bendich © Humana Press Inc., Totowa, NJ

Table 1
Prospective Trials Linking Nutrients and Bone Health

Nutrient	Reference	Patient population	Daily dose, duration	Major findings
Calcium and vitamin D	(69)	3270 elderly women living in nursing homes; mean age 84 yr	1.2 g calcium and 800 IU vitamin D, 18 mo	Reduced hip fractures and all nonvertebral fractures
	(70)	Extension to 36 mo of the study reported above (69)		Reduced hip fractures and all nonvertebral fractures
	(71)	176 men and 213 women aged 65 yr and older	0.5 g calcium and 700 IU vitamin D, 36 mo	Reduced nonvertebral fractures; reduced bone loss
Proteins	(31)	82 elderly patients with recent hip fracture (mean age 81 yr)	20 g protein, 32 d	Reduced length of stay in hospital; reduced bone loss at 1 yr
	(32)	59 elderly patients with recent hip fracture (mean age 82 yr)	20 g protein, 32 d	Reductions in mortality (at 6 mo), rate of complications, length of stay in hospital
	(33)	62 elderly patients with recent hip fracture (mean age 82 yr)	20 g protein, 38 d	Reductions in mortality (at 7 mo), rate of complications, length of stay in hospital
	(34)	17 elderly patients with recent hip fracture (mean age 75 yr)	125 mL/h of nasoenteral tube feeding (various nutrients; approx 800 kcal) for 16 d	Reduced mortality at 6 mo
Zinc	(91)	59 postmenopausal women (mean age 66 yr)	Zinc (15 mg) plus manganese (5 mg) and copper (2.5 mg), 24 mo	Increase in bone mineral density (BMD)
	(92)	8 postmenopausal women with rheumatoid arthritis	Beta-alanyl-L-histidinato Zinc (300 mg), 6 mo	Increase in BMD
Ascorbic acid		No studies reported		
Copper		No studies reported		
Vitamin A (excess)		No studies reported		
Magnesium	(129)	24 young healthy men	15 mmol Mg, 30 d	Reduced biochemical markers of bone turnover
	(130)	54 postmenopausal women (mean age 58 yr)	250–750 mg Mg, 6 mo, followed by 250 mg, 18 mo	Increase in BMD

Among the factors that affect bone health, nutrition plays a crucial role. Because calcium is a major substrate for bone mineralization, many studies concerning nutrition and osteoporosis focus on dietary calcium. Presently, it is well established that increased calcium intake lowers the bone remodeling rate, which increases BMD *(2,3)*. Although data regarding calcium supplements (without vitamin D) and the incidence of fractures are mixed *(3–6)*, an adequate calcium intake is recommended by all clinical guidelines as a baseline treatment for osteoporosis *(7–9)*.

1.1. Recommended Daily Intakes of Calcium

The recommended daily calcium intake from all sources (where "all sources" means total diet and supplements) is as follows: prepubertal children (ages 4–8 yr)—800 mg; adolescents (ages 9–18 yr)—1300 mg; premenopausal women—1000 mg; men after adolescence and until the age of 50 yr—1000 mg; postmenopausal women—1500 mg; men over the age of 50 yr—1500 mg; women 18 yr and older who are pregnant or lactating—same as nonpregnant women, i.e., 1000 mg.

1.2. Other Factors Influencing Bone Health

Besides calcium, many nutritional factors can influence bone health (Table 1). Similarly, the immune system's health is strongly influenced by nutritional status as established by the wider literature. However, the links between nutritional intakes, immunity, and bone have scarcely been studied. Recently, we have shown a positive association between total lymphocyte count (TLC) and femur BMD in a sample of elderly women with hip fractures *(10)*. The interest in hip fractures is emphasized by the prognostic role exerted by both BMD *(11)* and TLC *(12)*. The positive association was confirmed in a second sample of women with hip fractures, but it was not found in men with hip fractures *(13)*, showing an intriguing, although unexplained, sex specificity. The association was independent of age, weight, height, body mass index, erythrocyte sedimentation rate, fracture type (cervical or trochanteric), and time between surgery and laboratory analyses. Unfortunately, our work was not controlled for physical exercise, a variable that can influence both TLC (as stated by Pedersen in Chapter 19 on exercise and immune function) and BMD *(14–17)*. The first hypothesis to explain our data was based on the role of dietary protein intakes *(1)*, because TLC was described as a specific marker of protein nutritional status *(18–21)*. However, data about serum albumin, a protein nutrition status biochemical marker, in the same women were inconsistent *(13)*, which is consistent with the conflicting results published on the association between serum albumin and BMD *(22–25)*, and no data were available about patients' other biochemical markers, body composition, or dietary intakes. Moreover, TLC is a widely employed nutritional status marker *(26–31)*, but it is influenced by many nutrients *(32)*, apart from proteins. Several of these nutrients also influence bone and may link bone health to the immune system.

The main nutrients known to influence both immunity and bone turnover are reviewed in Sections 2.–8.

2. PROTEINS

Several lines of evidence support the role of dietary proteins in bone health and protein malnutrition in the genesis of low BMD and fragility fractures. Experimental studies showed decreased BMD in rats fed a low-protein diet and reduced bone strength resulting from isocaloric protein undernutrition *(33–34)*. In humans, protein intake was positively associated with BMD measured at various sites *(35–37)*. Moreover, low protein intake was recently associated with accelerated bone loss *(38)* and predicted hip fracture occurrence in a large prospective study *(39)*, in agreement with the well-known high prevalence of protein malnutrition in patients with hip fractures *(40)*. The risk of hip fracture was inversely associated with serum albumin levels in both a prospective study *(22)* and a case-control study *(41)*. Serum albumin was also positively associated with functional recovery after hip fracture *(42,43)*. Interest in this field was emphasized by some clinical trials showing beneficial effects of protein dietary supplements in patients with hip fractures: attenuation of proximal femur bone loss *(44)*, increase in muscle strength *(45,46)*, shorter duration of hospital stay *(44–46)*, reduced mortality *(45–47)* and reduced complication rates *(45–46)*. Protein supplements acted on bone independently of other dietary components *(46)*. The role of dietary proteins in bone health was not universally recognized, because concern existed about the known urinary calcium loss resulting from a high protein intake, which could potentially upset calcium balance and lead to bone loss *(48–50)*. Bone calcium may also be involved in buffering the increased acid load resulting from excessive dietary protein intake. However, a negative calcium balance was often observed with extremely high levels of dietary proteins, rarely seen in clinical practice, and the studies showing calcium waste owing to dietary proteins were short-term *(51)*. Moreover, no clinical study showed negative effects on bone resulting from high protein intake, and epidemiologic observations were weak supports for the positive association between high dietary protein intake and hip fracture *(52)*. On the contrary, the literature consistently indicates that low protein intake is detrimental in bone health and strongly suggests the relevancy of protein supplements to both prevent bone loss and fractures and ameliorate the prognosis after hip-fracture. The mechanism by which a low dietary protein intake may impair bone strength was not elucidated, but an effect on the structure and function of bone-related proteins is plausible, as suggested by experimental studies in ovariectomized rats *(53)* and evaluations of osteoporotic bones *(54)*: the lack of amino acids would lead to alterations in the synthesis of bone proteins. Another suggested mechanism of action involves various hormones (insulin-like growth factor [IGF]-I, leptin, and growth hormone) that are modulated by dietary proteins *(10,44,55,56)*.

Protein malnutrition exerts strong negative effects on the immune system. The immune deficiencies result in an enhanced susceptibility to many types of infections *(57)* that further aggravate both malnutrition and immune impairment *(58–60)*. Low levels of immune responses in cells of the macrophage-lymphocyte series are consistently related to protein malnutrition *(61–64)*, and several alterations have been described in detail: thymic atrophy *(65–67)*, spleen weight reduction *(57)*, and percentage of splenic macrophages expressing Ia (the murine equivalent of major histocompatibility complex [MHC] class II molecules) *(57)*, increased splenic T-suppressor cells *(57)*, decreased lymphocyte proliferation *(67–69)*, lymphopenia *(65)*, impaired cell- and antibody-mediated cytotoxicity *(70,71)*, decreased phagocyte function, and reduced antigen-presenting cell function *(64)*. Some changes in cytokine production have also been reported *(61,62)*, including impaired interleukin (IL)-2 production *(69)*, low levels of IL-2 receptors *(69)*, impaired tumoricidal response to IL-2 *(72)*, and low levels of interferon (IFN)-γ *(69)*. Low secretory immunoglobulin (Ig)A antibody production *(61,62,73)*, low antibody response to vaccine *(68)*, and impaired complement system function *(61,62)* have also been observed. In Western societies, protein malnutrition is often found in the elderly *(68,74)*, who show reduced immune responsiveness, particularly in cell-mediated immunity. Interestingly, the decline in immune function parallels the degree of protein malnutrition *(75)*, suggesting a causal role of dietary deficiencies. The specific role of malnutrition in the genesis of immunity impairment was confirmed by studies of nutrient supplementation showing increased TLC *(76–78)*, CD4 cells *(79)*, CD4-CD8 ratio *(79)*, T-lymphocyte responsiveness to mitogenic stimulation with Concanavalin A (Con A) *(79)*, and correction of hypocomplementemia *(80)*. Consistently, patients treated with nutrient supplements show fewer infections *(59,76,81)* and higher immune responses after vaccination *(59)*.

3. VITAMIN D

Vitamin D's critical role in bone health is well established and can be seen in the development of rickets in children and osteomalacia in adults resulting from the frank deficiency of the vitamin's active metabolite. Well-known examples of this condition are vitamin D-dependent rickets type I, owing to mutations in the 25-(OH)D1-hydroxylase gene, which renders it nonfunctional, leading to poor synthesis of $1,25-(OH)_2$ vitamin D, and vitamin D-dependent rickets type II, caused by mutations in the vitamin D receptor gene. Serum 25-(OH) D is the best indicator of vitamin D status, the classic threshold for defining vitamin D deficiency leading to rickets or osteomalacia is 12 ng/mL (30 nmol/L). However, many studies indicate that even a less severe deficiency, classified as *vitamin D insufficiency*, exerts a detrimental role in bone health: it does not lead to frank osteomalacia, but it contributes to the genesis of osteoporosis. The role of vitamin D insufficiency was suggested on a theoretical basis, because it causes secondary hyperparathyroidism and, consequently, bone loss. The theoretical hypothesis was mainly confirmed by three randomized controlled trials showing the antifracture efficacy of vitamin D (and calcium) supplements in the elderly *(82–85)*. The threshold level for serum 25-(OH) D defining vitamin D insufficiency was not precisely established. The main criterion suggests that the threshold be set at the 25-(OH) vitamin D level that minimizes parathyroid hormone (PTH) secretion *(85)*. Using this criterion, the threshold is between 20 and 32 ng/mL (50–80 nmol/L). Using this threshold, individuals can be divided into three groups on the basis of their vitamin D status, defined by serum 25-(OH) D levels: frank deficiency, leading to rickets or osteomalacia (fewer than 12 ng/mL or 30 nmol/L); insufficiency, contributing to the onset of osteoporosis (between 12 and 20–32 ng/mL or between 30 and 50–80 nmol/L); and normality (higher than 20–32 ng/mL or 50–80 nmol/L). The recommended daily vitamin D intake from all sources (where "all sources" means total diet and supplements) are as follows: men and women under 50 yr: 400 IU (10 μg) and men and women older than 50 yr: 800 IU (20 μg).

Apart from its role in bone and calcium metabolism, $1,25-(OH)_2$ vitamin D exerts general effects on cell proliferation and differentiation. Cell regulation strongly involves the immune system, where $1,25-(OH)_2$ vitamin D can behave as a paracrine factor, because it can be produced by monocytes *(86)*. The vitamin D receptor is found in significant concentrations in T-lymphocyte and macrophage populations *(87)*, showing the highest concentrations in the immature cells of the thymus and the mature CD8+ T lymphocytes.

Several immunomodulatory actions resulting from 1,25-$(OH)_2$ vitamin D have been reported at both the cellular and the molecular levels: suppressor cell activity enhancement *(88)*; inhibition of the secretion of both IL-2 and IFN-γ by helper T cells, and inhibition of their proliferation *(88–90)*; inhibition of the secretion of IL-1, IL-6, and tumor necrosis factor (TNF)-α by antigen-presenting cells *(88–89)*; inhibition of MHC class II molecule expression *(88)*; and enhancement of the production of transforming growth factor (TGF)-β and IL-4 *(87)*. Although 1,25-$(OH)_2$ vitamin D has no apparent effects on B lymphocytes, the T-cell suppression indirectly inhibits antibody production *(89)*. The final effect of the actions mentioned above is a strong immunomodulation, with intriguing clinical applications. In animal models, 1,25-$(OH)_2$ vitamin D prevents the development of experimental autoimmune encephalomyelitis, whereas vitamin D deficiency increases the disease's severity *(88,91)*. Vitamin D reduces the incidence of experimental diabetes and attenuates murine lupus *(88,90)*. The hormone also prolongs graft survival in experimental transplantation models *(88,90)*. In humans, immunomodulatory actions were reported in scleroderma *(88)*, and antiproliferative actions were observed in psoriasis *(88)*. The availability of vitamin D analogues sharing the immunological effects of the parent compound but decreased actions on calcium and bone metabolism provides a fertile area of research that may yield a new therapeutic tool in several diseases *(87)*. Moreover, vitamin D deficiency was suggested to play a role in the development of some autoimmune diseases in humans, because geographic areas with low vitamin D supplies correlate with regions with high incidence of multiple sclerosis, arthritis, and diabetes *(91)*.

4. ZINC

In experimental models, zinc exerted favorable effects in bone health both in vivo and in vitro. The prolonged oral administration of zinc prevented bone loss in the femur of ovariectomized rats *(92,93)* and in both the femur and the lumbar spine of rats on strenuous exercise *(94)*. Consistently, zinc deficiency in growing rats caused osteopenia in femoral cancellous bone *(95)*. Zinc supplementation enhanced protein synthesis in cultured bone tissue from both fractured and unfractured bones *(96,97)*, inhibited the differentiation of osteoclasts antagonizing the action of many resorbing factors *(98)*, enhanced the production of anabolic growth factors by cultured femur bone tissue, and strengthened their anabolic action *(99)*. In humans, the zinc ion levels in serum and bone tissue of patients with senile osteoporosis were lower than in healthy controls *(100)*. In women at various ages, zinc intake was positively correlated with forearm bone mineral content *(101)*. In women who were premenopausal, higher zinc intakes were associated with higher BMD levels measured at the lumbar spine *(102)*. Moreover, in a prospective study in a large sample of men, a low zinc intake was associated with a doubled risk of fractures *(103)*. Other authors have reported results of the effects of zinc supplementation in humans, showing preliminary encouraging data: bone loss in calcium-supplemented, older women who were postmenopausal was further reduced by concomitant administration of trace elements, including zinc *(104)* and, in a small sample of women who were postmenopausal with rheumatoid arthritis, zinc treatment improved periarticular osteoporosis *(105)*.

5. ASCORBIC ACID

Ascorbic acid was implicated in bone health, because it is involved in collagen formation, its deficiency is associated with abnormal bone development and limb fractures in experimental models *(106)*, and its serum concentration is low in elderly patients with hip fractures *(107)*. However, conflicting results were reported in several epidemiologic studies investigating the relationship between ascorbic acid intake, or its serum levels, and BMD or risk of fracture *(108–114)*. Presently, the exact role of dietary ascorbic acid in osteoporosis genesis cannot be established in the general population. It was suggested that dietary vitamin C intake may have a beneficial role in some groups of women who are postmenopausal, particularly those who are smokers. Because smoking increases the concentration of free radicals involved in bone resorption *(115)*, vitamin C's protective action in smokers, which is suggested by two survey studies *(111,115)*, may result from its antioxidant action.

6. COPPER

Copper, through its role as a cofactor for lysyl oxidase, is essential for collagen cross-links and may contribute to bone strength. Impaired mechanical bone strength was shown in copper-deficient rats *(116)*, and a relationship between copper deficiency and experimental osteoporosis was suggested: bone loss after ovariectomy was slightly more severe in copper-deficient rats *(117)* and copper supplementation prevented bone loss resulting from ovariectomy *(118)*. These data agree with a previous observation in lambs, showing increased susceptibility to fractures associated with a copper-deficient diet, which was partially reversed by copper supplementation *(119)*. In humans, bone abnormalities associated with copper deficiency were described in premature infants on hyper-alimentation *(120)*, and low serum copper levels were found in elderly patients with hip fractures *(121)*. However copper's role in osteoporosis genesis and treatment in humans has not been fully established.

7. VITAMIN A

Severe skeletal lesions, including osteopenia, fractures, deformities, and growth arrest, were produced in animals by toxic vitamin A levels (retinol, or its more potent metabolite, retinoic acid) *(122–124)*. The effect is likely to be related to a direct action exerted by vitamin A on bone, because in vitro studies have shown that vitamin A can selectively inhibit collagen synthesis *(123)*, stimulate osteoclast-like cell formation *(125)* and osteoclast proliferation *(126)*, enhance mature osteoclasts' bone-resorbing activity *(125)*, and increase calcium release from bone *(123)*. However, other mechanisms, such as the antagonism of vitamin D enhancement of intestinal calcium absorption, may also be operating *(127)*. In humans, anecdotal reports of accidental poisoning suggest that vitamin A may produce detrimental effects on bone *(128)*, and the possibility has been raised that long-term high vitamin A intake could contribute to osteoporosis and fracture risk *(129)*. Recently, the results of a prospective epidemiologic study involving a total of 72,337 postmenopausal women whose cases were followed for 18 yr were published. This study showed a significant association between a diet high in retinol and the risk of osteoporotic hip fractures *(130)*. The data strengthened a previous report of a cross-sectional study and of a case-control study performed in Sweden *(131)*, showing lower levels of BMD and higher incidence of hip fractures in women with high dietary retinol intakes. These findings may explain why the highest incidences of osteoporotic fractures are found in northern Europe, where the dietary vitamin A intake is unusually high. Moreover, vitamin A in fortified milk may explain the unexpected association between high calcium intake and hip fractures, because milk is a substantial source of both nutrients in northern Europe *(132)*. Although this is a large population group, the differences in vitamin A intake between cohorts were relatively small and may be insufficient to affect circulating vitamin A levels. A recent epidemiological study has not confirmed this report: no significant association was found between fasting serum retinyl esters and BMD *(133)*. Moreover, short-term vitamin A supplementation (25,000 IU of retinol palmitate) did not affect bone turnover in healthy men in a prospective randomized study *(134)*. In conclusion, uncertainty exists concerning the role of vitamin A excess in bone loss and bone fragility genesis. It is likely that a delicate balance exists between ensuring that the elderly consume sufficient vitamin A and simultaneously cautioning against excessive retinol supplementation *(135)*.

8. MAGNESIUM

Increase in osteoclast bone resorption without changes in bone-forming surface or osteoblast number was observed in rats given a low-magnesium diet (2 mg magnesium/100 g chow) vs. rats given a normal diet (63 mg magnesium/100 g chow). Such changes in bone metabolism led to uncoupling of bone formation and bone resorption, resulting in bone loss *(136)*. In contrast, long-term excessive magnesium supplementation (200 mg magnesium/100 g chow) was deleterious for bones in rats, resulting in reduced strength of bones vs. those rats given a normal diet (50 mg magnesium/100 g chow) *(137)*. In humans, magnesium depletion was suggested to contribute to the malabsorption-associated osteoporosis *(138)* and alcoholism *(139)*. However, individuals with magnesium deficiency owing to malabsorption or alcoholism commonly have other deficiencies, including calcium deficiency; how much of their bone deficit results from magnesium depletion and how much to the other depletions is unclear. Some studies showed a positive association between dietary magnesium intake and BMD in women who are premenopasual *(140)*, women who were postmenopausal *(141,142)*, and elderly men and women *(143)*. In men, magnesium intake was also associated with lower bone loss over 4 yr *(144)*. High magnesium intake was part of a diet rich in potassium, fruit, and vegetables, contributing to an alkaline environment. This may buffer the acid load owing to other dietary components, saving bone mineral, which may act as a buffer base as well *(143)*. Magnesium supplementation in normal young men caused reductions in the biochemical markers of bone turnover *(145)*. A small, non-randomized, 2-yr clinical trial in women who were postmenopausal showed favorable effects of magnesium supplementation on BMD *(146)*.

Magnesium plays a key role in many immune functions involving both B and T cells *(147,148)*. Magnesium deficiency in rodents impaired antibody production and cell-mediated immunity and increased infection susceptibility *(147)*. Consistently, magnesium supplementation in mice enhanced immune responses *(149)*. In humans, magnesium deficiency was associated with both bacterial and fungal infections *(150)* and caused enhanced inflammatory responses *(151,152)*.

9. CONCLUSIONS

Several nutrients are relevant to the health status of both the immune system and bone tissue. However, the studies reviewed in this chapter have important limitations. Many studies examined only one nutritional factor. Caution is needed in their interpretation, because the role of each factor depends on complex interactions in each individual, because many nutrients are codependent and simultaneously interact with genetic and environmental factors. Moreover, for the majority of the nutrients, there are no large prospective randomized clinical trials that confirm their roles in bone and immune health suggested by some of the experimental or survey studies. Finally, the interactions between nutrition, immunity, and bone health have not been specifically addressed. Therefore, nutritional trials with simultaneous evaluation of both bone health and the immune system would be the most useful tool to improve our knowledge in this field.

10. "TAKE-HOME" MESSAGES

1. Osteoporosis, a condition of bone fragility leading to high incidences of fractures, is a multifactorial disease. Nutritional status is one of the major factors that can affect bone turnover and cause bone fragility.
2. Because nutritional status strongly influences the health of both bone tissue and the immune system, the links between nutrients, immunity, and osteoporosis deserve greater attention.
3. Apart from calcium and vitamin D, several nutrients, including proteins, zinc, ascorbic acid, copper, vitamin A, and magnesium, affect bone turnover and immune function in both experimental and survey studies.
4. Prospective trials showing beneficial effects in bone health are available for few nutrients: calcium, vitamin D, and proteins. Small studies have focused on zinc and magnesium, with encouraging, although preliminary, results.
5. The link between nutrition, immunity, and bone turnover has not been specifically addressed.
6. Nutritional trials with simultaneous evaluation of both the immune system and bone health are needed to improve our knowledge in the field.

REFERENCES

1. *Assessment of fracture risk and its application to screening for postmenopausal osteoporosis: report of a WHO study group.* WHO, Geneva, 1994.
2. Riis B, Thomsen K, Christiansen C. Does calcium supplementation prevent postmenopausal bone loss? N Engl J Med 1987;316:173–177.
3. Chevalley T, Rizzoli R, Nydegger V, et al. Effects of calcium supplements on femoral bone mineral density and vertebral fracture rate in vitamin-D-replete elderly patients. Osteoporos Int 1994;4: 245–252.
4. Recker R, Hinders S, Davies K, et al. Correcting calcium nutritional deficiency prevents spine fractures in eldelry women. J Bone Miner Res 1996;11:1961–1966.
5. Long-term effects of calcium supplementation on bone loss and fractures in postmenopausal women: a randomized controlled trial. Am J Med 1995;98:331–335.
6. Riggs B, O'Fallon W, Muhs J, O'Connor M, Kumar R, Melton L. Long-term effects of calcium supplementation on serum parathyroid hormone level, bone turnover, and bone loss in elderly women. J Bone Miner Res 1998;13:168–174.

7. Brown J, Josse R, and the Scientific Advisory Council of the Osteoporosis Society of Canada. 2002 clinical practice guidelines for the diagnosis and management of osteoporosis in Canada. CMAJ 2002;167(Suppl): 1S–57S.

8. *Physician's guide to prevention and treatment of osteoporosis developed by The National Osteoporosis Foundation.* Washington, 2003.

9. American Association of Clinical Endocrinologists. Medical guidelines for clinical practice for the prevention and management of postmenopausal osteoporosis. Endocr Pract 2001;7:293–312.

10. Di Monaco M, Di Monaco R, Manca M, Cavanna A. Positive association between total lymphocyte count and femur bone mineral density in hip-fractured women. Gerontology 2002;48:157–161.

11. Di Monaco M, Di Monaco R, Mautino F, Cavanna A. Femur bone mineral density is independently associated with functional recovery after hip fracture in elderly women. Arch Phys Med Rehabil 2002;83:1715–1720.

12. McIntosh E, Laurent L. Nutritional assessment of the hospitalized patient. Am Fam Physician 1983;27:169–175.

13. Di Monaco M, Vallero F, Di Monaco R, Mautino F, Cavanna A. Biochemical markers of nutrition and bone mineral density in the elderly. Gerontology 2003;49:50–54.

14. Di Monaco M, Di Monaco R, Manca M, Cavanna A. Handgrip strength is an independent predictor of distal radius bone mineral density in postmenopausal women. Clin Rheumatol 2000;19:473–476.

15. Kroger H, Tuppurainen M, Honkanen R, Alhava E, Saarikoski S. Bone mineral density and risk factors for osteoporosis: a population-based study of 1600 perimenopausal women. Calcif Tissue Int 1994; 55:1–7.

16. Wolff I, van Croonenborg J, Kemper H, Kostense P, Twisk J. The effect of exercise training programs on bone mass: a meta analysis of published controlled trials in pre- and postmenopausal women. Osteoporos Int 1999;9:1–12.

17. Kerr D, Ackland T, Maslen B, Morton A, Prince R. Resistance training over 2 years increases bone mass in calcium-replete postmenopausal women. J Bone Miner Res 2001;16:175–181.

18. Patterson B, Cornell C, Carbone B, Levine B, Chapman D. Protein depletion and metabolic stress in elderly patients who have a fracture of the hip. J Bone Joint Surg Am 1992;74:251–260.

19. Cerra F, Mazuski J, Chute E, et al. Branched chain metabolic support. A prospective, randomized, double-blind trial in surgical stress. Ann Surg 1984;199:286–291.

20. Bonkowsky H, Singh R, Jafri I, et al. A randomized, controlled trial of treatment of alcoholic hepatitis with parenteral nutrition and oxandrolone. II. Short-term effects on nitrogen metabolism, metabolic balance, and nutrition. Am J Gastroenterol 1991;86:1209–1218.

21. Hwang T, Mou S, Chen M. The importance of a source of sufficient protein in postoperative hypocaloric partial parenteral nutrition support. J Parenter Enteral Nutr 1993;17:254–256.

22. Thiebaud D, Burckhardt P, Costanza M, et al. Importance of albumin, 25OH-vitamin D and IGFBP-3 as risk factors in elderly women and men with hip fracture. Osteoporos Int 1997;7:457–462.

23. Coin A, Sergi G, Beninca P, et al. Bone mineral density and body composition in underweight normal elderly subjects. Osteoporos Int 2000;11:1043–1050.

24. Lunde A, Barrett-Connor E, Morton D. Serum albumin and bone mineral density in healthy older men and women: the Rancho Bernardo Study. Osteoporos Int 1998;8:547–551.

25. D'Erasmo E, Pisani D, Ragno A, Raejntroph N, Letizia C, Acca M. Relationship between serum albumin and bone mineral density in postmenopausal women and in patients with hypoalbuminemia. Horm Metab Res 1999;31:385–388.

26. Shaver H, Loper J, Lutes R. Nutritional status of nursing home patients. J Parenter Enteral Nutr 1980;4:367–370.

27. De Groot L, Beck A, Schroll M, Van Staveren W. Evaluating the DETERMINE Your Nutritional Health Checklist and the Mini Nutritional Assessment as tools to identify nutritional problems in elderly Europeans. Eur J Clin Nutr 1998;52:877–883.

28. Weinsier R, Hunker E, Krumdieck C, Butterworth C. Hospital malnutrition. A prospective evaluation of general medical patients during the course of hospitalization. Am J Clin Nutr 1979;32:418–426.

29. Elmore M, Wagner D, Knoll D, et al. Developing an effective adult nutrition screening tool for a community hospital. J Am Diet Assoc 1994;94:1113–1118.

30. Lansey S, Waslien C, Mulvihill M, Fillit H. The role of anthropometry in the assessment of malnutrition in the hospitalized frail elderly. Gerontology 1993;39:346–353.

31. Conlan D. Value of lymphocyte counts as a prognostic index of survival following femoral neck fractures. Injury 1989;20:352–354.
32. Chandra R, Sarchielli P. Nutritional status and immune response. Clin Lab Med 1993;13:455–461.
33. Morii H, Shioi A, Inaba M, et al. Significance of albumin in the pathogenesis of osteoporosis: changes in genetically analbuminemic rats and rats fed a low albumin diet. Osteoporos Int 1997;7S3:S30–S35.
34. Ammann P, Bourrin S, Bonjour J, Meyer J, Rizzoli R. Protein undernutrition-induced bone loss is associated with decreased IGF-I levels and estrogen deficiency. J Bone Miner Res 2000;15:683–690.
35. Geinoz G, Rapin C, Rizzoli R, et al. Relationship between bone mineral density and dietary intakes in the elderly. Osteoporos Int 1993;3:242–248.
36. Cooper C, Atkinson E, Hensrud D, et al. Dietary protein intake and bone mass in women. Calcif Tissue Int 1996;58:320–325.
37. Lacey J, Andderson J, Fujita T, Yoshimoto Y, Fukase M, Tsuchie G. Correlates of cortical bone mass among premenopausal and postmenopausal Japanese women. J Bone Miner Res 1991;6:651–659.
38. Hannan M, Tucker K, Dawson-Hughes B, Cupples L, Felson D, Kiel D. Effect of dietary protein on bone loss in elderly men and women: the Framingham Osteoporosis Study. J Bone Miner Res 2000;15:2504–2512.
39. Munger R, Cerhan J, Chiu B. Prospective study of dietary protein intake and risk of hip fracture in postmenopausal women. Am J Clin Nutr 1999;69:147–152.
40. Bonjour J, Schurch M, Rizzoli R. Nutritional aspects of hip fractures. Bone 1996;183S:139s–144s.
41. Huang Z, Himes J, McGovern P. Nutrition and subsequent hip fracture risk among a national cohort of white women. Am J Epidemiol 1996;144:124–134.
42. Di Monaco M, Di Monaco R, Manca M, Cavanna A. Serum albumin is an independent predictor of functional recovery after hip fracture: a retrospective study of 275 in-patients. In: Burckardt P (ed.). Nutritional Aspects of Osteoporosis. Academic Press, San Diego, CA, 2001, pp. 251–259.
43. Koval K, Maurer S, Su E, Aharonoff G, Zuckerman J. The effects of nutritional status on outcome after hip fracture. J Orthop Trauma 1999;13:164–169.
44. Schurch M, Rizzoli R, Slosman D, Vadas L, Vergnaud P, Bonjour J. Protein supplements increase serum insulin-like growth factor-I levels and attenuate proximal femur bone loss in patients with recent hip fracture. A randomized, double blind, placebo-controlled trial. Ann Intern Med 1998;128:801–809.
45. Delmi M, Rapin C, Bengoa J, Delmas P, Vasey H, Bonjour J. Dietary supplementation in elderly patients with fractured neck of the femur. Lancet 1990;335:1013–1016.
46. Tkatch L, Rapin C, Rizzoli R, et al. Benefits of oral protein supplementation in elderly patients with fracture of the proximal femur. J Am Coll Nutr 1992;11:519–525.
47. Sullivan D, Nelson C, Bopp M, Puskarich-May C, Walls R. Nightly enteral nutrition support of elderly hip fracture patients: a phase I trial. J Am Coll Nutr 1998;17:155–161.
48. Sebastian A, Harris S, Ottaway J, Todd K, Morris R. Improved mineral balance and skeletal metabolism in postmenopausal women treated with potassium bicarbonate. N Engl J Med 1994;330:1776–1881.
49. Anand C, Linkswiler H. Effect of protein intake on calcium balance of young men given 500 mg calcium daily. J Nutr 1974;104:695–700.
50. Margen S, Chu J, Kaufmann N, Calloway D. Studies in calcium metabolism. I. The calciuretic effect of dietary protein. Am J Clin Nutr 1974;27:584–589.
51. Buclin T, Cosma M, Appenzeller M, et al. Diet acids and alkalis influence calcium retention in bone. Osteoporos Int 2001;12:493–499.
52. Abelow B, Holford T, Insogna K. Cross-cultural association between dietary animal protein and hip fracture: a hypothesis. Calcif Tissue Int 1992;50:14–18.
53. Higashi Y, Takenaka A, Takahashi S, Noguchi T. Effect of protein restriction on the messenger RNA contents of bone-matrix proteins, insulin-like growth factors and insulin-like growth factor binding proteins in femur of ovariectomized rats. Br J Nutr 1996;75:811–823.
54. Oxlund H, Barckman M, Ortoft G, Andreassen T. Reduced concentrations of collagen cross-links are associated with reduced strength of bone. Bone 1995;17:365S–371S.
55. Casanueva F, Dieguez C. Neuroendocrine regulation and actions of leptin. Front Neuroendocrinol 1999;20:317–363.
56. Tannenbaum G, Gurd W, Lapointe M. Leptin is a potent stimulator of spontaneous pulsatile growth hormone GH secretion and the GH response to GH-releasing hormone. Endocrinology 1998;139:3871–3875.

57. Nimmanwudipong T, Cheadle W, Appel S, Polk H. Effect of protein malnutrition and immuno-modulation on immune cell population. J Surg Res 1992;52:233–238.
58. Ulijaszek S. Transdisciplinarity in the study of undernutrition-infection interactions. Coll Antropol 1997;21:3–15.
59. Chandra R. Nutrition, immunity and infection: from basic knowledge of dietary manipulation of immune responses to practical application of ameliorating suffering and improving survival. Proc Natl Acad Sci 1996;93;14304–14307.
60. Scrimshaw N, SanGiovanni J. Synergism of nutrition, infection and immunity: an overview. Am J Clin Nutr 1997;66:464S–477S.
61. Chandra R, Kumari S. Nutrition and immunity: an overview. J Nutr 1994;124:1433S–1435S.
62. Chandra R. Nutrition and the immune system: an introduction. Am J Clin Nutr 1997;66:460S–463S.
63. Kishino Y, Moriguchi S. Nutritional factors and cellular immune response. Nutr Health 1992;8:133–141.
64. Conzen S, Janeway C. Defective antigen presentation in chronically protein-deprived mice. Immunology 1988;63:683–689.
65. McMurray D. Cell-mediated immunity in nutritional deficiency. Prog Food Nutr Sci 1984;8:193–228.
66. Slobodianik N, Pallaro A, Roux M, Rio M. Effect of low-quality dietary protein on the thymus of growing rats. Nutrition 1989;5:417–418.
67. Deitch E, Xu D, Qi L, Specian R, Berg R. Protein malnutrition alone and in combination with endotoxin impairs systemic and gut-associated immunity. J Parenter Enteral Nutr 1992;16:25–31.
68. Lesourd B. Nutrition and immunity in the elderly: modification of immune responses with nutritional treatments. Am J Clin Nutr 1997;66:478S–484S.
69. Mengheri E, Nobili F, Crocchioni G, Lewis J. Protein starvation impairs the ability of activated lymphocytes to produce interferon gamma. J Interferon Res 1992;12:17–21.
70. Lieberman M, Reynolds J, Redmond H, Leon P, Shou J, Daly J. Comparison of acute and chronic protein-energy malnutrition on host antitumor immune mechanisms. J Parenter Enteral Nutr 1991;15:15–21.
71. Watson R, Lim T. Thymosin fraction 5: effects on T cell functions in mice immunosuppressed by severe dietary protein deficiency. Int J Immunopharmacol 1986;8:545–552.
72. Lieberman M, Reynolds J, Goldfine J, Shou J, Daly J. Protein-calorie malnutrition inhibits antitumor response to interleukin-2 immunotherapy. Surgery 1990;108:452–458.
73. McGee D, McMurray D. Protein malnutrition reduces the IgA immune response to oral antigen by altering cell and suppressor T-cell functions. Immunology 1988;64:697–702.
74. Roebothan B, Chandra R. Relationship between nutritional status and immune function of elderly people. Age Ageing 1994;23:49–53.
75. Kawakami K, Kadota J, Iida K, Shirai R, Abe K, Kohno S. Reduced immune function and malnutrition in the elderly. Tohoku J Exp Med 1999;187:157–171.
76. Rapp R, Young B, Twyman D, et al. The favorable effect of early parenteral feeding on survival in head-injured patients. J Neurosurg 1983;58:906–912.
77. Cappell M, Iacovone F. The safety and efficacy of percutaneous endoscopic gastrostomy after recent myocardial infarction: a study of 28 patients and 40 controls at four university teaching hospitals. Am J Gastroenterol 1996;91:1599–1603.
78. Georgiannos S, Renaut A, Goode A. Short term restorative nutrition in malnourished patients: pros and cons of intravenous and enteral alimentation using compositionally matched nutrients. Int Surg 1997;82:301–306.
79. Sacks G, Brown R, Teague D, Dickerson R, Tolley E, Kudsk K. Early nutrition support modifies immune function in patients sustaining severe head injury. J Parenter Enteral Nutr 1995;19:387–392.
80. Sakamoto M, Fujisawa Y, Nishioka K. Physiologic role of the complement system in host defense, disease, and malnutrition. Nutrition 1998;14:391–398.
81. Chandra R. Nutrition and immunology: from the clinic to cellular biology and back again. Proc Nutr Soc 1999;58:681–683.
82. Chapuy M, Arlot M, Duboeuf F, et al. Vitamin D3 and calcium to prevent hip fractures in elderly women. N Engl J Med 1992;327:1637–1642.
83. Chapuy M, Arlot M, Delmas P, Meunier P. Effect of calcium and cholecalciferol treatment for three years on hip fractures in elderly women. BMJ 1994;308:1081–1082.

84. Dawson-Hughes B, Harris S, Krall E, Dallal G. Effect of calcium and vitamin D supplementation on bone density in men and women 65 years of age or older. N Engl J Med 1997;337:670–676.

85. Meunier P. Vitamin D insufficiency: reappraisal of its definition threshold and bone consequences. In: Burckhardt P, Dawson-Hughes B, Heaney R (eds.). Nutritional Aspects of Osteoporosis. Academic, San Diego, 2001, pp. 167–172.

86. Casteels K, Bouillon R, Waer M, Mathieu C. Immunomodulatory effects of 1,25-dihydroxyvitamin D3. Curr Opin Nephrol Hypertens 1995;4:313–318.

87. Deluca H, Cantorna M. Vitamin D: its role and uses in immunology. FASEB J 2001;15:2579–2585.

88. Lemire J. 1,25-Dihydroxyvitamin D3: a hormone with immunomodulatory preperties. Z Rheumatol 2000;59S1:24–27.

89. Muller K, Bendtzen K. 1,25-Dihydroxyvitamin D3 as a natural regulator of human immune functions. J Investig Dermatol Symp Proc 1996;1:68–71.

90. Lemire J. Immunomodulatory actions of 1,25-dihydroxyvitamin D3. J Steroid Biochem Mol Biol 1995;53:599–602.

91. Cantorna M. Vitamin D and autoimmunity: is vitamin D status an enviromental factor affecting autoimmune disease prevalence? Proc Soc Exp Biol Med 2000;223:230–233.

92. Segawa Y, Tsuzuike N, Tagashira E, Yamaguchi M. Preventive effects of beta-alanyl-L-histidinato zinc on the deterioration of bone metabolism in ovariectomized rats. Biol Pharm Bull 1993;16:486–489.

93. Kishi S, Segawa Y, Yamaguchi M. Histomorphological confirmation of the preventive effect of beta-alanyl-L-histidinato zinc on bone loss in ovariectomized rats. Biol Pharm Bull 1994;17:862–865.

94. Seco C, Revilla M, Hernandez E, et al. Effects of zinc supplementation on vertebral and femoral bone mass in rats on strenous treadmill training exercise. J Bone Miner Res 1998;13:508–512.

95. Eberle J, Schmidmayer S, Erben R, Stangassinger M, Roth H. Skeletal effects of zinc deficiency in growing rats. J Trace Elem Med Biol 1999;13:21–26.

96. Igarashi A, Yamaguchi M. Increase in bone protein components with healing rat fractures: enhancement by zinc treatment. Int J Mol Med 1999;4:615–620.

97. Igarashi A, Yamaguchi M. Stimulatory effect of zinc acexamate administration on fracture healing of the femoral-diaphyseal tissues in rats. Gen Pharmacol 1999;32:463–469.

98. Yamaguchi M. beta-Alanyl-L-histidinato zinc and bone resorption. Gen Pharmacol 1995;26:1179–1183.

99. Igarashi A, Yamaguchi M. Increase in bone growth factors with healing rat fractures: the enhancing effect of zinc. Int J Mol Med 2001;8:433–438.

100. Atik O. Zinc and senile osteoporosis. J Am Geriatr Soc 1983;31:790–791.

101. Angus R, Sambrook P, Pocock N, Eisman J. Dietary intake and bone mineral density. Bone Miner 1988;43:265–277.

102. New S, Bolton-Smith C, Grubb D, Reid D. Nutritional influences on bone mineral density: a cross-sectional study in premenopausal women. Am J Clin Nutr 1997;65:1831–1839.

103. Elmstahl S, Gullberg B, Janzon L, Johnell O, Elmstahl B. Increased incidence of fractures in middle-aged and elderly men with low intakes of phosphorus and zinc. Osteoporos Int 1998;8:333–340.

104. Strause L, Saltman P, Smith K, Bracker M, Andon M. Spinal bone loss in postmenopausal women supplemented with calcium and trace minerals. J Nutr 1994;124:1060–1064.

105. Sugiyama T, Tanaka H, Kawai S. Improvement of periarticular osteoporosis in postmenopausal women with rheumatoid arthritis by beta-alanyl-L-histidinato zinc: a pilot study. J Bone Miner Metab 2000;18:335–338.

106. Tsunenari T, Fukase M, Fujita T. Bone histomorphometric analysis for the cause of osteopenia in vitamin C-deficient rat (ODS rat). Calcif Tissue Int 1991;48:18–27.

107. Falch J, Mowe M, Bohmer T. Low levels of serum ascorbic acid in elderly patients with hip fracture. Scand J Clin Lab Invest 1998;58:225–228.

108. Morton D, Barrett-Connor E, Schneider D. Vitamin C supplement use and bone mineral density in postmenopausal women. J Bone Miner Res 2001;16:135–140.

109. Schnaid E, MacPhail A, Sweet M. Fractured neck of femur in black patients: a prospective study. J Bone Joint Surg Br 2000;82:872–875.

110. Leveille S, LaCroix A, Koepsell T, Beresford S, Van Belle G, Buchner D. Dietary vitamin C and bone mineral density in postmenopausal women in Washington State, USA. J Epidemiol Community Health 1997;51:479–485.

111. Simon J, Hudes E. Relation of ascorbic acid to bone mineral density and self-reported fractures among USA adults? Am J Epidemiol 2001;154:427–433.

112. Michaelsson K, Holmberg L, Mallmin H, et al. Diet and hip fracture risk: a case-control study. Study Group of the Multiple Risk Survey on Swedish Women for Eating Assessment. Int J Epidemiol 1995;24:771–782.

113. Wang M, Luz Villa M, Marcus R, Kelsey J. Associations of vitamin C, calcium and protein with bone mass in postmenopausal Mexican American women. Osteoporos Int 1997;7:533–538.

114. Hall S, Greendale G. The relation of dietary vitamin C intake in bone mineral density: results from the PEPI study. Calcif Tissue Int 1998;63:183–189.

115. Melhus H, Michaelsson K, Holmberg L, Wolk A, Ljunghall S. Smoking, antioxidant vitamins, and the risk of hip fracture. J Bone Miner Res 1999;14:129–135.

116. Jonas J, Burns J, Abel E, Cresswell M, Strain J, Paterson C. Impaired mechanical strength of bone in experimental copper deficiency. Ann Nutr Metab 1993;37:245–252.

117. Yee C, Kubena K, Walker M, Champney T, Sampson H. The relationship of nutritional copper to the development of postmenopausal osteoporosis in rats. Biol Trace Elem Res 1995;48:1–11.

118. Rico H, Roca-Botran C, Hernandez E, et al. The effect of supplemental copper on osteopenia induced by ovariectomy in rats. Menopause 2000;7:413–416.

119. Whitelaw A, Armstrong R, Evans C, Fawcett A. A study of the effects of copper deficiency in Scottish blackface lambs on improved hill pasture. Vet Rec 1979;104:455–460.

120. Allen T, Manoli A II, LaMont R. Skeletal changes associated with copper deficiency. Clin Orthop 1982;168:206–210.

121. Conlan D, Korula R, Tallentire D. Serum copper levels in elderly patients with femoral-neck fractures. Age Ageing 1990;19:212–214.

122. Forsyth K, Watson R, Gensler H. Osteotoxicity after chronic dietary administration af 13-cis-retinoic acid, retinyl palmitate or selenium in mice exposed to tumor initiation and promotion. Life Sci 1989;45:2149–2156.

123. Hough S, Avioli L, Muir H, et al. Effects of hypervitaminosis A on the bone and mineral metabolism of the rat. Endocrinology 1988;122:2933–2939.

124. Soeta S, Mori R, Kodaka T, Naito Y, Taniguchi K. Histological disorders related to the focal disappearance of the epiphyseal growth plate in rats induced by high dose of vitamin A. J Vet Med Sci 2000;62:293–299.

125. Kaji H, Sugimoto T, Kanatani M, Fukase M, Kumegawa M, Chihara K. Retinoic acid induces osteoclast-like cell formation by directly acting on hemopoietic blast cells and stimulates osteopontin mRNA expression in isolated osteoclasts. Life Sci 1995;56:1903–1913.

126. Colucci S, Grano M, Mori G, et al. Retinoic acid induces cell proliferation and modulates gelatinases activity in human ostoclast-like cell lines. Biochem Biophys Res Commun 1996;227:47–52.

127. Johansson S, Melhus H. Vitamin A antagonizes calcium response to vitamin D in man. J Bone Miner Res 2001;16:1899–1905.

128. Sowers M, Wallace R. Retinol, supplemental vitamin A and bone status. J Clin Epidemiol 1990;43:693–699.

129. Binkley N, Krueger D. Hypervitaminosis A and bone. Nutr Rev 2000;58:138–144.

130. Feskanich D, Singh V, Willet W, Colditz G. Vitamin A intake and hip fractures among postmenopausal women. JAMA 2002;287:47–54.

131. Melhus H, Michaelsson K, Kindmark A, et al. Excessive dietary intake of vitamin A is associated with reduced bone mineral density and increased risk of hip fracture. Ann Intern Med 1998;129:770–778.

132. Whiting S, Lemke B. Excess retinol intake may explain the high incidence of osteoporosis in northern Europe. Nutr Rev 1999;57:192–195.

133. Ballew C, Galuska D, Gillespie C. High serum retinyl esters are not associated with reduced bone mineral density in the Third National Health and Nutrition Examination Survey, 1988–1994. J Bone Miner Res 2001;16:2306–2312.

134. Kawahara T, Krueger D, Engelke J, Harke J, Binkley N. Short-term vitamin A supplementation does not affect bone turnover in men. J Nutr 2002;1169–1172.

135. Promislow J, Goodman-Gruen D, Slymen D, Barrett-Connor E. Retinol intake and bone mineral density in the elderly: the Rancho Bernardo Study. J Bone Miner Res 2002;17:1349–1358.

136. Rude R, Kirchen M, Gruber H, Stasky A, Meyer M. Magnesium deficiency induces bone loss in the rat. Miner Electrolyte Metab 1998;24:314–320.
137. Riond J, Hartmann P, Steiner P, et al. Long-term excessive magnesium supplementation is deleterious whereas suboptimal supply is beneficial for bones in rats. Magnes Res 2000;13:249–264.
138. Rude R, Olerich M. Magnesium deficiency: possible role in osteoporosis associated with gluten-sensitive enteropathy. Osteoporos Int 1996;6:453–461.
139. Abbott L, Nadler J, Rude R. Magnesium deficiency in alcoholism: possible contribution to osteoporosis and cardiovascular disease in alcoholics. Alcohol Clin Exp Res 1994;18:1076–1082.
140. New S, Bolton-Smith C, Grubb D, Reid D. Nutritional influences on bone mineral density: a cross-sectional study in premenopausal women. Am J Clin Nutr 1997;65:1831–1839.
141. Angus R, Sambrook P, Pocock N, Eisman J. Dietary intake and bone mineral density. Bone Miner 1988;4:265–277.
142. Tranquilli A, Lucino E, Garzetti G, Romanini C. Calcium, phosphorus and magnesium intakes correlate with bone mineral content in postmenopausal women. Gynecol Endocrinol 1994;8:55–58.
143. Tucker K, Hannan M, Chen H, Cupples L, Wilson P, Kiel D. Potassium, magnesium and fruit and vegetable intakes are associated with greater bone mineral density in elderly men and women. Am J Clin Nutr 1999;69:727–736.
144. Tucker K, Hannan M, Kiel D. The acid-base hypothesis: diet and bone in the Framingham Osteoporosis Study. Eur J Nutr 2001;40:231–237.
145. Dimai H, Porta S, Wirnsberger G, et al. Daily oral magnesium supplementation suppresses bone turnover in young adult males. J Clin Endocrinol Metab 1998;83:2742–2748.
146. Stendig-Lindberg G, Tepper R, Leichter I. Trabecular bone density in a two year controlled trial of peroral magnesium in osteoporosis. Magnes Res 1993;6:155–163.
147. Galland L. Magnesium and immune function: an overview. Magnesium 1988;7:290–299.
148. Yangou M, Hadjipetrou-Kourounakis L. Effect of magnesium deficiency on interleukin production by Fisher rats: effect of interleukins on reduced in vitro lymphocyte responses to concanavalin A and lipopolysaccharide. Int Arch Allergy Appl Immunol 1989;89:217–221.
149. Stankiewicz M, Migdalska A, Bankowska E, Jeska E. Complement activation, phagocytosis, tumor growth and parasitic infection after magnesium supplementation in diet of mice. Magnesium 1989;8:87–93.
150. Johnson S. The multifaceted and widespread pathology of magnesium deficiency. Med Hypotheses 2001;56:163–170.
151. Malpuech-Brugere C, Nowacki W, Daveau M, et al. Inflammatory response following acute magnesium deficiency in the rat. Biochim Biophys Acta 2000;1501:91–98.
152. Mak I, Dickens B, Komarov A, Wagner T, Phillips T, Weglicki W. Activation of the neutrophil and loss of plasma glutathione during Mg deficiency: modulation by nitric oxid synthase inhibition. Mol Cell Biochem 1997;176:35–39.

16 HIV Infection

Marianna K. Baum
and Adriana Campa

1. INTRODUCTION

HIV has become a major threat to populations throughout the world. The number of fatalities from this pandemic surpasses those of any war in the history of humankind. During 2001, more than 5 million people worldwide were newly infected with the virus. It is estimated that during the next 10 yr, if there are no effective treatments, more than 20 million people will die from this epidemic *(1)*. During the last 20 yr, HIV has been extensively studied, including the relationship between HIV infection and nutrition. Nutritional status affects the course of the infection from the onset, during latency, and its progression to AIDS, as well as throughout the course of opportunistic infections *(2–19)*. Nutritional therapy is critical in settings where antiretroviral therapies are not available *(19)*, as well as an adjunct to the combination antiretroviral drugs to support and maintain both the acquired and the innate nonspecific aspects of host defenses *(20)*.

Infections, no matter how mild, have a deleterious effect on nutritional status, and, in turn, nutrient deficiency, especially when sufficiently severe, impairs resistance to infection. Nutritional deficiency further burdens the already compromised immune system in the patient with HIV. The synergistic interaction between infection, nutritional status and immune function is particularly evident in patients with AIDS, who exhibit impaired immune function and altered nutritional status *(20)*. Micronutrient deficiencies, which influence immune function, are prevalent even before the development of HIV symptoms. Several studies indicate that alterations in nutritional status are widespread among various HIV-infected cohorts *(3,9,21,22)*. Decreased plasma levels of zinc, selenium, and vitamins B_6, B_{12}, A, and E are evident and are functionally relevant in maintaining the immune response integrity *(21,23–25)*.

Adequate nourishment is critical for individuals who are HIV positive. The gut is a major target for AIDS-related diseases, with conditions such as diarrhea, oral and esophageal candidiasis, dysphagia, and odynophagia further complicating the nutritional imbalances in patients who are infected with HIV. Nutrient deficiencies, whether derived from insufficient diet, anorexia, malabsorption, or increased nutrient requirements, lower host defenses, leaving the host susceptible to a range of opportunistic infections. Nutritional supplementation is needed to overcome nutritional deficiencies and ease the immune suppression caused by HIV *(26)*.

From: *Diet and Human Immune Function*
Edited by: D. A. Hughes, L. G. Darlington, and A. Bendich © Humana Press Inc., Totowa, NJ

Both macronutrients and micronutrients are important in managing HIV infection. Calorie-yielding nutrients are critical to prevent and treat wasting, which is still the most common AIDS-defining symptom in many countries *(27)* and strongly associated with rapid disease progression and death *(28–30)*.

2. THE HIV VIRUS

The nutritional interactions between HIV and its human host are apparent early in the viral life cycle. HIV is shaped like a sphere filled by viral protein and two identical RNA strands within its core. In the outer envelope, virally encoded glycoproteins (gp) 41 and 120 protrude from a bilayer of host-derived phospholipids. Glycoprotein 120 binds to the receptors on the host CD4+ T lymphocytes, macrophages, and follicular dendritic cells to enter these cells. After a complex process of cellular penetration, viral RNA is transcribed by reverse transcriptase enzymes into provirus DNA and subsequently incorporated into the host cell's nuclear DNA *(20)*.

Once inside the host cells, the virus replicates rapidly and is disseminated into the blood and tissues. The initial infection causes flu-like symptoms within 2–6 wk of infection. Within approx 3 mo, the initial high viral load is curtailed by host HIV-antibodies, and the disease enters a latency state. This stage can persist for many years, depending on numerous internal and external factors, and affects both the virus and the human host. Viral factors that can affect the course of the disease include the strain and subtype of the virus, its virulence, regulatory or structural genes, and the magnitude of viral sequestration into sanctuaries (macrophages, dendritic cells, lymph nodes, and other tissues). Host factors that affect the progression of the disease include age, gender, lifestyle, coexisting disease conditions, exposure to infections, alcohol, tobacco and drug use, and nutritional status at the onset and during the course of the disease *(20)*.

The latency period, although clinically asymptomatic, is marked by hypermetabolism, which is caused by an intense generation of additional HIV copies and the continuous effort of the immune system to eradicate the virus and maintain the function and number of circulating immune cells, particularly CD4+ T lymphocytes. The hypermetabolism is also evidenced by increased energy expenditure and fat oxidation rates *(31)*, as well as accelerated depletion of vitamins and minerals *(3)*.

As HIV disease progresses, there are measurable CD4+ T cell losses, as well as an increase in viral burden (the amount of virus present in the host) associated with clinical evidence of disease progression *(32)*. This progression is also accompanied by a loss of body weight: 5% loss predicts the onset of opportunistic infections and progression toward AIDS, and 10% involuntary loss of body weight is an AIDS-defining condition (wasting syndrome) *(30)*.

Chronic diarrhea in HIV disease is usually caused by secondary infectious agents, such as cryptosporidia, microsporidia, salmonella, and cytomegalovirus *(33,34)*. Diarrhea contributes to the loss of body weight in HIV infection with concomitant losses of sodium, potassium, bicarbonate, proteins, fats, vitamins, and minerals. In addition, anorexia, abnormal taste sensation, oral lesions, and the numerous medications that are usually consumed by patients with HIV infection, contribute to a decrease in food intake. Wasting syndrome is usually initiated by secondary infections, which occur as a consequence of low CD4+ T-cell count (CD4 cell counts) and increased viral burden, which are accompanied by the secretion of proinflammatory cytokines and hypermetabolism.

Depletion of lean body mass by 10% or more is critical, because lean body mass represents balanced and readily available mixtures of amino acids.

Although nutritional interventions can prevent or alleviate the added immunosuppressive burden imposed by malnutrition on the immune suppression already caused by HIV, the secondary infections must be treated before nutritional repletion of lean body mass is possible. Although adequate or aggressive nutrition—as might be needed to counteract nutrient deficiencies produced by HIV progression—will not cure HIV, when combined with antiretroviral medications, it is a critical life-prolonging therapy component.

3. MACRONUTRIENTS AND HIV/AIDS

Malnutrition in HIV-1 infection is characterized by protein-energy malnutrition accompanied by micronutrient abnormalities, which may persist even after administering effective antiretroviral treatments. Although there is a low prevalence of wasting among individuals infected with HIV who receive the most recent antiretroviral therapies (35–37), nutritional abnormalities persist and some, such as dyslipidemias, may be directly related to the use of specific types of antiretroviral drugs. Even a modest weight loss of 5% of total weight has been associated with a shorter survival time, independent of CD4 cell counts (38,39).

3.1. Wasting

Both forms of undernutrition, starvation and wasting, may exist or coexist in a patient living with HIV. Starvation may be caused by anorexia produced by medications, opportunistic infections, proinflammatory cytokines, and psychosocial factors, or may be produced by an inability to eat adequate amounts of food because of economic factors, fatigue, neurological factors, and opportunistic diseases related to diarrhea and malabsorption. Wasting in HIV is manifested by rapid weight loss, secondary to systemic infections and tumors, and is frequently accompanied by a hypermetabolic state. In wasting or cachexia, as defined by Kotler (40), rapid wasting of some muscle groups is visible and, when sustained, leads to protein depletion.

Macronutrient status refers to the proportion of protein and fat compartments in the body. In the early studies, low serum proteins, hemoglobin, and muscle wasting provided evidence of protein deficiency in the patients with AIDS (41). Kotler and colleagues, using a four-compartment model, found that the body cell mass was disproportionately depleted when compared to fat mass (42). In further studies, Kotler's group demonstrated that approximately half of the weight difference between groups of men with and without HIV infection could be ascribed to differences in skeletal muscle mass (43).

The most common dyslipidemias reported before the advent of the highly active antiretroviral therapy (HAART) were hypocholesterolemia and hypertriglyceridemia (44). After the HAART initiation, weight loss, especially in women, has been characterized by a more predominant loss of body fat (37,45). With the successful institution of HAART, wasting is rare, but continuous, although slow, loss of lean body mass, along with other nutritional alterations, has been reported, such as truncal obesity with persistent muscle wasting, buffalo hump, and marked hypertriglyceridemia and hypercholesterolemia, sometimes accompanied by hypertension and abnormal glucose tolerance (36,37).

High calorie and protein diets are used to forestall wasting and promote caloric repletion in patients with HIV. Findings from studies on the effectiveness of these treatments
are contradictory, mostly because of disease stage and the type of the treatment. Keithley
and colleagues *(46)* followed 90 people with HIV who were asymptomatic for 1 yr, and
supplemented them with either standard (Ensure Plus) or immune-enhanced (Advera)
formulas and compared them to a control group. Among the three groups, they found no
significant differences in body weight, bioelectrical impedance analysis, daily caloric
intake, or serum albumin *(46)*. In contrast, results of other hypercaloric feeding studies
that included appetite stimulants indicate that weight gain is possible but that the weight
gained is predominantly fat *(37)*. To restore body cell mass and achieve gains in skeletal
muscle, the physician and the patient must carefully monitor body weight to evaluate
changes, as well as establish effective prophylactic and therapeutic nutritional support
that provides calorie and protein replenishment, in conjunction with anabolic agents,
resistance exercise programs, and cytokine inhibitors *(37,47)*. Early diagnosis and treatment of wasting improves quality of life, reduces frequency of opportunistic diseases,
and decreases events requiring hospitalization *(47,48)*.

4. MICRONUTRIENT DEFICIENCY AND HIV/AIDS

The immune system requires several essential micronutrients to effectively resist
infectious agents. Insufficient intakes or stores of these micronutrients may inhibit the
ability to resist infections. Several vitamins and minerals may play a significant role in
HIV disease progression. Micronutrients that are relevant for maintaining immune function and are associated with HIV-1 disease progression are the B vitamins, iron, and
antioxidant nutrients, including vitamins A, C, and E and trace minerals selenium and
zinc *(2–19,21,26,49,50)*.

4.1. HIV and the Water-Soluble Vitamins

Several of the water-soluble vitamins have been linked with immune defects. Thiamin,
Riboflavin, and niacin deficiencies, which are part of the coenzymes in the tricarboxylic
acid (TCA) cycle, are manifested by lack of energy, a symptom common in HIV-infection. These deficiencies are aggravated by hypermetabolism during the course of the
disease, malabsorption, and anorexia. Deficiencies of the energy-releasing vitamins thiamin, riboflavin, and niacin are present in individuals with HIV, even in early asymptomatic states *(3)*.

Low plasma levels of vitamins B_6 and B_{12} are widespread in HIV infection *(3)*. Approximately half of the patients with HIV/AIDS have deficient vitamin B_6 levels, which are
associated with decreased natural killer (NK) cell activity; one fourth have deficient
vitamins B_2 and B_{12} levels; and two thirds have deficient folate levels *(51)*. Patients who
are HIVpositive require supplementation of B vitamins in multiples of the recommended
dietary allowance (RDA) to achieve normal plasma levels.

4.1.1. VITAMIN B_6

Vitamin B_6 deficiency is prevalent in individuals who are HIV positive, even those
who appear to have an adequate vitamin B_6 dietary intake. Decreased lymphocyte mitogen responsiveness and reduced NK-cell cytotoxicity were noted in subjects who were
vitamin B_6 deficient when compared to those whose vitamin B_6 status was normalized

(52). In addition, there is a strong association between vitamin B_6 levels and altered neuro-psychiatric function, and this deficiency may be an important cofactor contributing to the level of depression in individuals who are HIV infected *(53).* Both deficiency and excessive supplementation of vitamin B_6 significantly alter antibody production, specifically with immunoglobulin (Ig)G and IgE isotypes. Under deficiency conditions, alanine aminotransferase activity decreases, and cathepsin B activity is suppressed, inhibiting antibody production *(54).*

In individuals who are HIVnegative, vitamin B_6 deficiency decreases cell-mediated responses, including depression of interleukin (IL)-2 production and lymphocyte proliferation. In HIV infection, vitamin B_6 deficiency also diminishes the cellular immune response, delayed type hypersensitivity (DTH), lymphocyte proliferation, CD4+ lymphocyte cell numbers, and NK-cell activity *(55).*

4.1.2. VITAMIN B_{12}

Vitamin B_{12} deficiencies occur more commonly in persons with HIV disease or AIDS than in those without HIV. The prevalence of vitamin B_{12} deficiency has been estimated to be between 12% and 30% in several cohorts with HIV *(3,16,56,57).* Harriman and colleagues *(56)* found low vitamin B_{12} levels in 15% of an unselected sample of 121 persons with AIDS and 7% of 27 people with HIV without AIDS. In a Miami, Florida, cohort of HIV-positive men who had sex with men (MSM), 12% had overly low plasma vitamin B_{12} levels, despite being in the early stages of HIV disease and consuming adequate diets *(3).* In a sample of 49 patients with HIV who were symptomatic and referred for neurological evaluation, Kieburtz and colleagues *(58)* reported a 20% prevalence of vitamin B_{12} deficiency. This deficiency was associated with both peripheral neuropathy and myelopathy. The majority of the patients with a vitamin B_{12} deficiency with peripheral neuropathy who were treated with cyanocobalamin showed a therapeutic improvement *(58).* The low plasma vitamin B_{12} levels are related to abnormalities in plasma-binding proteins in the early stages of the disease, to frequent diarrhea, and to intestinal malabsorption in later stages of HIV infection.

During an 18-mo observational study of HIV+ homosexual men in Miami, a significant association was found between vitamin B_{12} deficiency and a decline in CD4 cell count ($p = 0.037$), whereas vitamin B_{12} normalization was significantly associated with higher CD4 cell count ($p = .006$). These findings were unaffected by zidovudine use. In this study, deficient plasma vitamin B_{12} levels significantly predicted accelerated HIV disease progression as determined by CD4 cell count ($p = .04$) and the AIDS index ($p = .005$) *(21).* HIV-1 seropositive drug users with low plasma levels of vitamin B_{12} exhibited a dramatically increased risk for HIV-1-related mortality (RR = 8.33, $p < .009$), independent of CD4 cell count <200 at baseline and CD4 over time *(5).* In accordance with these findings, other investigators have reported a nearly twofold increase in risk of progression to AIDS in subjects with HIV-1 infection with low serum vitamin B_{12} concentrations *(16).* Tamura and coworkers *(59)* reported that normalization of vitamin B_{12} deficiency to adequate plasma levels by supplementing methyl-cobalamin was associated with an increase in CD4/CD8 ratio and restoration of NK-cell activity. Partial restoration of NK-cell activity occurred after only 14 d of treatment, and complete normalization was obtained after 1–2 yr of the methyl-cobalamin therapy. The effect of cobalamin on morbidity and mortality could be related to cobalamin's ability to modify productive HIV-1 infection *(60),* possibly by DNA methylation *(61).*

Research by Herbert and colleagues *(62)* has detailed some of the mechanisms involved in vitamin B_{12} malabsorption in HIV infection. By assessing levels of holotrascobalamin II, they found evidence of negative vitamin B_{12} balance and vitamin B_{12} deficiency in 52 of 95 patients who were HIV positive, 79 of whom had normal serum vitamin B_{12} levels (above 250 pg/mL). Negative vitamin B_{12} balance was found in patients with serum levels as high as 500–749 pg/mL, evidenced by low levels of cobalamin binding.

Cognitive changes in HIV and AIDS, commonly referred to as AIDS dementia complex, are evidenced by cognitive, behavioral, and motor function abnormalities. Although AIDS dementia is most commonly seen in end-stage AIDS, neurologic symptoms are the first evidence of AIDS in 10% of patients *(63)*. A significant association was found between low serum vitamin B_{12} levels and cognitive deficits in information processing speed and visual-spatial problem-solving skills *(50)*. Serum vitamin B_{12} levels alone were not 100% sensitive or specific. Some patients who had neurologic symptoms of vitamin B_{12} deficiency and responded to vitamin B_{12} therapy had normal vitamin B_{12} levels, and conversely, not all patients with low vitamin B_{12} levels received benefit from replenishment therapy *(64)*. Because vitamin B_{12} deficiency is strongly related to the development of abnormalities of the fetal nervous system, vitamin B_{12} supplementation should be encouraged for pregnant women with HIV *(65)*.

As with other nutrient deficiencies in patients with HIV, vitamin B_{12} deficiency could result from decreased intake, or possibly malabsorption, resulting from direct infection of the ileum. Compared to patients with HIV with normal serum vitamin B_{12} levels, those with decreased vitamin B_{12} serum levels had metabolic and clinical disturbances, including low hemoglobin, leukocytes, and CD4/CD8 ratio. Several investigators *(4,16,50,55)* proposed that change in vitamin B_{12} concentration is a strong predictor of HIV disease progression to AIDS and that HIV disease progression may be delayed by vitamin B_{12} supplementation.

4.1.3. FOLATE

Reports regarding folate status in patients who are HIV positive are inconsistent. Several studies have reported folate deficiency, whereas others found high folate levels in patients with HIV. High levels of supplementation in the normal or high folate groups might explain this discrepancy. Herbert and colleagues *(62)* reported that 33% of patients who are HIV infected in their study had low serum folate, suggesting negative folate balance; 18% had low red cell folate, suggesting tissue folate depletion; and 4% had evidence of severe tissue depletion. The significance of either the high or the low folate levels in HIV infection, however, has not been elucidated.

4.1.4. VITAMIN A

The relationship between vitamin A deficiency and increased morbidity and mortality from infectious diseases has been documented since early in the last century *(66–69)*. Cross-sectional studies of vitamin A status and infectious disease in developing countries have demonstrated an increased incidence of respiratory infections and diarrhea in children with hypovitaminosis A *(69)*. Supplementation with vitamin A decreases mortality in measles *(66)*, reduces the morbidity from malaria *(72)*, and diminishes acute lower respiratory infections *(68)*. Fawzi and colleagues *(73)* performed a meta-analysis of several clinical trials of vitamin A supplementation and concluded that such supplementation reduced infant and child mortality by approx 30%. Another recent meta-analysis of randomized controlled trials indicated that vitamin A supplementation significantly reduced the incidence of croup by 47%, otitis media by 74%, and the duration of diarrhea, pneumonia, hospital stays, and fever. Vitamin A supplementation also had a beneficial effect on morbidity associated with measles (74). The differences in vitamin A efficacy in reducing total mortality and complications from measles across various studies most likely result from the effectiveness of vitamin A supplementation in populations suffering from varying nutritional deficiencies, as well as other infectious diseases (75).

Vitamin A deficiency is associated with epithelial damage in the respiratory tract, the gastrointestinal (GI) tract, the urinary tract, the vagina, and possibly the inner ear, increasing susceptibility to infections (76). In addition, vitamin A deficiency impairs the cytolytic activity of NK cells, reduces mitogen-stimulation response by lymphocytes, alters cytokine responses, and reduces serologic response to vaccines (77–79). Moreover, the inflammatory and acute-phase response to infections may alter the transport and metabolism of vitamin A and produce increased excretion of retinol, aggravating the nutritional deficiency (79). Deficiency of β-carotene, a provitamin A with antioxidant activity, may impair the antioxidant defenses needed to prevent oxidative damage during infection (80).

Vitamin A deficiency is prevalent in HIV-1 infection, as reported by several investigators (3,13,81,82), and vitamin A status is associated with disease progression and mortality (13,15,21,23). An observational study of women who were HIV seropositive in Rwanda found that vitamin A deficiency is associated with a rapid progression to AIDS, compared to those with normal vitamin A status (83). Maternal vitamin A deficiency has also been associated with increased HIV mother-to-child transmission (81) and more rapid HIV disease progression in infants born to these infected mothers, independent from maternal viral load and CD4 cell count during pregnancy (84). Although a U.S. study found no association between vitamin A deficiency and vertical HIV-1 transmission (85), it has been hypothesized that vitamin A deficiency in nutritionally deprived populations may have a role in mother-to-child HIV-1 transmission by impairing membrane integrity and allowing increased HIV vaginal shedding and higher HIV load in breast milk (86,87).

4.1.4.1. VITAMIN A SUPPLEMENTATION IN HIV

Although the observational studies largely indicated a strong relationship between vitamin A deficiency, mother-to-child HIV-1 transmission, increased HIV-1 disease progression, and mortality, vitamin A supplementation trials have been inconsistent. Fawzi and colleagues (19,88) conducted a randomized double-blind placebo-controlled trial to investigate the effects of vitamin A or multivitamin supplementation on HIV-1 disease progression and on birth outcomes in 1075 pregnant women in Tanzania. Compared to multivitamin supplementation (the B vitamins and vitamins E and C), which decreased the risk of fetal death, low birth weight, preterm birth, and small size for gestational age, vitamin A supplementation did not affect any of these parameters. In addition, multivitamin supplementation increased CD4 and CD8 cell counts in the pregnant women in a sustained manner, whereas vitamin A had no effect on T-cell counts. Another report from this trial demonstrated that neither the multivitamins nor vitamin A supplementation had an effect on the risk of vertical transmission of HIV-1 in utero, during the intrapartum, or during the early breast-feeding periods *(89)*. A more recent report by these investigators, however, showed that vitamin A supplementation increased the risk of HIV-1 transmission if the supplementation was conducted throughout the breast-feeding period (RR = 1.38, 95% CI (1.09–1.76) p = .009), although supplementation with the B vitamins and vitamins C and E reduced transmission through breast-feeding *(88)*.

In accordance with this study, a South African investigation of vitamin A supplementation conducted by Coutsoudis and colleagues *(90)* in 728 pregnant women with HIV infection also did not find a decline in risk of mother-to-child HIV transmission. Women receiving vitamin A supplementation, however, were less likely to have a preterm delivery, and when those supplemented women delivered a preterm infant, the infants were less likely to be vertically infected than those born from infected women in the placebo group. Moreover, the vitamin A supplementation was associated with improved weight retention after pregnancy in women whose baseline CD4+ count was less than 200 cells/ μL, and serum retinol 0–20 μ/dL.

A recent report of a large controlled clinical trial in Malawi supports the findings from Tanzania and South Africa. The trial in Malawi included 697 pregnant women who were HIV-1 seropositive to determine whether vitamin A supplementation could prevent anemia, low birth weight, growth failure, HIV vertical transmission, and mortality. The vitamin A-supplemented group delivered higher birth weight infants and had fewer low-birth-weight and anemic infants at 6 wk postpartum compared to those who were given placebo. Vitamin A supplementation also did not affect mother-to-child HIV transmission perinatally in this trial *(91,92)*.

A large database review combining the vitamin A supplementation trials in pregnant women who were HIV-1 seropositive concluded that vitamin A supplementation does not have an advantage in preventing mother-to-child HIV-1 transmission *(93)*, although the majority of the studies have demonstrated benefits in other pregnancy outcomes, such as birth weight and infant morbidity and mortality *(94–96)*.

4.2. HIV and Vitamin E

Vitamin E is essential for adequate functioning of the immune system, as well as for its immunostimulatory properties *(97)*. Studies in both human and animal models have shown that supplementation with vitamin E equivalent to 2 to 10 times the recommended levels significantly increases humoral and cell-mediated immune responses to antigens and enhances phagocytic functions *(98,99)*. More specifically, high doses of vitamin E, along with a nutritionally adequate diet, have repeatedly enhanced in vitro and in vivo antibody production, phagocytosis, lymphoproliferative responses of the T helper (Th)1 type, and resistance to viral diseases *(99)*.

In patients with AIDS, malnutrition and wasting are common and frequently of multifactorial origins, including anorexia, malabsorption, impaired digestion, urinary losses, and altered metabolism. Any or all of these conditions may produce vitamin E deficiency reported in the late stages of HIV infection *(29,100)*. In a recent study using a murine AIDS-induced mouse model, the effects of dietary vitamin E supplementation on immune dysfunctions were examined. In this study, infected mice treated with vitamin E showed an increase in secretion of IL-2 and interferon (IFN)-γ and an improvement in mitogenesis of splenocyte and NK-cell activities compared with infected untreated mice. In addition, vitamin E supplementation was associated with a reduction in levels of IL-4, IL-

5, IL-6, and tumor necrosis factor (TNF)-α, cytokines of the Th2 subtype. This suggests that vitamin E supplementation may normalize some of the immune abnormalities observed in this animal model of retroviral infection *(101)*.

Another mechanism by which vitamin E may enhance immune function is through its antioxidant properties. Rapidly proliferating cells of the immune system are highly susceptible to peroxides *(98)*. Vitamin E acts as a free-radical scavenger and prevents the lipid peroxidation of cell membranes. Vitamin E also modulates the production of prostaglandin E_2 (PGE_2) in the body. Elevated PGE_2 levels decrease the differentiation of T and B lymphocytes and increase the differentiation of PGE_2-receptor-bearing T cells into T-suppressor cells. PGE_2 also inhibits NK cell activation, which is a major source of IFN-γ. In animal studies, downregulation of PGE_2 by vitamin E has increased IL-2 and IFN-γ production, two important cytokines in the Th1 subtype response *(102,103)*.

Other proposed actions of vitamin E on the immune system are the result of its direct interaction with microphages, causing upregulation of IL-1 and IL-2 and, through its antioxidant properties, reducing TNF-α levels. Thus, in addition to its role as a free-radical scavenger, the effect of vitamin E on the regulation of various cytokines that favors the Th1 cytokine response is believed to play a major role in inhibiting HIV-1 replication.

In HIV infection, high doses of vitamin E have reduced the CD8+ T-cell number, increase the CD4+/CD8+ ratio and total lymphocyte count, and stimulate cytotoxic and NK-cell activity, phagocytosis of macrophages, and the mitogenic response *(24)*. Low serum vitamin E levels in individuals who are HIV-1 infected have been correlated with a higher degree of lipid peroxidation *(104)*, increased p24 antigenemia *(105)*, decreased plasma levels of polyunsaturated fatty acids (PUFAs), and increased plasma IgE levels *(106)*. Tang and colleagues *(26)* found that subjects in the highest quartile of serum tocopherol levels demonstrated a significant decrease in risk of progression to AIDS compared to the lower three quartiles combined and that high serum vitamin E levels were strongly associated with current use of multi- or single-vitamin E supplements. These combined findings indicate that vitamin E supplementation may be beneficial in delaying HIV disease progression. Vitamin E supplementation trials in HIV-1 individuals infected with HIV should be considered because of the nontoxic nature of this vitamin, its potential therapeutic effects, and the known response of serum levels to supplementation.

4.3. HIV and Iron

In infection, iron is sequestered from plasma into storage depots and is not used for synthesis of hemoglobin, consequently resulting in anemia *(107)*. Anemia is a common symptom of HIV infection and a prognostic marker of future disease progression or death, independent of CD4 count and viral load *(108)*. The etiology of anemia in HIV infection, however, is not only related to iron deficiency but also multifactorial, including deficiencies of protein; vitamins A, E, and B_{12}; folic acid; or a combination of them *(109)*, as well as a consequence of infections, neoplasms, blood loss, and medications. Low hemoglobin levels in patients with HIV are also associated with enhanced cellular immune activation, evidenced by increased IFN-γ, neopterin, and β2-microglobulin and with changes of iron metabolism. Thus, endogenous release of cytokines may be another underlying cause of anemia in HIV infection *(108)*.

The low hemoglobin level observed in HIV infection is paradoxically associated with high plasma ferritin levels, as well as iron accumulation in bone marrow, liver, macrophages, and brain and muscles cells (110). Elevated serum ferritin levels have been associated with more frequent infections and shorter survival times in patients with HIV infection (111). In reticulocytopenia, common in HIV-associated anemia, endogenous erythropoietin is low and a blunted erythropoietin feedback mechanism may contribute substantially to the prevalence of anemia in patients with HIV (112). Iron deficiency, however, is a common cause of anemia in HIV infection, particularly in children, because of the high prevalence of HIV infection in developing countries coinciding with high prevalence of malnutrition, primarily iron deficiency. In addition, in HIV infection, iron absorption and metabolism may be hindered by damage to the GI system by opportunistic infections, impaired hematopoietic processes, and intractable diarrhea characteristic of AIDS (109).

Treating severe anemia in patients with HIV-1 infection is critical, because recovery from anemia is associated with increased length of survival in these patients (113). Oral or parenteral therapy for anemia in children with iron deficiencies with HIV infection has resulted in an improved hemoglobin production (114). Blood transfusions and iron supplementation to treat HIV-related anemia without clear indication of iron deficiency, however, may activate HIV expression and facilitate disease progression. These observations are also supported by in vitro studies, which indicate that iron-mediated oxidative stress is likely to contribute to viral cytopathogenicity (115). Sappy and colleagues (116) demonstrated that nuclear factor (NF)-κB, a proviral transcription regulator, when activated by iron, could enhance the production of reactive iron species involved in oxidative stress, which may play an important role in enhancing HIV disease progression. This is consistent with the findings of Delanghe and colleagues (117), who described high levels of HIV RNA in haptoglobin 2 in two subjects who exhibited increased serum iron, higher transferrin saturation, and increased serum ferritin level. The oxidant nature of iron and its potential depressing effect on the immune system makes treatment with erythropoietin preferable to iron supplementation for HIV-related anemia, unless the patients have a clear evidence of iron deficiency.

Iron deficiency has been hypothesized to act synergistically with antiretroviral agents in inhibiting HIV-1 replication (118). To support this hypothesis, an in vitro study demonstrated that iron-chelating agents, such as deferoxamine, inhibit proliferation of HIV-infected mononuclear blood cells. Iron-chelating agents render iron catalytically inactive, an effect that may enhance the action of antiretroviral agents in HIV-infected individuals (119). In addition, iron withdrawal from participants with β-thalassemia is associated with protection against progression to AIDS (120). Additional evidence indicates that an inadvertent simultaneous administration of low doses of oral iron with dapsone to prevent Pneumocystis carinii pneumonia in patients with HIV infection was associated with excess mortality (121). These concerns have created a dilemma about the practice of supplementing iron for anemia in individuals with HIV infection who are not among the vulnerable groups for developing iron-deficiency anemia (122). Although iron supplementation is the treatment of choice for iron-deficiency anemia, in HIV infection, the risks of supplementation must be weighed against the benefits (115). If there is a clear indication of iron deficiency using erythrocyte protoporphyrin, serum ferritin, and transferrin saturation assays, iron should be supplemented. Low hemoglobin, hematocrit, and serum iron are not sufficient indicators of iron deficiency in HIV infection. Recombinant human erythropoietin therapy, frequently used to treat anemia in HIV infection, may be a more effective and safer means of improving hemoglobin than either blood transfusions or iron supplementation *(108)*.

4.4. HIV and Selenium

The prevalence of selenium deficiency varies among various cohorts with HIV-1 infection between 7% and 33% and increases as the disease advances to AIDS *(9,22)*. Selenium status is predictive of HIV-related prognosis and survival *(5,17)*. In a cohort of chronic drug users with HIV-1 infection only selenium deficiency was an independent predictor of survival (RR = 10.8; 95% CI [2.37–49.2], $p < .002$) when joint effect of nutritional deficiencies that had singly predicted mortality was evaluated. This significant effect of selenium persisted when controlling for CD4 count <200 cells/mm^3 at baseline and CD4 count over time *(5)*. Among a cohort of MSM with HIV infection the odds ratio (OR) was 7.2 for the risk of low plasma selenium and mortality when controlled for age, race, and CD4 cell count <200 at baseline. Moreover, selenium deficiency was associated with a decreased length of survival of 31.4 mo, compared with 57.4 mo for those with normal plasma selenium levels *(9)*. Selenium deficiency in children with HIV-1 infection was associated with immune dysfunction *(123)* and decreased survival *(22)*. Selenium deficiency was also associated with increased vaginal HIV shedding in a study in Kenya *(124)*. Moreover, in our cohort of drug users with HIV infection in Miami, selenium status was significantly correlated with manifestations of herpes and with candida infections *(125)*. In addition, low plasma selenium levels constituted a significant risk for mycobacterial disease (RR = 3, $p = .015$), after controlling for antiretroviral treatment and CD4 cell count in a multivariate model *(126)*. These studies are particularly significant because these diseases have been associated with HIV-1 disease progression. The dramatic association of selenium status with HIV-related mortality and morbidity may be related to selenium's role not only in maintaining immune competence but also in modulating viral expression and protecting against the oxidative damage caused by the infection *(127–131)*.

4.4.1. Selenium and Immunity in HIV

The relationship between nutritional status and immunity is well-recognized *(132)*. In animal models, selenium deficiency impairs the ability of phagocytic neutrophils and macrophages to destroy antigens. In patients with HIV-1 infection, selenium deficiency has been significantly correlated with total lymphocyte counts. Plasma selenium levels have been positively correlated with CD4 cell counts and CD4/CD8 ratio and inversely correlated with β_2-microglobulin and thymidine-kinase activity *(133)*, whereas Spallholz *(134)* demonstrated a close relationship between selenium status and humoral immune response.

Selenium has an important role in affecting cytokine response. In in vitro models, selenium regulates IL-2 levels, a Th1 cytokine, which is responsible for the earliest and most rapid expansion of T lymphocytes. Moreover, the enhancement of IL-2 production by selenium is dose dependent. The process occurs through the increased expansion of high-affinity receptors *(135)*. In addition, selenium status also modulates TNF-α production, which is related to anorexia, cachexia, and Kaposi's sarcoma *(136)*. Selenium supplementation suppresses TNF-α-induced HIV replication. Although the role of selenium in the virus-TNF-α interaction has not been fully explained, selenoprotein synthesis in the glutathione and thioredoxin systems is implicated *(137)*. In addition, Look and colleagues *(133)* demonstrated in patients with HIV-infection that plasma selenium levels are inversely correlated with levels of soluble TNF-α type II receptors. Thus, selenium supplementation may potentially prevent some of the adverse effects of high TNF-α circulating levels observed in anorexia, wasting, and Kaposi's sarcoma. Additional evidence for a selenium-cytokine interaction has been provided by studies suggesting that selenium decreases neuropathogenesis through suppression of IL-induced HIV-1 replication, neuronal apoptosis, and a reduction of blood brain barrier damage *(133,137–139)*.

4.4.2. SELENIUM SUPPLEMENTATION

Studies of selenium supplementation have demonstrated the effectiveness of selenium as a chemopreventive agent and its low toxicity when used daily at nutritional levels (50–200 μg/d). A long-term double-blind placebo-selenium supplementation trial (200 μg selenium/d) in healthy study participants demonstrated a 51% reduction in total cancer mortality and a 41% reduction in total cancer incidence, including several sites, as compared to the placebo group *(140)*. In other studies, nutritional supplementation of selenium significantly reduces the incidence of primary liver cancer in China *(141)* and provides significantly greater resistance to Aflatoxin B1-induced carcinogenic damage in lymphocytes from healthy human subjects administered daily selenium *(142)*.

The evidence associating the high risk of HIV-related mortality with selenium deficiency underscores the importance of maintaining adequate selenium status in HIV infection *(5)*. Selenium acts as a chemopreventive agent *(143–145)*, suggesting that selenium supplementation may help to increase the enzymatic defense systems *(146)*. Selenium's immunostimulatory properties have been documented in animal supplementation studies *(147)* and in elderly subjects *(148)*, as well as in patients with chronic uremia, psoriatic lesions, and gut-failure syndrome *(149–151)*. Although studies in HIV/AIDS patients are limited and have only been conducted in small numbers of individuals, an improvement in general health has been described after daily selenium (80–400 μg) supplementation *(152–154)*, without apparent adverse effects *(152,153)*.

In a case study in a child with HIV/AIDS, Kavanaugh-McHugh and colleagues *(155)* described complications similar to some of the features of Keshan Disease in China *(156)*, a disease associated with selenium deficiency. After supplementating the child with selenium (4 μg/kg), the deficiency symptoms improved *(155)*.

Chronic HAART, rather than decreasing the importance of antioxidant chemoprevention, has created new research challenges for the role of antioxidants in HIV-1 disease. Low selenium levels have been associated with hyperglycemia in drug users with HIV infection receiving HAART therapy *(157)*, whereas thrompocytopenia is significantly related to selenium deficiency but not to HAART *(158)*. Lipodystrophy, hyperlipidemias, and insulin resistance in patients receiving HIV protease inhibitors *(159)* may increase the long-term risk of oxidative damage associated with development of atherosclerosis and coronary heart disease *(160)*. Supplementation of antioxidants, including selenium, may prove to be an important part of the ammunitions used to fight the catastrophic sequelae of the HIV disease and AIDS.

4.5. HIV and Zinc

The trace element zinc has long been recognized as an important factor for maintaining a healthy immune system. Zinc deficiency reduces generation of T cells, depresses humoral and cell-mediated immunity, and leads to lymphopenia and thymic atrophy, reduced capacity of macrophages to take up and kill parasites, and increased susceptibility to a greater number of infections *(161,162)*. Many of these immune responses generally correlate with the degree of zinc deficiency *(162–166)*, because adequate levels of zinc are necessary to activate lymphocytes *(167–169)*.

Zinc is the structural component of several essential proteins, including the hormone thymulin, which is needed for the formation of T lymphocytes *(170)*. In animals and humans, zinc deficiency results in a rapid and marked atrophy of the thymus, impaired cell-mediated cutaneous sensitivity, and lymphopenia. Primary and secondary antibody responses are reduced in zinc deficiency, particularly for those antigens that require T-cell support, such as antibody response, and the generation of splenic cytotoxic T cells after immunization *(171)*. Zinc deficiency also produces the stress axis that results in a chronic production of glucocorticoids, which induce apoptosis in precursor lymphoid cells, sharply reducing the numbers of T and B cells to decrease their production and spare nutrients for vital tissues *(172)*. Studies in zinc-deficient mice showed, however, that although the lymphoid compartment is rapidly depleted, the myeloid compartment remains intact with neutrophils and macrophages, which are the first line of defense, being spared *(172)*.

4.5.1. ZINC DEFICIENCY AND CYTOKINES

Zinc deficiency has marked effects on the balance of Th1 and Th2 functions and their expression of cytokines. Cytokines associated with the Th1 subset of T-cell lymphocytes, IFN-γ and IL-2, were decreased, whereas those produced by Th2 cells (IL-4, IL-6, and IL-10) were not affected in a human model of mild zinc deficiency (plasma levels < 1.00 μg/mL). In addition, gene expression of IL-2 and IL-2 gene receptors and binding of NF-κB to DNA were also decreased *(173)*. Prasad *(173)* hypothesized that decreased activation of NF-κB and subsequent reduction in gene expression may cause the observed IL-2 reduction. In addition, zinc deficiency also reduced IL-4 secretion, resulting in significantly elevated TNF-α levels, implicated in the pathophysiology of cachexia and wasting in AIDS *(174–176)*.

Zinc supplementation resulted in a significant increase of IL-2 production and decreased incidence of documented bacteriologic infections *(173)*. Zinc supplementation inhibited TNF-α production *(176)*. These studies indicate an important role of adequate zinc status in preventing HIV disease progression *(177)*. Zinc supplementation, as an adjuvant therapy to HAART, particularly in patients with zinc deficiency, may speed recovery of the immune response when given in a nutritional but sustained dose through its effect on cytokine production over time. Thus, at least one of the mechanisms through which zinc deficiency depresses some aspects of the immune response is that zinc deficiency promotes the shift from Th1 to Th2. Supplementing zinc to zinc-deficient individuals increases the Th1-type cytokines, thereby reversing this shift.

4.5.2. ZINC STATUS AND HIV-1

Patients with AIDS exhibit clinical symptoms similar to those associated with zinc deficiency, including dysregulation of immune function, impaired taste and appetite, decreased food intake, GI malfunction with diarrhea, alopecia, epithelial lesions, hypogonadism, and hypospermia *(167,178)*. Levels of zinc in ranges indicative of zinc deficiency are prevalent in male and female drug users with HIV and are widespread in other HIV-1 infected cohorts *(5–7,21)*. Such low levels of plasma zinc have been linked with faster HIV-1 disease progression, independent of baseline CD4 cell count, lymphocyte levels, age, and calorie-adjusted dietary intake *(179,180)*.

In cohort studies in Miami, Florida, among MSM men who are HIV seropositive, those who became zinc deficient during the study decreased their mean CD4 cell count by a mean of 111, whereas those participants who increased their plasma zinc status from deficient to adequate, significantly increased $(p < .01)$ their CD4 cell count by a mean of 61 *(21)*. Multivariate analyses of zinc status in relation to mortality indicated that zinc inadequacy increased the risk of mortality by almost fivefold in this cohort (RR = 4.98; 95% CI [1.3–19]) and a negative dose-response relationship was observed between plasma zinc and mortality (RR = 0.94; 95% CI [0.90–0.98]), suggesting an approx 6% decrease in mortality risk with every increase of 1 µg/dL in plasma zinc level *(181)*.

In drug users who are infected with HIV, plasma zinc levels indicative of zinc deficiency independently increased the risk for HIV-related mortality by a factor of nearly three (RR = 2.91, 95% CI [1.04–8.18], $p = .04$) *(21)*. When dietary zinc intake was treated as a continuous variable, a dose-response relationship between dietary zinc and mortality was found *(182)*. The risk of dying from HIV-related disease decreased by 33% for every 1 mg/d increase in dietary zinc intake, and this relationship was independent of antiretroviral therapy and CD4 cell count at baseline and over time. The relative risk for mortality for those with an intake under the median (9.34 mg zinc/d) was 11 times greater (95% CI [1.14–106.3], $p = .038$), after adjusting for CD4 cell count as a time-dependent variable *(183)*.

Through its alterations of cellular immunity, zinc deficiency can also influence intracellular HIV-1 replication *(184,185)*. Although zinc deficiency causes immune system dysregulation, zinc also promotes multimerization and enhances enzymatic activity of viral integrase and its "zinc fingers" *(186)*. Zinc is also a component of HIV-1 nucleocapsid proteins *(187–189)*. In addition, HIV-1 transactivating protein (Tat) has a unique cysteine-rich region with zinc-binding properties *(190)* and has a high binding affinity to zinc. Reports from an observational study found an association between faster disease progression and increased mortality in men with HIV-1 infection with daily zinc intakes higher than the daily RDA for zinc *(15,23)*. This cohort, however, had relatively high intakes of zinc compared with other HIV seropositive cohorts, such as drug users and children, and changes on zinc intake or plasma zinc status over time were not considered. An earlier study indicated that excessive zinc intakes (300 mg/d, 20× the RDA) resulted in a significant immune impairment in healthy adult men *(171)*.

In summary, the current evidence indicates that an adequate amount of zinc is essential for maintaining integrity of the immune system and that individuals with HIV-1 infection are susceptible to zinc deficiency. The association between zinc deficiency and poor survival in individuals with HIV-1 infection indicates the need for studies that would develop an optimal zinc therapy.

5. CONCLUSIONS

The primary aim in the treatment of individuals with HIV infection is to bring the infecting retrovirus under control. Antiretroviral treatment should be provided when possible to minimize HIV replication. Prevention is necessary, as well as elimination of secondary infections characteristic of AIDS when they occur. Because a cure is not available, despite the best existing antiretroviral therapy, interventions for the malnutrition that develops concomitantly are important, because malnutrition imposes additional immunosuppressive burden on the already immunocompromised patients with HIV infection. Nutritional interventions must be individualized for each patient, considering the stage of the infection, type of treatment, exposure to opportunistic diseases, and his or her specific circumstances.

The following "Take-Home" messages summarize the individual nutrient deficiencies that are likely to contribute to the pathophysiology and progression of the HIV disease. More research is needed before specific recommendations for effective therapies with macronutrients and micronutrients can be established.

6. "TAKE-HOME" MESSAGES

1. HIV-1 infection is characterized by protein-energy malnutrition and micronutrient abnormalities, which may persist even after administering effective antiretroviral treatments.
2. Poor nutritional status facilitates HIV disease progression and mortality. Nutritional repletion should be an adjuvant to antiretroviral therapy.
3. Wasting occurs in advanced HIV infection, caused by the HIV and opportunistic infections, accompanied by hypermetabolism. Body weight must be closely monitored to detect a 5% to 10% decline; prophylactic nutritional support and regular resistance exercise program must be started early in the disease; later in the disease, calories and protein must be replenished, along with appetite stimulants and anabolic agents; and a regular resistance exercise program must be continued.
4. Vitamins B_1, B_2, B_3, and B_6 deficiencies are accompanied by lack of energy, fatigue, and neuropsychologic abnormalities (vitamin B_6). In hypermetabolic states, the requirement for these vitamins increases.
5. Vitamin B_{12} deficiency is associated with faster disease progression and mortality and neurologic abnormalities, which improve with vitamin B_{12} repletion.
6. Vitamin A deficiency is associated with croup, otitis media, measles, faster HIV disease progression, and mortality.
7. Iron-deficiency anemia is treated with erythropoietin. If iron deficiency is diagnosed (with erythrocyte protoporphyrin, serum ferritin, and transferrin saturation), iron should be supplemented. Low hemoglobin, hematocrit, and serum iron are not sufficient indicators of iron deficiency in HIV infection.
8. Selenium and zinc deficiency are associated with immunodeficiency, oxidative stress, increased HIV-related morbidity, and mortality.

REFERENCES

1. Joint United Nations Programme on HIV/AIDS. Report of HIV/AIDS Epidemic, 2002. A global overview of the epidemic. UNAIDS, Geneva, 2002, pp. 22–41.

2. Baum MK, Mantero-Atienza E, Shor-Posner G, et al. Association of vitamin B_6 status with parameters of immune function in early HIV-1 infection. J Acquir Immun Defic Syndr 1991;4:1122–1132.

3. Beach RS, Mantero-Atienza E, Shor-Posner G, et al. Specific nutrients abnormalities in asymptomatic HIV infection. AIDS 1992;6:701–708.

4. Baum MK. Nutritional alterations in high-risk groups in relationship to HIV-1 disease progression. Nutrition 1996;12:124–126.

5. Baum MK, Shor-Posner G, Lai S, et al. High risk of HIV-related mortality is associated with selenium deficiency. J Acquir Immune Defic Syndr Hum Retrovirol 1997;15:370–374.

6. Baum MK, Shor-Posner G, Zhang G, et al. HIV-1 infection in women is associated with severe nutritional deficiencies. J Acquir Immune Defic Syndr Hum Retrovirol 1997;16:272–278.

7. Baum MK, Shor-Posner G. Micronutrient status in relationship to mortality in HIV-1 disease. Nutr Rev 1998;56(S1–S2):58–62.

8. Baum MK, Shor-Posner G, Campa A. Zinc status in human immunodeficiency virus infection. J Nutr 2000;130:1421S-1423S.

9. Baum K. Role of micronutrients in HIV-infected intravenous drug users. J Acquir Immune Defic Syndr Hum Retrovirol 2000;25:S49–S52.

10. Shor-Posner G, Baum MK. Nutritional alterations in HIV-1 seropositive and seronegative drug users. Nutrition 1996;12:555–556.

11. Semba RD, Graham NMH, Waleska T, et al. Increased mortality associated with Vitamin A deficiency during Human Immunodeficiency Virus Type 1 infection. Arch Intern Med 1993;153:2149–2153.

12. Smit E, Graham NMH, Tang A, et al. Dietary intake of community based HIV-1 seropositive and seronegative injecting drug users. Nutrition 1996;12:496.

13. Semba RD, Caiaffa WT, Graham NMH, et al. Vitamin A deficiency and wasting as predictors of mortality in human immunodeficiency virus-infected injection drug users. J Infect Dis 1995;171: 1196–1202.

14. Huang CM, Ruddel M, Ronald JE. Nutritional status of patients with acquired immunodeficiency syndrome. Clin Chem 1988;34:1957–1959.

15. Tang AM, Graham NMH, Saah AJ. Effects of micronutrient intake on survival in human immunodeficiency virus type 1 infection. Am J Epidemiol 1996;143:1244–1256.

16. Tang AM, Graham NM, Chandra RK, Saah AJ. Low serum B_{12} concentrations are associated with faster human immunodeficiency virus type 1 (HIV-1) disease progression. J Nutr 1997;127:345–351.

17. Constans J, Pellegrin JL, Sergeant C, et al. Serum selenium predicts outcome in HIV infection. J Acquir Immun Defic Syndr 1995;3:392.

18. Fawzi WW, Hunter DJ. Vitamins in HIV disease progression and vertical transmission. Epidemiology 1998;9:457–466.

19. Fawzi WW, Msamanga GI, Spiegelman D, et al. Randomized trial of effects of vitamin supplements on pregnancy outcomes and T cell counts in HIV-1 infected women in Tanzania. Lancet 1998;351: 1477–1482.

20. Beisel WR. AIDS. In: Gershwin ME, German JB, Keen CL (eds.). Nutrition and Immunology: Principles and Practices. Humana, Totowa, NJ, 2000, pp. 389–403.

21. Baum MK, Shor-Posner G, Lu Y, et al. Micronutients and HIV disease progression. AIDS 1995;9: 1051–1056.

22. Campa A, Shor-Posner G, Indacochea F, et al. Mortality risk in selenium deficient HIV-positive children. J Acquir Immune Defic Syndr Hum Retrovirol 1999;20:508–513.

23. Tang AM, Graham NM, Kirby AJ, McCall LD, Willet WC, Saah AJ. Dietary micronutrient intake and risk of progression to acquired immunodeficiency syndrome (AIDS) in human immunodeficiency virus type 1 (HIV-1)-infected homosexual men. Am J Epidemiol 1993;138:937–951.

24. Tang AM, Graham NMH, Semba RD, et al. Association between serum viatmin A and E levels and HIV-1 disease progression. AIDS 1997;11:613–620.

25. Semba RD, Tang AM. Micronutrients and the pathogenesis of human immunodeficiency virus infection. Br J Nutr 1999;81:181–189.

26. Tang AM, Smith E. Selected vitamins in HIV infection: a review. AIDS Patient Care STD 1998;12: 263–273.

27. Centers for Disease Control and Prevention. AIDS-Defining Criteria. Morbidity and Mortality Weekly Report, August 14, 1987 (Suppl 3S–15S).
28. Chlebowski RT, Grosvenor MB, Bernhard NH, et al. Nutritional status, gastrointestinal dysfunction, and survival in patients with AIDS. Am J Gastroenterol 1989;84:1288–1294.
29. Kotler DP, Tierney AR, Wang J, et al. The magnitude of body cell mass depletion determines the timing to death from wasting in AIDS. Am J Clin Nutr 1989;50:444–447.
30. Stuttmann U, Ockenga J, Selber O, et al. Incidence and prognostic value of malnutrition and wasting in human immunodeficiency virus-infected outpatients. J Acquir Immune Defic Syndr 1995;8: 239–246.
31. Hommes MJT, Romi FA, Endert E, Saierweomg JP. Resting energy expenditure and substrate oxidation in human immunodeficiency virus (HIV)-infected asymptomatic HIV: HIV affects host metabolism in the early asymptomatic stage. Am J Clin Nutr 1991;54:311–315.
32. Pantaleo G, Graziosi C, Fauci AS. The immunopathogenesis of human immunodeficiency infection. N Engl J Med 1993;328:327–335.
33. American Gastroenterological Association. AGA Technical Review: Malnutrition and cachexia, chronic diarrhea, and hepatobiliary disease in patients with human immunodeficiency virus infections. Gastroenterology 1996;111:1724–1752.
34. Lambi BB, Federman M, Pleskow D, Wanke CA. Malabsorption and wasting in AIDS patients with microsporidia and pathogen-negative diarrhea. AIDS 1996;10:739–744.
35. Simply stated...are people still wasting? Res Initiat Treat Action 1998;4:15.
36. Roubenoff R, Grinspoon S, Skolnik PR, et al. Role of cytokines and testosterone in regulating lean body mass and resting energy expenditure in HIV-infected men. Am J Physiol Endocrinol Metab 2002;283:E138–E145.
37. Kotler DP. Nutritional alterations associated with HIV infection. J Acquir Immune Defic Syndr 2000;25(Suppl 1):S81–S87.
38. Gilbert C, Launer C, Bartsch G, et al. Body weight and percent weight change as predictors of mortality in Abstract 35th Interscience Conference on Antimicrobial Agents and Chemotherapy (ICAAC), San Francisco, CA, September 1995.
39. Palenicek JP, Grahm NM, He YH, et al. Weight loss prior to clinical AIDS as a predictor of survival. J Acquir Immune Defic Syndr 1995;10:366–372.
40. Kotler DP. Body cell mass and survival in the AIDS patient. In: Herber D, Blackburn GL, Go VLW (eds.). Nutritional Oncology. Academic, London, 1999, pp. 547–560.
41. Kotler DP, Gaetz HP, Klein EB, et al. Enteropathy associated with the acquired immunodeficiency syndrome. Ann Intern Med 1984;101:421–428.
42. Kotler DP, Wang J, Pierson RN. Studies of body composition in patients with the acquired immunodeficiency syndrome. Am J Clin Nutr 1985;42:1255–1265.
43. Kotler DP, Tierney AR, Dilmanian FA, et al. Correlation between total body potassium and total body nitrogen in patients with acquired immunodeficiency syndrome. Clin Res 1991;39:649A.
44. Gutierrez-Rodriguez R, Campa A, Shor-Posner G, Baum MK. Estado del metabolismo de los lipidos en la infeccion por VIH-1 y SIDA (Lipid metabolism status in HIV-1 infection and AIDS). Diagnostico 1998;37:336–343.
45. Grinspoon S, Corcoran C, Stanley T, Rabe J, Wilkie S. Mechanisms of androgen deficiency in human immunodeficiency virus-infected women with the wasting syndrome. J Clin Endocrinol Metab 2001;86:4120–4126.
46. Keithley JK, Swanson B, Zeller JM, et al. Comparison of standard and immune-enhancing oral formulas in asymptomatic HIV-infected persons: a multicenter randomized controlled clinical trial. JPEN J Parenter Enteral Nutr 2002;26:6–14.
47. Steinhart CR. HIV-associated wasting in the era of HAART: a practice-based approach to diagnosis and treatment. AIDS Read 2001;11:557–560, 566–569.
48. Solomon J, De TP, Melchior JC. Nutrition and HIV infection. Br J Nutr 2002;87(Suppl):S111–S119.
49. Baum, MK. Casetti, L. Bonvehi P. Inadequate intake and altered nutrition status in early HIV-1 infection. Nutrition 1994;10:16–20.
50. Beach RS, Morgan R, Wilkie F, et al. Plasma vitamin B_{12} level as a potential cofactor in studies of human immunodeficiency virus type-1 related cognitive changes. Arch Neurol 1992;49:501–506.

51. Glade MJ. Nutrient supplementation in HIV/AIDS, Forum on Therapeutic Nutrition: 2000 Clinical Practice Update. Conference Summary 2000, Palisades, NY.

52. Robson LC, Schwartz RM. Perkins WD. The effects of vitamin B$_6$ deficiency on the lymphoid system and immune responses. In: Tryfiates CP (ed.). Vitamin B$_6$ Metabolism and Role in Growth. Food and Nutrition, Westport, CT, 1980, pp. 205–222.

53. Shor-Posner G, Feaster D, Blaney NT, Baum MK. Impact of vitamin B$_6$ status on psychological distress in a longitudinal study of HIV infection. Intern J Psych Med 1994;24:209–222.

54. Inubushi T, Okada M, Matsui A. Effect of dietary vitamin B$_6$ contents on antibody production. Biofactors 2000;11:93–96.

55. Lee J, Yoshikawa K, Watson RR. Nutritional deficiencies in AIDS patients: a treatment opportunity. In: AIDS and Complementary and Alternative Medicine: Current Science and Practice (Standish LJ, Calabrese C, Galantino ML, eds.), Churchill Livingston, Bastyr Research, 2002, pp. 56–70.

56. Harriman GR, Smith PD, Horne MK. Vitamin B$_{12}$ malabsorption in patients with acquired immunodeficiency syndrome. Arch Intern Med 1989;149:2039–2041.

57. Partiel O, Falutz J, Veilleux M, Rosenblatt DS, Gordon K. Clinical correlates of subnormal vitamin B$_{12}$ levels in patients infected with the human immunodeficiency virus. Am J Hematol 1995;49:318–322.

58. Kieburtz KD, Giang DW, Schiffer RB. Abnormal vitamin B$_{12}$ metabolism in human immunodeficiency virus infection: association with neurological dysfunction. Arch Neurol 1991;48:312–314.

59. Tamura J, Kubota K, Murakami H. Immunomodulation by vitamin B$_{12}$: augmentation of CD8+ T lymphocytes and natural killer (NK) cell activity in vitamin B$_{12}$ deficient patient bymethyl-B$_{12}$ treatment. Clin Exp Immunol 1999;116:28–32.

60. Weinberg JB, Sauls DL, Misukonis MA, Shugars DC. "Inhibition of productive human immunodeficiency virus-1 infection by cobalamins." Blood 1995;86:1281–1287.

61. May BA. A novel antiviral strategy for HIV infection. Med Hypotheses 1993;40:93–94.

62. Herbert V, Fong W, Gulle V. Low holotranscobalamin II is the earliest serum marker for subnormal vitamin B$_{12}$ absorption in patients with AIDS. Am J Hematol 1990;34:132–139.

63. Navia BA, Price RW. The acquired immunodeficiency syndrome dementia complex as the presenter or sole manifestation of human immuno-deficiency virus infection. Arch Neurol 1987;44;65–69.

64. Lindenbaum J, Savage DG, Stabler SP. Diagnosis of cobalamin deficiency: II relative sensitivities of serum cobalamin, methylmalonic acid and total homocysteine concentrations. Am J Hematol 1990;34:99–107.

65. Frenkel EP, Yardley DA. Clinical and laboratory features and sequelea of deficiency of folic acid (folate) and vitamin B12 (cobalamin) in pregnancy and gynecology. Hematol Oncol Clin N Am 2000;14:1079–1100.

66. Ellison J. Intensive vitamin A therapy in measles. BMJ 1932;2:708–711.

67. West CE. Vitamin A and measles. Nutr Rev 2000;58:S46–S54.

68. Sempertegui F, Estrella B, Camaniero V, et al. The beneficial effects of weekly low-dose vitamin A supplementation on acute lower respiratory infections and diarrhea in Ecuatorian children. Pediatrics 1999;104:e1.

69. Sommer A, Tarwotjo I, Hussaini G, Susanto D. Increased mortality in children with mild vitamin A deficiency. Lancet 1983;2:585–588.

70. Sommer A, Tarwotjo I, Djunaedi E, et al. Impact of vitamin A supplementation on childhood mortality: a randomized controlled community trial. Lancet 1986;1:1169–1173.

71. Bloem MW, Wedel M, Egger RJ, et al. Mild vitamin A deficiency and risk of respiratory tract diseases and diarrhea in preschool and school children in Northeast Thailand. Am J Epidemiol 1990; 131:332–339.

72. Shankar AH, Genton B, Semba RD, et al. Effect of vitamin A supplementation on morbidity due to *Plasmodium falciparum* in young children in Papua New Guinea: a randomised trial. Lancet 1999;354:203–209.

73. Fawzi WW, Chalmers T, Herrera M, Mosteller F. Vitamin A supplementation and child mortality: a meta-analysis. JAMA 1993;269:898–903.

74. D'Souza RM, D'Souza R. Vitamin A for preventing secondary infections in children with measles— a systematic review. J Trop Pediatr 2002;48:72–77.

75. Villamor E, Fawzi WW. Vitamin A supplementation: implications for morbidity and mortality in children. J Infect Dis 2000;182(Suppl 1):S122–S133.

76. Whitney EN, Rolfes SR. The fat-soluble vitamins: A, D, E, and K. In: Understanding Nutrition (9th ed.). Wadsworth/Thomson Learning, Belmont, CA, 2002, pp. 354–385.

77. Semba RD. Vitamin A and immunity to viral, bacterial and protozoan infections. Proc Nutr Soc 1999;58:719–727.

78. Semba RD. Vitamin A, immunity and infection. Clin Infect Dis 1994;19:489–499.

79. Ross AC, Stephensen CB. Vitamin A and retinoids in antiviral responses. FASEB J 1996;10:979–985.

80. Watson R, Prabhala R, Plezia P, Alberts D. Effect of B-carotene on lymphocyte subpopulations in elderly humans: a dose-response relationship. Am J Clin Nutr 1991;53:90–94.

81. Semba RD, Miotti PG, Chiphangwi JD, et al. Maternal vitamin A deficiency and mother-to-child transmission of HIV-1. Lancet 1995;343:1593–1597.

82. Periquet BA, Jammes NM, Lambert WE, et al. Micronutrient levels in HIV-1-infected children. AIDS 1995;96:696–702.

83. Camp WL, Allen S, Alvarez JO, et al. Serum retinol and HIV-1 RNA viral load in rapid and slow progressors. J Acquir Immune Defic Syndr Hum Retrovirol 1998;18:21–26.

84. Rich KC, Fowler MG, Mofenson LM, et al. Maternal and infant factors predicting disease progression in human immunodeficiency virus type 1-infected infants. Women and Infants Transmission Study Group. Pediatrics 2000;105:e8.

85. Burger H, Kovacs A, Weiser B, et al. Maternal serum vitamin A levels are not associated with mother-to-child transmission of HIV-1 in the United States. J Acquir Immune Defic Syndr Hum Retrovirol 1997;14:321–326.

86. Semba RD. Overview of the potential role of vitamin A in mother-to-child transmission of HIV-1. Acta Paediatr Suppl 1997;421:107–112.

87. Fawzi W. Nutritional factors and vertical transmission of HIV-1. Epidemiology and potential mechanisms. Ann N Y Acad Sci 2000;918:99–114.

88. Fawzi WW, Msamanga GI, Hunter D, et al. Randomized trial of vitamin supplements in relation to transmission of HIV-1 through breastfeeding and early child mortality. AIDS 2002;16:1935–1944.

89. Fawzi WW, Msamanga G, Hunter D, et al. Randomized trial of vitamin supplements in relation to vertical transmission in HIV-1 in Tanzania. J Acquir Immune Defic Syndr 2000;23:246–254.

90. Coutsudis A, Pillay K, Spooner E, et al. Randomized trial testing the effect of vitamin A supplementation on pregnancy outcomes and early mother-to-child HIV-1 transmission in Durban, South Africa. South African Vitamin A Study Group. AIDS 1999;13:1517–1524.

91. Kumwenda N, Miotti PG, Taha TE, et al. Antenatal vitamin A supplementation increases birth weight and decreases anemia among infants born to human immunodeficiency virus-infected women in Malawi. Clin Infect Dis 2002;35:618–624.

92. French AL, Cohen MH, Gange SJ, et al. Vitamin A deficiency and genital viral burden in women infected with HIV-1. Lancet 2002;359:1210–1212.

93. Shey WI, Brocklehurst P, Sterne JA. Vitamin A supplementation for reducing the risk of mother-to-child transmission of HIV infection. Cochrane Database Syst Rev 2002:CD003648.

94. Villamor E, Mbise R, Spiegelman D, et al. Vitamin A supplements ameliorate the adverse effect of HIV-1, malaria, and diarrheal infections on child growth. Pediatrics 2002;109:E6.

95. Fawzi WW, Mbise RL, Hertzmark E, et al. A randomized trial of vitamin A supplements in relation to mortality among human immunodeficiency virus-infected and uninfected children in Tanzania. Ped Infect Dis J 1999;18:127–133.

96. Coutsoudis A, Bobat RA, Coovadia HM, Kuhn L, Tsai WY, Stein ZA. The effects of vitamin A supplementation on the morbidity of children born to HIV-infected women. Am J Public Health 1995;85:1076–1081.

97. Meydani SN, Barklund MP, Liu S, et al. Vitamin E supplementation enhances cell-mediated immunity in healthy subjects. Am J Clin Nutr 1991;53:976–977.

98. Tengerdy RP. The role of vitamin E in immune response and disease resistance. Ann N Y Acad Sci 1990;587:24–33.

99. Odeleye OE, Watson RR. The potencial role of immunologic abnormalities during acquired immune deficiency syndrome. Prog Food Nutr Sci 1991:15:1–19.

100. Pontes Monteiro J, Ferreira da Cunha D, Freire Carvaho Cunha S. Nutrition assessment of vitamin E in malnourished patients with AIDS. Nutrition 2000;16:339–343.
101. Wang Y, Huang DS, Liang B, Watson RR. Nutritional status and immune responses in mice with murine AIDS are normalized by vitamin E supplementation. J Nutr 1994;124:2024–2032.
102. Han SN, Wu D, Ha WK, et al. Vitamin E supplementation increases T helper 1 cytokine production in old mice infected with influenza virus. Immunology 2000;100:487–493.
103. Beharka AA, Wu D, Han SN, Meydani SN. Macrophage prostaglandin production contributes to the age-associated decrease in T cell function which is reverse by the dietary antioxidant vitamin E. Mech Ageing Dev 1997;93:59–77.
104. Malvy DJM, Richard MJ, Arnaud J, Favier A, Amedee-Manesme O. Relationship of plasma malondiadehyde, vitamin E and antioxidant micronutrients to human immunodeficiency virus-1 sero-positive. Clin Chim Acta 1994;224:89–94.
105. Constans J, Peuchant E, Pellegrin JL, et al. Fatty acids and plasma antioxidants in HIV-positive patients: correlation with nutritional and immunological status. Clin Biochem 1995;28:421–426.
106. Shor-Posner G, Miguez-Burbano MJ, Lu Y, et al. Elevated IgE level in relationship to nutritional status and immune parameters in early human immunodeficiency virus-1 disease. J Allergy Clin Immunol 1995;95:886–892.
107. Beisel WR. Nutrition and Infection. In: Linder MC (ed.) Nutritional Biochemistry and Metabolism (2nd ed.). Elsevier, New York, 1995, pp. 507–542.
108. Moyle G. Anaemia in persons with HIV infection: prognostic marker and contributor to morbidity. AIDS Rev 2002;4:13–20.
109. Semba RD, Gray GE. Pathogenesis of anemia during human immunodeficiency virus infection. J Investig Med 2001;49:225–239.
110. Gupta S, Imam A, Licorish K. Serum ferritin in acquired immune deficiency syndrome. J Clin Lab Immunol 1986;20:11–13.
111. De Monye C, Karcher DS, Boelaert JR, Gordeuk VR. Bone marrow macrophage iron grade and survival of HIV-seropositive patients. AIDS 1999;25:375–380.
112. Weiss G, Wachter H. Linkage of cellular immunity to iron metabolism. Immunol Today 1995;16:495–500.
113. Semba RD, Taha TE. Iron status and indicators of human immuno-deficiency virus disease severity among pregnant women in Malawi. Clin Infect Dis 2001;32:1496–1499.
114. Castaldo A, Tarallo L, Palomba E, et al. Iron deficiency and intestinal malabsorption in HIV disease. J Pediat Gastroenterol Nutr 1996;22:359–363.
115. Savarino A, Pescarmona GP, Boelaert JR. Iron metabolism and HIV infection: reciprocal interactions with potentially harmful consequences? Cell Biochem Funct 1999;17:279–287.
116. Sappey C, Boelaert JR. Iron chelation decreases NF-kappa B and HIV type-1 activation due to oxidative stress. AIDS Res Human Retrovir 1995;11:1049–1061.
117. Delanghe J, Langlosis M. Haptoglobin polymorphism, iron metabolism and mortality in HIV infection. AIDS 1998;12:1027–1032.
118. Afacan YE, Hasan MS, Jackson AO. Iron deficiency anemia in HIV infection: immunologic and virologic response. J Nat Med Assoc 2002;94:73–77.
119. Georgiou NA, van der Bruggen T, Oudshoorn M, Nottet HS, Marx JJ, van Asbeck BS. Inhibition of human immunodeficient virus type 1 replication in human mononuclear blood cells by iron chelators deferoxamine, deferiprone and bleomycin. J Infect Dis 2000;181:484–490.
120. Costagliola DG, de Montalembert M, Lefrere JJ, et al. Dose of deferrioxamine and evolution of HIV infection in thalassaemic patients. Br J Haematol 1994;87:849–852.
121. Jacobus DP. Randomization to iron supplementation of patients with advanced human immunodeficiency virus disease—an inadvertent but controlled study with results important for patient care. J Infect Dis 1996;153:1044–1045.
122. Clark TD, Semba RD. Iron supplementation during human immunodeficiency virus infection: a double-edge sword? Med Hypotheses 2001;57:476–479.
123. Bologna R, Indacochea F, Shor-Posner G, et al. Selenium and immunity in HIV-1 infected pediatric patients. J Nutr Immunol 1994;2:41–49.

124. Baeten JM, Mostad SB, Hughes MP, et al. Selenium deficiency is associated with shedding of HIV-1-infected cells in the female genital tract. J Acquir Immune Defic Syndr 2001;26:360–364.

125. Miguez-Burbano MJ, Campa A, Shor-Posner G, et al. Incidence of herpes infection in HIV-1 infected chronic drug users in relationship to selenium status. STI and The Millenium, a Joint Meeting of the ASTDA and the MSSVD, Baltimore, MD, May 3–6, 2000.

126. Shor-Posner G, Miguez MJ, Pineda LM, et al. Impact of selenium status on the pathogenesis of mycobacterial disease in HIV-1-infected drug users during the era of highly active antiretroviral therapy. J Acquir Immune Defic Syndr Hum Retrovirol 2002;29:169–173.

127. Taylor EW, Ramanathan CS, Nadimpalli RG, et al. Do some viruses encode selenoproteins? Assessment of the theory in the light of current theoretical, experimental and clinical data. Antiviral Res 1995;26:A271–A286.

128. Taylor EW, Ramanathan CS, Nadimpally RG. A general method for predicting new genes in nucleic acid sequences: application to the human immunodeficiency virus. In: Witten M (ed.). Computational Medicine, Public Health, and Biotechnology. Vol. 1. World Scientific, Singapore, 1996, pp. 285–309.

129. Taylor EW, Ramanathan CS. Theoretical evidence that the Ebola virus Zaire strain may be selenium-dependent: a factor in pathogenesis and viral outbreaks? J Orthomol Med 1996;10:131–138.

130. Taylor EW, Nadimpalli RG, Ramanathan CS. Genomic structure of viral agents in relation to the biosynthesis of seleno proteins. In: Scharauzer GN, Montagnier L (eds.). Proceedings of the first international symposium on "Human viral diseases: selenium, antioxidants and other emerging strategies of therapy and prevention," April 1996, Nonwiler, Germany. Biol Trace Elem Res 1997;56: 63–91.

131. Dworkin BM, Rosenthal WS, Wormser GP, et al. Abnormalities of blood selenium and glutathione peroxidase in patients with acquired immunodeficiency syndrome and AIDS-related complex. Biol Trace Elem Res 1988;20:86–96.

132. Scrimshaw NS, SanGiovanni JP. Synergism of nutrition, infecion, and immunity: an overview. Am J Clin Nutr 1997;66:464S–477S.

133. Look MP, Rocstroh JK, Rao GS, Kreuzer KA, Spengler U, Sauerbruch T. Serum selenium versus lymphocyte subsets and markers of disease progression and inflammatory response in human immunodeficiency virus-1 infection. Biol Trace Elem Res 1997;56:31.

134. Spallholz JE. Anti-inflammatory, immunologic and carcinostatic attributes of selenium in experimental animals. Adv Exp Med Biol 1981;135:43–62.

135. Roy M, Kiremidjian-Schumacher L, Wishe HI, Cohen MW, Stotzky G. Selenium supplementation enhances the expression of interleukin 2 receptor subunits and internalization of interleukin 2. Proc Soc Exp Biol Med 1993;202:295–231.

136. Haslett PA. Anticytokine approaches to the treatment of anorexia and cachexia. Sem Oncol 1998;25: 53–57.

137. Hori K, Hatfield D, Maldarelli F, Lee BJ, Close KA. Selenium supplementation suppresses tumor necrosis factor alpha-induced human immunodeficiency virus replication in vitro. AIDS Res Hum Retrovir 1997;13:1325–1332.

138. Moutet M, d'Alessio P, Mlette P, Dvaux V, Chaudiere J. Glutathione peroxidase mimics prevent TNF and neutrophil induced endothelial alterations. Free Radic Biol Med 1998;25:270–281.

139. Sappey C, Legrand-Poels S, Best-Belpomme M, Favier A, Rentier B, Piette J. Stimulation of glutathione peroxidase activity decreases HIV type 1 activation after oxidative stress. AIDS Res Human Retrovir 1994;10:1451–1461.

140. Clark LC, Combs GF, Turnbull BW, et al. The nutritional prevention of cancer with selenium 1983–1993: a randomized clinical trial. JAMA 1996;276:1957–1963.

141. Yu SY, Zhu YJ, Li WG, et al. A preliminary report on the intervention trials of primary liver cancer in high-risk populations with nutritional supplementation of selenium in China. Biol Trace Elem Res 1991;29:289–294.

142. Yu SY, Chu YJ, Li WG. Selenium chemoprevention of liver cancer in animals and possible human applications. Biol Trace Elem Res 1998;15:231–241.

143. Clark LC, Combs GS, Turnbull BW. The nutritional prevention of cancer with selenium 1983–1993: a randomized trial. FASEB J 1996;10:550.

144. Li JY, Taylor PR, Li B, et al. Nutrition intervention trials in Linxian, China: multiple vitamin/mineral supplementation, cancer incidence, and disease-specific mortality among adults with esophageal dysphasia. J Natl Cancer Inst 1993;85:1492–1498.

145. Blot WJ, Li JY, Taylor PR, et al. Nutrition intervention trials in Linxian, China: supplementation with specific vitamin/mineral combinations, cancer incidence, and disease-specific mortality in the general population. J Natl Cancer Inst 1993;85:1483–1492.

146. Delmas-Beauvieux MC, Peuchant E, Coucouron A, et al. The enzymatic antioxidant system in blood and glutathione status in human immunodeficiency virus (HIV)-infected patients: effects of supplementation with selenium or B-carotene. Am J Clin Nutr 1996;64:101–107.

147. Spallholz JE, Boylan LM, Larsen HS. Advances in understanding selenium's role in the immune system. Ann N Y Acad Sci 1990;587:123–139.

148. Peretz A, Neve J, Desmedt J, Duchateau J, Dramaix M, Famaey J-P. Lymphocyte response is enriched by supplementation of elderly subjects with selenium-enriched yeast. Am J Clin Nutr 1991;53:1323–1328.

149. Bonomini M, Forster S, De Risio F, et al. Effects of selenium supplementation on immune parameters in chronic uraemic patients on haemodialysis. Nephrol Dial Transplant 1995;10:1654–1661.

150. Harvima RJ, Jegerroos H, Kajander EO, et al. Screening of effects of selenomethionine-enriched yeast supplementation on various immunological and chemical parameters of skin and blood in psoriatic patients. Acta Derm Venereol 1993;73:88–91.

151. Peretz A, Neve J, Duchateau J, et al. Effects of selenium supplementation on immune parameters in gut failure patients on home parenteral nutrition. Nutrition 1991;7:215–221.

152. Cirelli A, Ciardi M, De Simone C, et al. Serum selenium concentration and disease progress in patients with HIV infection. Clin Biochem 1991;24:211–214.

153. Olmsted L, Schrauzer GN, Flores-Arce M, Dowd J. Selenium supplementation of symptomatic human immunodeficiency virus infected patients. Biol Trace Elem Res 1989;20:59–65.

154. Schrauzer GN, Sacher J. Selenium in the maintenance and therapy of HIV-infected patients. Chem Biol Interact 1994;91:199–205.

155. Kavanaugh-McHugh AL, Ruff A, Perlman E, Hutton N, Modlin J, Rowe S. Selenium deficiency and cardiomyopathy in acquired immunodeficiency syndrome. JPEN J Parenter Enteral Nutr 1991;15:347–349.

156. Alfthan G, Xu GL, Tan WH, et al. Selenium supplementation of children in a selenium-deficient area in China: blood selenium levels and glutathione peroxidase activities. Biol Trace Elem Res 2000;73:113–125.

157. Miguez-Burbano MJ, Shor-Posner G, Perez E, et al. Selenium and glucose homeostasis in the HAART era. XIII International HIV/AIDS Conference, Durban, South Africa, July 9–14, 2000. Abstract 8704.

158. Miguez-Burbano MJ, Burbano X, Campa A, et al. Selenium and platelet in the HAART era. Abstract accepted at FASEB 2001, March 31–April 4, Orlando, FL.

159. Carr A, Samaras K, Burton S, et al. A syndrome of peripheral lipodystrophy, hyperlipidaemia and insulin resistance in patients receiving HIV protease inhibitors. AIDS 1998;12:F51–F58.

160. Halliwell B. Oxidation of low-density lipoproteins: questions of initiation, propagation, and the effect of antioxidants. Am J Clin Nutr 1995;61:670S-677S.

161. Endre L, Beck F, Prasad A. The role of zinc in human health. J Trace Elem Exp Med 1990;3:337–375.

162. Fraker PJ, King L, Garvy B, Medina C. Immunopathology of zinc deficiency: a role for apoptosis. In: Klurfeld D (ed.). Human Nutrition—A Comprehensive Treatise (vol. 8). Plenum, New York, 1993, pp. 267–283.

163. Keen CL, Gershwin ME. Zinc deficiency and immune function. Ann Rev Nutr 1990;10:415–431.

164. Fraker PH, Haas SM, Luecke RW. Effect of zinc deficiency on the immune response of the young adult A/J mouse. J Nutr 1977;107:1889–1895.

165. Fernandes G, Nair M, Onoe K, Tanaka T, Floyd R, Good R. Impairment of cell mediated immunity function by dietary zinc deficiency in mice. Proc Natl Acad Sci USA 1979;76:457–461.

166. Wirth JJ, Fraker PJ, Kierszenbaum F. Zinc requirement for macrophage function: effect of zinc deficiency on uptake and killing of a protozoan parasite. Immunology 1989;68:114–114.

167. Odeh M. The role of zinc in acquired immunodeficiency syndrome. J Int Med 1992;231:463–469.

168. Chandra RK. Nutrition and the immune system: an introduction. Am J Clin Nutr 1997;66:460S-463S.

169. Fabris N, Mocchegiani E. Zinc, human diseases and aging. Aging (Milano) 1995;7:77–93.
170. Champion S, Imhof BS, Savagner P, et al. The embryonic thymus produces chemotactic peptides involved in the homing of hemopoietic precursors. Cell 1986;44:781–790.
171. Chandra RK. Trace element regulation of immunity and infection. J Am Coll Nutr 1985;4:5–16.
172. Fraker P. Impact of nutritional status on immune integrity. In: Gershwin ME, German JB, Keen CL (eds.). Nutrition and Immunology. Humana, Totowa, NJ, 2000, pp. 147–156.
173. Prasad AS. Effect of zinc deficiency on Th1 and Th2 cytokines shift. J Infect Dis 2000;182(Suppl 1):S62–S68.
174. Dowd PS, Kelleher J, Guillou PJ. T-lymphocyte subsets and interleukin-2 production in zinc deficient rats. Br J Nutr 1986;55:59–65.
175. Beutler B, Cerami A. Cachectin: more than a tumor necrosis factor. N Engl J Med 1987;316:479–485.
176. Flieger D, Riethmuller G, Ziegler-Heitbrock HWL. Zn^{2+} inhibits both tumor necrosis factor-mediated DNA fragmentation and cytolysis. Int J Cancer 1989;44:315–319.
177. Rosenberg ZF and Fauci AS. Immunopathogenic mechanisms of HIV infection: cytokine induction of HIV expression. Immunol Today 1990;11:176–180.
178. King JC, Keen CL. Zinc. In: Shils ME, Olson JA, Shike M, Ross AC (eds.). Modern Nutrition in Health and Disease (9th ed.). Lea and Febinger, Philadelphia, 1999, pp. 223–240.
179. Falutz J, Tsoukas C, Gold P. Zinc as a cofactor in human immunodeficiency virus-induced immuno-suppression. JAMA 1988;259:2850–2851.
180. Graham NMH, Sorenson D, Odaka N, et al. Relationship of serum copper and zinc levels to HIV-1 seropositivity and progression to AIDS. J Acquir Immune Defic Syndr 1991;4:976–980.
181. Lai H, Lai S, Shor-Posner G, et al. Plasma zinc, copper, copper/zinc ratio and survival in a cohort of HIV-1 infected homosexual men. J AIDS 2001;27:56–62.
182. Campa A, Baum K, Lai S, et al. Significant association between poor dietary zinc intake and zinc deficiency in HIV infected drug users. XIV International AIDS Conference, Barcelona, July 7–12, 2002, Abstract B10517.
183. Baum MK, Campa A, Lai S, et al. Zinc intake and mortality in HIV-1 infected drug users. XIV International AIDS Conference, Barcelona, July 7–12, 2002, Abstract and Poster ThPeB7323: 415.
184. Edeas MA, Peltier E, Claise C, et al. Immunocytochemical study of uptake of exogenous carrier-free copper-zinc superoxidase dismutase by peripheral blood lymphocytes. Cell Mol Biol 1996;42:1137–1143.
185. Sprietsma JE. Zinc-controlled Th1/Th2 switch significantly determines development of diseases. Med Hypotheses 1997;49:1–14.
186. Lee PS, Xiao J, Knutson JR, et al. Zn^{2+} promotes the self-association of human immunodeficiency virus type-1 integrase in vitro. Biochemistry 1997;36:173–180.
187. Berthoux L, Pechoux C, Ottman M, et al. Mutations in the N-terminal domain of human immunodeficiency virus type 1 nucleocapsid protein affect virion core structure and proviral DNA synthesis. J Virol 1997;71:6973–6981.
188. Darlix JL, Lapadat-Tapolsky M, de Rocquigny H, et al. First glimpses at structure-function relationships of the nuclecapsid protein of retroviruses. J Mol Biol 1995;254:523–537.
189. Zheng R, Jenkins TM, Craigie R. Zinc folds the N-terminal domain of HIV-1 integrase, promotes multimerization, and enhances catalytic activity. Proc Natl Acad Sci USA 1996;93:13659–13664.
190. Huang HW, Wang KT. Structural characterization of the metal binding site in the cysteine-rich region of HIV-1 Tat protein. Biochem Biophys Res Commun 1996;227:615–621.

17 Probiotics and Immunomodulation

*Kay J. Rutherfurd-Markwick
and Harsharnjit S. Gill*

1. INTRODUCTION

Probiotics are defined as live microbial food supplements that beneficially influence the health of the host *(1)*. Generally, this was considered to occur by improving the microbial balance *(2)*; however, it is becoming increasingly clear that probiotics elicit at least some of their health benefits from immunomodulation. The gastrointestinal (GI) tract fulfils many functions aside from digesting and absorbing nutrients. One of these other functions is the gut hosts a complex mixture of microbes that comprise our resident gut microflora, some of which may play a key role in maintaining human health. *Bifidobacterium* and *Lactobacillus* are strongly associated with optimum microbial balance in the gut, and it is for these two genera that the greatest body of evidence for health-promoting properties exists.

Interest in functional foods, particularly the use of probiotics by the general public for maintenance of general health, as well as the prevention of certain chronic diseases (e.g., cancer, diabetes, and allergies), gained momentum during the past decade. The rising cost of medical treatment; the increasing number of patients suffering from "Western diseases," such as allergies, autoimmune, inflammatory, and gut-related problems; the aging population; and the overall increasing interest of the general population in their own health are all key factors driving the surge of interest in probiotics for health.

Despite that man has consumed fermented food products for thousands of years and there is anecdotal evidence suggesting the health-promoting properties of such products, it is only now that a considerable volume of evidence supporting certain health benefits after the consumption of specific bacterial strains is mounting. The pathway to conclusively demonstrating a health benefit for a probiotic strain in humans is rather slow and arduous. Often, particularly if the bacterial strain to be tested is one not normally consumed by humans, it begins with evidence from animal trials, which aim to support a specific health claim and demonstrate safety of consumption. Conclusive evidence is then sought via a series of carefully controlled human clinical trials. Unfortunately, trials demonstrating the prevention of certain diseases or conditions, for example, traveler's diarrhea, can be extremely difficult to conduct for numerous reasons. This has added to problems in obtaining documented evidence of the efficacy of certain probiotics and functional foods and adds to the consumer's confusion, who often must make his or her

From: *Diet and Human Immune Function*
Edited by: D. A. Hughes, L. G. Darlington, and A. Bendich © Humana Press Inc., Totowa, NJ

purchasing decision based solely on the product's packaging information. Products are often sold with unsubstantiated or general health claims, and it is becoming increasingly clear in probiotics that all probiotic strains are **not** created equal. Also, there is controversy concerning the level of consumption of viable probiotic organisms required to confer health benefits in man: levels ranging from 10^6 colony-forming units (CFU) to 10^9 CFU at the time of consumption have been suggested, and various minimum standards have been set throughout the world *(3,4)*. Further controversy has arisen after reports that several probiotic products either did not contain the listed species or contained extra species or the levels of viable probiotics were less than one tenth of that stated on the package *(5)*. Because consumers are encouraged to consume probiotics on a daily basis, it is important that information detailing the probiotic strains (including accurate viability counts, dose, delivery medium, and safety) for which specific health benefits have been conclusively demonstrated, be made available to the consumer, as well as to health professionals who are likely to recommend such products.

Probiotics confer an array of health benefits; however, not all are fully proven through rigorous clinical trials. Research supporting the use of certain probiotic strains in the treatment of diarrheal diseases and lactose intolerance are well documented *(3)*. There is also a substantial body of evidence documenting specific probiotic strains' ability to modulate the immune system, although it is unclear if this translates into disease resistance *(6)*. Data supporting the use of probiotics to control inflammatory diseases, treat and prevent allergies, and prevent cancer are promising, and, no doubt, future research will soon be added in these areas.

2. INTESTINAL MICROFLORA AND THE ONTOGENY OF THE GUT IMMUNE SYSTEM

The GI tract provides a protective barrier between the internal environment and the constant challenge of externally derived food antigens and microorganisms. This includes the control of antigen transport by exclusion of antigens and elimination of foreign antigens, which have penetrated the mucosa, as well as the regulation of antigen-specific immune responses in the gut.

Colonization of the gut with healthy normal microflora, which begins immediately after birth, provides a source of microbial antigens that, along with dietary antigens, aid in the mucosal immune system's development and maturation. This is supported by observations that the spleen and lymph nodes (secondary lymphoid tissues) in germ-free animals are poorly developed because of the lack of antigenic stimulation *(7)*. The maturation process creates an environment in which inflammatory responses are maintained in a regulated, yet primed, state, hence promoting normal gut-barrier functions *(8)*. Therefore, exposure to bacterial and dietary antigens is essential both for the early education of the immune system and to ensure the development of a balanced immune system.

It is becoming clear that in our effort to sterilize food products and eliminate as many potentially pathogenic bacteria from both our food supply and our environment we have, in fact, also inadvertently eliminated several potentially beneficial bacteria, possibly even decreasing the diversity of bacteria colonizing the gut. In doing so, we have decreased the range of antigens to which our gut is exposed. This lack of exposure to microbial antigens results in inadequate priming of T helper type 1 (Th1) cell activity, thus leading to incorrect cytokine balance and a failure to fine-tune the T-cell repertoire in relation to epitopes that are cross-reactive between self and microorganisms *(9)*. These processes potentially predispose individuals to inflammatory diseases and allergies, which may provide an opportunity for the control or prevention of such diseases by supplementing the diet with probiotics or functional foods containing probiotics.

3. IMMUNOMODULATION

Numerous experimental studies have been carried out in both animals and humans to investigate the effects of probiotics on various aspects of immune function.

3.1. Effect on Nonspecific Immune Responses

Phagocytic cell and natural killer (NK) cell activities are key components of the nonspecific immune responses and, therefore, constitute the first line of host defense. Phagocytosis is a key mechanism by which pathogens are engulfed and eradicated from the human body. The phagocytosis process, which is carried out primarily by monocytes and macrophages (mononuclear phagocytes) and neutrophils (polymorphonuclear leukocytes), results in the induction of a series of intracellular events that result in the production of several microbicidal products, such as reactive oxygen (e.g., hydrogen peroxide and superoxide) and nitrogen species (e.g., nitric oxide [NO]), enzymes, tumor necrosis factor (TNF)-α, and interleukin (IL)-1. The role of NK cells is to protect against viral infections and tumor development.

Numerous animal studies have been conducted to investigate the effect of probiotic consumption on phagocyte function, and these indicate that the effects are often strain dependent. Phagocytic activity enhancement by mononuclear phagocytes and polymorphonuclear leukocytes after ingestion of probiotic bacteria has been reported, along with triggering of respiratory burst activity. Mice that were fed milk fermented with *Bifidobacterium longum, Lactobacillus acidophilus, L. casei rhamnosus,* or *L. helveticus* demonstrated enhanced alveolar macrophage function compared with control animals or animals that were fed streptococci-fermented milk *(10)*. Perdigon et al. *(11)* showed enhanced peritoneal macrophage function in mice that were fed milk fermented with *L. casei, L. acidophilus,* or both. Several other studies in which lactic acid bacteria (LAB) (*L. casei* and *L. acidophilus*) have been either orally fed or injected peritoneally also describe increases in macrophage function *(12–14)*. There is also evidence suggesting a dose-dependent effect of LAB on phagocytosis in mice, with reports indicating that mice fed 10^{11} CFU/d *L. rhamnosus* displayed significantly higher levels of peripheral blood leukocyte phagocytic activity compared to those fed 10^7 or 10^9 *(6,15)*. Increased lysosomal enzyme secretion *(11,16)* by phagocytes after consumption of certain LAB strains has also been reported. These include reactive oxygen *(17)* and nitrogen species *(6)*. Perdigon and colleagues *(11,18)* also reported observing an increase in in vivo clearance of colloidal carbon, which is an indicator of phagocyte function of the reticuloendothelial system (RES), in mice fed *L. acidophilus, L. casei,* and *L. delbruekii bulgaricus* compared with *Streptococcus thermophilus*.

L. acidophilus (La1) *(19,20)*, *B. bifidus* Bb12 *(20)*, *L. rhamnosus* (GG) *(21)*, *L. rhamnosus* and *B. lactis (22–24)* all enhanced the level of phagocytosis in human clinical trials. In a group of human subjects given *Enterococcus fascium* for 6 wk, Mikes et al.

(25) noted the increased ability of the neutrophils to produce oxygen radicals after incubation with zymosan or phorbol myristate acetate. Increased expression levels of certain receptors involved in phagocytosis, particularly the complement receptor 3 (CR3) have also been reported *(21,26)*. There are comparatively few studies that have investigated the effects of probiotic consumption in humans on NK cell activity; however, there is some evidence to suggest that some strains may positively enhance NK cell numbers or activity. Regular consumption of yogurt for 28 d leads to a progressive increase in peripheral blood NK cell numbers *(27)*. Increased NK cell numbers were also observed in patients suffering from Dukes A colorectal cancer who were administered *L. casei*. Consumption of *L. rhamnosus* or *B. lactis* for 3 wk enhances the NK cell activity level in the elderly by 101% and 62%, respectively, and increases the proportion of CD56+ lymphocytes (NK cells) in the peripheral circulation *(24,28,29)*.

3.2. Effect on Specific Immune Responses

Humoral and cell-mediated immunity are the two broad categories that comprise the specific immune response. Humoral immunity is mediated via antibodies produced by plasma cells (mature B cells). The antibodies specifically bind to antigenic epitopes on the surface of pathogenic bacteria and kill these pathogens with the aid of complement or prime them for phagocytosis by phagocytic cells. Cell-mediated immunity is carried out by T lymphocytes. After exposure to antigen or pathogens, specific T lymphocytes proliferate and produce cytokines. These cytokines then influence other immune cell activities, e.g., augmenting the ability of macrophages to kill intracellular pathogens and tumor cells. In addition, specific T-cell subsets act as helper cells (CD4+) for antibody production, as mediators of delayed type hypersensitivity (DTH) or as cytotoxic cells (CD8+) against virus-infected cells and cancer cells. Several studies in experimental animals and humans have reported that ingestion of specific strains of LAB leads to stimulation of humoral or cell-mediated immune function by increasing circulating antibody levels or influencing cytokine production *(6)*.

3.2.1. ANIMAL STUDIES

As with other bacteria, probiotic bacteria ingestion is likely to stimulate production of local antibodies against the probiotic bacteria itself and, in some cases, against other antigens. LAB consumption stimulates local/mucosal and systemic antibody responses. Perdigon and Alverez *(18)* investigated the effect of feeding mice a range of different LAB and showed they were capable of significantly enhancing circulating antibody responses against sheep red blood cells with *Lactobacilli* stains eliciting a superior response to *Streptococci*. Mice fed *L. rhamnosus* HN001 and orally immunized with ovalbumin and cholera toxin showed significantly higher antibody responses against these antigens than did the control animals *(6)*. Similarly, mice given LAB showed significant increases in specific mucosal and serum antibody responses after challenge with *Salmonella typhimurium* or *Shigella sonnei* *(30,31)*.

3.2.2. HUMAN STUDIES

In human trials, volunteers who consumed fermented milk supplemented with *L. acidophilus*, *Bifidobacterium* Bb12, and *Streptococcus thermophilus* for 3 wk showed significantly higher serum levels of IgA against an *S. typhi* Ty21 vaccine than did the controls *(32)*. Children suffering from acute rotavirus diarrhea demonstrated an increase in specific mucosal and serum antibody responses (to rotavirus) after administration of *Lactobacillus* GG *(33,34)*. Another human trial testing the effects of *Lactobacillus* GG observed a similar increase in immunoresponsiveness to an oral rotavirus vaccine *(35)*.

3.3. Probiotics and Cytokine Production

Immune cells produce cytokines to regulate cell growth, activation, differentiation, inflammation, and immunity *(36)*. Of key importance are the T helper cells, which can be differentiated into Th1 and Th2 cells based on their cytokine profiles. Th1 cells selectively produce interferon (IFN)-γ, IL-2, and IL-12, whereas Th2 cells produce IL-4, IL-5, IL-6, IL-10, and IL-13. Th1 cells promote cell-mediated immunity, whereas Th2 cells stimulate antibody production and are also associated with allergic responses.

Several animal studies have shown enhancement of IFN-γ production by blood and spleen (Th1-type response) cells after probiotic supplementation *(27,37)*. IFN-γ has a role in mediating macrophage and NK cell activation and is, therefore, a key factor in host defense against intracellular pathogens, as well as tumors. IFN-γ is also involved in regulating other cytokines, such as IL-4, IL-5, and IL-10. LAB consumption is also reported to increase IFN-α production in humans *(22,38)*. However, there have been conflicting reports regarding the effects of ingestion of yogurt supplemented with *Lactobacillus* and *Streptococci* on IFN-γ levels in human serum, with one study reporting increased levels *(39)* and others reporting no effects *(40,41)*. However, the half-life of IFN-γ in the serum is short, and it is usually secreted in low amounts (42); therefore, a negative result is not conclusive proof that no effect is actually occurring.

Several lactobacilli strains have been demonstrated to stimulate TNF-α, IL-6, and IL-10 expression by human peripheral mononuclear cells (in vitro and in vivo) *(40,43–45)*. There are conflicting reports on the effect of the ingestion of probiotics on IL-2 production in humans, with several reports demonstrating that blood lymphocytes have enhanced IL-2 responses after stimulation with T-cell mitogens *(40,46,47)*, whereas other studies failed to demonstrate any such effect *(48,49)*. Whether this simply resulted from different strains being used or some other reason is not clear. Differences in LAB's ability to influence Th1 and Th2 cytokine production have been reported *(6)*.

4. IMMUNOREGULATION

4.1. Antiallergy Effects

Early life exposure to environmental microbes, including the gut microflora, is important for preventing allergic-type immunoresponses. It has been suggested that as we continue to live in increasingly hygienic environments, we are no longer exposed to these environmental factors, thus leading to poorly developed immunoregulatory mechanisms, which, in turn, can result in the overexpression of Th2-type allergic responses—the so-called "Hygiene Hypothesis." This is supported by the work of Alm et al. *(50)*, who compared the incidence of skin-test-positive allergies and clinical atopy in children raised in comparatively clean westernized environments in Scandinavia, compared with their counterparts raised in more traditional environments (restricted use of vaccination, antibiotics and antipyretics, and a diet high in organic produce and fermented vegetables). They showed that the children from the traditional environments, who report a low use of antibiotics and a high consumption of lactobacilli containing fermented products, exhibited a lower incidence of allergic responses than those from the westernized environments.

The idea that appropriate microflora, such as lactobacilli, can reduce the risk of developing allergic responses is further supported by studies showing that children who are nonallergic are more likely to have lactobacilli as part of their normal gut microflora than their allergic counterparts *(51,52)*. Results from several clinical studies suggest that having an appropriate gut microflora can control the overexpression of atopy in allergen-sensitized individuals, as well as limit allergy development. In 1996, Sutas et al. *(53)* demonstrated that probiotics, in this case *L. rhamnosus* GG, can reduce the immunogenicity of potentially harmful food antigens. They showed a decrease in the level of IL-4 production by peripheral blood mononuclear cells in atopic infants who are allergic to cow's milk when they were fed *L. rhamnosus* GG hydrolyzed casein compared to that observed in infants fed unhydrolyzed casein. In a similar study, Majamaa and Isolauri *(54)* showed that consumption of an extensively hydrolyzed formula containing *Lactobacillus* GG by infants with atopic eczema and cow's milk allergy reduced the severity of the eczema.

In a trial comparing the effects of *Lactobacillus* GG consumption by adult subjects who are milk hypersensitive compared to control subjects, there was a significant downregulation in numerous milk-induced immunoinflammatory responses in the subjects who were milk hypersensitive, whereas in the control subjects, significant stimulation of the immune system occurred *(21)*. A recent study investigating the effects of *Lactobacillus* GG consumption on IL-10 production in atopic children over time (5 d to 4 wk) demonstrated a significant increase in serum IL-10 concentrations between before-, early-, and late-phase samples *(55)*.

Clearly, some studies have demonstrated the beneficial effects of probiotic supplementation in the treatment and prevention of allergic responses, such as eczema and milk allergies. However, other trials, including an investigation into the effects of *L. acidophilus* yogurt on asthma, failed to show any health benefit *(47)*. The research on the effects of probiotic consumption on allergies is relatively new, but it is gaining momentum, and more data should become available in the coming years.

4.2. Antiinflammatory Bowel Disease

Inflammatory bowel disease (IBD), ulcerative colitis, and Crohn's disease are chronic intestinal diseases of unknown etiology. The key factors influencing onset are believed to be genetic disposition, an immunological disturbance, and a triggering event. There is some evidence suggesting that certain members of the intestinal microflora could be the trigger. Healthy individuals are tolerant of their own microflora, but in patients with IBD, this tolerance has been lost *(56)*. This is supported by experiments in animal models of colitis, which showed that the interaction between the resident gut microflora and the mucosal immune system was important *(57,58)*.

Several human clinical trials have been conducted to investigate probiotic use in patients suffering from various forms of IBD, and, although at an early stage, the results are promising. Malin et al. *(59)* showed that some of the characteristic changes in gut immune responses found with IBD can be reversed by altering the intestinal microflora via probiotic supplementation. Specific probiotic strains are at least as effective at pre-

Table 1
Efficacy of Probiotic Supplementation (Randomized, Controlled Clinical Trials) in Patients
with Inflammatory Bowel Disease

Condition	Treatment group (Probiotics)	Control	n	Treatment duration	Relapse (%): (probiotic vs control group)
Crohn's disease	Escherichia coli Nissle 1917	Placebo	28	12 mo	30 vs 70 ($p < 0.05$)
	Saccharomyces boulardi + Mesalamine	Mesalamine	28	6 mo	6.3 vs 37.5 ($p < 0.05$)
	VSL#3	Mesalamine	28	12 mo	20 vs 40 ($p < 0.05$)
Ulcerative colitis	E. coli Nissle 1917	Mesalamine	120	12 mo	67 vs 73 NS
	S. boulardi + Mesalamine	Mesalamine	31	12 mo	30 vs 35 NS
Pouchitis	VSL#3	Placebo	40	9 mo	15 vs 100 ($p < 0.05$)
	VSL#3	Placebo	40	12 mo	10 vs 40 ($p < 0.05$)

VSL#3 (L. casei, L. plantarum, L. delbruecki subsp. bulgaricus); Mesalamine, 5-aminosalicylic acid; NS, not significant. Adapted from ref. 115.

venting relapse in patients with ulcerative colitis as is Mesalamine (5-aminosalicylic acid) (see Table 1). Treatment of patients suffering from chronic relapsing pouchitis with a mixture of different probiotic strains (predominantly Lactobacillus strains) resulted in all 20 subjects remaining in remission, compared to only 3 of the 20 controls (60). Although current evidence is promising, more research is clearly required to confirm the role that probiotics may play in IBD management.

4.3. Diabetes

The ability of certain strains of lactic acid bacteria to modulate autoimmune responses, such as seen in type 1 diabetes (insulin-dependent diabetes mellitus [IDDM]) has also been demonstrated. The feeding of Lactobacillus casei in the type 2 diabetes (non-insulin-dependent diabetes mellitus [NIDDM]) mouse model, KK-A^y, reduced plasma glucose levels and downregulated IFN-γ and IL-2 production (61). L. casei supplementation also prevented the development of type 1 diabetes in NOD mice (62); mice fed L. casei exhibited a decrease in the production of IFN-γ and the proportion of CD8+ cells compared with the control mice.

4.4. Rheumatoid Arthritis

It has been suggested that consumption of probiotics may have a beneficial effect in patients with rheumatoid arthritis (RA) (63). Consumption of a vegetarian diet or uncooked vegan diets, each rich in lactobacilli, by patients with RA induced significant changes in the composition of the fecal microflora and alleviated clinical symptoms of RA (64,65). Delayed onset and reduced severity of collagen-induced arthritis in lactobacilli-fed mice has also been reported (66). How the change in fecal microflora or the increased consumption of lactobacilli affects RA is unclear. As yet, insufficient evidence is available to state conclusively that probiotic consumption alleviates RA symptoms.

Table 2
Effect of Lactic Acid Bacteria on Diarrhea in Infants, Traveler's Diarrhea, and Antibiotic-
Associated Diarrhea in Humans

Condition	Treatment group (probiotics vs control)	Results NS or P value	Reference
Diarrhea in infants	Yogurt vs milk ($n = 45$)	S ($p < 0.05$)	(117)
	Lactobacillus GG vs placebo ($n = 71$)	S ($p < 0.001$)	(118)
	Bifidobacterium bifidum, S. thermophilus ($n = 55$)	S ($p = 0.035$)	(76)
	Lactobacillus GG vs oral rehydration ($n = 61$)	S ($p < 0.01$)	(75)
	Lactobacillus GG vs oral rehydration ($n = 123$)	S ($p = 0.03$)	(119)
	L. reuteri vs placebo ($n = 40$)	NS ($p = 0.07$)	(120)
Escherichia coli-induced diarrhea	Lactinex vs placebo ($n = 45$)	NS	(85)
Travelers' diarrhea	Lactinex vs placebo ($n = 50$)	NS	(121)
	L. acidophilus, B. bididum, L. Bulgaricus, S. thermophilus vs placebo ($n = 94$)	S ($p = 0.019$)	(87)
	Lactobacillus GG vs placebo ($n = 756$)	NS ($p = 0.065$)	(86)
Antibiotic-associated diarrhea	Lactinex vs placebo ($n = 79$)	NS	(91)
	Lactinex vs placebo ($n = 38$)	NS	(96)
	B. longum vs placebo ($n = 10$)	S ($p < 0.025$)	(122)

S, significant; NS, not significant.
Adapted from ref. *116*.

There is no doubt that further evidence on this subject will be forthcoming in the near future (*see also* Chapter 14 on Rheumatoid Arthritis).

5. ROLE OF PROBIOTICS IN DISEASE PREVENTION AND TREATMENT

Currently, investigation into the use of probiotics for the prophylaxis and treatment of diseases has primarily focused on diarrheal diseases. Several studies have also studied the effects on cancer (*see* Section 5.2.). Studies investigating probiotics' effects on controlling cholesterol levels and reducing septic complications in surgical and patients in the intensive care unit have, thus far, failed to support a role for probiotics in these areas *(67)*.

5.1. Gastrointestinal Tract—Antiinfection Effects

Probiotics mediate protection against numerous GI pathogens (*see* Table 2). Several mechanisms have been proposed to explain this protection, including immunostimulation, production of antimicrobial factors (such as bacteriocins) *(68–70)*, and competition for adhesion binding sites in the intestine *(71–73)*. Both animal and human studies support the immune system's role in protecting against certain forms of diarrhea, showing that immune activation is associated with the level of protection. Probiotic supplementation is also effective against travellers' diarrhea and antibiotic-associated diarrhea (*see* Table 2), although the role of the immune system in these cases is not clear *(74)*.

A study in mice investigating the efficacy of live vs dead *L. rhamnosus* on immune function showed that although dead bacteria enhanced some aspects of immune function, they did not enhance gut mucosal antibody responses to cholera toxin vaccine *(15)*. Dead bacteria are more easily removed from the intestinal mucosa and are, therefore, considered to be less efficient at stimulating the immune system than live bacteria *(42)*. That probiotics can effectively prevent and treat intestinal viral infections suggests that the mechanism of action may likely be via stimulation of the gut-associated lymphoid tissue (GALT), resulting in increased humoral antigen responses *(3,74)*.

Probiotics are beneficial in the treatment of diarrheal disease in children via stimulation of the immune system; in particular, rotavirus infection in infants, where probiotic supplementation reduced the duration of rotavirus shedding *(34,75)*, increased the levels of antirotavirus IgA-secreting cells *(33)*, reduced the increase in gut permeability (which is normally associated with rotavirus infection), and reduced the duration of diarrhea *(75,77)* and length of hospital stay *(77)*. In a follow-up study, Kaila et al. *(78)* demonstrated the need for the probiotic strain to be viable to interact with the mucosal immune system. Here, the trial was repeated using heat-inactivated *Lactobacillus* GG, and, although the duration of diarrhea was reduced, no enhancement in serum IgA levels was observed.

Several well-designed trials have also shown that probiotic supplementation can reduce diarrhea incidence in children. One study conducted in hospitalized children has shown that consumption of infant formula supplemented with *Bifidobacteria* and *S. thermophilus* reduced diarrhea incidence and reduced rotavirus shedding *(76)*; *L. rhamnosus* GG reduced diarrhea incidence in underprivileged children who were not breastfed as infants *(79)*. This may be associated with the fact that bottle-fed infants reportedly have 10-fold lower levels of *Bifidobacteria* in their faeces than breast-fed infants *(80)* and, coincidently, higher levels of various putrefactive bacteria, such as *Streptococci* and *Enterobacteriaceae (81)*.

5.1.1. Traveler's Diarrhea

Probiotics are believed to elicit at least some of their protective effects by stabilizing the indigenous gut microflora *(82)*. Several studies investigating the use of probiotics for the prevention of travelers' diarrhea and antibiotic-associated diarrhea, conditions, which result in changes in the gut microflora, have attempted to demonstrate the effectiveness and clinical benefits in the maintenance of a stable microflora by probiotic supplementation. However, with regard to traveler's diarrhea, the benefits are not consistent. Several trials failed to show any benefit from probiotic supplementation in preventing traveler's diarrhea *(83–85)*. A study in Finnish tourists traveling to Turkey conducted by Oksanen et al. *(86)* showed a reduction in diarrhea incidence in *Lactobacillus*-treated volunteers traveling to one location but not another. The study with the most definitive result was that of Black et al. *(87)*, who demonstrated that consumption of probiotic capsules (*L. acidophilus*, *B. lactis*, *L. bulgaricus*, and *S. thermophilus*) conferred 39% protection against diarrhea to Danish tourists visiting Egypt, although no change in the duration of the diarrhea was observed. Obviously, because trials have been conducted on several populations in different geographic locations, testing a range of different agents, it is impossible to extrapolate the results. Problems associated with compliance and assessing and documenting the diarrhea severity add to this dilemma. Therefore, it is difficult at this time to recommend the consumption of probiotics for the prevention of traveler's diarrhea.

5.1.2. ANTIBIOTIC-ASSOCIATED DIARRHEA

In animals, antiinfection studies against *S. typhimurium* have shown that feeding yogurt supplemented with live LAB increased the rate of survival compared to control animals *(88)*. Ingestion of *L. rhamnosus* and *B. lactis* also significantly enhances survival rate after *S. typhimurium* challenge in mice *(89,90)*.

Trials aimed at demonstrating the efficacy of probiotics in treating antibiotic-associated diarrhea have also given varying results. Numerous probiotic agents reduce the effects of antibiotic-associated diarrhea, including *L. acidophilus*, *L. bulgaricus (91)*, *L. rhamnosus* GG *(92,93)*, *Enterococcus faecium* SF68, and *S. boulardii (94,95)*. Reported benefits include decreased changes in stool consistency, reduced changes in bowel habits, and reduced length of time such changes are observed when associated with antibiotic use. However, other trials using some of the same probiotic strains (*L. acidophilus*, *L. bulgaricus*, and *S. boulardii*) failed to demonstrate any benefit of consumption on antibiotic-associated diarrhea *(96,97)*. Again, comparing the results from the trials is difficult because of the differences between them, which include different study populations, different probiotic strains and doses, and different definitions for the assessment of diarrhea. However, this also emphasizes that caution is required before advocating the use of probiotics for treatment of antibiotic-associated diarrhea.

5.2. Anticancer Effects

5.2.1. ANIMAL STUDIES

Several animal studies have examined the effect of LAB on both chemically induced tumors and the incidence of cancer in animals inoculated with tumor cells or transplanted with tumors. These studies suggest there is a link between immune function and LAB-mediated antitumor activity *(42)*.

Oral administration of numerous LAB strains significantly reduced the incidence of aberrant crypt foci (ACF; early precursors of colon cancer) or tumors in rodents. *B. longum* consumption reduced the incidence of ACF in at least five studies. Other strains also resulting in significant reduction in ACF or tumor incidence included *L. acidophilus* and *Lactobacillus* GG, whereas other strains, such as *B. fragilis* and *Bifidobacterium*, had no effect *(98)*.

Streptococci consumption inhibited the development of transplanted epitheliomas in rats. Restoration of phagocytic activity and intracellular killing were associated with this effect *(99)*. Consumption of heat-killed *L. casei* YIT9018 inhibited growth of inoculated Lewis lung carcinoma cells in mice and enhanced NK cell activity *(98)*. However, in a trial by Kato et al. *(100)* using both viable and heat-killed *L. casei* YIT9018, inhibition of secondary tumor growth of colon 26 tumor cells was only achieved with the viable bacteria. Feeding yogurt and fermented milk containing probiotics to animals reportedly resulted in tumor inhibition and proliferation *(101)*. In this case, probiotics are believed to inhibit carcinogen production by inhibiting microbial growth, stimulating the immune system of the host, and preventing the conversion of procarcinogens to carcinogens *(4)*.

5.2.2. HUMAN STUDIES

Studies in humans are relatively rare, but in one study, oral consumption of *L. casei* Shirota by patients with colon cancer increased T helper and NK cell *(102)*. In another human study, patients who had undergone a superficial bladder tumor transurethral

Table 3
Beneficial Lactic Acid Bacteria and Other Beneficial Microorganisms

Beneficial probiotics (specific strains of the following lactic acid bacteria)	Other beneficial microorganisms
Bifidobacterium longum	Escherichia coli Nissle 1917
B. bifidus	
B. lactis	S. boulardii
Lactobacillus acidophilus	
L. bulgaricus	
L. casei	
L. delbruekii bulgaricus	
L. helveticus	
L. rhamnosus	
Streptococcus thermophilus	
Enterococcus fascium	

resection were fed *L. casei* daily for a year. After this period, the incidence of tumor recurrence was significantly less than that of the control group *(103)*. *L. casei*'s prophylactic effect on superficial bladder tumors was confirmed in a later double-blind placebo-controlled trial, where tumor classification was more frequently downgraded in the treated group than the controls *(104)*.

Epidemiological studies relating cancer incidence to consumption of fermented milk products indicate that although high consumption may protect against breast cancer *(105–107)*, it is also correlated with a higher incidence of ovarian cancer *(108)*.

6. MECHANISMS BY WHICH PROBIOTICS MODULATE IMMUNE FUNCTION

Probiotics are believed to stimulate the immune system via adherence to intestinal cells and interactions with the GALT. This interaction probably occurs in the small intestine, where the LAB/probiotic strains (10^9 CFU) outnumber the indigenous flora ($10^{2–3}$ CFU). Thus, there is a higher likelihood that the LAB or their products will be in contact with immunocompetent cells. Microflora/LAB can interact directly with immunocompetent epithelial cells or indirectly via dendritic cells or the Peyer's patches. Dendritic cells also present bacterial antigens to immunocompetent cells. The Peyer's patches, which contain macrophages and antigen-presenting cells, B cells, and T cells, are designed to take up microbes and other particles present in the small intestinal lumen, hence serving as inductive sites for mucosal immune responses *(109,110)*. Because of this Peyer's patch function, probiotic bacteria may not have to colonize the small intestine to stimulate an immune response.

It is likely that probiotic bacteria are taken up across the mucosa of the small intestine and then ingested by macrophages, which, in turn, leads to the production of cytokines and other factors, which modulate cell-mediated immune function *(82,110)*. It is believed that LAB cell wall components are primarily responsible for immunostimulation and that differences in cell wall composition account for the different levels of immunostimulation observed with different probiotics *(6)*. Muramyl dipeptide (MDP), a peptidoglycan constituent of LAB, stimulates production of IL-1 by macrophages *(112,113)*; IL-1, IL-6, and TNF-α by monocytes; and IL-4 and IFN-γ by lymphocytes *(114)*. Cytokines play a key role in regulating immunoinflammatory responses at both the local and the systemic levels. It is the probiotic-induced stimulation of these cytokines and other mediators that are likely to result in the enhancement of several cell-mediated effector functions, such as enhanced phagocyte function and IFN-γ production *(6)*. One way in which probiotics may help to reduce inflammatory responses, such as those seen in Crohn's disease and food allergies, is by promoting the production of antiinflammatory cytokines and reducing the production of proinflammatory cytokines, hence strengthening the gut mucosal barrier *(82)*.

7. CONCLUSIONS

Many animal studies and human clinical trials have been conducted to establish the efficacy of probiotic strains in stimulating the immune system and preventing or treating various diseases. There is sufficient evidence from animal studies to conclude that certain probiotic strains can modulate both specific and nonspecific immune responses, such as antibody production, phagocyte and NK cell function enhancement, and cytokine production modulation. There are initial studies that suggest similar effects in humans, depending on the health status of the individual. It is via immune system stimulation that the majority of health benefits ascribed to probiotic bacteria are likely to be achieved. There is strong evidence supporting the prophylactic and therapeutic benefits of certain LAB strains in viral diarrhea, particularly in infants, although evidence supporting a role in the prevention of other forms of diarrhea is less clear. Evidence is building that supports probiotic use for the management of numerous gut conditions, including colitis, Crohn's disease, and IBD and allergy and cancer prevention and treatment. Research in these areas is ongoing, and more conclusive evidence will, no doubt, be forth coming.

There are several gaps in our knowledge, which require extensive research to fill. Theses include technological questions involving the stability, shelf-life, and efficacy of probiotic strains in different delivery media. There are also numerous factors that affect the immunomodulatory efficiency of probiotics. These include the strain, viability, dose, and age of the target population. One of the major problems is that few studies with convincing evidence have been conducted with adequate trial design and proper controls. Trials must be conducted for each potential probiotic strain, determining the efficacy of each, along with dose-response effects in different target populations, such as the elderly or children. The relevance of the biomarkers and assays currently used to assess immunomodulation and how these relate to a health outcome is also unknown, and it is important to ascertain whether the parameters measured translate into a health benefit, such as increased disease resistance. Currently, the relationship between immunomodulation and health outcomes with probiotics remains to be unequivocally demonstrated in human populations. Long-term trials also must be conducted to show that the positive benefits seen are not just the result of a short-term adjuvant-type effect. The importance of safety studies cannot be overlooked, especially if probiotic use is to be advocated in at-risk groups, such as those suffering from autoimmune diseases or immunodeficiency. Also, little is known about the mechanisms by which probiotics modulate their effects. Knowledge gained in this area will lend greater credibility to probiotics' potential health benefits, as well as providing information that should assist in the development of better administration protocols and the ability to better identify new and better probiotic strains.

The importance of carefully conducted double-blind placebo-controlled studies to document the efficacy of each individual probiotic strain for each application cannot be over emphasized. Different probiotic strains clearly elicit different immune responses, and therefore, it is likely that in the future we will see the development of several probiotic products marketed with specific health benefits.

8. "TAKE-HOME" MESSAGES

1. Consumption of a range of microorganisms, primarily lactic acid bacteria, has numerous beneficial health effects (Table 3).
2. Specific strains of probiotic bacteria are capable of stimulating both nonspecific and specific immune functions, although it is unclear if this translates into disease resistance.
3. Consumption of certain probiotic strains has prophylactic and therapeutic benefits in viral diarrhea.
4. Data supporting the use of probiotics for the treatment or control of several diseases, including cancer, allergies, and IBD are promising, but further research is needed.
5. Further studies are needed to increase our understanding of probiotics' mechanisms of action on the immune system.
6. Properly controlled clinical trials conducted in target populations are required.
7. Consumers should be provided with information detailing the effective dose, viability counts, safety, and delivery medium for probiotic strains for which specific health claims are made.

REFERENCES

1. Schrezenmeir J, de Vrese M. Probiotics prebiotics and synbiotics—approaching a definition. Am J Clin Nutr 2001;72(Suppl 2):361S–364S.
2. Fuller R. Probiotics in man and animals. Appl Bacteriol 1989;66:365–378.
3. Saavedra JM. Clinical applications of probiotic agents. Am J Clin Nutr 2001;73(Suppl):1147S–1151S.
4. Lourens-Harringh A, Viljoen BC. Yoghurt as probiotic carrier food. Intl Dairy J 2001;11:1–17.
5. Hamilton-Miller JMT, Shah S, Smith T. "Probiotic" remedies are not what they seem. Br Med J 1996;312:55–56.
6. Gill HS. Stimulation of the immune system by lactic cultures. Intl Dairy J 1998;8:535–544.
7. Berg RD. The indigenous gastrointestinal microflora. Trends Microbiol 1996;4:430–435.
8. Cebra JJ. Influences of microbiota on intestinal immune system development. Am J Clin Nutr 1999;69(Suppl):1046S–1051S.
9. Rook GAW, Stanford JL. Give us this day our daily germs. Immunol Today 1998;19:113–116.
10. Goulet J, Saucier L, Moineau S. Stimulation of the non-specific immune response of mice by fermented milks. In: National Yogurt Association (ed.). Yogurt: Nutritional and Health Properties. Kirby Lithographics, McLean, VA, 1989, pp. 187–200.
11. Perdigon G, de Macias ME, Alvarez S, Oliver G, de Ruiz Holgado AP. Systemic augmentation of the immune response in mice by feeding fermented milks with *Lactobacillus casei* and *Lactobacillus acidophilus*. Immunology 1988;63:17–23.
12. Sato K, Saito H, Tomioka H. Enhancement of host resistance against Listeria infection by *Lactobacillus casei*: activation of liver macrophages and peritoneal macrophages by *Lactobacillus casei*. Microbiol Immunol 1988;32:689–698.
13. Kato I, Yokokura T, Mutai M. Macrophage activation by *Lactobacillus casei* in mice. Microbiol Immunol 1983;27:611–618.

14. Perdigon G, Nader de Macias MEN, Alvarez S, Oliver G, Pesce de Ruiz Holgado AA. Enhancement of immune responses in mice fed with *Streptococcus thermophilus* and *Lactobacillus acidophilus*. J Dairy Sci 1987;70:919–926.

15. Gill HS, Rutherfurd KJ. Viability and dose-response studies on the effects of the immunoenhancing lactic acid bacterium *Lactobacillus rhamnosus* in mice. Br J Nutr 2001;86:285–289.

16. Paubert-Braquet M, Gan XH, Gaudichon C, et al. Enhancement of host resistance against *Salmonella typhimurium* in mice fed a diet supplemented with yogurt or milks fermented with various *Lactobacillus casei* strains. Intern J Immunotherapy 1995;11:153–161.

17. Balasubramanya NN, Lokesh BR, Ramesh HP, Krishnakantha TP. Effect of lactic microbes on super-oxide anion generating ability of peritoneal macrophages and tissue histopathology of murines. Indian J Dairy Biosci 1995;6:28–33.

18. Perdigon G, Alvarez S. Probiotics and the immune state. In: Fuller R (ed.). Probiotics. Chapman and Hall, London, 1992, pp. 146–176.

19. Schriffrin EJ, Rochat F, Link-Amster H, Aeschlimann JM, Donnet-Hughes A. Immunomodulation of human blood cells following the ingestion of lactic acid bacteria. J Dairy Sci 1994;74:491–497.

20. Schiffrin EJ, Brassart D, Servin A, Rochat F, Donnet-Hughes A. Immune modulation of blood leuko-cytes in humans by lactic acid bacteria: criteria for strain selection. Am J Clin Nutr 1997;66:515S–520S.

21. Pelto L, Isolauri E, Lilius EM, Nuutila J, Salminen S. Probiotic bacteria down-regulate the milk-induced inflammatory response in milk-hypersensitive subjects but have an immunostimulatory effect in healthy subjects. Clin Exp Allergy Immunol 1998;28:1474–1479.

22. Arunachalam K, Gill HS, Chandra RK. Enhancement of natural immune function by dietary consumption of *Bifidobacterium lactis* (HN019). Eur J Clin Nutr 2000;54:1–5.

23. Gill HS, Rutherfurd KJ. Probiotic supplementation to enhance human natural immunity: effects of a newly characterized immunostimulatory strain (*Lactobacillus rhamnosus* HN001) on leucocyte phago-cytosis. Nutr Res 2001;21:183–189.

24. Gill HS, Cross ML, Rutherfurd KJ, Gopal PK. Dietary probiotic supplementation to enhance cellular immunity in the elderly. Br J Biomed Sci 2001;58:94–96.

25. Mikes Z, Ferenicik M, Jahnova E, Ebringer L, Ciznar I. Hypocholesterolemic and immunostimulatory effects of orally applied *Enterococcus faecium* M-74 in man. Folia Microbiologica 1995;40:639–646.

26. He F, Tuomola LA, Arvilommi H, Salmonen S. Modulation of humoral immune responses through intake of probiotics. FEMS Immunol Med Microbiol 2000;29:47–52.

27. De Simone C, Bianchi Salvadori B, Jirillo E, Baldinelli L, Bitonti F, Vesely R. Modulation of immune activities in humans and animals by dietary lactic acid bacteria. In: Chandan RC (ed.). Yogurt Nutri-tional and Health Properties. John Libbey Eurotext, London, 1989, pp. 201–213.

28. Gill HS, Rutherfurd KJ, Cross ML, Gopal PK. Enhancement of immunity in the elderly by dietary supplementation with the probiotic *Bifidobacterium lactis* HN019. Am J Clin Nutr 2001;74:833–839.

29. Gill HS, Rutherfurd KJ, Cross ML. Dietary probiotic supplementation enhances natural killer cell activity in the elderly: an investigation of age-related immunological changes. J Clin Immunol 2001;21:264–271.

30. Nader de Macias ME, Apella MC, Romero NC, Gonzalez SN, Oliver G. Inhibition of Shigella sonnei by *Lactobacillus casei* and *Lactobacillus acidophilus*. J Appl Bacteriol 1992;73:407–411.

31. Perdigon G, Nader de Macias MEN, Alvarez S, Oliver G, de Ruiz Holgado AA. Prevention of gas-trointestinal infection using immunobiological methods with milk fermented with *Lactobacillus casei* and *Lactobacillus acidophilus*. J Dairy Res 1990;57:255–264.

32. Link-Amster H, Rochat F, Saudan KY, Mignot O, Aeschlimann JM. Modulation of a specific humoral immune response and changes in intestinal flora mediated through fermented milk intake. FEMS Immunol Medical Microbiol 1994;10:55–64.

33. Kaila M, Isolauri E, Soppi E, Virtanen E, Laine S, Arvilommi H. Enhancement of the circulating antibody secreting cell response in human diarrhoea by a human Lactobacillus strain. Pediatr Res 1992;32:141–144.

34. Majamaa H, Isolauri E, Saxelin M, Vesikari T. Lactic acid bacteria in the treatment of acute rotavirus gastroenteritis. J Pediatr Gastro Nutr 1995;20:333–338.

35. Isolauri E, Joensus J, Suomalainen H, Luomala M, Vesikari T. Improved immunogenicity of oral D XRRV reabsorbant rotavirus vaccine by *Lactobacillus casei* GG. Vaccine 1995;13:310–312.

36. Roitt IM. In: Essential Immunology (8th ed.). Blackwell Science Ltd., London, 1991, p. 434.
37. Muscettola M, Massai L, Tanganelli C, Grasso G. Effects of lactobacilli on interferon production in young and aged mice. Ann NY Acad Sci 1994;717:226–232.
38. Kishi A, Uno K, Matsubara Y, Okuda C, Kishida T. Effect of the oral administration of *Lactobacillus brevis* subsp coagulans on interferon producing capacity in humans. J Am Coll Nutr 1996;15:408–412.
39. De Simone C, Vesely R, Bianchi Salvadori B, Jirillo E. The role of probiotics in modulation of the immune system in man and in animals. Intern J Immunotherapy 1993;9:23–28.
40. Halpern GM, Vruwink KG, Van De Water J, Keen CL, Gershwin ME. Influence of long-term yogurt consumption in young adults. Intern J Immunotherapy 1991;7:205–210.
41. Solis-Pereyra B, Aattouri N, Lemonnier D. Role of food in the stimulation of cytokine production. Am J Clin Nutr 1997;66:521S–525S.
42. Meydani SN, Ha WK. Immunologic effects of yogurt. Am J Clin Nutr 2000;71:861–872.
43. Solis Pereyra B, Lemonnier D. Induction of human cytokines by bacteria used in dairy foods. Nutr Res 1993;13:1127–1140.
44. Miettinen M, Vuopio-Varkila J, Varkila K. Production of human tumor necrosis factor alpha interleukin-6 and interleukin–10 is induced by lactic acid bacteria. Infect Immunol 1996;64:5403–5405.
45. Aattouri N, Lemonnier D. Production of interferon induced by *Streptococcus thermophilus*: role of CD4+ and CD8+ lymphocytes. J Nutr Biochem 1997;8:25–31.
46. Wheeler JG, Bogle ML, Shema SJ, et al. Impact of dietary yoghurt on immune function. Am J Med Sci 1997;313:120–123.
47. Wheeler JG, Shema S, Bogle ML, et al. Immune and clinical impact of *Lactobacillus acidophilus* on asthma. Ann Allergy Asthma Immunol 1997;79:229–233.
48. Trapp CL, Chang CC, Halpern GM, Keen CL, Gershwin ME. The influence of chronic yogurt consumption on populations of young and elderly adults. Intern J Immunotherapy 1993;9:53–64.
49. Spanhaak S, Havenaar R, Schaafsma G. The effect of consumption of milk fermented by *Lactobacillus casei* strain Shirota on the intestinal microflora and immune parameters in humans. Eur J Clin Nutr 1998;52:899–907.
50. Alm J, Swartz J, Lilja G, Scheynius A, Pershagen G. Atopy in children of families with an anthroposophic lifestyle. Lancet 1999;353:1485–1488.
51. Bjorksten B, Naaber P, Sepp E, Mikelsaar M. The intestinal microflora in allergic Estonian and Swedish 2-year-old children. Clin Exp Allergy 1999;29:342–346.
52. Kalliomaki M, Kirjavainen P, Eerola E, Kero P, Salminen S, Isolauri E. Distinct patterns of neonatal gut microflora in infants in whom atopy was and was not developing. J Allergy Clin Immunol 2001;107:129–134.
53. Sutas Y, Hurme M, Isolauri E. Down-regulation of anti-CD3 antibody-induced IL-4 production by bovine caseins hydrolysed with *Lactobacillus GG*-derived enzymes. Scand J Immunol 1996;43:687–689.
54. Majamaa H, Isolauri E. Probiotics: a novel approach in the management of food allergy. J Allergy Clinl Immunol 1997;99:179–185.
55. Pessi T, Sutas Y, Hurme M, Isolauri E. Interleukin-10 generation in atopic children following oral *Lactobacillus rhamnosus* GG. Clin Exp Allergy 2000;30:1804–1808.
56. Duchmann R, Kaiser I, Hermann E, Mayet W, Ewe K, Meyer zum Buschenfelde KH. Tolerance exists towards resident intestinal flora but is broken in active inflammatory bowel disease (IBD). Clin Exp Immunol 1995;102:448–455.
57. Taurog JD, Richardson JA, Croft JT, et al. The germfree state prevents development of gut and joint inflammatory disease in HLA-B27 transgenic rats. J Exp Med 1994;180:2359–2364.
58. Madsen KL, Doyle JS, Jewell LD, Tavernini M, Fedorak RN. Lactobacillus species prevents colitis in interleukin 10 gene-deficient mice. Gastroenterology 1999;116:1107–1114.
59. Malin M, Suomalainen H, Saxelin M, Isolauri E. Promotion of IgA immune response in patients with Crohn's disease by oral bacteriotherapy with *Lactobacillus* GG. Ann Nutr Metab 1996;40:137–145.
60. Gionchetti P, Rizzello F, Venturi A, et al. Oral bacteriotherapy as maintenance treatment in patients with chronic pouchitis: a double-blind placebo-controlled trial. Gastroenterology 2000;119:305–309.
61. Matsuzaki T, Yamazaki R, Hashimoto S, Yokokura T. Antidiabetic effect of *Lactobacillus casei* in a non-insulin-dependent diabetes mellitus (NIDDM) model using KK-A^y mice. Endocrine J 1997; 44:357–365.

62. Matsuzaki T, Nagara Y, Kado S, et al. Prevention of onset in an insulin-dependent diabetes mellitus model NOD mice by oral feeding *Lactobacillus casei*. Acta Pathologica Microbiologica et Immunologica Scandinavica 1997;105:643–649.

63. Nenonen MT, Helve TA, Rauma AL, Hanninen OO. Incooked lactobacilli-rich vegan food and rheumatoid arthritis. Br J Rheumatol 1998;37:274–281.

64. Peltonen R, Nenonen M, Helve T, Hanninen O, Toivanen P, Eerola E. Faecal microbial flora and disease activity in rheumatoid arthritis during a vegan diet. Br J Rheumatol 1997;36:64–68.

65. Peltonen R, Kjeldsen-Kragh J, Haugen M, et al. Changes of faecal flora in rheumatoid arthritis during fasting and a one-year vegetarian diet. Br J Rheumatol 1994;33:638–643.

66. Kato I, Endo-Tanaka K, Yokokura T. Suppressive effect of the oral administration of lactobacillus casei on type II collagen-induced arthritis in DBA/1 mice. Life Sci 1998;63:635–644.

67. McNaught CE, MacFie J. Probiotics in clinical practice: a critical review of the evidence. Nutr Res 2001;21:343–353.

68. Barefoot SF, Klaenhammer TR. Purification and characterisation of the *Lactobacillus acidophilus* bacteriocin lactacin B. Antimicrob Agents Chemother 1984;26:328–334.

69. Zamfir M, Callewaert R, Cornea PC, Savu L, Vatafu I, De Vuyst L. Purification and characterization of a bacteriocin produced by *Lactobacillus acidophilus* IBB 801. J Appl Microbiol 1999;87:923–931.

70. Silva M, Jacobus N, Deneke C, Gorback S. Antimicrobial substance from a human Lactobacillus strain. Antimicrob Agents Chemother 1987;31:1231–1233.

71. Bernet MF, Brassart D, Neeser JR, Servin AL. *Lactobacillus acidophilus* LA1 binds to cultured human intestinal cells and inhibits cell attachment and cell invasion by enterovirulent bacteria. Gut 1994; 35:483–489.

72. Saxelin M. *Lactobacillus GG*—a human probiotic strain with thorough clinical documentation. Food Rev Int 1997;13:293–313.

73. Johansson M-L, Molin G, Jeppsson B, Nobaek S, Ahrne S, Bengmark S. Administration of different Lactobacillus strains in fermented oatmeal soup: in vivo colonisation of human intestinal mucosa and effect on the indigenous flora. Appl Environ Microbiol 1993;59:15–20.

74. Ouwehand AC, Kirjavainen PV, Shortt C, Salminen S. Probiotics: mechanisms and established effects. Intl Dairy J 1999;9:43–52.

75. Guarino A, Canani RB, Spagnuolo NI, Albano F, Benedetto L. Oral bacterial therapy reduces the duration of symptoms and of viral excretion in children with mild diarrhea. J Pediatr Gastroenterol Nutr 1997;25:516–519.

76. Saavedra JM, Bauman NA, Oung I, Perman JA, Yolken RH. Feeding of *Bifidobacterium bifidum* and *Streptococcus thermophilus* to infants in hospital for prevention of diarrhoea and shedding of rotavirus. Lancet 1994;344:1046–1049.

77. Guandalini S, Pensabene L, Zikri MA, et al. *Lactobacillus GG* administered in oral rehydration solution to children with acute diarrhoea: a multicenter European trial. J Paediatr Gastroenterol Nutr 2000; 30:54–60.

78. Kaila M, Isolauri E, Saxelin M, Arvilommi H, Vesikari T. Viable versus inactivated Lactobacillus strain GG in acute rotavirus diarrhea. Arch Dis Child 1995;72:51–53.

79. Oberhelman RA, Gilman RH, Sheen P, et al. A placebo-controlled trial of *Lactobacillus GG* to prevent diarrhea in undernourished Peruvian children. J Pediatr 1999;134:15–20.

80. Braun OH. Effect of consumption of human and other formulas on intestinal microflora in infants. In: Lebenthal E (ed.). Gastroenterology and Nutrition Infancy. Raven, New York, 1981, pp. 247–251.

81. Yuhara T, Isojima S, Tsuchiya F, Mitsuoka T. On the intestinal flora of bottle-fed infants. Bifidobacteria Microflora 1983;2:33–39.

82. Isolauri E. Probiotics in human disease. Am J Clin Nutr 2001;73:1142S–1146S.

83. Hilton E, Kolakowski P, Singer C, Smith M. Efficacy of *Lactobacillus GG* as a diarrheal preventative in travelers. J Travel Med 1997;4:41–43.

84. Katelaris PH, Salam I, Farthing MJ. Lactobacilli to prevent traveller's diarrhoea? N Engl J Med 1995;333:1360–1361.

85. Clements ML, Levine MM, Black RE, et al. Lactobacillus prophylaxis for diarrhoea due to enterotoxigenic *Escherichia coli*. Antimicrob Agents Chemother 1981;20:104–108.

86. Oksanen PJ, Salminen S, Saxelin M, et al. Prevention of traveler's diarrhoea by *Lactobacillus GG*. Ann Med 1990;22:53–56.
87. Black FT, Anderson PL, Orskov J, Orskov F, Gaarslev K, Laulund S. Prophylactic efficacy of lactobacilli on traveller's diarrhea. Travel Med 1989;8:333–335.
88. De Simone C, Jirillo E, Bianchi Salvadori B. Stimulation of host resistance by a diet supplemented with yogurt. Adv Biosci 1988;68:229–233.
89. Shu Q, Rutherfurd KJ, Fenwick SG, Prasad J, Gopal PK, Gill HS. Dietary *Bifidobacterium lactis* (HN019) enhances resistance to oral *Salmonella typhimurium* infection in mice. Microbiol Immunol 2000;44:213–222.
90. Gill HS, Shu Q, Lin H, Rutherfurd KJ, Cross ML. Protection against translocating *Salmonella typhimurium* infection in mice by feeding the immuno-enhancing probiotic *Lactobacillus rhamnosus* strain HN001. Med Microbiol Immunol 2001;190:97–104.
91. Gotz V, Romankiewica JA, Moss J, Murray HW. Prophylaxis against ampicillin-associated diarrhea with a Lactobacillus preparation. Am J Hosp Pharm 1979;36:754–757.
92. Siitonen S, Vapaatalo J, Salminen S, Gordin A, Saxelin M, Wikberg R, Kirkkola A-L. Effect of *Lactobacillus GG* yoghurt in prevention of antibiotic-associated diarrhea. Ann Med 1990;22:57–60.
93. Vanderhoof JA, Whitney DB, Antonson DL, Hanner TL, Lupo JV, Young RJ. *Lactobacillus GG* in the prevention of antibiotic-associated diarrhea in children. J Pediatr 1999;135:564–568.
94. Surawicz CM, Elmer GW, Speelman P, McFarland LV, Chin J, van Belle G. Prevention of antibiotic-associated diarrhea by *Saccharomyces boulardii*: a prospective study. Gastroenterology 1989;96:981–989.
95. McFarland LV, Surqwica CM, Greenberg RN, et al. Prevention of b-Lactam-associated diarrhoea by *Saccharomyces boulardii* compared to placebo. Am J Gastroenterol 1995;90:439–448.
96. Tankanow RM, Ross MB, Ertel IJ, Dickinson DG, McCormick LS, Garfinkel JF. A double-blind placebo-controlled study of the efficacy of Lactinex in the prophylaxis of amoxicillin-induced diarrhea. DICP Ann Pharmacother 1990;24:382–384.
97. Lewis SJ, Potts LF, Barry RE. The lack of therapeutic effect of *Saccharomyces boulardii* in the prevention of antibiotic related diarrhoea in elderly patients. J Infec 1998;36:171–174.
98. Parodi PW. The role of intestinal bacteria in the causation and prevention of cancer: modulation by diet and probiotics. Aust J Dairy Technol 1999;54:103–121.
99. Iannello D, Bonina L, Delfino D, Berlinghieri MC, Gismondo MR, Mastroeni P. Effect of oral administration of a variety of bacteria on depressed macrophage functions in tumour bearing rats. Ann Immunol 1984;135C:345–352.
100. Kato I, Endo K, Yokokura T. Effects of oral administration of *Lactobacillus casei* on antitumor responses induced by tumor resection in mice. Intern J Immunopharmacol 1994;16:29–36.
101. Kailasapathy K, Rybka S. *L. acidophilus* and Bifidobacterium spp—their therapeutic potential and survival in yogurt. Austr J Dairy Technol 1997;52:28–35.
102. Sawamura A, Yamaguchi Y, Toge T, et al. Enhancement of immuno-activities by oral administration of *Lactobacillus casei* in colorectal cancer patients. Biotherapy 1994;8:1567–1572.
103. Aso Y, Akaza H, Kotake T. Prophylactic effect of a *Lactobacillus casei* preparation on the recurrence of superficial bladder cancer. Urol Intern 1992;49:125–129.
104. Aso Y, Akaza H, Kotake T, Tsukamoto T, Imai K, Naito S, BLP Study Group. Preventive effect of a *Lactobacillus casei* preparation on the recurrence of superficial bladder cancer in a double-blind trial. Eur Urol 1995;27:104–109.
105. Le MG, Moulton LH, Hill C, Kramer A. Consumption of dairy products and alcohol in a case-control study of breast cancer. J Natl Cancer Inst 1986;77:633–636.
106. Van't Veer P, Dekker JM, Lamers JWJ, et al. Consumption of fermented milk products and breast cancer: a case-control study in The Netherlands. Cancer Res 1989;49:4020–4023.
107. Van't Veer P, van Leer EM, Rietdijk A, et al. Combination of dietary factors in relation to breast-cancer occurrence. Int J Cancer 1991;47:649–653.
108. Cramer DW, Harlow BL, Willett W, et al. Galactose consumption and metabolism in relation to the risk of ovarian cancer. Lancet 1989;2:66–71.

109. Claassen E, van Winsen R, Posno M, Boersma WJA. New and safe oral live vaccine based on Lacto-bacillus. In: Mestecky J, Russel MW, Jackson S, Michalek SM, Tlaskalova H, Sterzl J (eds.). Advances in Mucosal Immunology. Plenum, New York, 1995, pp. 1553–1558.
110. Isolauri E, Sutas Y, Kankaanpaa P, Arvilommi H, Salminen S. Probiotics: effects on immunity. Am J Clin Nutr 2001;73:444S–450S.
111. Iribe H, Koga T, Onoue K. Production of T cell-activating monokine of guinea pig macrophages induced by MDP and partial characterization of the monokine. J Immunol 1982;129:1029–1031.
112. Iribe H, Koga T, Onoue K, Kotani S, Kusumoto S, Shiba T. Macrophage-stimulating effect of synthetic muramyl dipeptide and its adjuvant-active and inactive analogs for the production of T cell activating monokines. Cell Immunol 1981;64:73–83.
113. Oppenheim JJ, Togawa A, Chedid L, Mizel S. Components of microbacteria and muramyl dipeptide with adjuvant activity induced lymphocyte activating factor. Cell Immunol 1980;50:71–81.
114. Tufano MA, Cipollaro De Lero G, Innielo R, Galdiero M, Galdiero F. Protein A and other surface components of *Staphylococcus aureus* stimulate production IL-1a, IL-6, TNF, and IFN-g. Eur Cytokine Net 1991;2:361–366.
115. Marteau P, Boutron-Ruault MC. Nutritional advantages of probiotics and prebiotics. Br J Nutr 2002;87(Suppl 2):S153–S157.
116. Hove H, Norgaard H, Brobech Mortensen P. Lactic acid bacteria and the human gastrointestinal tract. Eur J Clin Nutr 1999;53:339–350.
117. Boudraa G, Touhami M, Pochart P, Soltana R, Mary JY, Desjeux JF. Effect of feeding yogurt versus milk in children with persistent diarrhea. J Pediatr Gastroenterol Nutr 1990;11:509–512.
118. Isolauri E, Juntunen M, Rautanen T, Sillanaukee P, Koivula T. A human lactobacillus strain (*Lactobacillus casei* sp strain GG) promotes recovery from acute diarrhea in children. Pediatrics 1991;88: 90–97.
119. Shornikova AV, Isolauri E, Burkanova L, Lukovnikova S, Vesikari T. A trial in the Karelian Republic of oral rehydration and *Lactobacillus GG* for treatment of acute diarrhea. Acta Paediatr 1997;86: 460–465.
120. Shornikova AV, Casas IA, Isolauri E, Mykkanen H, Vesikari T. *Lactobacillus reuteri* as a therapeutic agent in acute diarrhea in young children. J Pediatr Gastroenterol Nutr1997;24:399–404.
121. Pozo-Olano JDD, Warram JH, Gomez RG, Cavazos MG. Effect of a lactobacilli preparation on traveler's diarrhea. Gastroenterology 1978;74:829–830.
122. Colombel JF, Cortot A, Neut C, Romond C. Yogurt with *Bifidobacterium longum* reduces erythromycin induced gastrointestinal effects. Lancet 1987;2:43.

18 Dietary Fat, Immunity, and Cancer

Kent L. Erickson, Darshan S. Kelley,
and Neil E. Hubbard

1. INTRODUCTION

There are few data and a paucity of studies that have investigated the relationship among dietary fat, the immune system, and cancer in humans; few valid conclusions can be made from those studies. However, there have been some studies in patients with cancer where the addition of n–3 fatty acids to the diet have improved immune parameters and have lengthened survival *(1,2)*. For example, non-Hodgkin's lymphoma, a cancer that occurs frequently in individuals with suppressed immune status, may be altered by dietary fat. Evaluation of women in the Nurses' Health Study showed that high dietary intakes of beef, pork, and lamb, as well as intakes of *trans*-unsaturated fat, were associated with an increased risk of non-Hodgkin's lymphoma *(3)*. In this chapter, we discuss the relationship of these topics separately *vis-a-vis* the dietary fat's effects on the immune system and its effects on the components of the malignant process. Mechanisms of dietary fat effects on cancer can then be loosely correlated with possible alterations in specific parameters of immune function that are involved in defending against tumors and their spread.

Dietary fat can have diverse effects on human health based on the amounts consumed and, perhaps more important, on the types consumed. Dietary fat may also differentially affect certain tissues and organs, depending on their development stage. The fatty acid composition of human tissues varies, depending on the types of fatty acids that are consumed in the diet; that composition has recently been used as a biomarker for correlating risk with disease. In addition, some dietary fatty acids can be transformed into potent biological mediators that initiate or alter numerous processes in the body. For example, linoleic acid, a common component of some vegetable oils, can be converted by mammalian tissues into arachidonic acid, a major precursor for the potent proinflammatory and protumorigenic agent, prostaglandin E_2 (PGE_2). Indeed, physiologic levels of PGE_2 can change depending on the tissue content of its precursor fatty acid. Because PGE_2 has been linked to alterations in the immune system and, more recently, to specific pathological processes, including cancer, dietary fat intake has played an increasing role in human disease. Those studies include measuring tissue fatty acid composition, determining dietary fat intake, modifying dietary fat during disease processes, and using specific fatty acids as adjuvants to treat disease. In this chapter, we focus

From: *Diet and Human Immune Function*
Edited by: D. A. Hughes, L. G. Darlington, and A. Bendich © Humana Press Inc., Totowa, NJ

on the recent work concerning the effects of dietary fat on the immune system. Therefore, the focus will be on dietary n–3 fatty acids that decrease PGE_2. In addition, numerous studies concerning dietary fat alterations of malignancy have been published in the last several years. Those studies involve several fatty acid types. Although major cancer research efforts involve numerous animal studies that compliment the epidemiologic studies and initiated clinical trials, their results are not discussed in this chapter because of space limitations. Links between dietary fat-induced alterations in immune function and resultant effects on cancer are discussed. Based on the studies presented herein, a case can be made for a beneficial effect of algal and fish oils in the diet to decrease cancer risk, resulting from either displacement of fats from other animal sources or via specific physiologic effects owing to the fatty acids in algal/fish oils.

2. DIETARY FAT AND IMMUNITY

The immune system functions by an intricate network of signals that are generated from extrinsic sources or intrinsically. Some of those intrinsic signals can be produced from metabolized dietary essential fatty acids. This provides a link between dietary fat and the alteration of immune function. Section 2.1. describes studies involving supplementation with n–3 fatty acids to modify the immune system. Usually, individuals were fed experimental diets or supplements and then several immune system parameters were evaluated, usually with blood samples or skin responses. Isolated immune system cells were then evaluated ex vivo using several different assays for function, such as chemotaxis or phagocytosis.

2.1. Dietary n–3 Fatty Acids and Immune and Inflammatory Responses

n–3 Polyunsaturated fatty acid sources used in human feeding trials have been flaxseed or linseed oil as sources of α-linolenic acid (ALA); fish and fish oils as sources of eicosapentaenoic acid (EPA) and docosahexaenoic acid (DHA); purified EPA and DHA esters; or DHA triglycerides from genetically engineered algae. There are only a few human studies with both flaxseed and fish oils, although there are several dozen studies with fish oils only.

2.1.1. ALPHA-LINOLENIC ACID

In one study, flaxseed oil was added to the diets of healthy men to increase ALA intake from 1 to 18 g/d *(4)*. Feeding the ALA diet for 8 wk significantly decreased peripheral blood mononuclear cells (PBMN) proliferation and the delayed type hypersensitivity (DTH) skin response *(4)*. The number of circulating white blood cells, granulocytes, monocytes, lymphocytes, and their subsets were not altered by the increased ALA intake. Other indices that did not change include the serum concentrations of immunoglobulin (Ig)G, IgA, C3, C4; B-cell proliferation; or ex vivo secretion of interleukin (IL)-2 and IL-2R. In another study, two diets based either on sunflower oil or flaxseed oil with 30% energy from fat were fed to young healthy men *(5)*. Ex vivo production of IL-1β and tumor necrosis factor-α (TNF-α) was significantly reduced in the flaxseed oil group within 4 wk of beginning this diet, although it remained unchanged in the sunflower oil group. In a third study, a modest level of 4 g/d ALA was provided for 12 wk to healthy men *(6)*. No change was found in neutrophil chemotaxis and superoxide production.

Thus, large amounts of ALA intake (10–15 times normal) inhibit both the in vivo and ex vivo indices of immune response, whereas moderate intakes do not have such inhibitory effects.

2.1.2. FISH CONSUMPTION

In one study, 500 g/d of salmon containing 2.3 g EPA and 3.6 g/d DHA was fed to 9 healthy young men *(7)*. The energy from fat was 24% and 27% for the salmon and control diets. Feeding the salmon diet for 40 d did not have any effect on numerous immune response indices, including DTH, PBMN proliferation, and serum Ig. In another study, feeding 120–188 g/d or 1.23 g EPA and DHA/day in fish without supplemental vitamin E to a group of elderly men and women for 24 wk significantly reduced DTH, lymphocyte proliferation, and the ex vivo production of the cytokines IL-1β, IL-6, and TNF-α *(8)*. None of these indices was inhibited in the group that received one fourth the amount of fish. More studies are needed to establish whether there are any risks associated with increased fish consumption. From the available data, 2–3 servings of fish/week should be safe, even without vitamin E supplementation, but that amount may not substantially alter immune response.

2.1.3. FISH OILS, EPA, AND DHA

Several studies have examined the effects of fish oil supplementation on ex vivo neutrophil and monocyte chemotaxis, superoxide production, phagocytosis, lymphocyte and monocyte cytokine production, lymphocyte proliferation, and in vivo immune response indices. The amount of fish oil supplemented ranged from 2 to 30 g/d (EPA and DHA 0.55–8.0 g/d) for periods of 4 to 52 wk. Many of these studies were longitudinal, without parallel control groups, in which the fish oils were added to the usual diets. This increased not only EPA and DHA intakes but also total fat intake. Only a few studies included placebo controls and held total fat intake constant. Some studies supplemented with variable amounts of vitamin E, which affects many immune response indices, whereas others did not. Most of the results indicate either inhibition or no effect of fish oil supplementation on the immune response variables tested.

2.1.3.1. EFFECTS OF EPA AND DHA ON IN VIVO INDICES OF IMMUNE STATUS

Three studies with EPA and/or DHA have examined their effects on the number of circulating white cells *(9–11)*. One study supplemented 2.4 g EPA + DHA/day to groups of women for 12 wk; α-tocopherol was supplemented at 6 mg/d. There was no change in the total number or the percentage of circulating white blood cells (WBC). In another study, a supplemental mixture of 3.2 g/d EPA and DHA was provided to adult men and women *(11)*. An additional 200 mg/d α-tocopherol was provided. No change in the numbers of circulating WBC was observed. In a third study, an additional 6 g/d DHA and 10 mg/d α-tocopherol were provided to healthy men *(10)*. Supplementation reduced the number of circulating WBC and circulating granulocytes by 25%. DHA's effects on the number of circulating granulocytes contrasted arachidonic acid, which caused a 25% increase *(10)*. DHA supplementation also did not alter serum IgG or C3 antibody titer against influenza vaccination, IL-2R, or DTH *(10)*.

Table 1
EPA and DHA Alteration of Neutrophil and Monocyte Functions*

Function	Amount of EPA and DHA (g/d)	Duration (wk)	subjects	Effect	Comments	Reference
Neutrophil chemotaxis	14.4	3	8	25–59% decrease	No placebo group	(28)
PMN chemotaxis	8.6	3	8/group	30–50% decrease	No placebo group	(16)
Monocyte superoxide production	6	6	9	47–60% decrease	No placebo group	(13)
PMN chemotaxis	5.4	6	7	70% decrease	No placebo group	(25)
Monocyte chemotaxis	4	8	5	57–70% decrease	No placebo group	(26)
Monocyte hydrogen peroxide production	4, EPA vs DHA vs corn oil	7	19/group	No change	Cells stored frozen before use	(29)
PMN chemotaxis and superoxide production	2.2	12	8/group	No change	Placebo controlled	(6)
PMN superoxide production	2.2	4	6/group	45–55% decrease	Placebo controlled	(12)
Monocyte hydrogen peroxide production	0.6	12	16/group	No change	Placebo controlled	(15)

*All subjects were adults 21 yr or older.
PMN, polymorphonuclear leukocyte; EPA, eicosapentaenoic acid; DHA, docosahexaenoic acid.

348

2.1.3.2. EFFECT OF EPA AND DHA ON NEUTROPHIL AND MONOCYTE RESPIRATORY BURST AND PHAGOCYTOSIS, AND CHEMOTAXIS

Two studies have reported an approx 50% reduction in ex vivo neutrophil and monocyte superoxide production when healthy human volunteers supplemented their diets with 0.65 to 5.8 g/d EPA and DHA for 4 to 12 wk *(12,13)*. Another study found a 64% reduction in neutrophil phagocytosis after 3.6 g/d EPA supplementation for 6 wk *(14)*.

Several studies have been published recently regarding the effects of EPA and DHA on neutrophil and monocyte chemotaxis (*see* Table 1). The EPA and DHA supplement in these studies ranged from 0.65 to 14.4 g/d for 3 to 12 wk. Neutrophil or monocyte chemotaxis was decreased in most of the studies with EPA and DHA intake of 1.3 g/d or more. One study that reported no inhibition of chemotaxis by EPA and DHA was based on supplementation of only 0.65 g/d for 12 wk *(15)*. Another study found that neutrophil chemotaxis was inhibited within 3 wk of a high dose of 8.7 g/d EPA and DHA, even if the subjects consumed 9 or 45 IU/d extra vitamin E *(16)*. There was no difference in the chemotaxis rate based on the two levels of vitamin E intake. The amount of vitamin E intake in this study may not be adequate to protect against the high intake of EPA and DHA. In the short-term studies, EPA and DHA intakes of fewer than 1 g/d did not inhibit neutrophil and monocyte chemotaxis; however, long-term studies must be conducted before firm conclusions can be made. Certainly, higher amounts of these fatty acids can inhibit neutrophil chemotaxis by 3 wk.

2.1.3.3. EPA AND DHA INHIBITION OF CYTOKINE PRODUCTION BY MONOCYTES

Numerous studies have been conducted to investigate the effects of feeding EPA and DHA to human volunteers and then examining ex vivo cytokine production (*see* Table 2). The amount of EPA and DHA intake ranged from 0.6 to 6.0 g/d for 4 to 52 wk; vitamin E supplementation ranged from 0 to 200 mg/d. Seven of these studies *(5,8,9,17–20)* reported a significant reduction in the concentration of the three proinflammatory cytokines—IL-1, IL-6, or TNF-α,—secreted by monocytes after stimulation with lipopolysaccharide (LPS). The remaining seven studies failed to find a reduction in monokine secretion. Four weeks was the shortest period in which EPA and DHA supplementation reduced TNF-α and IL-1 secretion. On the other hand, supplementation with approximately the same amount of those fatty acids for 6 mo or more did not inhibit the production of those cytokines *(21)*. This most likely resulted from investigators not examining cytokine secretion at any time before 6 mo; they also supplemented with 54 mg/d vitamin E. In another study, similar levels of EPA and DHA plus 200 mg/d vitamin E were given as a supplement for 12 wk; no reduction in IL-1 and TNF-α secretion was observed *(11)*. Besides the studies that used a mixture of n–3 fatty acids, two studies supplemented with DHA alone *(19,22)*. One study supplemented with 700 mg/d DHA for 12 wk but did not detect alteration in IL-1, IL-6, and TNF-α secretion *(22)*. In the other study, after 6 g/d DHA for 90 d, IL-1 and TNF-α secretions were reduced by 45% and 30% *(19)*. These results suggest that higher, but not lower, concentrations of both EPA and DHA can inhibit cytokine secretion. A possible reason for the discrepancies regarding the effect of EPA and DHA on monocyte cytokine secretion may be the genetic polymorphisms of the subjects. A recent study reported that TNF-α secretion inhibition by EPA and DHA was dependent on the polymorphism in the TNF-α gene *(20)*.

Table 2
Inhibition of Monocyte Cytokine Production by EPA and DHA*

Cytokine	Amount of EPA and DHA (g/d)	Duration (wk)	No. of subjects	Effect	Comments	Reference
IL-1, TNF-α	6, DHA	13	7 DHA; 4 control	30–45% decrease	10 mg/d vitamin E	(19)
IL-1, TNF-α	5.2	24	15–20 group	Decrease	Compared MS patients with healthy subjects	(18)
IL-1, TNF-α	4.6	6	9	20–60% decrease	No placebo group	(17)
IL-1, TNF-α	3.2	12	81 group	No change	205 mg/d vitamin E	(11)
IL-1, TNF-α	2.7	4	15 group	70–80%	No placebo group	(5)
IL-1, TNF-α	2.4	12	6 older; 6 younger	No change	Older > younger 6 mg/d vitamin E	(9)
TNF-α	1.8	12	111/6 groups	No change or depending on phenotype	TNF-α gene polymorphism affected response	(20)
IL-1, IL-6, TNF-α	1.2	24	11	No change	High fish and low fish diets	(8)
IL-1, IL-6, TNF-α	2.4	7	8–9 group	70–80% decrease	Cellular IL-1, but not secreted IL-1 or TNF-α	(9)
IL, IL-1Ra, TNF-α	1.1, 2.1 and 3.1	52	14–15/group	No change	Serum cytokines determined at 26 and 52 wk only; 5.4 IU/d vitamin E	(21)
TNF-α, IL-1, IL-6	0.6	12	16/group	No change	Placebo controlled	(15)

*All subjects were adults greater than 21 yr of age.
EPA, eicosapentaenoic acid; IL, interleukin; TNF, tumor necrosis factor; DHA, docosahexaenoic acid.

350

2.1.3.4. EFFECT OF EPA AND DHA ON LYMPHOCYTE AND MACROPHAGE FUNCTIONS

Natural killer (NK) cell activity was examined in three studies after supplementing EPA and/or DHA *(11,19,22)* and in one study where EPA-triglyceride was infused *(23)*. One study used 6 g/d DHA and found a significant reduction in NK cell activity after 12, but not 8, wk of supplementation *(19)*. The other two reports come from the same laboratory. In one, 3.2 g/d EPA and DHA and 200 mg/d vitamin E supplementation for 12 wk did not inhibit NK cell activity *(11)*. However, NK cell activity was significantly decreased even with 1 g/d EPA and DHA supplementation for 12 wk, whereas 0.7 g/d DHA supplementation for the same period did not inhibit NK cell activity *(22)*. Infusing 30 mL of EPA-triglyceride 24 h before isolation reduced NK cell activity by more than 50% *(23)*. Together, these studies suggest that EPA and DHA may inhibit NK cell activity.

Lymphocyte proliferation, IL-2 and interferon (IFN)-γ production or all were decreased in five of the nine studies in which the diets were supplemented with a mixture of EPA and DHA or DHA alone. The intake of EPA and DHA ranged from 1.2 to 5.2 g/d for 6 to 24 wk. Two studies *(19,22)* that reported no alteration of lymphocyte proliferation or cytokine production used 0.7 g or 6 g/d DHA supplementation for 12 wk. This indicates that the inhibition of lymphocyte proliferation and cytokine production may be caused by EPA and not DHA. The third study, which reported no effect, supplemented 3.2 g/d EPA and DHA for 12 wk *(11)*. The lack of inhibition observed in this study most likely resulted from the additional 200 mg/d of vitamin E. Another study showed that supplementing 200 mg/d vitamin E for 8 wk reversed the inhibition of lymphocyte proliferation caused by 15 g/d fish oil supplementation for 10 wk *(24)*. The fourth study found no inhibition of lymphocyte proliferation by fish oils, supplemented 4.6 g/d EPA and DHA for 6 wk. It is possible that more than 6 wk of fatty acid supplementation are required to inhibit lymphocyte functions, because all other studies reporting inhibition supplemented the fatty acids for 7–24 wk. Thus, the lowest concentration of EPA and DHA that inhibited lymphocyte functions was 1.2 g/d for 24 wk *(8)*, whereas the highest concentration that did not inhibit was 3.2 g/d for 12 wk *(11)*. The differences might result from fatty acid and antioxidant composition of the basal diet, duration of feeding, the EPA/DHA ratio, or the assay methods used.

Without additional vitamin E, supplementation with 1.3 to 8.0 g/d EPA and DHA for 4 wk or more reduced several neutrophil functions, including chemotaxis, chemiluminescence, superoxide production, and phagocytosis *(12–14,16,25–28)*. Monocyte chemotaxis and superoxide production were also decreased in some of these studies *(13,27)*. Monocyte chemotaxis and superoxide production were not reduced in one study that used a low concentration of fish oil (EPA and DHA 0.55 g/d) for 12 wk *(15)*. In another study, supplementation with 4 g/d EPA or DHA for 7 wk did not inhibit monocyte phagocytosis *(29)*. The effect of fish oil supplementation on IL-1β and TNF-α production has been examined in several studies. Many of these found a 25–75% decrease in the in vitro secretion of cytokines when 2.4 g/d or more EPA and DHA were supplemented in the diets for 4 wk or more *(5,10,17,19)*. Thus, cytokine production by lymphocytes is altered by fish oils.

2.1.3.5. POSSIBLE REASONS FOR REPORTED DIFFERENCES

Several differences in the study protocols and the methods used could have contributed to the discrepancies in results from different studies. Factors related to the study protocol include antioxidant nutrient content of the diets; total fat and fatty acid composition; ratio of n–6 and n–3 PUFA; amount and duration of supplementation; ratio of EPA and DHA (EPA is more inhibitory than DHA); the age, sex, and health status of the subjects; and inclusion of a placebo group. Methods and cells used for assessments have varied greatly. For example, isolated PBMN or whole blood cultured in autologous sera or fetal calf serum have been used with numerous agents to stimulate the cells and to monitor their responses. The most critical factor is the ratio of the amounts of n–3 PUFA and vitamin E, because the latter blocks the inhibition by n–3 PUFA and the duration of supplementation.

3. DIETARY FAT AND CANCER

Dietary fat is easily the most controversial and misunderstood macronutrient in the human diet. Its negative connotation began in the 1940s when it was shown to promote cancer in animal models. It was later correlated with increased risk of heart disease. With the history of being linked to two major killers in the human population, it was easy to suspect dietary fat as the culprit in all cancers and perhaps other diseases. However, several investigations have shown that not all fats are created equal! Numerous animal studies and studies involving cultured human tumor cells routinely show that n–6 fatty acids can have a promotional effect and n–3 fatty acids an inhibitory effect on several aspects of tumorigenesis and tumor cell proliferation. However, attempts to extend those findings to humans have produced results that were not as clear-cut. A summary of dietary fat effects on cancers of select sites is presented in Table 4. Studying dietary fat effects on cancer has more to do with the correct selection of human populations, choice of biomarkers, design of questionnaires, and statistical analyses than tumor biology. Limitations of questionnaires can be the completeness of the questionnaire, the ability of the respondent to recall accurately, and the accuracy of the database used to calculate dietary fat levels in the foods. Hopefully, several decades of effort in developing, evaluating, and refining methods of dietary assessment have laid the groundwork for further assessments of the role of dietary fat in cancer etiology that will emerge from the more than 30 large prospective studies that are currently underway (30).

3.1. Breast Cancer

In the most recent evaluation of breast cancer risk, with the large and lengthy epidemiologic data from the Nurses' Health Study, there was no correlation with the amount and type of dietary fat (see Table 5) (31). High intakes of fat and specific types of fat, including animal, saturated, polyunsaturated, and trans-unsaturated, had been postulated to increase breast cancer risk. In the Nurses' Health Study, approx 89,000 women free of cancer in 1980 have been followed for several years. The relative risk of invasive breast cancer with increased fat intake was ascertained by food-frequency questionnaires. A total of nearly 3,000 women were diagnosed as having breast cancer during the period of the study. Comparing women obtaining 30% to 35% of energy from fat with women consuming 20% of energy from fat, there was no evidence that lower intake of total fat or specific major types of fat was associated with a decreased risk of breast cancer (31).

In a recent pooled analysis of cohort studies, eight prospective studies that met predefined criteria were analyzed (32). Those studies were selected because they had at least

Table 3
DHA and EPA Alteration of Lymphocyte Functions*

Function	Amount of EPA and DHA (g/d)	Duration (wk)	No. of subjects	Effect	Comments	Reference
Proliferation	7	10	34	80% decrease	200 mg/d vitamin E	(24)
Proliferation	6, DHA	13	7 DHA; 4 control	No change	10 mg/d vitamin E	(10)
NK-cell activity	6, DHA	13	7 DHA; 4 control	20% decrease No change 8 wk	10 mg/d vitamin E	(19)
IL-2 and IFN-α secretion	5.2	24	15–20/group	25–30% decrease	400 mg/d vitamin E	(18)
IL-2 and IFN-α secretion	3.2	12	8/group	No change	205 mg/d vitamin E	(11)
Proliferation	3.2	12	8/group	No change	205 mg/d vitamin E	(11)
NK-cell activity	3.2	12	8/group	No change	205 mg/d vitamin E	(11)
IL-2 secretion	2.4	12	6	30% decrease	6 mg/d vitamin E	(9)
Proliferation	2.4	12	6	36% decrease	High fish and low fish diets	(9)
Proliferation	1.2	24	11	24% decrease		(8)
NK-cell activity	1, DHA	12	8/group	48% decrease	Reduction reversed within 4 wk	(22)
Proliferation	2 or 4	7	8/group	20–35% decrease wk 2 and 4	Placebo controlled	(9)

*All subjects were adults greater than 21 yr of age.
EPA, eicosapentaenoic acid; DHA, docosahexaenoic acid; NK, natural killer; IL, interleukin; IFN, interferon.

353

Table 4
Summary of Dietary Fat Effects on Cancer at Select Sites

Cancer site	Dietary fat	Effect	Comments	References
Breast	Various	No effect	Cohort and case-control studies	(31,32)
Prostate	EPA, DHA	Reduction	2 studies	(44,45)
Lung	Various	No effect	Cohort studies	(46)
Colorectal	n–3	Reduction	No effect of other fats	(47)
Esophagus	n–3	Reduction	Food patterning study	(49)
Distal Stomach	Fat of red meat	Induction	Food patterning study	(50)

EPA, eicosapentaenoic acid; DHA, docosahexaenoic acid.

200 incident breast cancer cases, assessed usual intake of foods and nutrients, and had a validation tool of the diet assessment method. The relative risk for increments of 5% of energy for saturated, monounsaturated, or polyunsaturated fat was compared with an equivalent amount of energy from carbohydrates or other types of fat. In the pooled database, more than 7,300 incident invasive breast cancer cases occurred in the more than 350,000 women. The data in this study were suggestive of only a weak positive association of breast cancer with substitution of saturated fat for carbohydrate consumption; none of the other types of fat examined was significantly associated with breast cancer risk relative to an equivalent reduction in carbohydrate consumption (32).

Some smaller cohort studies have shown a correlation between certain fats and increased or decreased risk of breast cancer. Therefore, the relationship of dietary fat and breast cancer risk remains somewhat unresolved. Both of the large studies described thus far grouped fats into major categories; other studies have attempted to evaluate the effects of specific fatty acids. Based on findings from numerous studies with animals, as well as human and animal breast cancer cell lines, several specific fatty acids have been hypothesized to have antitumorigenic effects in humans. Conjugated linoleic acid (CLA), present in milk products and meat from ruminants, is one such candidate, because it has anticarcinogenic activity against breast cancer in animal and cell lines in vitro. However, few epidemiologic studies have directly assessed the chemoprevention of those fatty acids. One study evaluated the relationship between CLA intake and breast cancer incidence (33). Intake data were derived from a 150-item food-frequency questionnaire and linked to an existing database with analytic data on specific fatty acids. After 6 yr of follow-up and 941 incident cases of breast cancer, based on statistical analysis for energy-adjusted intakes of CLA-containing food groups, the authors could not confirm the anticarcinogenic property of CLA reported for animal, as well as human, tumors in vitro.

In two other studies, measurements of CLA content in the serum (34) and in the breast adipose tissue (35) were used to assess correlation of CLA with breast cancer. In one study with women who were postmenopausal (34), dietary CLA and serum CLA were significantly lower in the women with breast cancer compared with the controls. However, in another study, where CLA levels in the breast adipose tissue were determined in women with or without breast cancer, no association was observed between adipose tissue CLA and breast cancer risk (35). The authors believe that before any lack of association could be concluded, additional studies based on similar approaches should be conducted in more heterogeneous populations or countries. However, it is unknown

Table 5
Select Epidemiological Studies of Diet and Breast Cancer

Study	Fat type	Result	Comment	References
Nurses' Health Study	All fat types and amounts	No effect	Almost 89,000 women	(31)
Pooled cohort studies[a]	Saturated	Small induction	More than 350,000 women	(32)
	Mono- and polyunsaturated	No effect		
Netherlands cohort study	Conjugated linoleic acid	No effect		(33)

[a]Adventist Health Study, Canadian National Breast Screening Study, New York State Cohort, New York University Women's Health Study, Nurses' Health Study, Iowa Women's Health Study, Netherlands Cohort Study, Sweden Mammography Cohort

whether dietary CLA or other fatty acids, or the amount, affects breast development in puberty and thus, alters risk of breast cancer later in life. That should be determined, because animal studies indicate that dietary CLA can alter breast development, which, in turn, can lead to a significantly decreased incidence of breast cancer (36).

The other fatty acids that may prove to be major players in dietary fat alterations of breast cancer risk are n–3 fatty acids. Long-chain n–3 fatty acids also consistently inhibit the growth of human breast cancer cells in both culture and grafts in immunosuppressed mice (37). Large cohort studies, however, have failed to confirm a protective effect for n–3 fatty acids against breast cancer risk. Alpha-linolenic acid may have a protective effect in breast cancer (38). A case-control study conducted in a homogeneous population in France used fatty-acid levels in adipose breast tissue as a biomarker of past qualitative dietary intake of fatty acids. Biopsies of adipose breast tissue at the time of diagnosis were obtained from women with invasive nonmetastatic breast carcinoma; women with benign breast disease served as controls. No association was found between fatty acids (saturated, monounsaturated, or long-chain polyunsaturated n–6 or n–3) and the disease, except for ALA, which showed an inverse association with breast cancer risk (38).

Therefore, based on epidemiological studies only, dietary fat changes as part of a regimen to decrease breast cancer risk would not be warranted. However, dietary fat changes to alter cardiovascular disease risk should not increase breast cancer risk. In fact, it has recently been shown that fish and n–3 fatty acid intake is inversely correlated with coronary heart disease risk in women (39).

3.2. Prostate Cancer

Although there have been fewer human studies of diet and prostate cancer with a large sample size compared to breast cancer, the results from studies with animals, as well as human prostate cancer cell lines in vitro, provide compelling evidence for epidemiological studies. The relationship of dietary fat to prostate cancer risk has recently been reviewed (40). Correlations between animal products and prostate cancer have been noted in numerous observational studies; however, it is not clear whether the high fat content of these foods or some other component accounts for those associations. In the Health Professionals Follow-Up Study, more than 50,000 men contributed detailed

Table 6
Select Epidemiological Studies of Dietary Fat and Prostate Cancer

Study	Fat type	Result	Comment	References
Health Professional's Follow-up Study	Red meat and dairy products	Increased risk of metastatic prostate cancer	51,529 men	(41)
Case-control, New Zealand	Monounsaturated n–3	Decreased risk	317 cases; 480 controls	(43)
Swedish study	Fish consumption	Decreased risk	6272 men	(45)

dietary data by completing a semiquantitative food-frequency questionnaire (*see* Table 6) *(41)*. A high intake of both red meat and dairy products was associated with a statistically significant twofold elevation in risk of metastatic prostate cancer, compared with low intake of both products; however, most of the excess risk could be explained by known nutritional components of these foods.

Like breast cancer, n–6 fatty acids promote, and n–3 fatty acids inhibit, prostate tumor development in animal models. In one case-control study that focused on n–3 and n–6 fatty acids, prostate cancer risk was increased in men in the highest compared to the lowest quartile of ALA consumption. Positive associations were also observed with higher levels of linoleic acid and total n–6 fatty acids. In contrast to animal studies, ALA was positively associated with prostate cancer risk *(42)*.

Another study, with 317 patients with prostate cancer and 480 controls, focused on dietary patterns associated with consumption of vegetable oils rich in monounsaturated fatty acids (MUFA) and risk of prostate cancer *(43)*. A food-frequency questionnaire was used to collect data for consumption of MUFA-rich vegetable oils. The group of participants who consumed high levels of MUFA-rich vegetable oils per day also had a diet relatively high in n–3 fish oils. Increasing MUFA-rich vegetable oil intake was associated with a progressive reduction in prostate cancer risk. That risk was not associated with intake of total MUFA or the major animal food sources of MUFA. This finding may be explained by the protective effect of an associated dietary pattern high in antioxidants and fish oils, an independent protective effect of MUFA-rich vegetable oils unrelated to the MUFA component, or a combination of these factors. A closely related study with the same population focused on the association of n–3 polyunsaturated fatty acid intake derived from marine foods, such as EPA and DHA, with the risk of prostate cancer *(44)*. Reduced prostate cancer risk was associated with high erythrocyte levels of those fatty acids. In a study of more than 6,000 men, those who ate no fish had a twofold to threefold higher frequency of prostate cancer than those who ate moderate or high amounts *(45)*. These observations are consistent with in vitro experiments. These fatty acids may possibly act by inhibition of arachidonic acid-derived eicosanoid biosynthesis *(44)*.

In contrast to breast cancer, prostate cancer is altered by n–3 fatty acids in humans. It is unknown whether the effects resulted from a better quality of life with less comorbidity or direct n–3 fatty acid effects in animal and in vitro studies. Numerous ongoing prospective studies of dietary fat and prostate cancer should provide much-needed answers about whether dietary fat should be modified to reduce risk *(40)*.

3.3. Other Cancers

Lung cancer rates are often highest in countries with the greatest fat intakes *(46)*. In several case-control studies, positive associations have been observed between lung cancer and total and saturated fat intakes, particularly in nonsmokers *(46)*. Recently, eight prospective cohort studies were analyzed for any association between fat and lung cancer *(46)*. Among the participants who were followed for up to 16 yr, no associations were observed between intakes of total or specific types of fat and lung cancer risk among never, past, or current smokers. These data do not support an important relationship between fat and lung cancer risk *(46)*. Smoking still remains one of the greatest risk factors for lung cancer.

Dietary fat may be an important risk factor in colorectal cancer. Mortality data for colorectal cancer for 24 European countries was correlated with the consumption of animal, but not vegetable, fat *(47)*. There was an inverse correlation with fish and fish oil consumption and colorectal cancer, when expressed as a proportion of total or animal fat. This correlation was significant, either based on intakes in the current time period or up to 23 yr before cancer mortality. These effects were observed only in countries with a high animal fat intake. Thus, fish oil was associated with protection against the promotional effects of animal fat in colorectal carcinogenesis. However, in another cohort study, where the relationships between consumption of total fat, major dietary fatty acids, cholesterol, meat, or eggs and the incidence of colorectal cancers were studied, total fat, as well as saturated, monounsaturated, or polyunsaturated fatty acids, were not significantly associated with colorectal cancer risk *(48)*.

The relationship between nutrient intakes and adenocarcinoma of the esophagus and distal stomach in a population-based case-control study showed significant interaction between dietary fat intake, but not intakes of other nutrients, and cancer for both sites *(49)*. Moreover, they observed positive associations between saturated fat intake and risk of esophageal adenocarcinoma and distal stomach cancer. Risk of esophageal adenocarcinoma was inversely associated with dairy product, fish, all vegetables, citrus fruit and juice, and dark bread intakes and was positively associated with gravy intake. Risk of distal stomach adenocarcinoma was positively associated with red meat intake *(50)*.

3.4. Fatty Acids in Cancer Treatment

Long-chain polyunsaturated fatty acids may increase the sensitivity of mammary tumors to several cytotoxic drugs. In one prospective study, fatty acids stored in breast adipose tissue were correlated with the response to combinations of four drugs used for chemotherapy in patients with localized breast carcinoma. The level of n–3 polyunsaturated fatty acids in adipose tissue was higher in patients with complete or partial response to chemotherapy than in patients with no response or with tumor progression. Among n–3 polyunsaturates, only DHA was significantly associated with tumor response, and it proved to be an independent predictor for chemosensitivity. Those results suggested that in breast cancer, DHA may increase the response of the tumor to the cytotoxic agents used *(51)*.

4. CONCLUSIONS

Because published studies to date have not focused on dietary fat effects on immunity in the cancer patient or how dietary fat alters specific tumor immunity in humans, we have focused on dietary fat and immune status or response, as well as dietary fat and cancer risk. Select fatty acids, notably those of the n–3 family, selectively decrease some lymphocyte, neutrophil, and macrophage functions, but not all. Even when the same lymphocyte function or cytokine profiles were assessed after dietary fat manipulation, different and sometimes divergent results were reported by different investigators. Although an extensive number of animal studies, as well as in vitro studies with human tumors, have shown pronounced effects of dietary fats and specific fatty acids in reducing tumorigenesis at several sites, case-control and cohort studies have demonstrated an effect of altering tumorigenesis at fewer sites. Whether any of those changes are related to altered tumor immunity is unknown. Intervention studies are clearly needed to resolve which fats alter tumorigenesis at which sites. Those types of studies are extremely difficult, given the often long duration between dietary alteration and clinical detection of a tumor. Nevertheless, reduction of fat consumption and an increase of n–3 fatty acids may be prudent, because no detrimental effects have been reported with respect to immunity and cancer and, in some cases, beneficial effects.

5. "TAKE-HOME" MESSAGES

1. No studies to date on dietary fat and immunity in the cancer patient.
2. Moderate intakes of ALA do not inhibit indices of immune response.
3. High concentrations of EPA and DHA can inhibit neutrophil and monocyte functions that may depend on added levels of vitamin E.
4. EPA and DHA may decrease proinflammatory cytokine production. Differences reported may result from genetic polymorphisms of the individuals. Cytokine production by lymphocytes is altered more by fish oil than cytokines produced by macrophages.
5. Although various tumors in animals, as well as human tumors in vitro, can be altered by either dietary fat or specific fatty acids, epidemiologic studies demonstrate an effect at fewer sites.

REFERENCES

1. Gogos CA, Ginopoulos P, Salsa B, Apostolidou E, Zoumbos NC, Kalfarentzos F. Dietary omega-3 polyunsaturated fatty acids plus vitamin E restore immunodeficiency and prolong survival for severely ill patients with generalized malignancy: a randomized control trial. Cancer 1998;82:395–402.
2. Tashiro T, Yamamori H, Takagi K, Hayashi N, Furukawa K, Nakajima N. n–3 versus n–6 polyunsaturated fatty acids in critical illness. Nutrition 1998;14:551–553.
3. Zhang S, Hunter DJ, Rosner BA, et al. Dietary fat and protein in relation to risk of non-Hodgkin's lymphoma among women. J Natl Cancer Inst 1999;91:1751–1758.
4. Kelley DS, Branch LB, Love JE, Taylor PC, Rivera YM, Iacono JM. Dietary alpha-linolenic acid and immunocompetence in humans. Am J Clin Nutr 1991;53:40–46.
5. Caughey GE, Mantzioris E, Gibson RA, Cleland LG, James MJ. The effect on human tumor necrosis factor alpha and interleukin 1 beta production of diets enriched in n–3 fatty acids from vegetable oil or fish oil. Am J Clin Nutr 1996;63:116–122.
6. Healy DA, Wallace FA, Miles EA, Calder PC, Newsholm P. Effect of low-to-moderate amounts of dietary fish oil on neutrophil lipid composition and function. Lipids 2000;35:763–768.
7. Kelley DS, Nelson GJ, Branch LB, Taylor PC, Rivera YM, Schmidt PC. Salmon diet and human immune status. Eur J Clin Nutr 1992;46:397–404.
8. Meydani SN, Lichtenstein AH, Cornwall S, et al. Immunologic effects of national cholesterol education panel step-2 diets with and without fish-derived N–3 fatty acid enrichment. J Clin Invest 1993;92:105–113.

9. Meydani SN, Endres S, Woods MM, et al. Oral (n–3) fatty acid supplementation suppresses cytokine production and lymphocyte proliferation: comparison between young and older women. J Nutr 1991;121:547–555.

10. Kelley DS, Taylor PC, Nelson GJ, Mackey BE. Dietary docosahexaenoic acid and immunocompetence in young healthy men. Lipids 1998;33:559–566.

11. Yaqoob P, Pala HS, Cortina-Borja M, Newsholme EA, Calder PC. Encapsulated fish oil enriched in alpha-tocopherol alters plasma phospholipid and mononuclear cell fatty acid compositions but not mononuclear cell functions. Eur J Clin Invest 2000;30:260–274.

12. Thompson PJ, Misso NL, Passarelli M, Phillips MJ. The effect of eicosapentaenoic acid consumption on human neutrophil chemiluminescence. Lipids 1991;26:1223–1226.

13. Fisher M, Levine PH, Weiner BH, et al. Dietary n–3 fatty acid supplementation reduces superoxide production and chemiluminescence in a monocyte-enriched preparation of leukocytes. Am J Clin Nutr 1990;51:804–808.

14. Fisher M, Upchurch KS, Levine PH, et al. Effects of dietary fish oil supplementation on polymorpho-nuclear leukocyte inflammatory potential. Inflammation 1986;10:387–392.

15. Schmidt EB, Varming K, Moller JM, Bulow Pedersen I, Madsen P, Dyerberg J. No effect of a very low dose of n–3 fatty acids on monocyte function in healthy humans. Scand J Clin Lab Invest 1996;56: 87–92.

16. Luostarinen R, Siegbahn A, Saldeen T. Effects of dietary supplementation with vitamin E on human neutrophil chemotaxis and generation of LTB4. Ups J Med Sci 1991;96:103–111.

17. Endres S, Ghorbani R, Kelley VE, et al. The effect of dietary supplementation with n–3 polyunsaturated fatty acids on the synthesis of interleukin-1 and tumor necrosis factor by mononuclear cells. N Engl J Med 1989;320:265–271.

18. Gallai V, Sarchielli P, Trequattrini A, et al. Cytokine secretion and eicosanoid production in the peripheral blood mononuclear cells of MS patients undergoing dietary supplementation with n–3 polyunsaturated fatty acids. J Neuroimmunol 1995;56:143–153.

19. Kelley DS, Taylor PC, Nelson GJ, et al. Docosahexaenoic acid ingestion inhibits natural killer cell activity and production of inflammatory mediators in young healthy men. Lipids 1999;34:317–324.

20. Grimble RF, Howell WM, O'Reilly G, et al. The ability of fish oil to suppress tumor necrosis factor alpha production by peripheral blood mononuclear cells in healthy men is associated with polymorphisms in genes that influence tumor necrosis factor alpha production. Am J Clin Nutr 2002;76:454–459.

21. Blok WL, Deslypere JP, Demacker PN, et al. Pro- and anti-inflammatory cytokines in healthy volunteers fed various doses of fish oil for 1 year. Eur J Clin Invest 1997;27:1003–1008.

22. Thies F, Nebe-von-Caron G, Powell JR, Yaqoob P, Newsholme EA, Calder PC. Dietary supplementation with eicosapentaenoic acid, but not with other long-chain n–3 or n–6 polyunsaturated fatty acids, decreases natural killer cell activity in healthy subjects aged >55 y. Am J Clin Nutr 2001;73:539–548.

23. Yamashita N, Maruyama M, Yamazaki K, Hamazaki T, Yano S. Effect of eicosapentaenoic and docosahexaenoic acid on natural killer cell activity in human peripheral blood lymphocytes. Clin Immunol Immunopathol 1991;59:335–345.

24. Kramer TR, Schoene N, Douglass LW, et al. Increased vitamin E intake restores fish-oil-induced suppressed blastogenesis of mitogen-stimulated T lymphocytes. Am J Clin Nutr 1991;54:896–902.

25. Lee TH, Hoover RL, Williams JD, et al. Effect of dietary enrichment with eicosapentaenoic and docosahexaenoic acids on in vitro neutrophil and monocyte leukotriene generation and neutrophil function. N Engl J Med 1985;312:1217–1224.

26. Payan DG, Wong MY, Chernov-Rogan T, et al. Alterations in human leukocyte function induced by ingestion of eicosapentaenoic acid. J Clin Immunol 1986;6:402–410.

27. Schmidt EB, Pedersen JO, Varming K, et al. n–3 fatty acids and leukocyte chemotaxis. Effects in hyperlipidemia and dose-response studies in healthy men. Arterioscler Thromb 1991;11:429–435.

28. Sperling RI, Benincaso AI, Knoell CT, Larkin JK, Austen KF, Robinson DR. Dietary omega-3 polyunsaturated fatty acids inhibit phosphoinositide formation and chemotaxis in neutrophils. J Clin Invest 1993;91:651–660.

29. Halvorsen DS, Hansen JB, Grimsgaard S, Bonaa KH, Kierulf P, Nordoy A. The effect of highly purified eicosapentaenoic and docosahexaenoic acids on monocyte phagocytosis in man. Lipids 1997;32: 935–942.

30. Willett WC. Diet and cancer: one view at the start of the millennium. Cancer Epidemiol Biomarkers Prev 2001;10:3–8.
31. Holmes MD, Hunter DJ, Colditz GA, et al. Association of dietary intake of fat and fatty acids with risk of breast cancer. JAMA 1999;281:914–920.
32. Smith-Warner SA, Spiegelman D, Adami HO, et al. Types of dietary fat and breast cancer: a pooled analysis of cohort studies. Int J Cancer 2001;92:767–774.
33. Voorrips LE, Brants HA, Kardinaal AF, Hiddink GJ, van den Brandt PA, Goldbohm RA. Intake of conjugated linoleic acid, fat, and other fatty acids in relation to postmenopausal breast cancer: the Netherlands Cohort Study on Diet and Cancer. Am J Clin Nutr 2002;76:873–882.
34. Aro A, Mannisto S, Salminen I, Ovaskainen ML, Kataja V, Uusitupa M. Inverse association between dietary and serum conjugated linoleic acid and risk of breast cancer in postmenopausal women. Nutr Cancer 2000;38:151–157.
35. Chajes V, Lavillonniere F, Ferrari P, et al. Conjugated linoleic acid content in breast adipose tissue is not associated with the relative risk of breast cancer in a population of French patients. Cancer Epidemiol Biomarkers Prev 2002;11:672–673.
36. Ip C, Banni S, Angioni E, et al. Conjugated linoleic acid-enriched butter fat alters mammary gland morphogenesis and reduces cancer risk in rats. J Nutr 1999;129:2135–2142.
37. Stoll BA. N–3 fatty acids and lipid peroxidation in breast cancer inhibition. Br J Nutr 2002;87:193–198.
38. Klein V, Chajes V, Germain E, et al. Low alpha-linolenic acid content of adipose breast tissue is associated with an increased risk of breast cancer. Eur J Cancer 2000;36:335–340.
39. Hu FB, Bronner L, Willett WC, et al. Fish and omega-3 fatty acid intake and risk of coronary heart disease in women. JAMA 2002;287:1815–1821.
40. Moyad MA. Dietary fat reduction to reduce prostate cancer risk: controlled enthusiasm, learning a lesson from breast or other cancers, and the big picture. Urology 2002;59:51–62.
41. Michaud DS, Augustsson K, Rimm EB, Stampfer MJ, Willet WC, Giovannucci E. A prospective study on intake of animal products and risk of prostate cancer. Cancer Causes Control 2001;12:557–567.
42. Newcomer LM, King IB, Wicklund KG, Stanford JL. The association of fatty acids with prostate cancer risk. Prostate 2001;47:262–268.
43. Norrish AE, Jackson RT, Sharpe SJ, Skeaff CM. Men who consume vegetable oils rich in monounsaturated fat: their dietary patterns and risk of prostate cancer (New Zealand). Cancer Causes Control 2000;11:609–615.
44. Norrish AE, Skeaff CM, Arribas GL, Sharpe SJ, Jackson RT. Prostate cancer risk and consumption of fish oils: a dietary biomarker-based case-control study. Br J Cancer 1999;81:1238–1242.
45. Terry P, Lichtenstein P, Feychting M, Ahlbom A, Wolk A. Fatty fish consumption and risk of prostate cancer. Lancet 2001;357:1764–1766.
46. Smith-Warner SA, Ritz J, Hunter DJ, et al. Dietary fat and risk of lung cancer in a pooled analysis of prospective studies. Cancer Epidemiol Biomarkers Prev 2002;11:987–992.
47. Caygill CP, Charlett A, Hill MJ. Fat, fish, fish oil and cancer. Br J Cancer 1996;74:159–164.
48. Jarvinen R, Knekt P, Hakulinen T, Rissanen H, Heliovaara M. Dietary fat, cholesterol and colorectal cancer in a prospective study. Br J Cancer 2001;85:357–361.
49. Chen H, Tucker KL, Graubard BI, et al. Nutrient intakes and adenocarcinoma of the esophagus and distal stomach. Nutr Cancer 2002;42:33–40.
50. Chen H, Ward MH, Graubard BI, et al. Dietary patterns and adenocarcinoma of the esophagus and distal stomach. Am J Clin Nutr 2002;75:137–144.
51. Bougnoux P, Germain E, Chajes V, et al. Cytotoxic drugs efficacy correlates with adipose tissue docosahexaenoic acid level in locally advanced breast carcinoma. Br J Cancer 1999;79:1765–1769.

V   Environmental Stressors

19 Exercise, Cytokines, and Lymphocytes

Nutritional and Metabolic Aspects

Bente K. Pedersen

1. INTRODUCTION

Recent studies suggest that the beneficial effects of exercise may, in part, be mediated by exercise-induced changes in cytokine responses, which, in turn, have several effects, including effects on metabolism and on the cellular immune system *(1)*. The mechanisms underlying exercise-induced immune changes also include neuroendocrinological factors *(2)*. Thus, nutritional intervention may influence the immune response to exercise on several levels. When the immune system is studied at rest in trained vs. untrained humans, few differences are found. However, the so-called natural immunity mediated by natural killer (NK) cells is slightly enhanced in trained subjects *(2)*. Whereas little changes are found in trained vs. untrained subjects at rest, an acute bout of exercise induces dramatic immune system changes. Regarding lymphocyte changes (number and function), the findings are highly consistent. The intensity and duration of the exercise affect the magnitude of changes, whereas the mode of exercise has little influence *(2)*. However, if the exercise includes an eccentric component and thereby muscle damage and cell infiltration, this has some effect, which is described later. In general, both moderate and intense exercise (even if only for a few minutes) induce mobilization of lymphocytes to the blood. After intense exercise (more than 70% of VO_{2max}) of long duration (more than 45 min), immune impairment occurs *(2)*. The nature of these changes, the mechanisms of action, and the influence of nutritional intervention are described in this chapter.

2. EFFECTS OF EXERCISE

Recent studies show that several cytokines can be detected in plasma during and after strenuous exercise *(1,2)*. However, in relation to exercise interleukin (IL)-6 is produced in larger amounts than any other cytokine examined. The IL-6 increase is followed by increases in other antiinflammatory cytokines, such as IL-1 receptor antagonist (IL-1ra), tumor necrosis factor-α (TNF-α) receptors, and IL-10. It has recently been demonstrated that contracting skeletal muscles produce IL-6. Initially, it was believed that the cytokine response to exercise represented a reaction to exercise-induced muscle injury. Thus, we found that peak IL-6 was associated with prolonged muscle damage using an eccentric

From: *Diet and Human Immune Function*
Edited by: D. A. Hughes, L. G. Darlington, and A. Bendich © Humana Press Inc., Totowa, NJ

exercise model in which the creatine kinase (CK) level peaked at day 4 after exercise *(3)*. However, later studies from our group using exercise models in which CK peaked 1 d after exercise failed to show an association between peak IL-6 and peak CK levels *(4,5)*. Furthermore, using an eccentric exercise model, we recently demonstrated that CK levels increased up to 1000-fold, with only a fourfold increase in plasma-IL-6 during subsequent days *(6)*. The latter findings suggest that the huge increase in IL-6 plasma levels in exercise models where the CK level does not change or is enhanced a few-fold only is related to mechanisms other than muscle damage. Also, a recent study *(7)* failed to find an association between increases in IL-6 and biochemical markers for muscle damage. The latter study *(7)* showed that training reduced the myoglobin increase and decreased delayed onset muscle soreness in response to a bout of eccentric exercise, whereas the IL-6 increase was not influenced by a training effect. It is most likely that the huge and immediate IL-6 increase in response to long-duration exercise is independent of muscle damage, whereas muscle damage is followed by repair mechanisms, including macrophage invasion into the muscle, leading to IL-6 production by the macrophages. The IL-6 production in relation to muscle damage occurs later and is less intense compared to the IL-6 production related to muscle contractions.

The finding of markedly increased IL-6 levels after strenuous exercise has consistently been found in many studies *(4,5,8–17)*. A twofold increase in plasma IL-6 was demonstrated after 6 min of intense exercise *(18)*. In treadmill running, the IL-6 level in blood was significantly enhanced 30 min after the start of running, with IL-6 peaking in the end of 2.5 h of running *(4)*. In other studies, in which IL-6 was not measured during the running but at several time points after, maximum IL-6 levels were found immediately after the exercise, followed by a rapid decline. Thus, after a marathon run, maximum IL-6 levels (100-fold increase) were measured immediately after the 3–3.5 h race *(5,16)*.

In contrast, using a prolonged eccentric one-legged exercise model lasting 1 h *(14)* or a two-legged high-intensity eccentric exercise leg model lasting 30 min *(3)*, the IL-6 level did not peak until 1–1.5 h after exercise. In another study, subjects performed five bouts of one-legged eccentric exercise. The plasma IL-6 concentration peaked 90 min after exercise and remained elevated for 4 d *(15)*. It is clear that IL-6 kinetics differ from those induced by concentric muscle contractions and those induced by eccentric exercise associated with muscle damage *(3,5,14,16)*. In relation to concentric exercise, the IL-6 increase is related to exercise duration *(4)*, and there is a logarithmic relationship between the increase in IL-6 and exercise duration. The IL-6 levels decline after the concentric exercise to reach prevalues within a few hours. In contrast, eccentric exercise induces only a modest increase in plasma IL-6, and the IL-6 level peaks some time after exercise cessation and remains elevated for several days.

Data from the Copenhagen Marathon race (1996, 1997, and 1998, $n = 56$) suggest that there is a correlation intensity between exercise intensity and plasma IL-6 increase *(19)*. Furthermore, a correlation between peak IL-6 levels and heart rate was demonstrated *(4)*. An animal study suggested that the increase in epinephrine (adrenaline) during stress was responsible for the increase in IL-6 *(20)*. However, recent data from our group showed that when epinephrine was infused to volunteers, which closely mimicked the increase in plasma-epinephrine during 2.5 h of running exercise, plasma-IL-6 increased only fourfold during the infusion but 30-fold during the exercise *(21)*. Thus, epinephrine plays only a minor role in the exercise-induced plasma IL-6 increase. A study was performed to test the hypothesis that inflammatory cytokines were produced in skeletal muscle in response to intense long-duration exercise *(16)*. Muscle biopsies and blood samples were collected before and after a marathon race. The levels of IL-6 and IL-1ra proteins were markedly increased after the exercise. IL-6 plasma levels decreased, whereas IL-1ra increased further 2 h after exercise. A comparative polymerase chain reaction (PCR) technique was established to detect mRNA for cytokines in skeletal muscle biopsies and peripheral blood mononuclear cells (PBMN). Before exercise, mRNA for IL-6 could not be detected in muscle or PBMN. In contrast, mRNA for IL-6 was detected in muscle biopsies after exercise but not in the PBMN samples *(16)*.

Starkie et al. *(22)* observed that the intracellular levels of IL-6 and IL-1ra protein in circulating monocytes were not augmented in response to exercise and concluded that these cells did not contribute to the exercise-induced plasma IL-6 increases. That blood cells do not contribute to the exercise-induced increase in IL-1β and IL-6 plasma levels was further substantiated by a quantitative PCR approach. Quantification of the IL-6 mRNA level in PBMN during exercise demonstrated no change in the IL-1β and IL-6 mRNA levels, despite an increase in the plasma level of the protein *(23)*. The presence of IL-6 mRNA in muscle in response to exercise was confirmed in a rat exercise model, using the quantitative competitive RT-PCR method *(24)*. In this model, rats were subjected to electrically stimulated eccentric or concentric contractions of one hind leg, whereas the other leg remained at rest. Both the eccentric and the concentric contractions resulted in elevated IL-6 mRNA levels in the exercised muscle, whereas the level in the resting leg was not elevated. The presence of similar IL-6 mRNA levels in both concentric and eccentric exercised muscle indicates that the cytokine production cannot be as closely related to muscle damage as first believed. However, local IL-6 production is connected with exercising muscle—and does not result from systemic effect—because IL-6 mRNA was elevated only in the muscle from the exercising leg and not in the resting leg.

Recently, we demonstrated that the net IL-6 release from contracting skeletal muscles could more than account for the exercise-induced increase in arterial plasma concentrations *(25)*. Moreover, by obtaining arterial-femoral venous differences in an exercising leg, we found that exercising muscles released IL-6. In addition, during the last 2 h of exercise, the release per unit time was approx 17-fold higher than the amount accumulating in the plasma.

3. CARBOHYDRATE INGESTION AND IL-6

Several studies have reported that carbohydrate ingestion attenuates plasma IL-6 elevations during both running and cycling *(12,26)*. In contrast, researchers from Melbourne, Australia *(22)*, reported that plasma IL-6 was unaffected by carbohydrate ingestion during cycling. However, in that study, the subjects were highly endurance trained and plasma IL-6 increased only twofold, even without carbohydrate ingestion. This increase is markedly less than that previously observed in moderately trained subjects *(26)*. Recently, the same group reported that carbohydrate ingestion did attenuate the plasma IL-6 increase found in response to both cycling and running *(27)*. In the latter experiment, subjects had similar aerobic fitness to those previously reported *(26)*. Furthermore, IL-6 gene expression in the muscles was investigated. However, the IL-6 mRNA level was not affected by carbohydrate ingestion. These data indicate that the blood glucose level influences either IL-6 translation and/or release of IL-6 *(27)*.

3.1. Muscle-Derived IL-6 May Act as a Hormone

During the past 30 yr, there has been intense research to unravel the mechanisms that regulate the release of glucose from the liver to the blood during physical exercise, so that the blood glucose level is maintained despite increased glucose uptake in working skeletal muscles *(28)*. Research has demonstrated that exercise-induced changes in insulin and/or glucagons *(28)*, cortisol *(29)*, epinephrine *(30)*, or adrenergic neural stimulation *(31,32)* cannot, by themselves, account for the exercise-induced increase in hepatic glucose production. Indeed, it has been concluded that the possibility exists that a yet unidentified factor released from contracting muscle cells may contribute to the increase in hepatic glucose production *(30)*. Elevated plasma IL-6 response was found when subjects exercised in a glycogen-depleted state *(33)*.

Recent data demonstrate that although epinephrine does not play an important role in stimulating IL-6 release *(21)*, glycogen content of muscle is a determining factor for IL-6 production *(34,35)*. Thus, in a recent study, one leg was glycogen-depleted by exercise, before two-legged knee-extensor exercise. In the latter design, both legs were exposed to the same blood-glucose and hormones concentrations. IL-6 gene expression, IL-6 release *(35)*, and heat shock protein (HSP) 72 expresion *(36)* in muscle were faster and greater in the leg and had low glycogen compared to the control leg *(35,36)*. In another study, the IL-6 transcription rate in muscle nuclei isolated from muscle biopsies obtained before, during, and after exercise was fast and further enhanced when muscle glycogen content was low *(34)*. We have also recently shown that cultured human primary muscle cells are capable of increasing IL-6 mRNA when incubated with the calcium ionophore, ionomycin (Keller et al., unpublished data). Therefore, it is likely that myocytes produce IL-6 in response to muscle contraction and that IL-6 production by such tissue accounts for the exercise-induced increase in plasma levels of this cytokine. Recently, we demonstrated that 3 h of nondamaging exercise was sufficient to induce both IL-6 and HSP72 gene transcription. Antioxidant treatment blunted the exercise-induced HSP72 expression but not the IL-6 response, suggesting that, in contracting muscle, IL-6 is not mediated via an HSP72-dependent pathway (Fischer et al., unpublished data).

The biological roles of muscle-derived IL-6 have been investigated in studies where human-recombinant IL-6 was infused into healthy volunteers to closely mimic the IL-6 concentrations observed during prolonged exercise. We have demonstrated that physiological IL-6 concentrations clearly induce lipolysis. Although we have yet to determine the precise biologic action of muscle-derived IL-6, our data support the hypothesis that the role of IL-6 release from contracting muscle during exercise is to act in a hormone-like manner to mobilize extracellular substrates and/or augment substrate delivery during exercise. Another possible biological role of IL-6 is to inhibit the production of TNF-α and, thereby, inhibit TNF-induced insulin resistance. Of note, Wallenius et al. *(37)* have recently demonstrated that IL-6-deficient mice develop obesity and glucose intolerance, whereas chronic treatment of these animals with IL-6 partially attenuates these metabolic perturbations.

The biological roles of IL-6 are still not clear. However, accumulating evidence exists to suggest that contracting muscle produces and releases IL-6 that is further enhanced if muscle glycogen is low. IL-6's role is to induce lipolysis, but it is less clear whether it also contributes to maintaining glucose homeostasis during exercise. In addition, IL-6 may

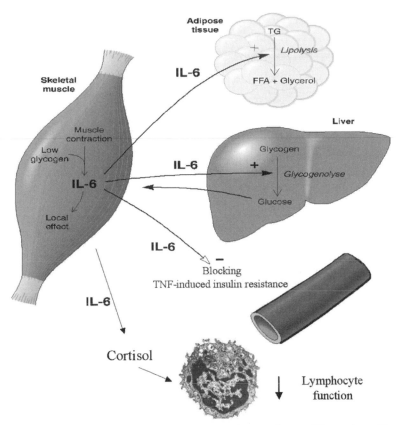

Fig. 1. The biologic roles of muscle-derived interleukin(IL)-6 are still not clear. However, accumulating evidence exists that contracting muscles produce and release IL-6 and that this release is further enhanced if muscle glycogen content is low. The role of IL-6 is to induce lipolysis, whereas it is less clear if IL-6 also contributes to maintain glucose homeostasis during exercise. In addition, IL-6 may inhibit tumor necrosis factor (TNF)-induced insulin resistance. Furthermore, IL-6 stimulates cortisol production. Thereby, IL-6 is an important player in exercise-induced immune impairment.

inhibit TNF-induced insulin resistance. Furthermore, IL-6 stimulates cortisol production, a powerful immunosuppressant. Therefore, muscle-derived IL-6 indirectly mediates exercise-induced immune impairment (*see* Fig. 1).

3.2. Carbohydrate Supplementation of Muscle-Derived IL-6

3.2.1. Possible Clinical Effects on Metabolism

Based on the link between muscle glycogen and muscle-derived IL-6 and the finding that carbohydrate supplementation diminishes the IL-6 response to exercise, it is obvious that IL-6-related effects will also be influenced if subjects have had a high carbohydrate intake before exercise or a high carbohydrate-rich drink intake during exercise.

Thus, carbohydrate supplementation inhibits IL-6-induced lipolysis. Furthermore, given that IL-6 inhibits TNF production, it is most likely that exercise induces suppression of TNF gene activation locally in the muscle, and, when it is released in high amount to the circulation, IL-6 may mediate suppression of TNF in other tissues, e.g., adipose

Physical exercise and IL-6 inhibit
the production of TNF

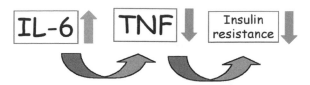

Fig. 2. Exercise induces suppression of endotoxin-induced tumor necrosis factor (TNF) production. The mechanism may include muscle-derived interleukin (IL)-6. Thereby, exercise may induce inhibition of TNF-induced insulin resistance.

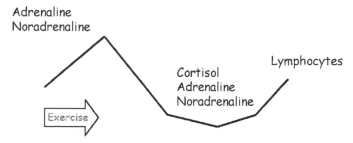

Fig. 3. Relationship between hormones and lymphocyte changes in response to exercise.

tissue. TNF mediates insulin resistance by downregulating the GLUT4-receptor and by inhibiting the insulin receptor function *(38)*. Thus, in theory, carbohydrate supplementation during exercise may, in principal, abrogate the beneficial effect of exercise on insulin resistance (*see* Fig. 2).

3.2.2. POSSIBLE CLINICAL EFFECTS ON IMMUNE FUNCTION

The lymphocyte concentration in blood increases during exercise and falls below preexercise values after intense long-duration exercise *(39)*. The acute exercise effect on lymphocytes is mediated by catecholamines, particularly epinephrine *(21)*. However, the postexercise lymphocyte decline is mediated by both epinephrine and cortisol (Fig. 3). The latter hormone is particularly interesting if the exercise's duration is long. IL-6 mediates the increase in cortisol *(40)*. Further support for the latter is based on a study from our group, in which IL-6 was infused to normal healthy volunteers in low concentrations to mimic the exercise effect on IL-6 plasma concentration. IL-6 induced a clear increase in cortisol. Thus, in theory, if IL-6 is inhibited, postexercise immune impairment will be less pronounced.

4. CHANGES IN LYMPHOCYTE NUMBER AND FUNCTION IN RELATION TO AN ACUTE BOUT OF EXERCISE

Several reports describe exercise-induced changes in subsets of blood mononuclear cells (PBMN) *(41)*. Increased lymphocyte concentrations likely result from the recruitment of all lymphocyte subpopulations to the vascular compartment: CD4+ T cells, CD8+ T cells, CD19+ B cells, CD16+ NK cells, and CD56+ NK cells. During exercise, the CD4/CD8 ratio decreases, reflecting the greater increase in CD8+ lymphocytes than CD4+ lymphocytes. CD4+ and CD8+ cells contain both CD45RO+ memory and CD45RA+ virgin or naive cells and "true" naive cells are identified by the absence of 45RO and the presence of CD62L (42). Data from Gabriel et al. (43) show that the recruitment is primarily of CD45RO+. We have recently found that CD45RO+ and CD45RO-CD62L cells are mobilized to the circulation, suggesting that memory, but not naive lymphocytes, are rapidly mobilized to the blood in response to acute physical exercise (44).

We further demonstrated that in response to exercise, lymphocytes lacking the CD28 molecule are mobilized to the circulation and telomere lengths in CD4+, and CD8+ lymphocytes were significantly shorter compared to cells isolated at rest (44). This demonstrates that old activated cells are recruited to the blood. Thus, the initial increase in CD4+ and CD8+ cells after exercise does not result from repopulation by newly generated cells but may be a redistribution of activated cells, in agreement with kinetics of CD4+ repopulation after anti-HIV treatment (45) and chemotherapy (46) and CD4 and CD8 repopulation after bone marrow transplantation (47). Although the number of all lymphocyte subpopulations increases, the percentage of CD4+ cells declines, primarily resulting from NK cells increasing more than any other lymphocyte subpopulations. Accordingly, the relative fraction of lymphocyte subpopulations changes, and this contributes to the exercise-induced alterations in in vitro immune assays in which a fixed number of PBMN is studied. The acute recruitment of lymphocytes to the blood is mediated by epinephrine (2).

After intense long-duration exercise, NK and B cells' functions are suppressed. Thus, the NK and lymphokine-activated killer (LAK) cell activity (the ability of cytotoxic cells to lyse a certain number of tumor target cells) is inhibited (41,48–50). Furthermore, B-cell function is inhibited (51), and the local production of secretory IgA in saliva decreases in response to exercise (52). Although the results are heterogeneous, most studies find that both concentric and eccentric exercise induce decreased proliferative responses to mitogens (53).

There are few studies that document immune system responses in vivo, in relation to exercise. Bruunsgaard et al. investigated whether an in vivo impairment of cell-mediated immunity and specific antibody production could be demonstrated after intense long-duration exercise (triathlon race) (54). The cellular immune system was evaluated as a skin-test response to seven recall antigens, whereas the humoral immune system was evaluated as the antibody response to pneumococcal polysaccharide vaccine (this vaccine is generally T-cell independent) and tetanus and diphtheria toxoids (both of which are T-cell dependent). The skin-test response was significantly lower in the group that performed a triathlon race compared to triathlete controls and untrained controls who did not participate in the triathlon. No differences in specific antibody titres were found between the groups. Thus, in vivo cell-mediated immunity was impaired in the first days after prolonged, high-intensity exercise, whereas there was no impairment of the in vivo antibody production measured 2 wk after vaccination.

5. ROLE OF CARBOHYDRATES

Earlier research had established that a reduction in blood glucose levels is linked to hypothalamic-pituitary-adrenal activation, an increased release of adrenocorticotrophic hormone and cortisol, an increased plasma growth hormone, a decreased insulin, and a variable effect on blood epinephrine level *(55)*. Given the link between stress hormones and immune responses to prolonged and intensive exercise *(56)*, carbohydrate compared to placebo ingestion should maintain plasma glucose concentrations and attenuate increases in stress hormones, thereby diminishing changes in immunity. The new observation is that IL-6 links the effect of low blood glucose and low glycogen concentration in the muscle to the effect on cortisol, which may influence exercise's effect on the immune system.

The hypothesis that carbohydrate may influence exercise-induced immune changes has been tested in several studies by Nieman et al. *(12,57,58)* using double-blind placebo-controlled randomized designs. Carbohydrate beverage ingestion before, during (about 1 L/h), and after 2.5 h of exercise was associated with higher plasma glucose levels, an attenuated cortisol and growth hormone response, fewer perturbations in blood immune cell counts, lower neutrophil and monocyte phagocytosis and oxidative burst activity, and a diminished proinflammatory and antiinflammatory cytokine response. Overall, the hormonal and immune responses to carbohydrate compared to placebo ingestion were diminished. Some immune variables were affected slightly by carbohydrate ingestion (e.g., neutrophil and monocyte function), whereas others were strongly influenced (e.g., plasma cytokine concentrations and blood cell counts).

The clinical significance of these carbohydrate-induced effects on the endocrine and immune systems awaits further research. Currently, the data indicate that athletes who ingest carbohydrate beverages before, during, and after prolonged and intense exercise should experience lowered physiologic stress. Research to determine whether carbohydrate ingestion will improve host protection against viruses in endurance athletes during intensified training or after competitive endurance events is also warranted (*see* Fig. 4).

6. DO OTHER NUTRIENTS INFLUENCE EXERCISE-INDUCED IMMUNE CHANGES?

Because the mechanisms underlying exercise-induced immune changes are multifactorial and include altered metabolism during exercise, as well as a pronounced neuroendocrinologic response, many theories have been developed. Thus, it is suggested that the decline in plasma-glutamine concentrations, as a result of muscular activity, will inhibit lymphocyte function *(59)*. Furthermore, as a consequence of the catecholamine-induced and growth hormone-induced immediate changes in leukocyte subsets, the relative proportion of these subset changes and activated leukocyte subpopulations may be mobilized to the blood. Free oxygen radicals and prostaglandins (PG) released by the elevated number of neutrophils and monocytes may influence the function of lymphocytes and contribute to the impaired function of the latter cells. Thus, nutritional supplementation with glutamine, antioxidants, and PG inhibitors may, in principle, positively influence exercise-associated immune function.

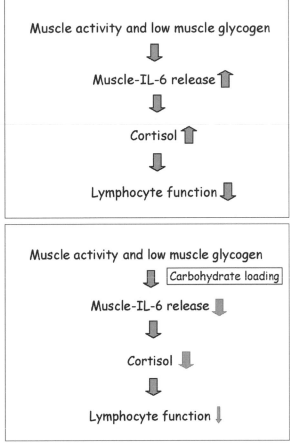

Fig. 4. Carbohydrate loading: IL-6 is produced in and released from working muscle. The IL-6 production is further enhanced if muscle-glycogen content is low. IL-6 stimulates the release of cortisol, which suppresses lymphocyte function. Carbohydrate loading does not influence the IL-6 mRNA increase in the muscle but inhibits the release of IL-6 from working muscle. Thereby, the plasma cortical increase during exercise is less pronounced and, consequently, the exercise-induced immune impairment is less pronounced.

6.1. Does Glutamine Supplementation Abolish Exercise-Induced Immune Changes?

Skeletal muscle is the major tissue involved in glutamine production and releases glutamine into the bloodstream at a high rate. Therefore, skeletal muscle may play a vital role in maintaining the key process of glutamine use in the immune cells. Consequently, the activity of the skeletal muscle may directly influence the immune system. It has been hypothesized (the so-called "glutamine-hypothesis") that under intense physical exercise or in relation to surgery, trauma, burns, and sepsis, the demands on muscle and other organs for glutamine is such that the lymphoid system may be forced into a glutamine debt, which temporarily adversely affects its function. Thus, factors that directly or indirectly influence glutamine synthesis or release could, theoretically, influence lymphocyte and monocyte functions *(60,61)*. After intense long-term exercise and other physical stress disorders, the glutamine concentration in plasma declines *(62–65)*.

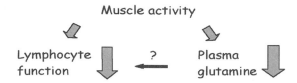

Fig. 5. Glutamine supplementation The glutamine hypothesis suggests that the exercise-induced decrease in plasma-glutamine causes impaired lymphocyte function. However, there is a substantial amount of evidence to decline this hypothesis, because glutamine supplementation abolishes the exercise-induced decrease in plasma glutamine without changing exercise-induced immunosuppression.

Glutamine in vitro enhances lymphocyte proliferation and LAK cell activity but has no effect on NK cell activity *(66)*. Furthermore, in in vitro experiments, glutamine stimulates IL-2 and IFN-γ production without influencing IL-1β, IL-6, or TNF production *(67)*. Glutamine added to in vitro assays did not abolish postexercise decline in proliferative responses and did not normalize the low lymphocyte proliferation in patients who were HIV seropositive *(66)*.

A study by Castell et al. *(68)* found that glutamine supplementation decreased the incidence of upper respiratory tract infections (URTI) after a marathon. In contrast, Mackinnon et al. *(69)* found no differences in plasma-glutamine levels in swimmers who did or did not develop URTI after intensified swimming training. In four placebo-controlled glutamine intervention studies *(70–73)*, glutamine abolished the postexercise decline in plasma glutamine without influencing postexercise impairment of NK and LAK cell function or mitogen-induced proliferative responses or salivary IgA. Thus, the latter studies did not support the hypothesis that the postexercise decline in immune function is caused by a decrease in the plasma glutamine concentration *(74)* (*see* Fig. 5).

6.2. Does n–3 PUFA Supplementation Abolish Exercise-Induced Immune Changes?

There are two principal classes of polyunsaturated fatty acids (PUFA): the n–6 and the n–3 families *(75)*. The precursor of the n–6 family is linoleic acid, which is converted to arachidonic acid, the precursor of PGs and leukotrienes (LT), which have potent proinflammatory and immunoregulatory properties. The precursor of the n–3 family of PUFA is α-linolenic acid (ALA). If the n–6/n–3 ratio decreases by administration of a diet rich in n–3 fatty acids, the PGE_2-mediated immunosuppression may be abolished or reduced.

The possible interaction between intense acute exercise, immune function, and PUFA was examined in inbred female C57BI/6 mice *(76)*. The animals received either a natural ingredient diet or a diet supplemented with various oils, such as beef tallow, safflower, fish oil, or linseed oil for an 8-wk period. In the group receiving 18:3 (n–3) linseed oil, linseed oil abolished postexercise immunosuppression of the IgM plaque-forming cell response. The effect of linseed oil may be ascribed to a link between a diet rich in n–3 PUFA and abolishment of prostaglandin-related immunosuppression. In support of this hypothesis, when the PGE_2 production was inhibited in vitro by the PG-inhibitor indomethacin, exercise-induced suppression of NK-cell activity and B-cell function was partly abolished *(51,77)*.

Another study attempted to test if dietary modification of fatty acids influenced neutrophil and monocyte secretion after an in vivo inflammatory stress in older human subjects *(78)*. In vivo, neutrophil degranulation was assessed by plasma elastase concentrations and monocyte function was assessed by IL-1β secretion in vitro. In response to eccentric exercise, older subjects (>60 yr) taking placebo had no apparent elastase response, whereas those taking fish oil supplements responded with a significant increase (142%) in plasma elastase, which was similar to the responses of younger reference individuals. There was no effect of fish-oil on IL-1β secretion.

The possibility that n–3 fatty acids may diminish the exercise-induced increased concentration of cytokines was based on the finding that, in animal experiments, the increase in IL-1 and TNF after endotoxin application was reduced when the animals were pretreated with n–3 fatty acids (fish oil) *(79)*. However, n–3 fatty acids had no influence on the cytokine response to long-duration exercise (marathon) *(80)*, which may be explained by when one exercises, little or no increase is found in TNF or IL-6, whereas the antiinflammatory cytokine response is dramatic.

6.3. Does Antioxidant Supplementation Abolish Exercise-Induced Immune Changes?

During exercise, the enhanced oxygen use leads to production of reactive oxygen species, as indicated by the blood glutathione redox status. Antioxidants may, in theory, neutralize the reactive species that are produced by neutrophils during phagocytosis *(81,82)*.

In the early 1970s, Pauling *(83)* concluded from previously published studies that vitamin C supplementation decreases the incidence of the common cold *(83)*. However, the majority of studies carried out thereafter have not found that regular vitamin C supplementation (>1 g/d) has any marked effect on common cold incidence *(82)*. The results of three placebo-controlled studies that examined the effect of vitamin C supplementation on common cold incidence in subjects under heavy physical stress were analyzed *(84)*. In one study, the subjects were schoolchildren at a skiing camp in Swiss Alps, in another they were military troops training in Northern Canada, and in the third they were participants in a 90-km running race. In each of the three studies, a considerable reduction in common cold incidence in the group supplemented with vitamin C was found. These studies indicate that vitamin C may reduce the risk of obtaining an infection after extreme exercise. In the third study, Peters et al. *(85)* evaluated Vitamin C's effect on URTI incidence during the 2-wk period after the 90-km Comrades Ultramarathon. The URTI incidence was 68% in the placebo group, which was significantly more than in the vitamin C supplementation group, where only 33% reported URTI when taking a 600-mg vitamin C supplementation daily for 3 wk before the race. In another study, Peters et al. *(86)* found that vitamin A supplementation had an insignificant effect on URTI incidence in marathoners.

Vitamin C supplementation for 2 wk before treadmill running for 1.5 or 2.5 h running did not influence leukocyte subsets, NK-cell activity, lymphocyte proliferative responses, neutrophil phagocytosis and activated burst, catecholamines, and cortisol *(87,88)*. In a recent double-blind placebo controlled study by Nielsen et al. *(89)*, N-acetylcysteine, an antioxidant (6 g/d for 3 d), had no effect on ergometer-rowing-induced suppression of lymphocyte proliferation or NK-cell activity.

In a study of the age-related response of neutrophils and muscle damage to eccentric exercise, Cannon et al. *(90)* examined subjects who were younger than 30 yr and older than 55 yr. The subject groups were further divided in a double-blind placebo-controlled protocol, which examined the influence of 48 d of dietary vitamin E supplementation before the exercise. All subjects were monitored for 12 d after exercise. Dietary supplementation with vitamin E eliminated the differences between the two age groups, primarily by increasing the responses of the older individuals.

The same group investigated the influence of damaging eccentric exercise on in vitro production and plasma concentrations of cytokines and their relationship to muscle breakdown. In a double-blind placebo-controlled study, they examined the effect of vitamin E supplementation for 48 h on the exercise-induced acute phase response. The volunteers were either young (average age 25 yr) or elderly (average age 65 yr) sedentary men. They performed 45 min of eccentric exercise (downhill treadmill). Twenty-four hours after this single session of eccentric exercise, endotoxin-induced secretion of IL-1β was augmented in cells obtained from the placebo subjects, but no significant increase was observed in cells from the vitamin E-supplemented subjects *(90)*.

The finding by Cannon et al. *(91)* that IL-1β and TNF secretion was increased the morning after exercise without any changes in mononuclear cell numbers indicates that the monocytes are activated in relation to eccentric exercise. The effect of vitamin E on IL-1β and IL-6 could not be ascribed to PGE_2 changes *(91)*. Oxygen radicals enhance endotoxin-induced IL-1 production *(92)* and, furthermore, the concentrations of these reactants increase with exercise *(93)*. Thus, vitamin E's effects on IL-1β secretion are consistent with a mechanism involving oxygen radicals. Antioxidants' effects on plasma cytokines have recently been evaluated. Few studies have examined antioxidants' effect on plasma cytokines. In a study by Petersen et al. *(88)*, treatment of healthy subjects with vitamin C (500 mg/d) and vitamin E (400 IU/d) had no effect on the exercise-induced increase in plasma-IL-6 and other cytokines. Runners completing the 90-km Comrades Ultramarathon experienced strong increases in concentrations of plasma IL-6, IL-10, IL-1ra, and IL-8. These increases were attenuated in runners ingesting 1500 mg but not 500 mg vitamin C supplements for 1 wk before the race and on race day *(94)*.

In another study, subjects performed a prolonged (90 min) intermittent shuttle-running test 14 d after receiving 400 mg vitamin C. Postexercise serum creatine kinase activities and myoglobin concentrations were unaffected by supplementation. Furthermore, although plasma IL-6 increased immediately after exercise in both groups, values in the supplemented groups were lower *(95)*. Unpublished data from our group (Fischer et al.) demonstrate that IL-6 release from contracting skeletal muscles (3 h) was diminished in groups receiving vitamin C (500 mg/d) and vitamin E (400 IU/d) for 4 wk. Thus, data are accumulating to suggest that some combinations of antioxidant vitamins may lower plasma cytokine levels after exercise. The clinical significance is not yet known.

7. CONCLUSIONS

Recent research demonstrates that exercise induces the working muscle to produce and release IL-6. The latter cytokine has important metabolic effects, and the IL-6 production is tightly regulated by muscle glycogen and blood glucose levels. Carbohydrate supplementation diminishes the systemic concentration of IL-6. A biologic consequence of carbohydrate loading during exercise may be that lipolysis during exercise is inhibited, although the clinical significance of this is not known. Furthermore, IL-6 is a major cortisol inducer, which induces immunosuppression. Thus, if IL-6 production and/or release is inhibited, the consequence is that plasma cortisol does not increase and that immune changes in response to exercise are diminished. It has also been demonstrated that carbohydrate loading during exercise attenuates the exercise effects on lymphocyte function. With regard to other dietary supplements, although the effect of glutamine supplementation has been extensively investigated, it is clear that the exercise-induced decrease in plasma glutamine can be abolished without any influence on exercise-induced lymphocyte changes. Regarding to other supplements, the available data do not yet allow firm conclusions to be made.

8. "TAKE-HOME" MESSAGES

1. Exercise induces recruitment of lymphocytes to the blood, which is followed by low lymphocyte numbers and impaired lymphocyte function.
2. Although the initial recruitment of lymphocytes to the blood is mediated by increased catecholamine level during exercise, the long-term effects are likely to be mediated by increased cortisol levels, which are stimulated by the exercise-induced IL-6 increase.
3. Low glycogen level is an important stimulus for muscle-derived IL-6, and carbohydrate loading during exercise diminishes the IL-6 response to exercise. Thereby, carbohydrate loading abolishes the cortisol increase and, consequently, the exercise-induced immune changes are less pronounced. The clinical significance of carbohydrate loading during exercise is, however, not known.
4. Accumulating evidence concludes that although the exercise-induced decline in glutamine level is abolished by glutamine supplementation, it has no effect on exercise-induced immune changes.
5. Regarding other supplements, such as treatment with antioxidants or n–3 PUFA (fish oil), the available data do not allow firm conclusions at this time.

ACKNOWLEDGMENT

This work was supported by The National Research Foundation grant no. 504-14.

REFERENCES

1. Pedersen BK, Steensberg A, Schjerling P. Exercise and interleukin-6. Curr Opin Hematol 2001;8: 137–141.
2. Pedersen BK, Hoffman-Goetz L. Exercise and the immune system: regulation, integration and adaption. Physiol Rev 2000;80:1055–1081.
3. Bruunsgaard H, Galbo H, Halkjaer-Kristensen J, Johansen TL, MacLean DA, Pedersen BK. Exercise-induced increase in interleukin-6 is related to muscle damage. J Physiol (London) 1997;499:833–841.
4. Ostrowski K, Hermann C, Bangash A, Schjerling P, Nielsen JN, Pedersen BK. A trauma-like elevation in plasma cytokines in humans in response to treadmill running. J Physiol (London) 1998; 508:949–953.
5. Ostrowski K, Rohde T, Asp S, Schjerling P, Pedersen BK. The cytokine balance and strenuous exercise: TNF-alpha, IL-2beta, IL-6, IL-1ra, sTNF-r1, sTNF-r2, and IL-10. J Physiol (London) 1999;515: 287–291.
6. Toft AD, Jensen LB, Bruunsgaard H, et al. The cytokine response to eccentric exercise in young and elderly humans. Am J Physiol Cell Physiol 2002;283:C289–C295.
7. Croisier JL, Camus G, Venneman I, et al. Effects of training on exercise-induced muscle damage and interleukin 6 production. Muscle Nerve 1999;22:208–212.

8. Northoff H, Berg A. Immunologic mediators as parameters of the reaction to strenuous exercise. Int J Sports Med 1991;12(Suppl 1):S9–S15.

9. Sprenger H, Jacobs C, Nain M, et al. Enhanced release of cytokines, interleukin-2 receptors, and neopterin after long-distance running. Clin Immunol Immunopathol 1992;63:188–195.

10. Ullum H, Haahr PM, Diamant M, Palmo J, Halkjaer Kristensen J, Pedersen BK. Bicycle exercise enhances plasma IL-6 but does not change IL-1alpha, IL-1beta, IL-6, or TNF-alpha pre-mRNA in BMNC. J Appl Physiol 1994;77:93–97.

11. Drenth JP, van Uum SH, van Deuren M, Pesman GJ, van der ven Jongekrug J, van der Meer JW. Endurance run increases circulating IL-6 and IL-1ra but downregulates ex vivo TNF-alpha and IL–1beta production. J Appl Physiol 1995;79:1497–1503.

12. Nehlsen-Canarella SL, Fagoaga OR, Nieman DC. Carbohydrate and the cytokine response to 2.5 hours of running. J Appl Physiol 1997;82:1662–1667.

13. Castell LM, Poortmans JR, Leclercq R, Brasseur M, Duchateau J, Newsholme EA. Some aspects of the acute phase response after a marathon race, and the effects of glutamine supplementation. Eur J Appl Physiol 1997;75:47–53.

14. Rohde T, MacLean DA, Richter EA, Kiens B, Pedersen BK. Prolonged submaximal eccentric exercise is associated with increased levels of plasma IL-6. Am J Physiol 1997;273:E85–E91.

15 Hellsten Y, Frandsen U, Orthenblad N, Sjodin N, Richter EA. Xanthine oxidase in human skeletal muscle following eccentric exercise: a role of inflammation. J Physiol (London) 1997;498:239–248.

16. Ostrowski K, Rohde T, Zacho M, Asp S, Pedersen BK. Evidence that IL-6 is produced in skeletal muscle during intense long-term muscle activity. J Physiol (London) 1998;508:949–953.

17. Toft AD, Ostrowski K, Asp S, et al. The effects of n–3 PUFA on the cytokine response to strenuous exercise. J Appl Physiol 2000;89:2401–2405.

18. Nielsen HB, Secher N, Perdersen BK. Lymphocytes and NK cell activity during repeated bouts of maximal exercise. Am J Physiol 1996;271:R222–R227.

19. Ostrowski K, Rohde T, Asp S, Schjerling P, Pedersen BK. Chemokines are elevated in plasma after strenuous exercise in humans. Eur J Appl Physiol 2001;84:244–245.

20. DeRijk RH, Boelen A, Tilders FJ, Berkenbosch F. Induction of plasma interleukin-6 by circulating adrenaline in the rat. Psychoneuroendocrinology 1994;19:155–163.

21. Steensberg A, Toft ADSP, Halkjaer-Kristensen J, Pedersen BK. Plasma interleukin-6 during strenuous exercise—role of adrenaline. Am J Physiol 2001;281:1001–1004.

22. Starkie RL, Angus DJ, Rolland J, Hargreaves M, Febbraio M. Effect of prolonged submaximal exercise and carbohydrate ingestion on monocyte intracellular cytokine production in humans. J Physiol (London) 2000;528:647–655.

23. Moldoveanu AI, Shephard RJ, Shek PN. Exercise elevates plasma levels but not gene expression of IL-1beta, IL-6, and TNF-alpha in blood mononuclear cells. J Appl Physiol 2000;89:1499–1504.

24. Jonsdottir I, Schjerling P, Ostrowski K, Asp S, Richter EA, Pedersen BK. Muscle contractions induces interleukin-6 mRNA production in rat skeletal muscles. J Physiol (London) 2000;528:157–163.

25. Steensberg A, van Hall G, Osada T, Sacchetti M, Saltin B, Pedersen BK. Production of IL-6 in contracting human skeletal muscles can account for the exercise-induced increase in plasma IL-6. J Physiol (London) 2000;529:237–242.

26. Nieman DC, Nehlsen-Canarella SL, Fagoaga OR, et al. Influence of mode and carbohydrate on the cytokine response to heavy exertion. Med Sci Sports Exerc 1998;30:671–678.

27. Starkie RL, Arkinstall MJ, Koukoulas I, Hawley JA, Febbraio MA. Carbohydrate ingestion attenuates the increase in plasma interleukin-6, but not skeletal muscle interleukin-6 mRNA, during exercise in humans. J Physiol 2001;533:585–591.

28. Kjaer M. Hepatic fuel metabolism during exercise. In: Hargreaves M (ed.). Exercise Metabolism. Human Kinetics Inc., Champaign, IL, 1995.

29. Cryer PE. Glucose counterregulation: prevention and correction of hypoglycemia in humans. Am J Physiol 1993;264:E149–E155.

30. Howlett K, Febbraio M, Hargreaves M. Glucose production during strenuous exercise in humans: role of epinephrine. Am J Physiol 1999;276:E1130–E1135.

31. Sigal RJ, Fisher SJ, Manzon A, et al. Glucoregulation during and after intense exercise: effects of alpha-adrenergic blockade. Metabolism 2000;49:386–394.

32. Sigal RJ, Purdon C, Bilinski D, Vranic M, Halter JB, Marliss EB. Glucoregulation during and after intense exercise: effects of beta-blockade. J Clin Endocrinol Metab 1994;78:359–366.
33. Gleeson M, Bishop NC. Special feature for the Olympics: effects of exercise on the immune system: modification of immune responses to exercise by carbohydrate, glutamine and anti-oxidant supplements. Immunol Cell Biol 2000;78:554–561.
34. Keller C, Steensberg A, Pilegaard H, et al. Transcriptional activation of the IL-6 gene in human contracting skeletal muscle: influence of muscle glycogen content. FASEB J 2001;15:2748–2750.
35. Steensberg A, Febbraio MA, Osada T, et al. Interleukin-6 production in contracting human skeletal muscle is influenced by pre-exercise muscle glycogen content. J Physiol (London) 2001;537:633–639.
36. Febbraio MA, Steensberg A, Walsh R, et al. Reduced glycogen availability is associated with an elevation in HSP72 in contracting human skeletal muscle. J Physiol 2002;538:911–917.
37. Wallenius V, Wallenius K, Ahren B, et al. Interleukin-6-deficient mice develop mature-onset obesity. Nat Med 2002;8:75–79.
38. Hotamisligil GS. The role of TNFalpha and TNF receptors in obesity and insulin resistance. Intern Med 1999;245:621–625.
39. McCarthy DA, Dale MM. The leucocytosis of exercise. A review and model. Sports Med 1988;6:333–363.
40. Steensberg A, Toft AD, Bruunsgaard H, Sandmand M, Halkjaer-Kristensen J, Pedersen BK. Strenuous exercise decreases the percentage of type 1 T cells in the circulation. J Appl Physiol 2001;91:1708–1712.
41. Pedersen BK. Exercise immunology. In: Pedersen BK (ed.). Exercise Immunology. R.G. Landes, Austin, TX, 1997, pp. 1–206.
42. Bell EB, Spartshott S, Bunce C. CD4+ T cell memory, CD45R subsets and the persistence of antigen— a unifying concept. Immunol Today 1998;19:60–64.
43. Gabriel H, Schmitt B, Urhausen A, Kindermann W. Increased CD45RA+CD45R0+ cells indicate activated T cells after endurance exercise. Med Sci Sports Exerc 1993;25:1352–1357.
44. Bruunsgaard H, Jensen MS, Schjerling P, et al. Exercise induces recruitment of lymphocyets with an activated phenotype and short telomeres in young and elderly humans. Life Sci 1999;65:2623–2633.
45. Kelleher AD, Carr A, Zaunders J, Cooper DA. Alterations in the immune response to human immuno-deficiency (HIV)-infected subjects treated with an HIV-specific protease inhibitor, ritonavir. J Infect Dis 1996;173:321–329.
46. Hakim FT, Cepeda R, Kaimei S, et al. Constraints on CD4 recovery postchemotherapy in adults: thymic insufficiency and spoptotic decline of expanded peripheral CD4 cells. Blood 1997;90:3789–3798.
47. Bengtsson M, Totterman TH, Smedmyr B, Festin R, Oberg G, Simonsson B. Regeneration of functional and activated NK and T subset cells in the marrow and blood after autologous bone marrow transplantation: a prospective phenotypic study with 2/3-color FACS analysis. Leukemia 1989;3:68–75.
48. Hoffman-Goetz L, Pedersen BK. Exercise and the immune system: a model of the stress response? Immunol Today 1994;15:382–387.
49. Brines R, Hoffman-Goetz L, Pedersen BK. Can you exercise to make your immune system fitter? Immunol Today 1996;17:252–254.
50. Pedersen BK. In: Pedersen BK (ed.). Exercise Immunology. R.G. Landes, Austin, TX, 1997, pp. 1–206.
51. Tvede N, Heilmann C, Halkjaer Kristensen J, Pedersen BK. Mechanisms of B-lymphocyte suppression induced by acute physical exercise. J Clin Lab Immunol 1989;30:169–173.
52. Mackinnon LT, Hooper S. Mucosal (secretory) immune system responses to exercise of varying intensity and during overtraining. Int J Sports Med 1994;15:S179–S183.
53. Nielsen HB, Pedersen BK. Lymphocyte proliferation in response to exercise. Eur J Appl Physiol 1997;75:375–379.
54. Bruunsgaard H, Hartkopp A, Mohr T, et al. In vivo cell mediated immunity and vaccination response following prolonged, intense exercise. Med Sci Sports Exerc 1997;29:1176–1181.
55. Nieman DC, Pedersen BK. Exercise and immune function: recent development. Sports Med 1999;27:73–80.
56. Pedersen BK, Bruunsgaard H, Klokker M, et al. Exercise-induced immunomodulation—possible roles of neuroendocrine factors and metabolic factors. Int J Sports Med 1997;18(Suppl 1):S2–S7.
57. Nieman DC, Henson DA, Garner EB, et al. Carbohydrate affects natural killer cell redistribution but not activity after running. Med Sci Sports Exerc 1997;29:1318–1324.

58. Nieman DC, Fagoaga OR, Butterworth DE, et al. Carbohydrate supplementation affects blood granulocyte and monocyte trafficking but not function after 2.5 hours of running. J Appl Physiol 1997;82: 1385–1394.
59. Newsholme EA, Parry Billings M. Properties of glutamine release from muscle and its importance for the immune system. JPEN J Parenter Enteral Nutr 1990;14(4 Suppl):63S–67S.
60. Newsholme EA. Biochemical mechanisms to explain immunosuppression in well-trained and overtrained athletes. Int J Sports Med 1994;15:S142–S147.
61. Newsholme EA. Psychoimmunology and cellular nutrition: an alternative hypothesis [editorial]. Biol Psychiatry 1990;27:1–3.
62. Parry Billings M, Budgett R, Koutedakis Y, et al. Plasma amino acid concentrations in the overtraining syndrome: possible effects on the immune system. Med Sci Sports Exerc 1992;24:1353–1358.
63. Keast D, Arstein D, Harper W, Fry RW, Morton AR. Depression of plasma glutamine concentration after exercise stress and its possible influence on the immune system. Med J Aust 1995;162:15–18.
64. Essen P, Wernerman J, Sonnenfeld T, Thunell S, Vinnars E. Free amino acids in plasma and muscle during 24 hours post-operatively—a descriptive study. Clin Physiol 1992;12:163–177.
65. Lehmann M, Huonker M, Dimeo F, et al. Serum amino acid concentrations in nine athletes before and after the 1993 Colmar ultra triathlon. Int J Sports Med 1995;16:155–159.
66. Rohde T, Ullum H, Palmo J, Halkjaer Kristensen J, Newsholme EA, Pedersen BK. Effects of glutamine on the immune system—influence of muscular exercise and HIV infection. J Appl Physiol 1995;79: 146–150.
67. Rohde T, MacLean DA, Pedersen BK. Glutamine, lymphocyte proliferation and cytokine production. Scand J Immunol. 2003;44:648–650.
68. Castell LM, Poortmans JR, Newsholme EA. Does glutamine have a role in reducing infections in athletes? Eur J Appl Physiol 1996;73:488–490.
69. Mackinnon LT, Hooper SL. Plasma glutamine and upper respiratory tract infection during intensified training in swimmers. Med Sci Sports Exerc 1996;28:285–290.
70. Rohde T, MacLean D, Pedersen BK. Effect of glutamine on changes in the immune system induced by repeated exercise. Med Sci Sports Exerc 1998;30:856–862.
71. Rohde T, Asp S, MacLean DA, Pedersen BK. Competitive sustained exercise in humans, lymphokine activated killer cell activity, and glutamine—an intervention study. Eur J Appl Physiol 1998;78: 448–453.
72. Krzywkowski K, Petersen EW, Ostrowski K, et al. Effect of glutamine and protein supplementation on exercise-induced decreases in salivary IgA. J Appl Physiol 2001;91:832–838.
73. Krzywkowski K, Petersen EW, Ostrowski K, Kristensen JH, Boza J, Pedersen BK. Effect of glutamine supplementation on exercise-induced changes in lymphocyte function. Am J Physiol Cell Physiol 2001;281:C1259–C1265.
74. Hiscock N, Pedersen BK. Exercise-induced immunodepression—plasma glutamine is not the link. J Appl Physiol 2002;93:813–822.
75. Calder PC. Fat chance of immunomodulation. Immunol Today 1998;19:244–247.
76. Benquet C, Krzystyniak K, Savard R, Guertin F. Modulation of exercise-induced immunosuppression by dietary polyunsaturated fatty acids in mice. J Tox Environm Health 1994;43:225–237.
77. Pedersen BK, Tvede N, Klarlund K, et al. Indomethacin in vitro and in vivo abolishes post-exercise suppression of natural killer cell activity in peripheral blood. Int J Sports Med 1990;11:127–131.
78. Cannon JG, Fiatarone MA, Meydani M, et al. Aging and dietary modulation of elastase and interleukin-1 beta secretion. Am J Physiol 1995;268:R208–R213.
79. Johnson JA 3rd, Griswold JA, Muakkassa FF. Essential fatty acids influence survival in sepsis. J Trauma 1993;35:128–131.
80. Toft AD, Thorn M, Ostrowski K, et al. N–3 polyunsaturated fatty acids do not affect cytokine response to strenuous exercise. J Appl Physiol 2000;89:2401–2406.
81. Babior BM. Oxidants from phagocytes: agents of defense and destruction. Blood 1984;64:959–966.
82. Hemila H. Vitamin C and the common cold. Br J Nutr 1992;67:3–16.
83. Pauling L. The significance of the evidence about ascorbic acid and the common cold. Proc Natl Acad Sci USA 1971;68:2678–2681.

84. Hemila H. Vitamin C and the common cold incidence: a review of studies with subjects under heavy physical stress. Int J Sports Med 1996;17:379–383.

85. Peters EM, Goetzsche JM, Grobbelaar B, Noakes TD. Vitamin C supplementation reduces the incidence of postrace symptoms of upper-respiratory-tract infection in ultramarathon runners. Am J Clin Nutr 1993; 57:170–174.

86. Peters EM, Cambell A, Pawley L. Vitamin A fails to increase resistance to upper respiratory in distance runners. S Afr J Sports Med 1992;7:3–7.

87. Nieman DC, Henson DA, Butterworth DE, et al. Vitamin C supplementation does not alter the immune response to 2.5 hours of running. Int J Sports Nutr 1997;7:173–184.

88. Petersen EW, Ostrowski K, Ibfelt T, et al. Effect of vitamin supplementation on cytokine response and on muscle damage after strenuous exercise. Am J Physiol Cell Physiol 2001;280:C1570–C1575.

89. Nielsen HB, Kharazmi A, Bolbjerg ML, Poulsen HE, Pedersen BK, Secher NH. N-acetylcysteine attenuates oxidative burst by neutrophils in response to ergometer rowing with no effect on pulmonary gas exchange. Int J Sports Med 2001;22:256–260.

90. Cannon JG, Orencole SF, Fielding RA, et al. Acute phase response in exercise: interaction of age and vitamin E on neutrophils and muscle enzyme release. Am J Physiol 1990;259:R1214–R1219.

91. Cannon JG, Meydani SN, Fielding RA, et al. Acute phase response in exercise. II. Associations between vitamin E, cytokines, and muscle proteolysis. Am J Physiol 1991;260:R1235–R1240.

92. Kasama TK, Kobayashi T, Fukushima M, et al. Production of interleukin 1-like factor from human peripheral blood monocytes and polymorphonuclear leukocytes by superoxide anion: the role of interleukin 1 and reactive oxygen species in inflamed sites. Immunol Immunopathol 1989;53:439–448.

93. Davies KJA, Packer L, Brooks GA. Free radicals and tissue produced by exercise. Biochem Biophys Res Commun 1982;107:1198–1205.

94. Nieman DC, Peters EM, Henson DA, Nevines EI, Thompson MM. Influence of vitamin C supplementation on cytokine changes following an ultramarathon. J Interferon Cytokine Res 2000;20:1029–1035.

95. Thompson D, Williams C, McGregor SJ, et al. Prolonged vitamin C supplementation and recovery from demanding exercise. Int J Sport Nutr Exerc Metab 2001;4:466–481.

20 Military Studies and Nutritional Immunology

Undernutrition and Susceptibility to Illness*

Karl E. Friedl

"From time immemorial famine and pestilence have been considered an inseparable pair, the twin fruits of war . . . Prominent among the diseases thus associated with famine have been scarlet fever, diphtheria, dysentery, typhoid, typhus, cholera, and tuberculosis. Not only have these at times become epidemic in periods of famine, but there is much evidence that their course becomes more severe. It has been rather generally assumed that both the increased incidence and the virulence in such cases are due, at least in part, to the prevailing state of undernutrition."

Human Biology of Starvation, p. 1002 (2).

1. INTRODUCTION

This chapter reviews research findings from military studies on the connection between nutritional status and immune function and provides some conclusions on what has been learned to date.

In the Army's new fighting concept, the Objective Force Warrior, small teams are expected to conduct sustained and continuous operations for at least 72 h and possibly more than 100 h. This new force will have many technological advantages, but, ultimately, the centerpiece is still a human operator subject to biological principles. Although we know how to design machines that may operate flawlessly for thousands of hours, we are just beginning to understand human limits and to develop reliable predictions of failure rates. A central focus of military medical research is to devise approaches to sustain physiological functions in the face of multiple environmental challenges. These challenges include physical and mental overload with limited opportunities for recovery,

*The views, opinions, and findings contained in this report are those of the author and should not be construed as an official Department of the Army position, policy, or decision. Portions of this chapter are derived from an earlier presentation on military requirements for nutritional immunology research and from the conclusions of that symposium that were summarized in the 708-page report on "Military Strategies for Sustainment of Nutrition and Immune Function in the Field," Committee on Military Nutrition Research, 1999 (1).

From: *Diet and Human Immune Function*
Edited by: D. A. Hughes, L. G. Darlington, and A. Bendich © Humana Press Inc., Totowa, NJ

as well as thermal, hypoxia, toxic chemical, and other environmental exposures, and psychological factors, such as uncertainty, isolation, separation, and anxiety. Singly, or in combination, these factors may degrade an individual's functional status in terms of mental performance, physical capabilities, and resistance to disease.

The Army has long looked to nutritional interventions as a main strategy to extend soldier's limits. This includes enhancing resistance to disease supported, in part, by the correlation between immune competence and nutritional status. Endpoints of immune function, such as mitogen-stimulated lymphocyte proliferation, have provided sensitive and dependable markers of nutritional status in past Army ration studies (3). It also results from an assumption that stresses of military training will have similar effects on immune functions as those reported in the literature resulting from psychologic stress.

Stress, the physiological response to external challenges or stressors, has been associated with a reduced resistance to infectious agents. It is important to note that this association has typically been demonstrated using psychologic stressors (4,5) and that data to support an effect from any other stressors working through mechanisms other than psychologic (i.e., anxiety-provoking or noxious stimuli) are thin. Nevertheless, there is a prevalent assumption that military training and operational settings produce alterations in immune function that increase risk for susceptibility to disease. Such a connection would have serious consequences in military environments because deployed forces face significant risks of infection, including indigenous diseases, such as typhus, malaria, and diarrheal diseases, that have rendered combat units ineffective in previous wars; contagious infections from malnourished refugees who may have a high prevalence of infectious disease (6); and biological warfare agents, such as anthrax that may be used against our forces.

Although vaccines to protect soldiers against militarily important diseases represent important investments and might be expected to mitigate any increase in susceptibility induced by stresses in the military environment, vaccine effectiveness may, itself, be substantially modulated by stress and nutritional status (7), and this area of research has been given relatively little attention. Moreover, recent studies suggest that there may be a connection between the administration of multiple vaccines over limited time courses to soldiers already under stress and the development of chronic multisymptom illnesses (8).

Traditionally defined stress responses, involving activation of the hypothalamic-pituitary-adrenal (HPA) axis, have distinct suppressive effects on immunological function that probably play an important and protective regulatory role against maladaptive hyperresponsiveness (9). If the HPA axis served as a single common pathway resulting in impaired function for all stressors affecting soldiers, interventions with a focus on modulating the effects of glucocorticoids could be relatively straightforward. However, in studies of the most challenging military training possible, such as specialized small unit field tactical training, adrenal axis activation is a transient and sometime negligible response (10,11). Furthermore, energy deficit is not a classical stressor as defined by Selye, because it does not necessarily stimulate an adrenal response, except in later phases of chronic semistarvation (11,12). Even the immune function responses to exogenous corticosterone in rats are far from clear, and the effects are moderated by physiologic states, such as fasting (13–15). Ultimately, stressor effects on immune parameters, such as lymphocyte proliferative response and natural killer (NK)-cell activity, may be mediated through common integrating pathways at the hypothalamic level, but the input is likely to be variable, depending on effects as diverse as glucose availability to the brain and endorphin or glucocorticoid inputs. These are important considerations in determining stressor effects on immune function, and these aspects of neuroimmunology are not yet charted. Until that work is completed, it would be of great value to the Army if a nutritional profile could be found that optimally supports muscle and brain physiologic mechanisms and that also provides soldiers protection against disease through mitigation of depressed immune system functions resulting from training stress. Therefore, the nutritional studies in military training environments discussed in this chapter were initiated with these premises as a backdrop: that military training environments represent stresses that may lead to immune alterations sufficient to place service personnel at risk for increased disease and that nutritional supplementation may mitigate this risk through manipulation of immune status.

2. STRESSORS AND POSSIBLE EFFECTS ON IMMUNE FUNCTION PARAMETERS

The Army's interest in nutrition and immune function was invigorated by a problem with high rates of *Streptococcal pneumonia* in otherwise healthy men who were participating in the intensive 8-wk Ranger training course *(16)*. Instead of simply leaving this disease outbreak to a short-term clinical solution, a young Army Captain, Robert Moore, designed a comprehensive study to investigate the associations between nutritional status and immunologic parameters *(17)*. Teamed with Dr. Tim Kramer, a field immunologist from the U.S. Department of Agriculture, this expanded to a wider investigation of military stressors and immune function *(18,19)*. It was surprising to discover the high prevalence of cellulitis and respiratory infections in initially healthy young men who were also among the fittest members of the military *(20)*. In contrast, results from studies of another and important stress model, Army basic training, had minimally negative or even beneficial effects on immunologic status, including infectious illness outcomes *(21,22)*. The results suggested the potential importance of energy balance as a stressor that was capable of degrading some aspects of immune function. The results also provided an apparent inconsistency with prevailing notions of the correlation between fitness and resistance to disease and required more careful testing.

Many countries have some form of specialized small unit field tactical training, usually referred to as "Ranger" or "commando" training *(17,23–26)*. The studies discussed in this section were conducted using classes from the following tactical training courses: 1-wk Norwegian Ranger course, 8-wk US Army Ranger course, and the 3-wk Special Forces Assessment and Selection (SFAS) course.

These training settings provided the stress models needed to examine immune function related to nutritional status. These research models provide specific and multiple stressors (including, at least, inadequate sleep, inadequate food intake, and prolonged physical workload) that far exceed any experimental parameter that a human ethics committee would permit a researcher to design; they are more similar and have more application to both military training and real-world military operations than a more restricted-variable laboratory model would be; and, because of the consistency and precision of the training regime, they provide a greater potential for consistent physiologic readings from study to study. However, these are also messy studies. That these studies were conducted in actual training environments imposes ethical difficulties for an intrusive scientist trying to establish appropriate control groups, obtain true baseline measures, and interpret the influence of the range of variables acting on the study.

Norwegian military cadets are required to participate in a 1-wk Ranger training course that typically involves no food and no organized sleep. By the end of the week, cadets are in a profound energy deficit produced by an estimated 8,000 to 10,000 kcal expenditure/ d, and they may have hallucinations, ataxia, and concentration problems from lack of sleep (25). They may also be cold, and they collapse from hypoglycemia. The US Army Ranger study, conducted in hot and humid conditions, provided stressors with partial food and sleep deprivation for 8 wk. Semistarvation occurred as a result of deliberate energy deficits averaging 1200 kcal/d during the 8 wk in men, starting at an average 15% body fat. Sleep, based on wrist-worn actigraphy, averaged 3.6 h/d for the 8 wk.

The responses in these two models are remarkably similar, although the 8-wk Ranger course energy-deficit responses progressed at a slower rate, which is consistent with the longer course of the study (17). It is important to note that neither of these models has a significant psychologic "anxiety" component. The participants became progressively fatigued and hungry and were eventually capable of only the most overtrained mental tasks; they were too fatigued for the luxury of reflective anxiety. This absence of a deliberate psychologic stress distinguishes these military training models from psychologic stressors encountered in combat (27,28) and from other studies that demonstrate impaired disease resistance in psychologically stressed humans and animals (4,5).

Detailed immune function studies have been conducted in both of these models. The detailed studies on Norwegian Rangers demonstrated a complicated series of changes in their 1-wk course (see Table 1). Monocytes remained activated throughout the course, whereas other immune functions were progressively suppressed. Granulocyte activity was stimulated at the beginning of the course and then suppressed (29,30). A similar rise in glucocorticoids was also observed during the first few days but subsequently declined (10), perhaps reflecting interactions between the hypophyseal-adrenal axis and immunologically important cytokines. Dr. Pal Wiik speculates that the priming of phagocyte response at the start of the course may have provided acute protection against infectious agents but may also contribute to inflammatory responses that lead to musculoskeletal injuries (13).

Lymphocyte mitogenic responses increased in some 1-wk course studies but demonstrated no change in others (29). These assessments were performed using a method of purified cells originally devised by Dr. Arne Boyum (31) that has become one of the most quoted methods in the field. In the 8-wk Ranger course, lymphocyte mitotic responses were measured with a whole blood method, with the handling of field specimens perfected by Dr. Tim Kramer (19). These 8-wk Ranger studies demonstrated a decline in proliferative responses to several different mitogens tested (pokeweed mitogen, phytohemagglutinin [PHA], concanavalin A [Con A], and tetanus toxoid) within the first 2 wk of the course (17,18). This suppression was consistent whether expressed per blood volume or adjusted for lymphocyte counts, with mean suppression through the middle of the course as large as 50% (18). Interleukin (IL)-2 and IL-2 receptor (IL-2R) from the cell supernatant followed a similar pattern and magnitude of change. At the end of the 8-wk course, without easing any of the deliberate stressors on the students, proliferative and

Table 1
Summary of Immunological Data in Norwegian (1 wk) and the United States (8 wk) Stressful Military Training Studies

Parameter	Norwegian Military Academy cadets (n = 20)		US Army Ranger candidates (n = 41)	
	Days 1–3	Days 4–7	4 wk	8 wk
Leucocyte studies				
Granulocyte count	+	+	+	+
Granulocyte function	+	–		
Monocyte count	+	+	–	–
Monocyte function	–	+		
Eosinophils	–	–		
Lymphocyte count			–	–
T-lymphocyte count				–
B-lymphocyte count	–	–		–
CD4+ helper T cells	–	–	–	+
CD8+ suppressor T cells	–	–	0	–
Natural killer cells	–	–		
Lymphocyte response to mitogens	–/+	–/+	–	–
Cytokine measurements				
Interleukin (IL)-2 cellular			–	–
IL-2R in vitro			–	0
IL-6 cellular	–	–	0	–
IL-6 plasma			+	–
GM-CSF	+	–		

GM-CSF, granulocyte-macrophage colony-stimulating factor.
Table derived from refs. *1, 18, 29, 30.*
– Decrease; + Increase

IL-2 responses began to normalize (*see* Fig. 1). This was observed in two separate studies that were conducted 1 yr apart and reflected an adaptation to the stressors. Toward the end of the course, the soldiers had reduced resting body temperatures and had developed other metabolic efficiencies, such as behavioral adaptations, involving a complete absence of fidgeting and other unproductive motion. In combination, the changes may have produced a reduction in energy deficit sufficient to provide some recovery in the immune function parameters. There are animal data to suggest that the recovery is not an adaptation of the immune system itself; underfed mice still demonstrate a reduced proliferative response at the end of an 8-wk calorie-restriction period *(32)*. It is also unlikely that the observed changes in immune function parameters are attributable to metabolic signals reflecting the progressive depletion of body fat stores and increasing reliance on body protein to feed the energy deficit, because the depletion of body fat was most severe during the terminal portion of the course *(33)*.

Increased infection rates have not been observed in the Norwegian course but are prominent in the US Ranger course *(18,20,29)*. In a 1989 class of students, a dozen young men were hospitalized for pneumonia, leading to one series of medical studies conducted on Ranger training *(16)*. A subsequent problem in a 1994 winter class, in which there were

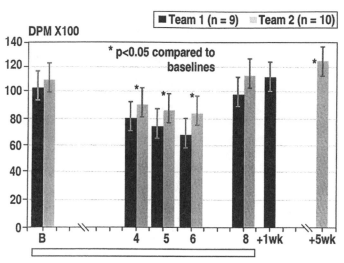

Fig. 1. T-lymphocyte proliferative response after in vitro stimulation with phytohemagglutinin in Ranger students with an average energy deficit of 1000 kcal/d during the 8-wk course *(18,42)*. Mean data are presented for two random teams of men followed through the Ranger course (indicated by the horizontal bar, denoted in weeks) that were also tested after the end of the course, at 1 wk (+1) or at 5 wk (+5) to study recovery. The suppressed responses in these men (−30% from B, baseline) were less than the 50% suppression seen at 4 and 6 wk in the original study without 400 kcal/d supplementation and net energy deficit of 1200 kcal/d (not shown). One week of increased intake during the course was not sufficient to restore the response, as noted in the sample at week 5 that followed a period of normal feeding.

hypothermia deaths, led to another series of studies on cold susceptibility in stressed men *(34)*.

Soft-tissue infections are common in Ranger students, and the largest proportion of infections occurs at the end of the course. In one study, one fourth of the graduating class required treatment with antibiotics for various types of infection *(17,18)*. Some of this relates to abrasion and insect bites that became infected after exposure to pathogens when the men waded through polluted rivers in the final phase of their training (the pollution was serious enough that eating fish from these rivers was deemed unsafe) *(20)*.

In other intensive military training, the incidence of infectious disease is not noticeably elevated, but this may reflect differences in pathogen exposures rather than differences in disease resistance. In the 3-wk SFAS course, another intensive military training program, we found no increase in illness rates, despite total daily energy expenditures, based on doubly labeled water methods, that exceeded those measured in Ranger students. Although adequate food was provided, the soldiers did not keep up with their extraordinary energy demands and they lost weight *(35)*. Parameters of immune function, such as mitogen-stimulated lymphocyte proliferation, were also markedly suppressed in this course.

Unfortunately, no single test has yet been demonstrated as a useful indicator of immune competence. Even the seemingly remarkable magnitude of suppression in proliferative response in these studies may not carry much weight in comparison to responses of profoundly immunocompromised hospitalized patients; thus, the interpretation of threshold values in these semiquantitative tests is in question.

Similarly, historically important semistarvation studies do not provide strong support for immune function changes, except during anergy at extreme levels in severely morbid patients, and as in the military field studies, conclusions from these studies are confounded by variations in exposures to pathogens.

In 1945, Dr. Ancel Keys and his colleagues conducted the Minnesota Study under the sponsorship of the Surgeon General of the Army to determine safe and effective approaches to nutritional rehabilitation of returning prisoners of war (2). The more important contribution was in uncovering physiologic consequences of underfeeding. Every conceivable measurement and observation of health was collected, as each man lost weight to his individual target weight of 24% body weight reduction over 24 wk. There was no difference in respiratory infections, with 1.1 colds per man in the experimental group during the 6 mo of semistarvation compared to 1.2 colds/man/6 mo for the workers who mixed with them, nor was severity different (2). However, this was a slower rate of weight loss than in Ranger students, who lost an average of 16% of their body weight in 8 wk, with the most extreme weight loss for one soldier at 25% of body weight in 8 wk (33). As the Rangers experienced more extreme energy deficits, their more extreme results should provide supporting evidence correlating energy deficits and immune dysfunctions and an increased risk of infection; yet, although results may suggest the possibility, they are not clear-cut. This leads us back to Dr. Pal Wiik's conclusion that the numerous changes in immunologic status may provide differential opportunities for protection against different classes of infectious agents (13). This observation gains additional support from another astounding scientific effort from the World War II era. A published report, based on smuggled writings of Jewish physicians studying themselves and their patients as they slowly were being starved to death for a 3-yr period in the Warsaw Ghetto, found that, in the face of this most severe energy deficit, susceptibility to some diseases increased and tuberculin tests were negative (36). The tests were negative even in individuals with active cases of tuberculosis, illustrating the severity of anergy. There was also an increase in typhus, diptheria, typhoid, virulent tuberculosis, and several tissue infections (36).

3. APPARENT ROLE OF ENERGY DEFICIT IN IMMUNOLOGIC FUNCTION: FEEDING INTERVENTIONS

Small feeding interventions have been investigated for their effects on immunologic function in both of the Ranger course models. Although not well-controlled laboratory models, these military courses, excluding uncontrollable meteorologic factors, follow highly reproducible training regimens from class to class, as indicated by consistent physiologic measures from year to year. For example, three different classes of students, studied at 1- to 5-yr intervals, yielded the same average daily sleep measurements, using wrist-worn actigraphs, of 3.4–3.6 h/night for the 8-wk periods (37,38). Many laboratory-based studies do not carry this level of precision and reproducibility.

The Norwegian Ranger model has been a unique test bed for experimental manipulations and interventions, with careful studies that allowed separation of sleep deprivation and energy-deficiency effects. Sleep deprivation plays a relatively small role in the pattern of endocrine and other physiologic responses, except for effects on mental status (39). In laboratory settings with sleep deprivation as the sole stressor, acute sleep deprivation models ranging from 24 to 64 h consistently produce increased NK activity, with no changes in proliferative responses to mitogens (40,41). In the 1-wk Ranger model, adding food (1200 kcal/d or an approx 15% reduction in the huge energy deficit) without increasing sleep produced small differences in the responses, including greater priming of granulocytes and a lower chemotactic response, but there were no differences in IL responses or several other parameters (13,30). The observed changes were not large to begin with, and the feeding intervention was modest compared with the huge energy deficit in this model, so perhaps it is not surprising that the effects were small.

In the US Rangers, a modest increase in food intake (+400 kcal/d) reduced the average daily energy deficit from 1200 to 1000 kcal/d (with approximately half of the increase presumably going to increased energy expenditure). This modest increase had a marked effect on physiological and immune parameters; most notably, it attenuated the suppression of lymphocyte proliferation responses and the concentrations of soluble IL-2R (18). During the 8-wk course, there were also periods of improved feeding without modification of other stressors, such as sleep restriction and high workload. One 9-d period of midcourse refeeding temporarily restored body weight, along with lymphocyte subset counts, but without acute recovery of the suppressed lymphocyte responses (18); lymphocyte responses were completely restored or even enhanced 1 mo after the end of the course with ad libitum feeding and adequate sleep (42) (see Fig. 1).

Serum IL-6 levels increased 2 wk into the course and then progressively fell to the lowest point at the end of the course. In the group with the supplemental intake, IL-6 changes paralleled the original pattern but were delayed by 2 wk. As a useful marker of overall stress status, the early rise in IL-6 may be expected as an acute-phase-type response, but the subsequent progressive reduction may also reflect important consequences for other immune function parameters that are affected by IL-6, such as IL-2R and T-cell proliferative responses. Infection rates were also dramatically reduced in the group with the feeding intervention. Rates dropped from approx 25% of the class with active infections during the second half of the course to few (2–8%) infections in the better fed group (18). The change is in the right direction for a possible association between energy deficit and immune dysfunction with increased risk of infection.

Energy intake was relatively well-controlled but, as noted in connection with the recovery of immune function parameters at the end of the 8-wk course, behavioral and physiologic adaptations may have begun to counterbalance inadequate intakes. The other side of the energy-balance equation, energy expenditure or exercise, has not been as well studied as intake or overall energy balance. There is no shortage of speculation on the effect of exercise as a stressor, distinct from its effect on energy balance, although this is not always given appropriate consideration in study design.

Like sleep deprivation, the most consistently reported immunological finding in acute exercise studies is an apparent increase in NK cells. This is generally described as part of the acute-phase response and may reflect redistribution of the concentration of immune cells. Pedersen et al. reviewed the studies involving hypoxia, head-up tilt, hyperthermia, and exercise and found a consistent response in NK increases and determined that, in more prolonged stress models, immune parameters were suppressed (43). Nieman took this further by reviewing infection and upper respiratory tract infections in runners. He described a J-shaped curve for infection rates, with the highest rates associated with prolonged stress (44). Although this would appear to align with studies showing apparent

Table 2
Summary of Contemporary US Army Field Studies of Nutrition and Immune Function

Study year	Study name	Model/objective(s)	References
1991	Ranger I	Stress associations with infectious disease	(11,17,18,20,33)
1992	Ranger II	Effects of modest increase in energy intake (+400 kcal/d) on immune function	(11,18,38,42)
1993	Jackson BCT	Basic training stressor associations with immune function in female recruits	(21)
1993	SFAS I	Stress associations with immune function with increased food availability	(35)
1994	Ranger cadre	Acute effects of high energy flux on immune function (carbohydrate, 8000 kcal/d)	(47)
1995	SFAS II	Placebo-controlled trial for effects of glutamine supplementation in high stress training	(48,49)
1995	Ranger III	Stress associations with immune function in cold weather training	(34,49)
1996	SFAS III	Placebo-controlled trial for effects of anti-oxidant beverage in high stress training	(50)
1997	Ranger IV	Placebo-controlled trial for effects of anti-oxidant food bar in high stress training and effect on vaccine efficacy	(7)

SFAS, Special Forces Assessment and Selection.

declines in NK- and T-cell function with prolonged stress, Nieman highlights that adjustments made for exercise-induced alteration in plasma volume and lymphocyte subsets abolish the differences. Nieman also found that making these adjustments for the lymphocyte counts in proliferation studies after acute bouts of intensive exercise abolished some of the apparent changes in response (45).

The primary conclusion to be drawn from most of the exercise literature is that modest exercise produces beneficial improvements in immune function and disease resistance and intensive or prolonged exercise may degrade immunocompetence, although the supporting evidence is slim (44,46). These observations are borne out in three other military field studies that included collaborations with Dr. Tim Kramer, who performed careful proliferation studies and other measures of immune function that also included careful prospective monitoring of illnesses and injuries (18,21,35,47,48) (see Table 2).

At one extreme, the SFAS course included extraordinarily high workloads for 3 wk (exceeding 5000 kcal/d). Even though adequate food was provided, the soldiers could not consume enough to maintain energy balance. Lymphocyte proliferation was suppressed but not to the levels observed in the 8-wk Ranger course, which suggests a stronger effect from energy deficit than from the total energy expenditure (35). Infections were not an important problem. A second study tested Ranger instructors during a rigorous 3-d physical challenge in hot humid conditions in the most demanding mountainous terrain of the US Army Ranger School. The testing involved extraordinarily high exercise demands but only modest energy deficits. A carbohydrate and electrolyte beverage provided to one group did not modify impairments in immune function compared to the results observed in a water-fed group; however, there was an unexplained greater impairment in a third aspartame-fed comparison group *(47)*.

At the other end of the spectra of physical intensity and energy balance is a study of women recruits attending an 8-wk Army basic training course. They expended an estimated 2600 kcal/d that, for many, involved a relatively large increase in regular physical activity over their previous habits. Although food was freely available, the recruits lost weight during their 8-wk basic training course, and the women with the greatest adiposity lost the most weight. Observations made midway through the course and at the end of the course demonstrated notable improvements in immune function parameters, including large increases in lymphocyte proliferative response. No significant problems with infectious illnesses were observed *(21)*. These beneficial changes occurred despite an apparent worsening of iron status in this group *(21)*.

One of the pitfalls of military field studies is that baseline measures may not depict a stable state, which may be the case in the study of women recruits. Subsequent improvements noted in the study, such as the notable improvement in immune function parameters, may reflect the alleviation of a preexisting condition or stressor rather than benefits provided by conditions of the study, such as regular exercise, improved sleep hygiene, and adequate and balanced nutrition. It is conceivable that the changes in the new recruits reflected measures initially impaired by the recruits' anxiety associated with the uncertainties of leaving home and entering basic training.

4. INVESTIGATIONS OF SPECIFIC AMINO ACID OR ANTIOXIDANT RATION COMPONENTS

There has been a long-standing search for a pan-immune booster based on various theories derived from observations in stress studies. For example, ROS increase in soldiers who are performing in demanding environments, and oxidative stress mechanisms have been proposed to be at the root of immune dysfunction *(51,52)*. Even the Ranger course studies were encouraged by the school commander in hopes that all it would take was an "iron pill" to moderate the high infection rates in Ranger students without reducing the deliberate stressors in the course believed to be essential to the training of infantry leaders *(17)*.

In the 1990s, Army research focused primarily on empiric studies testing some of these theories *(see* Table 2). These included experimental interventions involving glutamine, antioxidant nutrients, zinc, and carbohydrate supplements. The practical question driving Army material developers was "Is there a dietary supplement that substantially reduces susceptibility of soldiers to infection in stressful operational settings?"

One theoretically promising supplement tested in small unit field tactical training was glutamine. Glutamine is interesting as a single amino acid supplement for athletes for several reasons: observations of an association in its use with a decline in infection, the known importance in sustaining immune cells, and the connection to muscle metabolism *(53–55)*. Unfortunately, these remain interesting conjectures and no studies have demonstrated a benefit to glutamine supplementation on immune function or other physiologic functions *(53–56)*. The glutamine field study in Special Forces candidates tested SFAS course a convincingly high dose of oral glutamine (15 g/d) consumed in a drink, compared to placebo controls *(48,49)*. No tests of immune function were modified by the glutamine compared to placebo controls, although the course stressors suppressed functions in a highly predictable way based on the original SFAS study *(35)*. For example, blood lymphocyte proliferation, studied in the same manner as the previous studies, demonstrated, respectively, reductions of 21% and 22% from baseline testing for glycine control and glutamine test groups *(49)*. In the original study, a 20% reduction was observed, which highlights the reproducibility of the test when conducted in precisely the same way. Because traumatic injury, not infection, is the primary medical problem in the SFAS course, the most important endpoint of modified infection rates was not testable in this setting. No conclusive studies anywhere else indicate that oral glutamine will boost immune function in healthy stressed individuals.

In 1998, the Surgeon General of the Army, intrigued by claims of an "antioxidant revolution," asked whether soldiers should be provided with an antioxidant nutrient-containing "shaker" on mess hall tables, along with the salt and pepper. He asked if there was evidence compelling enough that the Army should move swiftly to provide every soldier with an opportunity to optimize his or her health by increasing vitamin C and E and β-carotene intakes several times more than the recommended dietary allowance (RDA). The Committee on Military Nutrition Research (CMNR) of the Institute of Medicine was asked to provide recommendations to the Army on this question. In light of another Army-sponsored review that was concurrently underway to determine Dietary Reference Intakes for antioxidant nutrients *(57)*, the panel focused on whether soldiers had a greater need for antioxidant nutrients than the general US population because of occupational and environmental stressors encountered in military life. The final report concluded that evidence was lacking for the need for special antioxidant supplementation of soldiers and that a greater health return might be expected from investments in smoking cessation, moderation of alcohol use, adequate exercise, maintenance of desirable weight, and consuming appropriate diets *(58)*. The panel provided these same recommendations when it considered the evidence for other nutritional supplements proposed to improve soldier immune function and disease resistance. If interventions were pursued, they encouraged the Army to explore the relationship of vitamin C, vitamin E, and β-carotene and immune function in soldiers under field and laboratory conditions *(1)*.

Field studies exploring the potential benefits of antioxidant cocktails were conducted in the Ranger course and in the SFAS course (*see* Table 2). Earlier studies with the SFAS course demonstrated a 20% decline in PHA-stimulated lymphocyte proliferation in the 3-wk physically intensive course that included an average 3.2 kg weight loss through inadequate intakes against an estimated 5000 kcal/d requirement *(35)*. In the same model, a group of 49 men were administered a liquid supplement containing antioxidant nutrients (500 mg vitamin C, 400 IU vitamin E, 15 mg β-carotene, and 100 µg selenium/d) and compared to a group of men (*n* = 57) receiving a nonsupplemented drink. There were no significant differences in immune function parameters, including mitogen-stimulated lymphocyte proliferation, delayed type skin hypersensitivity, or white cell subpopulations *(49,50)*. In an additional study, a food bar equivalent of this drink supplement was tested in Ranger students who were compared to peers receiving food bars without the antioxidants. The antioxidant supplement provided no significant advantage in any immune function outcome *(7)*. It should be noted that this Ranger course model was substantially different from previous Ranger studies because smaller energy deficit occurred, owing to changes in the feeding regimen instituted after the earlier studies documenting excessive weight losses. The results showed no significant effect of the antioxidant supplements. An interesting addition to this study was the administration of a hepatitis A vaccine to vaccine-naïve students midway through the course. The purpose was to determine if training stressors produced a deficient response in antibody production in students compared with their training cadre *(7)*. Unfortunately, inadequate sample sizes and variable responses failed to statistically support a trend to reduced titers in some of the students.

Despite the design and technical problems that may have confounded the negative findings in these field studies, other studies have suggested that in the absence of a specific nutrient deficiency, specific antioxidants may not produce the benefits that can be seen from other nutrients obtained from mixed carotenoids or tomato juice *(59,60)*. Any future Army studies in this area must consider the emerging understanding of the importance of other carotenoids (e.g., luteins and lycopenes) and yet-undefined phytochemicals and will likely involve a whole-foods approach to supplementation. Ultimately, with advances in food science and genetic engineering, soldiers may be provided the best of both worlds by receiving both key nutritional elements and protection against key pathogens through antigens introduced into specially engineered tomatoes *(61,62)*.

5. CONCLUSIONS

The existing data support the idea that beneficial changes in immune function parameters result from modest exercise and that negative effects on immune function occur from extreme and prolonged energy deficits. Studies of intensive military training provide an informative, but not sufficient, body of evidence for a connection between nutritional status as a key stressor and diminished resistance to disease.

The Army will continue to field interventions that are likely to make a substantial difference to soldier health and performance. To date, no such benefit from any single nutrient or vitamin has been demonstrated in military field studies based on testing of the most promising leads from published studies. Studies conducted in the past decade failed to demonstrate any advantage of glutamine or various antioxidant mixtures for stressed healthy soldiers. This may result from a failure to study models in which infection is an important problem, and because all the studies have been conducted in difficult-to-control field settings that do not permit definitive conclusions. It is important to stress this point, because justification for marketing some nutritional supplements is traceable to loose interpretations of findings from military stress studies, none of which has yet demonstrated a clear cause-and-effect relationship between any stressor or combination of stressors and change in functional status in resistance to disease. What many of the studies have shown is an effect on specific immune function parameters, the significance of which is largely unknown. A lesson learned is that new strategies should only be tested in military field settings once adequate laboratory tests indicate true promise. An important effect of energy balance has been suggested from several military studies, which is consistent with findings from other studies. Although alterations in specific immune function parameters were demonstrated, functional consequences of these changes have been more difficult to establish. Controlled laboratory studies to demonstrate the effect of specific military stressors on susceptibility to disease, particularly stress-related disease susceptibility, are still needed. To understand the potential role of nutrition in stress-related disease susceptibility, the nature of the stressors in any model must be more precisely defined. Finally, as noted by the CMNR, there is a critical need for the development of a practical marker of immune competence for use in field studies.

6. "TAKE-HOME" MESSAGES

1. The significance of high-stress military training effects on changes in immune function parameters remains equivocal, but there is evidence of an effect on infectious illness susceptibility, as well as diminished vaccine effectiveness.
2. Energy balance appears to be the most important determinant of immune competence in military field studies.
3. No specific supplements, including glutamine and antioxidant nutrients, have been demonstrated to correct stress-induced alterations in immune function measures.
4. A better understanding of the relationship between practical measures of immune function and disease resistance is needed.

ACKNOWLEDGMENT

Stephen Grate, DVM, is acknowledged for his valuable discussion and assistance with this review.

REFERENCES

1. Committee on Military Nutrition Research. Food and Nutrition Board. Institute of Medicine. Military Strategies for Sustainment of Nutrition and Immune Function in the Field. National Academy Press, Washington, DC, 1999.
2. Keys A, Brozek J, Henschel A, Mickelsen O, Taylor HL. The Biology of Human Starvation. University of Minnesota Press, Minneapolis, 1950, pp. 1002–1014.
3. Sauberlich HE. Implications of nutritional status on human biochemistry, physiology and health. Clin Biochem 1984;17:132–142.
4. Cohen S, AJ Tyrrell, AP Smith. Psychological stress and susceptibility to the common cold. N Engl J Med 1991;325:606–612.
5. Kiecolt-Glaser JK, Glaser R. Stress and immune function in humans. In: Ader R, Felten DL, Cohen N (eds.). Psychoneuroimmunology. Academic, Boston, 1991, pp. 849–864.
6. Centers for Disease Control. Famine-affected, refugee, and displaced populations: recommendations for public health issues. MMWR Morb Mortal Wkly Rep 1992;41:1–76.
7. Wood TR, Kennedy JS, Shippee R, Arsenault J. The Effects of a Nutrient-Enriched Bar on Host Defense Mechanisms and Immunogenicity of Hepatitis A Vaccine during U.S. Army Ranger Training. Technical Report T00-12. U.S. Army Research Institute of Environmental Medicine, Natick, MA, February 2000.
8. Hotopf M, David A, Hull L, Ismail K, Unwin C, Wessely S. Role of vaccinations as risk factors for ill health in veterans of the Gulf war: cross sectional study. BMJ 2000;320:1363–1367.
9. Kapcala LP, Chautard T, Eskay RL. The protective role of the hypothalamic-pituitary-adrenal axis against lethality produced by immune, infectious, and inflammatory stress. Ann NY Acad Sci 1995;771:419–437.
10. Opstad PK, Aakvaag A. The effect of a high calory diet on hormonal changes in young men during prolonged physical strain and sleep deprivation. Eur J Appl Physiol 1981;46:31–39.
11. Friedl KE, Moore RJ, Hoyt RW, Marchitelli LJ, Martinez-Lopez LE, Askew EW. Endocrine markers of semistarvation in healthy lean men in a multistressor environment. J Appl Physiol 2000;88: 1820–1830.
12. Mason JW. Specificity in the organization of neuroendocrine response profiles. In: Seeman P, Brown G (eds.). Frontiers in Neurology and Neuroscience Research. University of Toronto, Toronto, 1974, pp. 68–80.

13. Wiik P. Immune function studies during the Ranger training course of the Norwegian Military Academy. In: Military Strategies for Sustainment of Nutrition and Immune Function in the Field. National Academy Press, Washington, DC, 1999, pp. 185–202.

14. Wiik P, Skrede KK, Knardahl S, et al. Effect of in vivo corticosterone and acute food deprivation on rat resident peritoneal cell chemiluminescence after activation ex vivo. Acta Physiol Scand 1995;154: 407–416.

15. Roshol H, Skrede KK, Aero CE, Wiik P. Dexamethasone and methylprednisolone affect rat peritoneal phagocyte chemiluminescence after administration in vivo. Eur J Pharmacol 1995;286:9–17.

16. Riedo FX, Schwartz B, Glono S, et al., and the Pneumococcal Pneumonia Study Group. Pneumococcal pneumonia outbreak in a Ranger Training Battalion. Program and Abstracts of the Interscience Conference on Antimicrobial Agents and Chemotherapy, Abstract #48. American Society of Microbiology, Sept. 29, 1991, Chicago, IL.

17. Moore RJ, Friedl KE, Kramer TR, et al. Changes in soldier nutritional status and immune function during the Ranger training course. Technical Report No. T13-92, September 1992, U.S. Army Research Institute of Environmental Medicine, Natick, MA. 162 pp. AD-A257 437.

18. Kramer TR, Moore RJ, Shippee RL, et al. Effects of food restriction in military training on T-lymphocyte responses. Int J Sports Med 1997;18(Suppl):S84–S90.

19. Kramer TR. Application of whole-blood cultures to field study measurements of cellular immune function in vitro. In: Military Strategies for Sustainment of Nutrition and Immune Function in the Field. National Academy Press, Washington, DC, 1999, pp. 9–262.

20. Martinez-Lopez LE, Friedl KE, Moore RJ, Kramer TR. A prospective epidemiological study of infection rates and injuries of Ranger students. Mil Med 1993;158:433–437.

21. Westphal KA, Friedl KE, Sharp MA, et al. Health, performance, and nutritional status of U.S. Army women during basic combat training. Technical Report No. T96-2, May 1995, U.S. Army Research Institute of Environmental Medicine, Natick, MA.

22. Brunner IKM, Severs YD, Rhind SG, Shephard RJ, Shek PN. Immune function and incidence of infection during basic infantry training. Mil Med 2000;165:878–883.

23. Guezennec CY, Satabin P, Legrand H, Bigard AX. Physical performance and metabolic changes induced by combined prolonged exercise and different energy intakes in humans. Eur J Appl Physiol 1994;68:525–530.

24. Wittels P, Johannes B, Enne R, Kirsch K, Gunga HC. Voice monitoring to measure emotional load during short-term stress. Eur J Appl Physiol 2002;87:278–282.

25. Opstad PK. Medical Consequences in Young Men of Prolonged Physical Stress with Sleep and Energy Deficiency. Norwegian Defence Research Establishment Report No. 95/05586. Kjeller, Norway, 1995.

26. Consolazio CF, Johnson HL, Nelson RA, et al. The relationship of diet to the performance of the combat soldier minimal calorie intake during combat patrols in a hot humid environment (Panama). Technical Report No. 76, October 1979, Letterman Army Institute of Research, Presidio of San Francisco, CA.

27. Rose RM, Bourne PG, Poe RO, Mougey EH, Collins DR, Mason JW. Androgen responses to stress. II. Excretion of testosterone, epitestosterone, androsterone and etiocholanolone during basic combat training and under threat of attack. Psychosomatic Med 1969;31:418–436.

28. Bourne PG, Coli WM, Datel WE. Anxiety levels of six helicopter ambulance medics in a combat zone. Psychol Rep 1966;19:821–822.

29. Boyum A, Wiik P, Gustavsson E, et al. The effect of strenuous exercise, calorie deficiency and sleep deprivation on white cells, plasma immunoglobulins and cytokines. Scand J Immunol 1996;43: 228–235.

30. Wiik P, Opstad PK, Boyum A. Granulocyte chemiluminescence response to serum opsonized zymosan particles ex vivo during long-term strenuous exercise, energy and sleep deprivation in humans. Eur J Appl Physiol Occup Physiol 1996;73:251–258.

31. Boyum A, Lovhaug D, Tresland L, Nordlie EM. Separation of leucocytes: improved cell purity by fine adjustments of gradient medium density and osmolality. Scand J Immunol 1991;34:697–712.

32. Christadoss P, Talal N, Lindstrom J, Fernandes G. Suppression of cellular and humoral immunity to T-dependent antigens by calorie restriction. Cell Immunol 1984;88:1–8.

33. Friedl KE, Moore RJ, Martinez-Lopez LE, et al. Lower limits of body fat in healthy active men. J Appl Physiol 1994;77:933–940.

34. Young AJ, Castellani JW, O'Brien C, et al. Exertional fatigue, sleep loss, and negative energy balance increase susceptibility to hypothermia. J Appl Physiol 1998;85:1210–1217.

35. Fairbrother B, Shippee R, Kramer T, Askew W, Mays M. Nutritional and immunological assessment of soldiers during the Special Forces Assessment and Selection Course. Technical Report T95-22. U.S. Army Research Institute of Environmental Medicine, Natick, Massachusetts. Sept. 1995. AD A299 556.

36. Fliederman J. Clinical aspects of hunger disease in adults. In: Winick M (ed.). Hunger Disease—Studies by the Jewish Physicians in the Warsaw Ghetto. Wiley-Interscience Publication, New York, 1979, pp. 1–44.

37. Pleban RJ, Valentine PJ, Penetar DM, Redmond DP, Belenky GL. Characterization of sleep and body composition changes during Ranger training. Mil Psychol 1990;2:45–156.

38. Shippee R, Friedl K, Kramer T, et al. Nutritional and Immunological Assessment of Ranger Students with Increased Caloric Intake. Technical Report T95-5. U.S. Army Research Institute of Environmental Medicine, Natick, MA, 1994.

39. Opstad PK, Aakvaag A. The effect of sleep deprivation on the plasma levels of hormones during prolonged physical strain and calorie deficiency. Eur J Appl Physiol 1983;51:97–107.

40. Irwin M, McClintick J, Costlow C, Fortner M, White J, Gillin JC. Partial night sleep deprivation reduces natural killer and cellular immune responses in humans. FASEB J 1996;10:643–653.

41. Dinges DF, Douglas SD, Zaugg L, et al. Leukocytosis and natural killer cell function parallel neurobehavioral fatigue induced by 64 hours of sleep deprivation. J Clin Invest 1994;93:1930–1939.

42. Friedl KE, Mays MZ, Kramer TR, Shippee RL. Acute recovery of physiological and cognitive function in U.S. Army Ranger students in a multistressor field environment. In: The Effect of Prolonged Military Activities in Man—Possible Means of Rapid Recuperation. NATO Research and Technology Organization, Meeting Proceedings 42. March 2001. Neuilly-sur-Seine, Cedex, France, pp. 6.1–6.10.

43. Pedersen BK, Kappel M, Klokker M, Nielsen HB, Secher NH. The immune system during exposure to extreme physiologic conditions. Int J Sports Med 1994;15(Suppl):S116–S121.

44. Nieman DC. Exercise, infection, and immunity: practical applications. In: Military Strategies for Sustainment of Nutrition and Immune Function in the Field. National Academy Press, Washington, DC, 1999, pp. 363–389.

45. Nieman DC, Henson DA, Johnson R, Lebeck L, Davis JM, Nehlsen-Cannarella SL. Effects of brief, heavy exertion on circulating lymphocyte subpopulations and proliferative response. Med Sci Sports Exerc 1992;24:1339–1345.

46. Rhind SG, Shek PN, Shinkai S, Shephard RJ. Effects of moderate endurance exercise and training on in vitro lymphocyte proliferation, interleukin-2 (IL-2) production, and IL-2 receptor expression. Eur J Appl Physiol Occup Physiol 1996;74:348–360.

47. Montain SJ, Shippee RL, Tharion WJ, Kramer TR. Carbohydrate-electrolyte solution during military training. Effects on physical performance, mood state and immune function. Technical Report T95-13. U.S. Army Research Institute of Environmental Medicine, Natick, MA, 1995. AD A297 258.

48. Shippee R, Wood S, Anderson P, Kramer T, Nieta M, Wolcott K. Effects of glutamine supplementation on immunological responses of soldiers during the Special Forces Assessment and Selection Course (abstract). FASEB J 1995;9:A731.

49. Shippee RL. Physiological and immunological impact of U.S. Army Special Operations training—a model for the assessment of nutritional intervention effects on temporary immunosuppression. In: Military Strategies for Sustainment of Nutrition and Immune Function in the Field. National Academy Press, Washington, DC, 1999, pp. 163–184.

50. Kennedy JS, Wood SM, Shippee R, Arsenault J. Effects of a nutrient-enriched beverage on host defense mechanisms of soldiers completing the Special Forces Assessment and Selection school. Technical Report T00-10. U.S. Army Research Institute of Environmental Medicine, Natick, MA, 2000, AD A373 799.

51. Schmidt MC, Askew EW, Roberts DE, Prior RL, Ensign WY Jr, Hesslink RE Jr. Oxidative stress in humans training in a cold, moderate altitude environment and their response to a phytochemical antioxidant supplement. Wilderness Environ Med 2002;13:94–105.

52. Simon-Schnass I. Oxidative stress at high altitudes and effects of vitamin E. In: Marriott BM, Carlson SJ (eds.). Nutritional Needs in Cold and in High-Altitude Environments—Applications for Military Personnel in Field Operations, National Academy Press, Washington DC, 1996, pp. 393–418.

53. Newsholme EA. Biochemical mechanisms to explain immunosuppression in well-trained and over-trained athletes. Int J Sports Med 1994;15:S142–S147.
54. Parry-Billings M, Blomstrand E, McAndrew N, Newsholme EA. A communicational link between skeletal muscle, brain, and cells of the immune system. Int J Sports Med 1990;11(Suppl 2):S122–S128.
55. Scheltinga MR, Young LS, Benfell K, et al. Glutamine-enriched intravenous feedings attenuate extra-cellular fluid expansion after a standard stress. Ann Surg 1991;214:385–395.
56. Wagenmakers AJM. Supplementation with branched-chain amino acids, glutamine, and protein hydrolysates: rationale for effects on metabolism and performance. In: The Role of Protein and Amino Acids in Sustaining and Enhancing Performance. National Academy Press, Washington DC, 1999, pp. 309–329.
57. Food and Nutrition Board. Institute of Medicine. Dietary Reference Intakes for Vitamin C, Vitamin E, Selenium, and Carotenoids. National Academy Press, Washington, DC, 2000.
58. Committee on Military Nutrition Research. Food and Nutrition Board. Institute of Medicine. Letter Report: Antioxidants and Oxidative Stress in Military Personnel. Feb 11, 1999. Report to U.S. Army Medical Research and Material Command, Fort Detrick.
59. Kramer TR, Burri BJ. Modulated mitogenic proliferative responsiveness of lymphocytes in whole-blood cultures after a low-carotene diet and mixed-carotenoid supplementation in women. Am J Clin Nutr 1997;65:871–875.
60. Paetau I, Khachik F, Brown ED, et al. Chronic ingestion of lycopene-rich tomato juice or lycopene supplements significantly increased plasma concentrations of lycopene and related tomato carotenoids in humans. Am J Clin Nutr 1998;68:1187–1195.
61. Anderson AO. New technologies for producing systemic and mucosal immunity by oral immunization: immunoprophylaxis in Meals, Ready-to-Eat. In: Carlson-Newberry SJ and Costello RB (eds.). Emerging Technologies for Nutrition Research—Potential for Assessing Military Performance Capability. National Academy Press, Washington, DC, 1997, pp. 451–500.
62. Mason HS, Warzecha H, Mor T, Arntzen CJ. Edible plant vaccines: applications for prophylactic and therapeutic molecular medicine. Trends Mol Med 2002;8:324–329.

21

Air Pollution, Reactive Oxygen Species, and Allergic Bronchial Asthma

The Therapeutic Role of Antioxidants

Gennaro D'Amato

1. INTRODUCTION

Bronchial asthma is characterized by airway inflammation, airway hyperresponsiveness to several specific and nonspecific stimuli, and reversible airway obstruction with the appearance of respiratory symptoms, such as dyspnea, chest tightness, wheezing, and cough. Although the pathogenesis of bronchial asthma is not completely understood, it is evident that this clinical condition has a multifactorial etiology, and a body of evidence suggests that bronchial asthma has become more common worldwide in recent years *(1–2)*. There is a link between the increase in the prevalence of allergic airway diseases and the increase in air pollution. Several studies have shown the adverse effects of ambient air pollution on respiratory health *(3–10)*. Moreover, exposure to components of air pollution enhances the airway response to inhaled allergens in susceptible individuals and, in most industrialized countries, people who live in urban areas are more affected by allergic respiratory diseases than those who live in rural areas *(11,12)*. Road traffic, with its gaseous and particulate emissions, is currently, and likely to remain, the main contributor to air pollution in most urban settings *(13–16)*.

Although the nature and concentration of outdoor pollutants vary from one area to another, the most abundant pollutants in the urban atmospheres are nitrogen dioxide, ozone, and fine particulate matter. Sulfur dioxide is an additional concern in industrial areas, whereas in rural and in urban areas aeroallergens are carried and delivered by plant-derived particles, such as pollen grains or fungal spores. The interaction between air pollution and aeroallergens can favor both the appearance and the exacerbation of allergic respiratory diseases.

Reactive oxygen species (ROS) play an important role in the pathogenesis of inflammatory airway diseases, such as bronchial asthma, and dietary antioxidants have a protective effect in bronchial asthma.

From: *Diet and Human Immune Function*
Edited by: D. A. Hughes, L. G. Darlington, and A. Bendich © Humana Press Inc., Totowa, NJ

2. COMPONENTS OF AIR POLLUTION

2.1. Ozone

Ozone is the most important factor in so-called "summer smog," because it is the main component of photochemical oxidants. Ozone probably accounts for up to 90% of total oxidant levels in cities that enjoy a mild sunny climate, such as the Mediterranean area and California, where current safety standards for ozone levels are frequently exceeded. Ozone is generated at ground level by photochemical reactions involving ultraviolet (UV) radiation of atmospheric mixtures of nitrogen dioxide and hydrocarbons, derived mainly from vehicle emissions. Consequently, ozone trends depend on not only substrate supply (nitrogen dioxide emitted by cars) but also sunny weather that favors the transformation of nitrogen dioxide into ozone, thereby producing photochemical smog. Approximately 40–60% of inhaled ozone is absorbed in the nasal airways, and the remainder reaches the lower airways. However, ozone can affect both the upper and the lower respiratory tracts, and it induces more adverse effects in asthma sufferers than in healthy individuals.

Exposure to increased atmospheric ozone levels causes decrements in lung function and increased airway reactivity to nonspecific and specific bronchoconstrictor agents and is related to an increased risk of asthma exacerbation in susceptible patients with asthma (16–21). Atmospheric levels of ozone and nitrogen dioxide have been linked to increases in respiratory morbidity and in-hospital admissions for asthma in children and adults. Ozone can modulate the airway inflammation of diseases, such as bronchial asthma, by increasing the release of inflammatory mediators from bronchial epithelial cells (22). It has also been observed that ozone exposure has a priming effect on allergen-induced responses, as well as an intrinsic inflammatory effect in the airways of allergic asthmatics (23–25). Indeed, ozone produces an immediate dose-dependent increase in intracellular ROS, as well as in epithelial cell permeability, which could facilitate entry of inhaled allergens and toxins, causing an increase in the release of inflammatory cells and their products.

Because inhalation of ozone by healthy subjects increases airway responsiveness and airway inflammation, subjects with asthma were once expected to be more sensitive to the acute effects of ozone. Epidemiologic studies have provided evidence that high ambient ozone concentrations are associated with an increased rate of asthma attacks (17–19). Because ozone-induced airway inflammation may last several days and ozone-related asthma exacerbations often occur several days after exposure, it is feasible that ozone-induced enhancement of preexisting airway inflammation enhances susceptibility to asthma exacerbations.

Ozone decreases exercise tolerance in well-trained athletes without asthma (26–27). Repeated daily short-term exposure to ozone in healthy subjects attenuates the acute decreased lung function and inflammatory responses (28,29). It is important to establish whether the enhanced ozone-induced inflammatory responses of persons with asthma also become attenuated with repeated daily exposures, particularly because exposure to high ozone concentrations may occur for several consecutive days during smog episodes.

It has long been speculated that ozone and other pollutants may render allergic individuals more susceptible to antigens to which they are sensitized. Recently, it has been observed that the incidence of new diagnoses of asthma is associated with heavy exercise in communities with high concentrations of ozone; thus, air pollution and outdoor exercise could contribute to the development of asthma in children *(30)*.

The outcome of two controlled human exposure studies, described below, support investigations in which ozone exposure enhanced responses to inhaled antigens in animals. Indeed, by lowering the threshold concentration of allergen capable of inducing clinical symptoms, ozone can enhance the airway responsiveness of sensitized subjects. Molfino et al. *(23)* reported that a 1-h exposure to 0.12 ppm ozone when at rest caused a twofold reduction in the provocation concentration of inhaled antigen required to cause early bronchoconstriction in specifically sensitized subjects with asthma. In fact, the mean provocation dose of ragweed necessary to reduce forced expiratory volume in 1 s (FEV_1) by 20% in specifically sensitized asthmatic subjects was significantly reduced to approximately half the dose of allergen when the patients were preexposed to 0.12 ppm ozone for 1 h vs. preexposure to air. Jorres and coworkers *(25)*, using a higher effective dose (0.25 ppm inhaled through a mouthpiece with intermittent exercise) and a longer duration of exposure (3 h), found that 23 of 24 subjects with mild asthma required a lower provocation dose of allergen to cause a 20% decrease in FEV_1 after ozone exposure.

Atopic individuals have a hereditary tendency to produce immunoglobulin (Ig) E antibody to common inhalant allergens (e.g., house dust mite and grass pollen) that provoke no immune responses in nonatopic individuals. Devalia et al. *(31)* investigated the effect of previous ozone and nitrogen dioxide exposure on subsequent allergen-induced changes in the nasal mucosa of patients with seasonal allergic rhinitis or perennial allergic asthma. They found that exposure to these pollutants significantly increased the allergen-induced release of esinophil cationic protein (ECP) in nasal lavage. Esinophils are now considered to be the cells that mediate much of the pathology and disordered airway function that characterizes atopic and nonatopic asthma. Of the proteins secreted by esinophils, ECP and major basic protein (MBP) are particularly active in rendering the epithelium fragile and unstable. The results of Devalia et al.'s study suggest that ozone and nitrogen dioxide exposure may "prime" the esinophils to subsequent activation by inhaled allergens in patients who are atopic.

Taken together, the results of the studies described here are consistent with a dose-dependent effect and indicate that ozone concentration and exposure length are critical, with a possible threshold range 0.1 to 0.2 ppm.

2.2. Nitrogen Dioxide

Nitrogen dioxide, a precursor of photochemical smog, is found in outdoor air in urban and industrial regions and, in conjunction with sunlight and hydrocarbons, produces ozone. Automobile exhaust is the most significant source of outdoor nitrogen dioxide, although power plants and other power sources that burn fossil fuels also release nitrogen dioxide into the environment. The most significant exposure to nitrogen dioxide occurs indoors in conjunction with the use of gas cooking stoves and kerosene space heaters. Most ambient nitrogen dioxide is generated by burning fossil-derived fuels. Like ozone, nitrogen dioxide is an oxidant pollutant, although it is less chemically reactive and thus probably less potent. Outdoor levels of nitrogen dioxide are not usually associated with notable changes in bronchial function in patients with asthma. Controlled exposure studies of subjects with asthma have produced inconsistent results regarding the ability of nitrogen dioxide to enhance nonspecific airway responsiveness, with some evidence that only certain individuals show an increased sensitivity *(32–34)*. Limited data from epidemiological studies suggest that exposure to high levels of nitrogen dioxide may be associated with acute decrements in lung function in individuals with asthma *(35–37)*.

2.3. Sulfur Dioxide

Sulfur dioxide is primarily generated from the burning of sulfur-containing fossil fuel and is released into the atmosphere primarily as a result of industrial combustion of high sulfur containing coal and oil. Sulfur dioxide induces acute bronchoconstriction in subjects with asthma at concentrations well below those required to induce this response in healthy subjects *(38,40)*. In contrast to ozone, the bronchoconstrictor effect of inhaled sulfur dioxide in individuals with asthma occurs after brief periods of exposure, especially with oral breathing and high ventilatory rates, as in exercise. Although the data on responses of subjects with asthma to nitrogen dioxide exposure are inconsistent, there is no question that brief (i.e., <1 h) exposures to low concentrations of sulfur dioxide can induce bronchoconstriction in such subjects *(39,40)*. Unlike pollutants, such as nitrogen dioxide and ozone, sulfur dioxide has a rapid effect on the lung function of subjects with asthma, and significant responses are observed within 2 min, with a maximal response seen within 5 to 10 min. There can also be spontaneous recovery (30 min after challenge) and a refractory period of up to 4 h, whereas repeated exposure to low levels of sulfur dioxide results in tolerance to subsequent exposure. Pharmacological studies suggest a cholinergically mediated neural mechanism. However, the mechanisms by which sulfur dioxide can induce asthma have yet to be completely clarified.

Sulfur dioxide exposure augments responses to other environmental agents that exacerbate bronchospasm. In this context, exposure of guinea pigs to as little as 0.1 ppm sulfur dioxide enhanced allergic sensitization to inhaled ovalbumin, as measured by the development of bronchoconstriction by specific inhalation challenge testing and increased concentrations of specific antibodies in both bronchoalveolar lavage (BAL) fluid (fluid recovered after the delivery and reaspiration of saline, by bronchoscopy, from the lungs) and serum *(41)*.

2.4. Particulate Matter

Airborne particulate matter is a major component of urban air pollution and contains a mixture of solid and liquid particles of different origin, size, and composition, among which are pollen grains and other vegetable particles carrying allergens and mold spores. Inhalable particulate matter that can reach the lower airways is classed as PM10 (<10 μ in aerodynamic diameter) and PM2.5 (<2.5μ) *(42–45)*. Human lung parenchyma retains PM2.5, whereas particles >5 μ and <10 μ only reach the proximal airways, where they are eliminated by mucociliary clearance if the airway mucosa is intact *(42–44)*. Particulate matter is the most serious air pollution problem in many cities and towns, and it is the component of air pollution most consistently associated with adverse health effects. Particulate air pollution is significantly associated with enhanced mortality from respiratory and cardiovascular diseases, exacerbation of allergies, asthma, chronic bronchitis, respiratory tract infection, and hospital admissions in many geographical areas. Moreover, the World Health Organization (WHO) estimates that inhalation of particulate matter is responsible for 500,000 excess deaths each year worldwide *(3)*. Adverse health events have also been observed in a range of air concentrations considered safe according to WHO guidelines *(10)*.

One explanation for the acute respiratory effects associated with inhalable particulate matter *(46)* is that transition metals in the particles damage the airways by generating free radicals. In particular, iron, which generates hydroxyl radicals, is responsible for many of the adverse respiratory effects *(47,48)*. Other transition metals (chromium, cobalt, copper, manganese, nickel, titanium, vanadium, and zinc) derived from various urban or combustion source samples were also correlated to free-radical activation and lung injury in animal experiments *(49–51)*. In the context of inhalable particulate matter, the diesel exhaust particulate (DEP) accounts for most of the airborne particulate matter (up to 90%) in the atmosphere of the world's largest cities *(52–56)*. DEP is characterized by a carbonaceous core, in which 18,000 different high molecular weight organic compounds are adsorbed. Diesel engines generate approx 100 times more particles per mile compared with petrol (gasoline) engines of equivalent power. Although diesel engines emit far less carbon dioxide than petrol engines, they emit more than 10 times more nitrogen dioxide, aldehydes, and inhalable particulate matter than unleaded petrol engines and more than 100 times more engines fitted with catalytic converters *(52)*. Diesel exhaust particles exert their effects by way of specific activities of chemical agents, including polyaromatic hydrocarbons. The particles are deposited on the mucosa of the airways, and, by virtue of the hydrophobic nature of the aromatic hydrocarbons, this allows diffusion through cell membranes and the binding to cytosolic receptor complexes. Through the subsequent nuclear action, aromatic hydrocarbons can modify the growth and the differentiation programs of cells *(52)*.

Acute exposure to diesel exhaust causes nose and eye irritation, lung function changes, respiratory changes, headache, fatigue, and nausea, whereas chronic exposure is associated with cough, sputum production, and lung function decrements *(53,54)*. Experimental studies have shown that DEP causes respiratory symptoms and can modify the immune response in predisposed animals and humans *(55–60)*. In fact, DEP exerts an adjuvant immunological effect on IgE synthesis in atopic subjects, thereby influencing sensitization to airborne allergens. More than a decade ago, Rudell et al. *(58)* showed that healthy volunteers who were exposed to DEP had a greater number of alveolar macrophages, neutrophils, and T lymphocytes in BAL than did controls. In the wake of these and other observations *(57–60)*, recent studies have confirmed the enhancing effects of DEP on airway inflammation and demonstrated an atopy-enhancing effect of diesel exhaust *(56)*.

Diaz-Sanchez et al. *(56)* studied the effect of DEP on antigen responses in ragweed-sensitive subjects challenged (nasal provocation test) with either DEP or Amb a1 (the major ragweed allergen) or a combination of DEP and Amb a1. Provocation with ragweed led to an increase in both total and ragweed-specific IgE in nasal lavage fluid measured 18 h, 4 d, and 8 d postchallenge. The DEP challenge increased the concentration of ragweed-specific IgE 16-fold vs. concentrations observed after challenge with ragweed alone. The same group observed that combined exhaust particulate and ragweed allergen challenge markedly enhanced human in vivo nasal ragweed-specific IgE and shifted cytokine production to a T-helper (Th) 2 cell-type pattern *(56)*, which favors the development of allergic responses (*see* Chapter 1). All these results indicate that DEP plays a role in the enhanced allergic inflammatory response.

Human epithelial cells and macrophages phagocytoze the DEP, which stimulates the production of the inflammatory cytokines interleukin (IL)-6, IL-8, and GM-CSF. IL-8, which is increased in lung and nasal washes of subjects with asthma and/or rhinitis, stimulates chemotaxis of lymphocytes, neutrophils, and esinophils and causes histamine release, plasma leakage, smooth muscle contraction of the airways, and increased airway hyperresponsiveness (56–60).

The data on DEP are particularly interesting because of the increasing percentage of new cars with diesel engines in industrialized countries. In Europe, for example, approx 50% of all new cars are diesel powered, owing to their lower maintenance costs.

2.5. Aeroallergens

Respiratory diseases induced by allergens released from pollen grains are common (61), and their cost, in terms of impaired work fitness, sick leave, consulting physicians, and medications, is high. Individuals living in urban areas are more affected by plant-derived respiratory disorders than those living in rural areas. Various studies suggest that there is an interaction between air pollutants and allergens that exacerbates the development of atopy and the respiratory symptoms of allergic disease in urban areas (10,62). In a time-series study, Brunekreef et al. (63) found a strong association between the day-to-day variation in pollen concentrations and deaths from cardiovascular disease, chronic obstructive pulmonary disease, and pneumonia.

To prevent pollen allergy, an ideal but hardly feasible approach is to minimize the risk of contact with these agents by moving to a nonrisk area. A much easier alternative is to reduce inhalation of pollen allergens by remaining at home with the windows closed (64).

3. REACTIVE OXYGEN SPECIES, DIETARY ANTIOXIDANTS, AND BRONCHIAL ASTHMA

ROS plays an important role in the pathogenesis of various inflammatory airway diseases, such as bronchial asthma (65,66). ROS formation occurs continuously during normal metabolic processes in every cell. However, activated phagocytic cells, such as macrophages, neutrophils, and esinophils, produce larger amounts, particularly when stimulated by inhaled particles and other components of air pollution. When respiratory tissues are exposed to oxidative stress induced by air pollution, inflammation, or reduced concentration of antioxidants, increased levels of ROS can induce deleterious effects on the respiratory tissues (damage to DNA, lipids, proteins, and carbohydrates), leading to detrimental effects on cellular function and increased inflammatory reactions (65,66).

A protective role for dietary antioxidants in bronchial asthma has been proposed. In particular, it has been observed that there is an association between dietary intake or blood concentrations of dietary factors and response to air pollutants and that supplementation of the diet with antioxidants protects against effects of pollutants (67). Not surprisingly, most investigators have concentrated on the known oxidizing agents nitrogen dioxide and ozone. Effects of experimental exposure of healthy subjects to high concentrations of these gases have been reduced by prior treatment with high doses of vitamin C (e.g., 500 mg, 4 times a day for 3 d) (68–70). A few studies have focused on the protection afforded by antioxidants against the cocktail of substances comprising ambient air pollution. Bucca et al. (71) showed that vitamin C can reduce the adverse effects of ambient pollution on lung function and airway reactivity in traffic police. Romieu and colleagues *(72)* showed that vitamins C, E, and A provided some protection against reductions in lung function related to ozone in Mexico City street workers. Grievink et al. *(73)* showed that supplementation of the diet with the same vitamins (100 mg vitamin E and 500 mg vitamin C, daily for 15 wk) protected cyclists from postexercise ozone-related falls in lung function.

Recently, there has been considerable interest in the association between dietary intake of antioxidants and measurements of systemic oxidative stress and lung function/symptoms in the general population and in smokers. It is not known what active dietary constituents contribute to these protective effects, but it is often assumed that antioxidant nutrients contribute to this defense. A possible protective effect against either the development of obstructive respiratory symptoms or a decline in pulmonary function has been associated with dietary antioxidant *(74–76)* and/or fruit intake *(77,78)*, as well as with n–3 fatty acids and/or fish intake *(79)*. Antioxidants and foods rich in antioxidants are believed to protect the airways against oxidant-mediated damage *(80)*, whereas the n–3 fatty acids, mainly present in oily fish, are believed to have antiinflammatory effects through their influence on the metabolism of arachidonic acid *(81)*. Blueberries and spinach have high antioxidant capacities *(82,83)*, 20–50 times higher than those of some other fruits and vegetables, such as honeydew melon and cucumber, on a fresh-weight basis.

Epidemiological evidence is accruing to indicate that low intakes of antioxidant nutrients, such as vitamins C and E and β-carotene (provitamin A), may be associated with reduced lung function *(84–86)* and chronic respiratory symptoms *(87,88)*. Vitamin C is a versatile water-soluble antioxidant. It protects against lipid peroxidation by scavenging ROS in the aqueous phase before they can initiate lipid peroxidation. Vitamin E is the most important antioxidant for preventing lipid peroxidation. It resides in the lipid domain of biologic membranes and plasma lipoproteins, where it prevents lipid peroxidation of polyunsaturated fatty acids (PUFAs).

A significant amount of research has indicated that smokers have a higher requirement for vitamin C than nonsmokers *(89)*. Vitamin C concentrations are lower in smokers than in nonsmokers and are inversely related to cigarette consumption *(90)*. The lower vitamin C status of smokers most likely results from increased turnover of the vitamin as a result of increased oxidative stress *(91)*. In one study, vitamin C supplementation (2000 mg/d for 5 d) significantly reduced the levels of urinary F_2-isoprostanes, an indicator of oxidative stress that is elevated in smokers, whereas vitamin E had no effect *(92)*. It has been proposed that smokers require ≥ twofold to threefold the current recommended dietary allowance of 60 mg/d to maintain plasma vitamin C concentrations comparable with those of nonsmokers *(93)*.

It has been demonstrated that higher intakes of vitamin C and β-carotene, but not vitamin E, are associated with a higher FEV_1 and forced vital capacity (FVC) than is seen in individuals with low intakes of these antioxidants *(94)*. No consistent associations were observed with respiratory symptoms. This suggests that dietary vitamin C and β-carotene have a protective effect on lung function but not on respiratory symptoms. A recent population-based study of 3,714 men and 4,256 women supports a protective role for vitamin C against the risk of obstructive airways disease and corroborates the hypothesis that this vitamin may be an effective modifier for the adverse effects of smoking on the risk of obstructive airways disease *(95)*. However, a more recent study has demonstrated that vitamin E and β-cryptoxanthin, a carotenoid, are stronger correlates of lung function than vitamin C *(96)*.

Recently, it has been suggested that a beneficial effect may be achieved from a high intake of catechins, which are polyphenolic compounds from green tea and fruits, of preventing obstructive chronic bronchitis *(97)*.

Selenium supplementation to the diet of patients with asthma enhances the activity of the selenium-dependent enzyme glutathione peroxidase and improves clinical symptoms with regard to the assembled clinical evaluation made of each patient *(98)*. This improvement could, however, not be validated by significant changes in the separate clinical parameters of lung function and airway hyperresponsiveness. Using data from the Third National Health and Nutrition Examination Survey comprising a sample representative of the U.S. population in 1988–1994, Hu and Cassano *(99)* found that serum selenium had a stronger positive association with FEV_1 in smokers. Although data in patients with chronic obstructive pulmonary disease are not available, this finding might have implications for further research.

Another compound that might be interesting for the treatment of inflammatory reactions in the airways is ebselen [2-phenyl-1,2-benz-isoselenazol-3(2H)-one], a selenoorganic compound that has both antioxidant and antiinflammatory properties and also possesses thiol peroxidase activity. Ebselen exhibits its antioxidant activity mainly as a glutathione peroxidase mimic but has also acted as a scavenger of peroxynitrite *(100,101)*. However, ebselen used alone was not successful in reducing the effect of 50% oxygen on morphogenesis of mouse immature lung explants *(102)*. Further research is therefore required to assess the potential beneficial uses of this compound.

4. CONCLUSIONS

Evidence suggests that urbanization, with its high levels of vehicle emissions, and westernized lifestyle are linked to the rising incidence of respiratory allergic diseases, such as bronchial asthma, seen in most industrialized countries. Moreover, the increase in respiratory allergy parallels an increase in outdoor and indoor air pollution. Although outdoor pollutants' role in allergic sensitization of airways has yet to be elucidated, it is well-established that outdoor pollution exacerbates respiratory symptoms in subjects who are atopic and that some components, such as ozone and diesel exhaust particles, can induce the appearance of bronchial asthma.

Acute and chronic exposure to components of air pollution, such as nitrogen dioxide, ozone, sulfur dioxide, and inhalable particulate matter, either isolated or in various combinations, enhance airway responsiveness to aeroallergens in subjects who are atopic. In addition, by inducing airway inflammation, which increases airway epithelial permeability, pollutants overcome the mucosal barrier and "prime" allergic respiratory responses. In other words, the airway mucosal damage and the impaired mucociliary clearance induced by air pollution may facilitate the penetration and access of inhaled allergens to the cells of the immune system, thereby promoting airway sensitization. Consequently, an enhanced IgE-mediated response to aeroallergens and enhanced airway inflammation favored by air pollution could account for the increasing prevalence of allergic respiratory diseases in urban areas.

Oxidative stress can induce deleterious effects on the respiratory tissues, with production of ROS, which are generated as a consequence of inflammation or may arise directly by inhalation of oxidants from the environment (e.g., oxidant compounds in cigarette smoke or in outdoor air pollution).

Supplementation of diet by dietary factors has a protective role against the deleterious effects of air pollutants. In particular, foods rich in antioxidants protect the airways against oxidant-mediated damage.

5. "TAKE-HOME" MESSAGES

1. Exposure to air pollution components enhances the airway response to inhaled allergens in susceptible individuals, and, in most industrialized countries, people who live in urban areas are more affected by allergic respiratory diseases than those who live in rural areas.
2. ROS play an important role in the pathogenesis of inflammatory airway diseases, such as bronchial asthma. Therefore, a protective role for dietary antioxidants has been proposed.
3. There is now much literature supporting the beneficial influence of foods containing vitamin C on airway reactivity, and there is some evidence that foods containing vitamin E may protect against allergy.
4. Effects of experimental exposure to high concentrations of nitrogen dioxide and ozone in healthy subjects have been reduced by previous treatment with high doses of vitamin C.
5. Older adults with low blood concentrations of β-carotene have greater falls in peak flow rate in relation to rises in particulate pollution compared with those older adults with high blood concentrations.
6. Increased vitamin C intake may reduce the risk of obstructive airways disease in cigarette smokers.

REFERENCES

1. European Community Respiratory Health Survey. Variations in the prevalence of respiratory symptoms, self-reported asthma attacks and the use of asthma medications in the European Community Respiratory Health Survey (ECRHS). Eur Respir J 1996;9:687–695.
2. The International Study of Asthma and Allergy in Childhood (ISAAC). Steering Committee. Worldwide variation in prevalence of symptoms of asthma, allergic rhinoconjunctivitis and atopic eczema. Lancet 1998;351:1225–1232.
3. United Nations Environment Programme and WHO Report. Air pollution in the world's megacities. A report from the U.N. Environment Programme and WHO. Environment 1994;36:5–37.
4. American Thoracic Society. Health effects of outdoor air pollution. Part I. Am J Respir Crit Care Med 1996;153:3–50.
5. American Thoracic Society. Health effects of outdoor air pollution. Part II. Am J Respir Crit Care Med 1996;153:477–498.
6. Lebowitz MD. Epidemiological studies of the respiratory effects of air pollution. Eur Respir J 1996;9:1029–1054.
7. Holgate S, Samet JM, Koren HS, Maynard RL. Air pollution and health. Academic, London, 1999.
8. Boezen HM, van der Zee SC, Postma DS, et al. Effects of ambient air pollution on upper and lower respiratory symptoms and peak expiratory flow in children. Lancet 1999;353:874–878.
9. Künzli N, Kaiser R, Medina S, et al. Public health impact of outdoor and traffic-related air pollution: a European assessment. Lancet 2000;356:795–801.
10. Donaldson K, Lang Tran C, MacNee W. Deposition and effects of fine and ultrafine particles in the respiratory tract. In: D'Amato G, Holgate ST (eds.). The Impact of Air Pollution on Respiratory Health. Number 21. European Respiratory Monograph. Sheffield, UK, 2002, pp. 77–92.

11. Riedler J, Eder W, Oberfeld G, Schrener M. Austrian children living on a farm have less hay fever, asthma and allergic sensitization. Clin Exp Allergy 2000;30:194–200.

12. Braun-Fahrlander C, Gassner M, Grize L, et al. Prevalence of hay fever and allergic sensitization in farmers' children and their peers living in the same rural community. SCARPOL team. Swiss study on childhood allergy and respiratory symptoms with respect to air pollution. Clin Exp Allergy 1999;29:28–34.

13. Wjst M, Reitneir P, Dold S, et al. Road traffic and adverse effects on respiratory health in children. BMJ 1993;307:596–600.

14. Edwards J, Walters S, Griffiths RK. Hospital admissions for asthma in preschool children: relationship to major roads in Birmingham, United Kingdom. Arch Environ Health 1994;49:223–227.

15. D'Amato G, Liccardi G, D'Amato M, Cazzola M. The role of outdoor air pollution and climatic changes on the rising trends in respiratory allergy. Respir Med 2001;95:606–611.

16. Gielen MH, Van der Zee SC, Van Eijenen JH, Van Steen CJ, Brunekreef B. Acute effects of summer air pollution on respiratory health of asthmatic children. Am J Respir Crit Care Med 1997;155:2105–2108.

17. Bates DV, Sizto R. Relationship between air pollution levels and hospital admissions in southern Ontario. Can J Public Health 1983;74:117–133.

18. Balmes JR. The role of ozone exposure in the epidemiology of asthma. Environ Health Perspect 1993;101(Suppl 4):219–224.

19. White MC, Etzel RA, Wilcox WD, Lloyd C. Exacerbations of childhood asthma and ozone pollution in Atlanta. Environ Res 1994;65:56–68.

20. Thurston GD, Gwynn RC. Ozone and asthma mortality/hospital admissions in New York City. Am J Respir Crit Care Med 1997;155:A426.

21. Peters JM, Avol E, Gauderman WJ, et al. A study of twelve Southern California communities with differing levels and types of air pollution. II. Effects on pulmonary function. Am J Respir Crit Care Med 1999;159:768–775.

22. Bayram H, Sapsford RJ, Abdelaziz MM, Khair OA. Effect of ozone and nitrogen dioxide on the release of proinflammatory mediators from bronchial epithelial cells on non-atopic non-asthmatic subjects and atopic asthmatic patients in vitro. J Allergy Clin Immunol 2001;107:287–294.

23. Molfino NA, Wright SC, Katz I, et al. Effect of low concentration of ozone on inhaled allergen responses in asthmatic subjects. Lancet 1991;338:199–203.

24. Peden DB, Setzer RW, Devlin RB. Ozone exposure has both a priming effect on allergen induced responses as well as an intrinsic inflammatory action in the nasal airways of perennial allergic asthmatics. Am J Respir Crit Care Med 1995;151:1336–1345.

25. Jorres R, Nowak D, Magnussen H. Effect of ozone exposure on allergen responsiveness in subjects with asthma or rhinitis. Am J Resp Crit Care Med 1996;153:56–64.

26. Adams WC, Schelegle ES. Ozone and high ventilation effects on pulmonary function and endurance performance. J Appl Physiol 1983;55:805–812.

27. Foxcroft WJ, Adams WC. Effects of ozone exposure on four consecutive days on work performance and VO_2 max. J Appl Physiol 1986;61:960–966.

28. Devlin RB, Folinsbee LJ, Biscardi F, et al. Attenuation of cellular and biochemical changes in the lungs of humans exposed to ozone for five consecutive days. Am Rev Respir Dis 1993;147:A71.

29. Christian DL, Chen LL, Scannell CH, Ferrando RE, Welch BS, Balmes JR. Ozone-induced inflammation is attenuated with multi-day exposure. Am J Respir Crit Care Med 1996;153:A699.

30. McConnell R, Berhane K, Gilliland F, et al. Asthma in exercising children exposed to ozone: a cohort study. Lancet 2002;359:386–391.

31. Devalia JL, Rusznak C, Davies RJ. Allergen/irritant interaction—its role in sensitization and allergic disease. Allergy 1998;53:335–345.

32. Bauer MA, Utell MJ, Morrow PE, Speers DM, Gibb FR. Inhalation of 0.30 ppm nitrogen dioxide potentiates exercise-induced bronchoconstriction in asthmatics. Am Rev Respir Dis 1986;134:1203–1208.

33. Moshenin V. Airway responses to nitrogen dioxide in asthmatic subjects. J Toxicol Environ Health 1987;22:371–380.

34. Roger LJ, Horstman DH, McDonnell WF, et al. Pulmonary function, airway responsiveness and respiratory symptoms in asthmatics following exercise in NO_2. Toxicol Ind Health 1990;6:155–171.

35. Lebowitz MD, Holberg CJ, Boyer B, Hayes C. Respiratory symptoms and peak flow associated with indoor and outdoor air pollutants in the southwest. J Air Pollut Control Assoc 1985;35:1154–1158.
36. Goldstein IF, Lieber K, Andrews LR, et al. Acute respiratory effects of short-term exposures to nitrogen dioxide. Arch Environ Health 1988;43:138–142.
37. Tunnicliffe WE, Burge PS, Ayres JG. Effect of domestic concentrations of nitrogen dioxide on airway responses to inhaled allergen in asthmatic patients. Lancet 1994;344:1733–1736.
38. Linn WS, Avol EL, Peng RC, Shamoo DA, Hackney JD. Replicated dose-response study of sulfur dioxide in normal, atopic and asthmatic volunteers. Am Rev Respir Dis 1987;136:1127–1134.
39. Horstman D, Roger LJ, Kehrl H, Hazucha MJ. Airway sensitivity of asthmatics to sulfur dioxide. Toxicol Ind Health 1986;2:289–298.
40. Balmes JR, Fine JM, Sheppard D. Symptomatic bronchoconstriction after short-term inhalation of sulfur dioxide. Am Rev Respir Dis 1987;136:1117–1121.
41. Reidel F, Kramer M, Scheibenbogen C, Rieger CHL. Effects of SO_2 exposure on allergic sensitization in the guinea pig. J Allergy Clin Immunol 1988;82:527–534.
42. Churg A, Brauer M. Human lung parenchyma retains PM2.5. Am J Respir Crit Care Med 1997;155: 2109–2111.
43. Brain JD, Valberg PA. Deposition of aerosol in the respiratory tract. Am Rev Respir Dis 1979;120: 1325–1373.
44. Anderson M, Svartengren M, Philipson K, Camner P. Regional human lung deposition studied by repeated investigations. J Aerosol Sci 1994;25:567–581.
45. Salvi S, Holgate S. Mechanisms of particulate matter toxicity. Clin Exp Allergy 1999;29:1187–1194.
46. Seaton A, MacNee W, Donaldson K, Godden K. Particulate air pollution and acute health effects. Lancet 1995;345:176–178.
47. Smith KR, Aust AE. Mobilization of iron from urban particulates leads to generation of reactive oxygen species in vitro and induction of ferritin synthesis in human lung epithelial cells. Chem Res Toxicol 1997;10:828–834.
48. Ghio AJ, Hatch GE. Lavage phospholipid concentration after silica instillation in the rat is associated with complexed (Fe3+) on the dust surface. Am J Respir Cell Mol Biol 1993;8:403–407.
49. Donaldson K, Brown DM, Mitchell C, et al. Free radical activity of PM10: iron mediated generation of hydroxyl radicals. Environ Health Perspect 1997;105(Suppl 5):1285–1289.
50. Costa DL, Dreher KL. Bioavailable transition metals in particulate matter mediate cardiopulmonary injury in healthy and compromised animal models. Environ Health Perspect 1997;105(Suppl 5): 1053–1060.
51. Dreher KL, Jaskot RH, Lehmann JR, et al. Soluble transition metals mediate residual oil fly ash induced acute lung injury. J Toxicol Environ Health 1997;50:285–305.
52. Diesel Working Group. Diesel exhaust, a critical analysis of emissions, exposure and health effects. Health Effects Institute, Cambridge, MA, 1995.
53. Sydbom A, Blomberg A, Parnia S, Stenfors N, Sandstrom T, Dahlén SE. Health effects of diesel exhaust emissions. Eur Respir J 2001;17:733–746.
54. Nauss KM, Busby WF Jr, Cohen AJ, et al. Critical issue in assessing the carcinogenicity of diesel exhaust: a synthesis of current knowledge. In: Health Effects Institute's Diesel Working Group. Diesel Exhaust. A Critical Analysis of Emission, Exposure and Health Effects. Health Effects Institute, Cambridge, MA, 1995, pp. 13–18.
55. Takenaka H, Zhang K, Diaz-Sanchez D, Tsien A, Saxon A. Enhanced human IgE production results from exposure to the aromatic hydrocarbons from diesel exhaust: direct effects on B-cell IgE Production. J Allergy Clin Immunol 1995;95:103–115.
56. Diaz-Sanchez D, Tsien A, Fleming J, Saxon A. Combined diesel exhaust particulate and ragweed allergen challenge markedly enhances human in vivo nasal ragweed-specific IgE and skews cytokine production to a T helper cell 2-type pattern. J Immunol 1997;158:2406–2413.
57. Bayram H, Devalia JL, Sapsford RJ, et al. The effect of diesel exhaust particles on cell function and release of inflammatory mediators from human bronchial epithelial cells in vitro. Am J Respir Cell Mol Biol 1998;18:441–448.
58. Rudell B, Sandstrom T, Stjernberg N, Heldman KB. Controlled diesel exhaust exposure in an exposure chamber: pulmonary effects investigated with bronchoalveolar lavage. J Aerosol Sci 1990;21:S411–S414.

59. Brown JL, Frew AJ. Diesel exhaust particles and respiratory allergy. In: D'Amato G, Holgate ST (eds.). The Impact of Air Pollution on Respiratory Health. European Respiratory Monograph, 2002.

60. Frew A, Salvi S, Sandstrom T, Holgate ST. The effect of diesel particulates on normal and asthmatic airways. In: D'Amato G, Holgate ST (eds.). The Impact of Air Pollution on Respiratory Health. European Respiratory Monograph, 2002.

61. D'Amato G, Spieksma, Liccardi G, et al. Pollen-related allergy in Europe. Position Paper of the European Academy of Allergology and Clinical Immunology. Allergy 1998;53:567–578.

62. D'Amato G. Urban air pollution and plant-derived respiratory allergy. Clin Exp Allergy 2000;30: 628–636.

63. Brunekreef B, Hoek G, Fischer P, Spieksma FTHM. Relation between airborne pollen concentrations and daily cardiovascular and respiratory-disease mortality. Lancet 2000;355:1517–1518.

64. D'Amato G, Liccardi G, D'Amato M, Cazzola M. Outdoor air pollution, climate changes and allergic diseases. Eur Resp J 2002;20:763–776.

65. Henricks PAJ, Nijkamp FP. Reactive oxygen species as mediators in asthma. Pulm Pharnacol Therap 2001;14:409–421.

66. Vallyathan V, Shi X. The role of oxygen free radicals in occupational and environmental lung diseases. Environ Health Perspect 1997;105(Suppl 1):165–177.

67. Soutar A, Seaton A, Brown K. Bronchial reactivity and dietary antioxidants. Thorax 1997;52:166–170.

68. Chatham MD, Eppler JH, Saunder LR, Green D, Kulle TJ. Evaluation of the effects of vitamin C on ozone-induced bronchoconstriction in normal subjects. Ann NY Acad Sci 1987;498:269–279.

69. Mohsenin V. Effect of vitamin C on NO_2–induced airway hyperresponsiveness in normal subjects. Am Rev Respir Dis 1987;136:1408–1411.

70. Bielory L, Gandhi R. Asthma and vitamin C. Ann Allergy 1994;73:89–96.

71. Bucca C, Rolla G, Caria E, Arossa W, Bugiani M. Effects of vitamin C on airway responsiveness to inhaled histamine in heavy smokers. Eur Respir J 1989;2:229–233.

72. Romieu I, Meneses F, Ramirez M, et al. Antioxidant supplementation and respiratory functions among workers exposed to high levels of ozone. Am J Respir Crit Care Med 1998;158:226–232.

73. Grievink L, Zijlstra AG, Brunekreef B. Double-blind intervention trial on modulation of ozone effects on pulmonary function by antioxidant supplements. Am J Epidemiol 1999;149:306–314.

74. MacNee W. Oxidative stress and lung inflammation in airways disease. Eur J Pharmacol 2001;429: 195–207.

75. Britton JR, Pavord ID, Richards KA, et al. Dietary antioxidant vitamin intake and lung function in the general population. Am J Respir Crit Care Med 1995;151:1383–1387.

76. Grievink L, Smit HA, Ocké MC, et al. Dietary intake of antioxidant (pro)-vitamins, respiratory symptoms and pulmonary function: the MORGEN study. Thorax 1998;78:166–171.

77. Cook DG, Carey IM, Whincup PH, et al. Effect of fresh fruit consumption on lung function and wheeze in children. Thorax 1997;52:628–633.

78. Carey IM, Strachan DP, Cook DG. Effect of changes in fresh fruit consumption on ventilatory function in healthy British adults. Am J Respir Crit Care Med 1998;158:728–733.

79. Sharp DS, Rodriquez BL, Shahar E, et al. Fish consumption may limit the damage of smoking on the lung. Am J Respir Crit Care Med 1994;150:983–987.

80. Sridhar MK. Nutrition and lung health: should people at risk of chronic obstructive lung disease eat more fruit and vegetables? BMJ 1995;310:75–76.

81. Simopoulos AP. Omega-3 fatty acids in health and disease and in growth and development. Am J Clin Nutr 1991;54:438–463.

82. Cao G, Sofic E, Prior RL. Antioxidant capacity of tea and common vegetables. J Agric Food Chem 1996;44:3426–3431.

83. Prior RL, Cao G, Martin A, et al. Antioxidant capacity as influenced by total phenolic and anthocyanin content, maturity, and variety of Vaccinium species. J Agric Food Chem 1998;46:2686–2693.

84. Strachan DP, Cox BD, Erzinclioglu SW, et al. Ventilatory function and winter fresh fruit consumption in a random sample of British adults. Thorax 1991;46:624–629.

85. Schwartz J, Weiss ST. Relationship between dietary vitamin C intake and pulmonary function in the first national health and nutrition examination survey (NHANES 1). Am J Clin Nutr 1994;59:110–114.

86. Grievink L, van de Zee SC, Hoek G, et al. Modulation of the acute respiratory effects of air pollution by serum and dietary antioxidants: a panel study. Eur Respir J 1999;13:1439–1446.

87. Schwartz J, Weiss ST. Dietary factors and their relation to respiratory symptoms: the second national health and nutrition examination survey. Am J Epidemiol 1990;132:67–76.

88. Miedema I, Feskens EJM, Heederik D, et al. Dietary determinants of long-term incidence of chronic nonspecific lung diseases: the Zutphen study. Am J Epidemiol 1993;138:37–45.

89. Weber P, Bendich A, Schalch W. Vitamin C and human health—a review of recent data relevant to human requirements. Int J Vitam Nutr Res 1996;66:19–30.

90. Lykkesfeldt J, Prieme H, Loft S, Poulsen HE. Effect of smoking cessation on plasma ascorbic acid concentration. BMJ 1996;313:91.

91. Lykkesfeldt J, Loft S, Nielsen JB, et al. Ascorbic acid and dehydroascorbic acid as biomarkers of oxidative stress caused by smoking. Am J Clin Nutr 1997;65:959–963.

92. Reilly M, Delanty N, Lawson JA, et al. Modulation of oxidant stress in vivo in chronic cigarette smokers. Circulation 1996;94:19–25.

93. Smith JL, Hodges RE. Serum levels of vitamin C in relation to dietary and supplemental intake of vitamin C in smokers and nonsmokers. Ann NY Acad Sci 1987;498:144–152.

94. Repine JE, Bast A, Lankhorst I, and the Oxidative Stress Study Group. Oxidative stress in chronic obstructive pulmonary disease. Am J Respir Crit Care Med 1997;156:341–357.

95. Sargeant LA, Jaeckel A, Wareham NJ. Interaction of vitamin C with the relation between smoking and obstructive airways disease in EPIC Norfolk. European Prospective Investigation into Cancer and Nutrition. Eur Respir J 2000;16:397–403.

96. Schunemann HJ, Grant BJ, Freudenheim JL, et al. The relation of serum levels of antioxidant vitamins C and E, retinol and carotenoids with pulmonary function in the general population. Am J Respir Crit Care Med 2001;163:1246–1255.

97. Tabak C, Arts ICW, Smit HA, et al. Chronic obstructive pulmonary disease and intake of catechins, flavonols, and flavones. The MORGEN Study. Am J Respir Crit Care Med 2001;164:61–64.

98. Hasselmark L, Malmgren R, Zetterström O, et al. Selenium supplementation in intrinsic asthma. Allergy 1993;48:30–36.

99. Hu G, Cassano PA. Antioxidant nutrients and pulmonary function: the Third National Health and Nutrition Examination Survey (NHANES III). Am J Epidemiol 2000;151:975–981.

100. Sies H. Ebselen: a glutathione peroxidase mimic. Meth Enzymol 1994;234:476–484.

101. Sies H, Masumoto H. Ebselen as a glutathione peroxidase mimic and as a scavenger of peroxynitrite. Adv Pharmacol 1997;38:229–246.

102. Wilborn AM, Evers LB, Canada AT. Oxygen toxicity to the developing lung of the mouse: role of reactive oxygen species. Ped Res 1996;40:225–232.

22

Use of Drugs that Affect Nutrition and Immune Function

*Adrianne Bendich
and Ronit Zilberboim*

1. INTRODUCTION

The objectives of this chapter are to examine the effects of drug treatments on four major immune-related diseases and to determine the nutritional consequences of the drug-disease interaction in adults living in developed countries. The diseases discussed include HIV infection, diabetes (type 1 and type 2), rheumatoid arthritis, and osteoporosis. Osteoporosis is included because of the role of the osteoclast, which is a macrophage-derived cell involved in bone breakdown *(1)*. Insulin is a significant enhancer of bone formation, and, therefore, osteoporosis is often a consequence of diabetes *(2)*. Osteoporosis is also included after the discussion of rheumatoid arthritis (RA) because the major drug class used to treat RA, glucocorticoids, is a known cause of secondary osteoporosis *(3–5)*. Finally, organ transplant-associated osteoporosis demonstrates the links between a medical event (transplantation), immunotherapy, and nutritional effects *(6,7)*.

For each of the immune-related diseases, there is a brief overview of the disease and its major health consequences, with emphasis on the nutritionally related effects, followed by a description of the classes of drugs used to treat the disease. The nutritional effects are then described. If relevant, recommendations are also provided concerning potential nutritional interventions that could increase drug efficacy and/or reduce adverse side effects. Several excellent texts/chapters served as the major sources of information complied in this chapter *(8–25)*.

It is important to note that several immune-related diseases are diagnosed in midlife, and that the diseases, such as osteoporosis or type 2 diabetes, often do not occur independently of other chronic conditions *(10,23,26,27)*. It is estimated that 85% of adults older than 65 yr take some prescription drug before the diagnosis of a new disease, such as type 2 diabetes *(28)*. For the majority of chronic diseases, whether or not immune-related, there are cardinal features of disease that affect nutritional status. Usually, during the course of disease, there is an increase in metabolic rate that is often associated with fever; gastrointestinal (GI) tract impairment, resulting in decreased intake and/or absorption; increased excretion; and pain. Often, prolonged drug therapy affects the liver and its

From: *Diet and Human Immune Function*
Edited by: D. A. Hughes, L. G. Darlington, and A. Bendich © Humana Press Inc., Totowa, NJ

capacity to enhance fat absorption (and fat-soluble vitamin absorption), production of nutrient carrier proteins, and increase gut motility. Similarly, many drugs affect pancreatic function, causing alterations in protein breakdown, glucose use, and gastric emptying. Many chronic diseases (and several drugs used to treat the diseases) result in tissue destruction, possibly resulting from increases in oxidative damage; it is often difficult to determine which is the first event and which is the consequence *(9,10,17,19,21,22,24,25)*. Nevertheless, this chapter reviews the current knowledge on the interactions between certain immune-related diseases, current therapies, and nutritional consequences.

2. HIV INFECTION

HIV was first identified in 1984, after the recognition in 1981 of an unusually high number of infections caused by the pathogenic microorganism *Pneumocystis carinii* and the appearance of a rare form of cancer, Kaposi's sarcoma, in homosexual men in San Francisco and New York *(29)*. HIV infection was caused by one of two retroviral species designated HIV-1 and HIV-2. The virus infects immune system cells, resulting in severe immunosuppression that has been termed acquired immunodeficiency syndrome (AIDS) *(30–32)*. T lymphocytes with CD4 cell-surface receptors are the prime target of HIV infection. The major function of these T cells is to help develop immune responses. The balance within the immune system is derived from the signals between T helper (Th) cells and T-suppressor cells (CD8). When HIV destroys the Th cells, the balance is tipped toward immune suppression. Additionally, the capacity to mount a vigorous immune response to external pathogens is also diminished because of a lack of Th cells. Thus, a consequence of HIV infection is greater risk of other infections and a decreased capacity to recover from infection. Moreover, the immunosurveillance role of the immune system is also impaired, resulting in a greater risk for the development of precancerous and cancerous lesions. Antioxidant status, measured by dietary intake, serum levels of relevant molecules, or in vitro assays of radical quenching capacity, is particularly important in HIV infection. Free radicals can induce the HIV transcription factor-nuclear factor (NF) κB in vitro that results in the replication of the virus *(29,31,33)*.

Many opportunistic infection sites seen in HIV infection include the digestive system: mouth, stomach, intestine, colon, and rectum. These are common sites for bacterial and fungal, as well as other, viral infections in individuals with HIV infection. Hepatitis is also common, resulting in decreased liver function. Often, there is accompanying fever and other discomforts that can affect appetite and energy requirements. Finally, abdominal pain, nausea, vomiting, and/or diarrhea contribute to the weight loss and wasting seen in the end stages of AIDS *(32)*.

2.1. Drugs Used to Treat HIV Infection and AIDS

The primary objective of drug therapy is to halt viral replication. Two major drug targets are the enzymes that either permit the virus to enter the host cell's DNA or decrease the potential for the virus to replicate within the host's cells. Drugs targeted at HIV reverse transcriptase block the incorporation of the virus into host DNA. There are three major classes of antiretroviral drugs that block the reverse transcriptase enzyme; a fourth class of antiretrovirals interferes with the HIV protease enzyme. Drug treatment usually involves the simultaneous administration of at least two drugs. Some drug treatment is usually given to infected individuals from the onset of symptoms and continues indefinitely. Often, there are multiple changes in drugs because development of HIV drug resistance is common (*see* Table 1) *(8,29,34)*.

2.2. Drug/Disease Effects on Nutritional Status

Several drugs used to treat HIV and AIDS have similar adverse effects on the GI tract, resulting in nausea and diarrhea, loss of appetite, loss of sensation in the mouth, and changes in taste perception. Protease inhibitors cause dyspepsia and anorexia. Additionally, because multiple drug therapies are the normal treatment, the number of drugs consumed may affect appetite and induce nausea and other GI tract reactions, resulting in decreased food intake. More serious adverse effects include pancreatitis and liver dysfunction *(32,35)*.

Beisel *(29)* recently described the nutritional consequences of AIDS that remain relevant even when patients are asymptomatic. There is a continuing production of proinflammatory cytokines and a general state of increased metabolic activity that contribute to the weight loss seen as the disease progresses. Three major factors contribute to the "nutritionally acquired immune deficiency syndrome": reduced dietary intake, metabolic effects, and nutrient malabsorption. There is also an acceleration of loss of nutrients because of the persistent diarrhea seen with the disease, as well as in response to drug therapy. Both macronutrients and micronutrients are lost in diarrhea, including sodium, potassium, proteins, fat, and fat- and water-soluble vitamins.

There is an increased requirement for macronutrients and several micronutrients in individuals with HIV infection. When clinical studies are undertaken, these patients are almost always treated with a combination of the drugs listed in Table 1. Patients with HIV infection often have elevated triglycerides and may have higher circulating fatty acids. Certain amino acids that are immunomodulatory—arginine and glutamine—have been given to patients with HIV infection, with consequent beneficial effects, such as increases in lymphocyte counts and decreases in infections. Regarding micronutrients, there are consistent reports of significantly lower circulating levels of riboflavin, niacin, folate, and vitamins B_6 and B_{12}; vitamin B_6 and folate are important for optimal immune responses. Low serum vitamin A levels are predictive of poor long-term outcomes. Indicators of increased oxidative stress are well-documented, and selenium and vitamin C and E circulating levels are often reduced *(26,29–31,36–38)*.

Low zinc status is associated with depressed immune responses in non-HIV-infected adults and children. The mechanisms involved in zinc immunosuppression include its requirement for the synthesis of thymulin needed for the maturation of T cells in the thymus. Zinc is also required for the activation of several enzymes associated with immune cell replication. In HIV, in vitro studies have shown that zinc can block the activity of the HIV protease that is required for the synthesis of new viral particles. Also, other zinc-containing proteins can inactivate HIV replication in vitro. As mentioned, reactive oxygen-containing radicals can initiate HIV replication, and zinc is the mineral found in the antioxidant metallothionein and copper-zinc superoxide dismutase. Thus, it is not surprising that low zinc status in individuals with HIV infection and AIDS is predictive of poorer immune status than if zinc status is normal *(29)*. Several small studies have examined the effects of zinc status in HIV and AIDS and have also examined the effect of zinc supplementation (intravenous and oral administration) on drug therapy.

Table 1
Drugs Used to Treat HIV

Drug class/ mode of action	Specific drug	Drug common name	Drug composition and active metabolite
Nucleoside analogs The drug is converted to an active metabolite in the cells, and the metabolite inhibits the activity of the HIV reverse transcriptase: • Competing with the natural substrate • Incorporating into the viral DNA	Zidovudine (formerly AZT)	Retrovir	A pyrimidine nucleoside analog active against HIV Active metabolite zidovudine 5'-triphosphate (AztTP)
	Dianosine	Videx	A purine nucleoside analog active against HIV Active metabolite dideoxycytidine 5'-triphosphate (ddCTP)
	Zalcitabine	HIVID	A nucleoside analog of deoxycytidine Active metabolite dideoxycytidine 5'-triphosphate (ddCTP)
	Stavidine	Zerit	A thymidine nucleoside active against HIV Active metabolite stavudine triphosphate
	Lamivudine	Epivir	Lamivudine is the (-) enantiomer of a dideoxy analog of cytidine Active metabolite lamivudine triphosphate (L-TP)
Protease inhibitors Inhibition activity of HIV protease: • Prevents cleavage of viral polyproteins that are necessary for the maturation of the virus • Leads to the production of immature HIV particles that are noninfectious	Saquinavir Ritonavir Indinavir Amprenavir	Invirase Norvir Viracept Agenerase	A peptide-like substance saquinavir mesylate A peptidomimetic inhibitor of HIV protease Nelfinavir mesylate is an inhibitor of HIV protease Amprenavir binds to the active site of HIV-1 protease and prevents its processing mechanisms
	Indinavir	Crixivan	Indinavir binds to the HIV protease and inhibits its function
Nonnucleoside reverse transcriptase (RT) Nonnucleotide derivatives that inhibit the activities of RT	Nevirapine Delaviridine Efavirenz	Viramune Rescriptor Sustiva	Nevirapine binds directly to RT Blocks RNA and DNA dependent RT activities Noncompetitive inhibition of RT

Table 1
(Continued)

Drug class/ mode of action	Specific drug	Drug common name	Drug composition and active metabolite
Prophylactic drugs			
Against *Pneumocystis carinii*	Trimethoprim and sulfame-thoxazole	Bactrim	
Block two consecutive steps in the biosynthesis of nucleic acids and proteins that are needed for the bacteria			
Against *Mycobacterium avium*	Clarithromycin	Biaxin	
Inhibit protein synthesis by binding to ribosome of microorganisms			
Appetite enhancing/stimulation	Megestrol	Megace	A synthetic derivative of the naturally occurring progesterone
The exact mechanism by which megestrol acetate affects anorexia and cachexia is unkown			
Testosterone	Dronabinol	Marinol	Dronabinol is a cannabinoid
Complex effects on the central nervous system			
Growth hormone			
Increases the level of IGF-1, counterregulatory hormone			
Anabolic steroid with potent andro-genic properties; helps rebuild lean body mass			
Anabolic hormone; helps rebuild lean body mass			
Synthetic androgens	Nandrolone	Deca-durabolin, Durabolin	
Anabolic hormones with less andro-genic properties than testosterone; helps rebuild lean body mass			

From references (*21,23,37,61*).
IGF, insulin-like growth factor.

415

Specifically, zinc supplements enhanced the zidovudine efficacy as measured by reduction in secondary infections *(38)*. In contrast, there are also cross-sectional epidemiological data that suggest zinc supplementation is associated with decreased survival in patients who are supplemented with more than the current recommended daily intake level of 15 mg/d *(39)*.

3. DIABETES

Diabetes is a global term that encompasses several chronic conditions that result from impaired glucose use. Fewer than 1% of the US population suffers from the genetically inherited form of diabetes that is sometimes called juvenile diabetes and other times referred to as type 1 diabetes. Seven percent of the US population has adult-onset diabetes, or type 2 diabetes *(40–42)*. Unfortunately, there is a significant increase in the prevalence of type 2 diabetes in children and teens, often associated with obesity. Diagnosing diabetes requires measuring fasting blood glucose levels; adults with levels higher than 126 mg/dL are diabetic. Another common measurement used to monitor diabetes is the blood glycosylated hemoglobin (HbA1C) levels. HbA1C is formed when glucose binds to hemoglobin and is directly reflective of diabetes severity. Lipoproteins can also be glycosylated in a patient with diabetes; glycosylated low-density lipoprotein (LDL) are more prone to oxidation and incorporation into fatty streaks that can occlude blood vessels. In both type 1 and type 2 diabetes, there are numerous and cumulative debilities to many tissues and organs of the body. These disease consequences are outlined in Table 2 *(42–47)*. Hyperglycemia, both acute and chronic, is associated with depressed cellular immune responses that result in increased prevalence of bacterial and fungal infections in the patient with diabetes. Infections are often persistent, with the formation of ulcers and deep infections in the joints *(48–50)*.

Hyperglycemia is associated with increased oxidative stress and free-radical damage that could be the cause of many of the pathologies seen in diabetes *(51)*. The major cause of death in patients with diabetes is atherosclerotic cardiovascular disease *(52)*. As diabetes progresses, there is an overall decrease in antioxidant status, with decreased levels of vitamin C, glutathione, superoxide dismutase, and other antioxidants in the blood of patients with diabetes compared to non-diabetics that are age, gender, and dietary intake matched *(53)*. Reduced antioxidant status may be a major factor in the increased damage to both the microvasculature and the macrovasculature in patients with diabetes. There is an increase in the procoagulant factors in the blood, and hypertriglyceridemia and increased LDL with reduced HDL levels are common. Advanced glycation endproducts (AGEs) are triggers for many immune cells to produce inflammatory cytokines. AGE receptors are also found on endothelial and renal cells, where AGE binding results in inflammatory cytokines production, such as interleukin (IL-1, tumor necrosis factor (TNF) and insulin-like growth factor (IGF-1. Consequently, there is an increase in inflammation in the blood vessels throughout the body and loss of renal function *(54)*.

3.1. Type 1 Diabetes

Type 1 diabetes, an autoimmune disease, is caused by the self-destruction of the majority of the insulin-secreting cells of the pancreas *(55,56)*. Inappropriate destruction of islet cells results in an increased oxidative stress on the pancreas, and continued

Table 2
Biochemical Short- and Long-Term Consequences of Type 1 and Type 2 Diabetes

Biochemical consequences	Short-term consequences	Long-term consequences
Type 1 diabetes • Cellular and humoral immune changes in the peripheral blood, including altered glucose tolerance, reduced insulin secretion • Destruction and death of insulin producing pancreatic β cells • Eventually, there is no insulin secretion Type 2 diabetes • The mass of pancreatic β cells is 50% to 100% of normal cell mass • Basal insulin level is normal or elevated, but secretory responses to glucose are lower than normal • Insufficient insulin secretion with or without insulin resistance • Insulin secretory response to oral glucose varies from normal and differs between individuals depending on the extent of glucose intolerance • Blunted glucose potentiation (that normally occurs in response to gastrointestinal hormones)	Type 1 diabetes • Elevated levels of glucose in the blood • Formation of nonenzymatic glycation products in the blood, on nerves, and in blood vessels • Low level of vitamin C in the blood. • Elevated triglycerides Type 2 diabetes • Chronic insulin hypersecretion as evidenced by amyloid deposits produced by β cells • Evidence of insulin resistance in the peripheral tissues • Insulin resistance is linked with hypertension, hypertriglyceridemia, decreased HDL, and increased risk of atherosclerosis and cardiovascular diseases • Hypertriglyceridemia, probably resulting from a decrease in lipoprotein lipase activity; consequently, the plasma levels of VLDL are elevated and increased deposition of lipids possibly accelerate the atherosclerotic process	Type 1 and Type 2 diabetes • Cardiovascular diseases, including acceleration of atherosclerosis of coronary and peripheral arteries, cardiomyopathy, and cardiac neuropathy • Monckeberg sclerosis resulting from calcification of the media of large arteries • More frequent ischemic heart disease relative to general population • More frequent myocardial infraction with an increased lethal ventricular arrhythmias, possibly induced by more fibrosis complicated by reduced response to antiarrhythmic drugs • Autonomic neuropathy causes the alteration in the vagus nerve function and sympathetic activity, leading to cardiac arrhythmia. • Increased stiffness of diabetic ventricle may lead to congestive heart failure • Peripheral neuropathy: increased incidence of peripheral vascular disease; chronic foot ulcers involving both microvessels and macrovessels • Diabetic gastroenteropathy include dysphagia, nausea, vomiting, diarrhea, constipation, and fecal incontinence • The incidence of liver diseases is higher in people with diabetes with frequent viral hepatitis • Blindness and vision disability that develops in both type 1 and type 2 diabetes (although the onset and the rate may be different in the two types of diabetes)

417

(continued)

Table 2
(Continued)

Biochemical consequences	Short-term consequences	Long-term consequences
• Varied degree of insulin resistance resulting from several defects in insulin actions (that correlated with certain patterns of obesity); these changes may precede clinical evidence of diabetes	• Cardiac dysfunction (cardiomyopathy) originating from atherosclerotic changes in the coronary macrovessels	• Plasma glucose levels and hypertension are the major determinants of risk
	• Injury to the endothelial cells as a result of hyperglycemia, insulin resistance, increased plasma LDL, decreased HDL, abnormal platelet aggregation, and coagulation	• Cataract is considered an important ocular manifestation of diabetes
• Increased levels of plasma thiobarbituric acid-reactive substances (TBARS) a measure of ROS-induced lipid peroxidase damage		• Increased levels of glaucoma
	• Increased production of oxidants by the endothelial cells as a result of hyperglycemia via two mechanisms: nonenzymatic glycation of proteins and increased H_2O_2 production	• Diabetic nephropathy in type 1 (30–40%) and type 2 (5–10%)
• Increased lipid peroxidation in blood		• Clinical signs of diabetic nephropathy include hypertension, renal insufficiency, heavy albuminurea, and edema
	• Increased level of lipid peroxidation products, as well as antioxidant enzymes	• Formation of advanced glycosylation products, activation of protein kinase C, increasing growth factor, and production of cytokines
		• Morbidity resulting from infection
		• Once infected, the ability of diabetics to tolerate the infection is reduced; control over glucose levels is compromised
		• Noninfectious complications of diabetes include several abnormalities including xanthomas, sclerederma, and necrobiosis

From references (42–47).
HDL, high-density lipoproteins; VLDL, very low-density lipoproteins; LDL, low-density lipoproteins; ROS, reactive oxygen species.

418

adverse effects, resulting from the lack of insulin, further increase the potential for oxidative damage *(57–59)*. There are two major factors that are believed to be essential in the development of type 1 diabetes: genetic predisposition and a triggering factor that initiates the inappropriate recognition of the insulin-secreting pancreatic islet cell as nonself by T cells *(60)*. T cells then initiate B cells to develop autoantibodies to surface receptors and other molecules associated with insulin-secreting cells. Islet cells that have autoantibodies attached to the cellular membrane are targeted for destruction by other immune cells, such as cytotoxic T cells *(61)*.

Recent findings have shown that insulin has a direct stimulatory action on the bone-building cells, osteoblasts. With the lack of insulin seen in type 1 diabetes, it is not difficult to understand the presence of osteopenia in many patients *(62,63)*. Jain et al. examined the potential for beneficial effects of antioxidant supplementation in patients with type 1 diabetes. They have found a marked decrease in glycosylated hemoglobin and reduction in triglyceride levels after vitamin E supplementation *(57)*.

3.1.1. DRUGS USED TO TREAT TYPE 1 DIABETES

The initial major drug requirement difference between the two diabetes is the need for insulin immediately once there is a diagnosis of type 1 diabetes, because the autoimmune destruction of the islet cells of the pancreas that produce insulin has proceeded to the point of clinical recognition of the disease. The precipitous rise in circulating glucose levels is often the defining feature of the diagnosis; glucose is also excreted at high levels in the urine. Moreover, glucose does not enter the tissues appropriately, resulting in a lack of energy source in critical tissues and organs, such as the brain and retina *(45,46)*. Without insulin administration, the patient with type 1 diabetes will die in a few weeks or months. Thus, insulin is the drug that is administered daily to patients with type 1 diabetes. Type 1 diabetes often develops during childhood before the age of 10 yr. Even with the use of insulin, the nutritional management of the patient (who is usually young) is critical for optimal long-term treatment *(64,65)*.

There are several types of insulin (derived from human and nonhuman sources), routes of administration, and dosage forms that are available currently *(66)*. The overall goal is the normalization of blood glucose levels during waking hours, especially before and immediately after meals, as well as during the overnight fast (Table 3) *(34,66)*.

3.2. Type 2 Diabetes

Type 2 diabetes develops most frequently in midlife. Approximately 50% of individuals with type 2 diabetes are 65 yr old or older. The disease is characterized by a depressed response of target tissues to insulin, resulting in a higher than normal circulating level of glucose and a lower than normal level of glucose in tissues *(44,48,51,67)*. Additionally, patients with type 2 diabetes often have hyperlipidemia and hypertension and are also often obese. Increased body mass index (BMI), used to define obesity, is related to decreased insulin sensitivity in this disease *(42)*. There is an increased risk of type 2 diabetes in both men and women with increased central or visceral obesity (68). The long-term effects of type 2 diabetes include nephropathy, neuropathy, retinopathy, impaired cellular immunity, osteoporosis, and multiple adverse effects on the cardiovascular system *(4,43,52,69–76)*. Diet changes are often the first line of defense against the insulin resistance seen in type 2 diabetes. However, only approx 10% of adults can control their circulating glucose levels with lifestyle changes alone *(77)*.

Table 3
Drugs Used to Treat Type 1 Diabetes

Drug class	Insulin type	Drug mode of action	Specific drug	Indications for use and comments
Short-acting insulin	Insulin analog—chemically modified	Rapid acting, short duration	Lispro	Controls for meal, glucose rise, rapid control of high glucose levels. Effective in combinations with intermediate and long acting insulin. Frequency of hypoglycemia is reduced relative to regular insulin
	Crystalline zinc in a neutral buffer			Maintains good control when a long time elapses between meals
Intermediate-acting insulin	Complexed with zinc and protamine in a phosphate buffer		Neutral protamine Hagedon (NPH)	
	Pork insulin that is partly crystallized and partly amorphous. It is mixed in an acetate buffer that is gradually released in the subcutaneous tissues	Slower onset and longer acting (up to 24 h)	Lente (Novolin L), Iletin II	
Long-acting insulin	Alternate human insulin synthesized with the help of *Escherichia coli* that has been genetically altered by the addition of a human gene for the production of insulin	Slower onset with a longer duration and less intense duration (up to 28 h)	Humulin	

420

From references (34,66).

3.2.1. DRUGS USED TO TREAT TYPE 2 DIABETES

There are several drugs used to treat type 2 diabetes, although the patients receiving these drugs often require additional insulin as well *(8,78,79)*. Metformin, which is frequently the first drug used in the treatment of type 2 diabetes in adults, is the only oral hypoglycemic drug that is currently approved for the treatment of type 2 diabetes in children. Combination therapies are frequently prescribed. These include the addition of α-glucosidase inhibitors or thiazolidinediones, sulfonylurea agents in combination with the oral hypoglycemic drugs (Table 4) *(79,80)*.

3.3. Drug/Disease Effects on Nutritional Status

Insulin, which is the most commonly used drug for treatment of both types of diabetes, has a well-recognized side effect of increased weight gain. Thus, it is especially difficult for the patient who is overweight or obese to lose or even maintain weight during insulin therapy. Currently, patients with diabetes who are obese are also often given antiobesity drugs, including Xenical and Meridia. These drugs can reduce fat-soluble vitamin status and also reduce long-chain fatty acid levels that are important immunomodulators. The effects of weight reduction interventions on nutritional, as well as immunologic status can be numerous and particularly serious for the diabetic *(28,81)*.

Sulfonylureas have also been associated with increased weight gain and hypoglycemia *(82)*. α-glucosidase inhibitors compete with the native enzyme and slow the breakdown of starches, thereby slowing the rise in blood glucose after a meal. However, there are GI side effects, such as diarrhea, cramping, abdominal pain, and flatulence, that can affect compliance and also result in loss of fluids and micronutrients. Lowered serum levels of vitamins B_6 and B_{12} and folic acid are associated with increased serum homocysteine, a risk factor for cardiovascular and cerebrovascular diseases and diabetic neuropathy *(83–88)*. Although there has not been a clear association between serum homocysteine levels and drugs to treat diabetes, Metformin may induce vitamin B_{12} malabsorption, and this may result in higher homocysteine levels *(89)*.

Oxidative stress is increased in patients with diabetes *(53,90)*, and antioxidant nutrient status is often lower than optimal *(91)*. Ascorbic acid (vitamin C) and glucose enter cells through the glucose transporter, and elevated glucose levels competitively inhibit the movement of vitamin C into cells. Consequences of lower-than-optimal antioxidant status have been documented in the cardiovascular tissues and lipoproteins of patients with diabetes *(92)*. Vitamins E and C supplementation has beneficial effects on several immune parameters in patients with diabetes *(93)*. Vitamin E supplementation reduced protein glycosylation and platelet aggregation in patients with type 1 diabetes and improved glycemic control and insulin action in patients with type 2 diabetes *(94)*. Several studies have shown that vitamin E supplementation reduced the potential for LDL oxidation ex vivo. Recent data suggest that vitamin E reduces the synthesis and secretion of inflammatory cytokines from macrophages taken from patients with diabetes *(54)*.

Chromium supplementation in some studies in patients with diabetes decreased blood glucose by potentiating the action of insulin. However, there are data indicating that chromium absorption is decreased in patients with diabetes *(95,96)*.

Table 4
Drugs Used to Treat Type 2 Diabetes

Drug class	Specific drug	Drug common name	Drug mode of action	Indications for use and comments
Sulfonylureas (first generation)	Tolbutamide Acetohexamide Tolazamide Chlorpropamide	Diaben Diabewas	Insulinotropic, increases circulating insulin Insulin secretion from the islet is stimulated perhaps by increasing β-cell sensitivity to glucose 90–99% of the absorbed drug is bound to plasma proteins	Numerous drugs (niacin, thiazide diuretics, beta blockers, corticosteroids) reduce insulin sensitivity, thus decreased efficacy
Sulfonylureas (second generation)	Glipizide Glyburide (glibenclamide) Glyburide (miconized)	Glucotrol Daonil, Glubate, Libanil	Insulinotropic, increases circulating insulin Insulin secretion from the islet is stimulated perhaps by increasing β-cell sensitivity to glucose Absorbed drug only to nonionic sites (thus less likely to interact with other medications in comparison to the first generation)	Second-generation drugs control blood glucose without deleterious changes in the plasma lipoprotein levels Has no antidiuretic activity
Meglitinides	Repaglinide	Prandin	Insulinotropic, stimulated the release of insulin from the pancreas (requires functioning β cells)	Effective with Metformin; should not be taken with sulfonylureas

422

Table 4
(Continued)

Drug class	Specific drug	Drug common name	Drug mode of action	Indications for use and comments
Biguanides	Metformin	Glucophage, Glucovance (glyburide and Metformin)	Increases insulin-simulated glucose uptake, reduces hepatic glucose production, and increases insulin-simulated glucose uptake at the periphery	Used effectively with sulfonylureaes slightly anorectic; may reduce triglycerides
Carbohydrase inhibitors	Acarbose, Miglitol	Perecose, Glyset	Inhibition of α-glucosidases in the intestinal brush border, leading to delay in carbohydrate absorption	May be used in combination with sulfonylurea; may be used in combination with Metformin or insulin Due to its different mechanism of action, the effects of the combined drugs are additive
Thiazolidinediones	Rosiglitazone, Pioglitazone	Avandia, Actos	Enhances insulin sensitivity Lower blood glucose levels and decrease insulin level Increased the insulin content of pancreatic islets	Has been approved for use in combination with sulfonylureas or Metformin; slight weight increase

423

From refs. *(79,80)*.

4. RHEUMATOID ARTHRITIS

Rheumatoid arthritis (RA) is a chronic progressive autoimmune disease of unknown origin that, like type 1 diabetes, is associated with a genetic predisposition and an environmental trigger *(97–99)*. RA causes a deterioration of articular joints, causing pain, stiffness, swelling, and deformity that, with time, results in severe disability. The autoantibodies in RA are sometimes referred to as rheumatoid factor, and titers are used diagnostically. The autoantibodies are found in the joint fluids and are probably the initiators of the symmetric inflammation seen in peripheral joints. As with type 1 diabetes, age of onset may be in youth or young adulthood, resulting in juvenile RA. One percent of the population suffers from adult-onset RA; more than 2 million US adults are affected, 75% of whom are women. Oxidative damage to the joints and increased production of inflammatory cytokines are RA hallmarks. Patients with RA may also have symptoms of anemia that is unrelated to a lack of dietary intake of iron. Anemia of chronic disease (ACD) is associated with a reduction in red blood cell (RBC) iron. There is a redistribution of iron from inside the RBC to within the synovial fluid. The RBCs have receptors for the rheumatoid factor. Binding of rheumatoid factor to the receptor on the RBC triggers autoimmune destruction of the RBC and release of iron into the synovial fluid. RA-associated ACD causes an increase in oxidative damage in the joints exposed to free iron *(97,100)*.

4.1. Drugs Used to Treat RA

Aspirin and nonsteroidal antiinflammatory drugs (NSAIDs) are the first medications given to reduce RA inflammation. However, their efficacy is often inadequate. Corticosteroids are potent antiinflammatory drugs but do not stop the joint erosion, and their efficacy decreases with use. Disease-modifying drugs, such as gold compounds, are administered orally, intravenously, or intramuscularly, with varying levels of success and potential adverse reactions that include GI tract disturbances. Cytotoxic drugs are the next group of drugs given when RA continues to cause pain and joint erosion *(101)*. Methotrexate, a cytotoxic drug that is often used in RA treatment, reduces pain but does not affect disease progression. The progressive nature of RA results in the successive use of more toxic drugs that have serious side effects on overall health and nutritional status *(36,102,103)*. Additionally, as discussed in Section 5.2., the potential for the development of drug-induced osteoporosis is significantly increased by both corticosteroids and cytotoxic drugs (Table 5) *(34,36,98,102,104–108)*.

Newer drugs used to treat RA include etanercept (Enbrel) and infliximab (Remicade). These two drugs show indications of stopping the disease progression. Both drugs target TNF, an inflammatory cytokine produced by immune cells. The drugs bind to TNF before it can trigger inflammatory responses. These two drugs are not given orally; etanercept is given by injection, and infliximab is given by intravenous infusion *(36,108)*.

4.2. Drug/Disease Interactions and Nutritional Effects of RA

Most of the cytotoxic drugs, such as methotrexate, are folate antagonists and, therefore, will decrease folate status and increase homocysteine levels. Increasing folate intake can overcome some of these effects; however, there may be a decrease in drug efficacy

Table 5
Drugs Used to Treat Rheumatoid Arthritis

Drug class	Drug mode of action	Specific drug	Drug common name	Indications for use and comments
Nonsteroidal anti-inflammatory drugs (NSAIDs)	Antiinflammatory, analgesic, and anti-pyretic. Mode of action is not known, but its ability to inhibit prostaglandin synthesis from arachidonic acid may be involved. Their action in the early arachidonic acid cascade and the specific eicosanoids involved has not been identified	Indomethacin Ibuprofen Naproxen Diclofenac Piroxicam	Indocin Ec-naprosyn Naprosyn Cataflam, Voltaren Feldene	Joint pain
Immuno-suppressant drugs: glucocorticoids—adrenocortical steroids	Antiinflammatory effects; modify the body's immune response to diverse stimuli Glucocorticoids have the following effects: • Inhibit synthesis of most cytokines and several cell surface molecules that are required for immune function • Affect leukocyte movement, function, and humoral factors • Inhibit the recruitment of neutrophils and monocyte-macrophages to an inflammatory site • By inhibiting the release of arachidonic acid from phospholipids these inhibit prostaglandin and leukotriene synthesis	Cortone Prelone Depo-Medrol Decadron Celestone	Cortisone Prednisolone Methylprednis-olone Dexamethasone Betamethasone	These are short-acting compounds based on the duration of corticotrophin (ACTH) suppression. These drugs need to undergo biotransformation in the liver to become active compounds These are long-acting compounds. These drugs need to undergo biotrasformatins in the liver to become active compounds.
Disease-modifying antirheumatic drugs (DMARDs)	Antiinflammatory effects, as well as immunomodulatory properties. These drugs are considered weak in their immunomodulatory function relative to cytotoxic drugs	Gold compounds Antimalarial agents	Myochrysine	Predominant action is a suppressive effect on the synovitis of active rheumatoid disease Reduce number of monocytes and cytokine production Inhibition of lysosomal enzymes

425

Table 5
(Continued)

Drug class	Drug mode of action	Specific drug	Drug common name	Indications for use and comments
Disease-modifying antirheumatic drugs (DMARDs)		Penicillamine	Cuprimine	This is a chelating agent recommended for patients with excess copper. It also reduces excess of cystine and suppresses rheumatoid disease activity. Reduced function of T and natural killer cells and monocytes
Cytotoxic immuno-suppressive drugs	Cytotoxic drugs are used based on the premise that they downregulate immune functions; however, there is lack of evidence that the suppression of the immune system accounts for clinical effects	Cyclophosphamide	Cytoxan	Active alkylating metabolites interfere with the growth of rapidly dividing cells. The mechanism is believed to be through crosslinking to DNA
	Cytotoxic drugs suppress both cellular and humoral host defenses	Methotrexate	Methotrexate (formerly Amethopterin)	Decrease leukocyte trafficking. Considered effective as an antiinflammatory, as well as an immune suppressive agent
		Azathioprine	Imuran	Immunosuppressive antimetabolite. Mechanism in which it affects autoimmune disease is unknown. Inhibits the proliferation of T lymphocytes and antibody formation
		6-Mercapto-purine	Purinethol	Purine analog that interferes with nucleic acid biosynthesis
		Cholrambucil	Leukeran	Bifunctional alkylating agent that is active against selected neoplastic diseases
Novel drugs	Tumor necrosis factor (TNF) antagonist	Infliximab	Remicade	This compound is a monoclonal antibody containing regions that binds to tumor necrosis factor (TNF)
	Tumor necrosis factor (TNF) antagonist	Etanercept	Enbrel	This compound binds to TNF and blocks its interaction with cell-surface TNF receptors, thus preventing the biological activity of TNF

From references (34,36,98,102,104–108).

426

(106). Methotrexate also can cause mouth ulcers that can affect overall food consumption. Liver dysfunction and GI tract discomforts are common with NSAIDs, cytotoxic drugs, and corticosteroids.

Cyclosporine, another cytotoxic drug, reduces T-cell activity and is a potent immunosuppressive agent used for transplantation and RA therapy *(105)*. However, side effects include hyperglycemia, hypercholesterolemia, electrolyte disturbances, and renal insufficiency *(109)*. Newer NSAIDs that target only the type 2 cyclo-oxygenase enzyme (COX-2), may not cause as many GI tract problems as older drugs that targeted both COX-1 and COX-2. The TNF-targeted drugs can result in increased infections, because TNF is a normal immune cytokine involved in destruction of pathogens *(97)*.

Several dietary components inhibit COX-2 and/or reduce the formation of inflammatory prostaglandins—the products of COX-2 enzyme activity *(110,111)*. These include vitamin E and long-chain omega-3 (n–3) and omega-6 (n–6) fatty acids. Supplementation has resulted in pain reduction in some studies and reduction in pain medication use in others. In one study involving 49 patients with RA, supplementation with γ-linolenic acid (an n–6 fatty acid) and eicosapentaenoic acid (an n–3 fatty acid) for 1 yr resulted in decreased pain and tapering of NSAID use in 80% of patients, compared with 33% in the placebo group. Several studies have examined the effects of supplementation with n–3 fatty acids and have shown consistent reductions in tender joints and morning stiffness *(112)*.

5. OSTEOPOROSIS

Osteoporosis is defined as a progressive systemic skeletal disease characterized by low bone mass and deterioration of bone tissue architecture, with a consequent decrease in bone strength and increase in bone fragility and susceptibility to fracture *(2)*. There can also be a concomitant loss of bone from the jaw, resulting in dental complications, including tooth loss *(113)*. Clinical relevance of osteoporosis derives from the fractures that it produces. More than one third of adult women who are postmenopausal will suffer one or more osteoporotic fractures in their lifetime. The lifetime risk in men is approx 50% that in women. The decrease of the bone mineral density (BMD) is the most important cause of fracture risk. Postmenopausal osteoporosis is the primary cause of fractures and is linked to the loss of estrogen during menopause. Estrogen maintains the normal balance between bone formation and bone resorption that occurs throughout life. Estrogen also enhances calcium deposition in bone. The loss of estrogen is associated with an increased breakdown of bone tissue by osteoclasts that is not matched by an equivalent bone formation by the osteoblasts. Not only is there a loss of BMD, but also there can be a loss of structural integrity and bone strength. Among other considerations, calcium and vitamin D deficiencies are important risk factors for a decrease in BMD, consequently inducing osteoporosis *(114,115)*. In fact, calcium intake is considered inadequate in 90% of US adult women, and vitamin D intake is also low in the majority of adults > 65 yr *(116)*.

In addition to postmenopausal osteoporosis and the osteoporosis associated with aging in both women and men *(117)*, there are many cases of osteoporosis that result from treatment of other diseases, primarily from chronic inflammation (secondary osteoporosis) *(3,5,118–124)*.

Mechanistically, the cause of osteoporosis is the imbalance between bone formation and bone breakdown. The cell responsible for bone breakdown, the osteoclast, is derived from the macrophage and remains responsive to immune modulators and signals. As discussed in Section 5.2., several of the drugs that cause secondary osteoporosis are immunosuppressive *(1,125)*.

5.1. Drugs for Osteoporosis Treatment

Hormone replacement therapy (HRT) with estrogen and progesterone slows the loss of bone and reduces the risk of vertebral fractures in women who are postmenopausal *(126,127)*. Estrogen promotes osteoclast apoptosis, consequently restoring some of the balance between bone formation and bone destruction by the osteoclast *(128)*. The recent data from the HRT arm of the women's health initiative *(129)* showed a 34% decrease in hip fractures in women taking an estrogen-progesterone combination daily for an average of 5.2 yr; however, there were also increased risks of cardiovascular disease and breast cancer. Bisphosphonates, taken with adequate calcium and vitamin D, increase BMD at the spine and hip and reduce vertebral fractures significantly after 1 or more years of intervention *(130)*. Certain bisphosphonates also reduce the risk of glucocorticoid-induced osteoporosis. The mechanism of action includes the increase in osteoclast apoptosis. The bisphosphonate is incorporated into the bone, resulting in increased BMD that has been associated with fracture reduction. Selective estrogen receptor modulators (SERMS) also reduce the risk of vertebral fractures associated with increased BMD *(131)*. Calcitonin, a thyroid-secreted hormone, is important in the delivery of calcium from the blood to bone. Calcitonin decreases osteoclast activity and is effective in increasing BMD; unlike the other drugs described, this drug is not taken orally but delivered nasally *(132,133)*. There are no consistent data on the reduction of fractures with calcitonin and no dose-response relationship with respect to BMD. The side effects are minimal with this drug, resulting in studies using a combination of calcitonin with other drugs that can improve bone morphology *(134)*. Recently, small intermittent intravenous doses of parathyroid hormone (PTH) have been found to increase BMD dramatically and reduce fracture risk *(135)*. PTH reduces osteoblast apoptosis, prolongs osteoblast lifetime, and results in increased bone formation and BMD and reduction in fracture *(136,137)*. A summary of the drugs is outlined in Table 6 *(8,34,66,78,79,124,127, 130,133,136)*. For all antiosteoporosis drugs, calcium and vitamin D status needs to be optimal.

5.2. Glucocorticoids: Effects on Bone

Glucocorticoid drugs are used for many immune-related diseases to reduce inflammatory responses and/or immune response imbalances *(7)*. As discussed in Section 4.1., glucocorticoids, sometimes referred to as steroids, are often used to treat RA *(6,104,138)* (*see* Table 5). Glucocorticoids have many pharmacological actions. The primary effects are to inhibit T-cell-mediated immune responses that result in both antiinflammatory and antiadhesion responses by the immune cells. Regarding the effects on bone, the principal action is the reduction in bone formation associated with reduced osteoblast number and bone matrix synthesis, and reduced calcium absorption in the intestine and reabsorption in the kidney. Glucocorticoids also cause the development of hypogonadism in men. These increases in bone loss result in a condition termed glucocorticoid-induced

Table 6
Drugs Used to Treat Osteoporosis

Drug class	Drug mode of action	Specific drug	Drug common name	Indications for use and comments
Hormone replacement therapy (HRT)	Estrogen replacement therapy reduces bone resorption and retards postmenopausal bone loss. Circulating estrogens modulate the pituitary secretion of gonadotropins, luteinizing hormone (LH) and follicle-stimulating hormone (FSH) through a negative feedback mechanism. In postmenopausal women, a reduction in the elevated levels of these hormones is achieved through estrogen replacement therapy. Progesterone is given with estrogen to reduce the risk of endometrial cancer	Vivelle, Esclim, Climara	Estradiol	Postmenopausal symptoms
		Premarin	Conjugated estrogen	
		Ortho-Est, Ogen	Estropipate	
		Estratab	Esterified estrogen	
		Femhrt, Activella	Norethindrone/ estradiol	Progestin-estrogen combination. Used for treatment of vastomotor symptoms and prevention of osteoporosis. Concurrent administration of progestin with estrogen reduces the risk of endometrial cancer
		Ortho-Prefest	Estradiol/ norgestimate	Estrogen and progesterone mixture
		Prempro/ Premphase	Conjugated estrogen/ medroxpro- gesterone	Estrogen and progesterone in separate tablets for treatment of vasomotor symptoms, vulvar and vaginal atrophy; prevention of osteoporosis
Selective estrogen receptor modulators (SERMS)	Selective estrogen receptor modulator. This class is composed of a large number of molecules that bind to estrogen receptors, thus activating estrogenic pathways and blockade of others	Nolvadex	Tamoxifen	This is a first-generation estrogen modulator. It prevents bone loss but causes endometrial hyperplasia
		Evista	Raloxifene	This compound decreases resorption of bone. In women, it reduces biochemical markers of bone turnover in serum and urine to levels before menopause. All these changes result in increased bone mineral density

Table 6
(Continued)

Drug class	Drug mode of action	Specific drug	Drug common name	Indications for use and comments
				It has an effect on lipid metabolism; it decreases total and low-density lipoproteins cholesterol
Antiresorptive (bisphosphonates)	Bisphosphonates inhibit osteoclast-mediated bone resorption and modulate bone metabolism Actonel is an analog of pyrophosphate. These compounds are attractive for women who do not wish to take estrogen	Actonel	Risedronate	This compound has an affinity for hydroxyapatite crystals in bones and acts as antiresorptive. It changes the surface of the bone and thus reduces active resorption
		Fosamax	Alendronate	Specifically adheres under osteoclasts and inhibits its activity not through adherence to the bone surface, but through its modulation of the resorption process
		Skelid	Tiludronate	Bone-resorption inhibitor. Exact mechanism of action is not clear. This compound adsorbs to calcium phosphate and may directly block calcium phosphate dissolution
		Aredia	Pamidronate	
		Didronel	Etidronate	This compound regulates bone metabolism. This is a first-generation bisphosphonate, and there is some concern over the possibility that at therapeutic doses it may impair mineralization, thus a long-term negative effect
Calcitonin	Calcitonin acts primarily in bone; however, it has direct effects on renal function, as well as actions on the gastrointestinal tract	Miacalcin, Calcimar	Calcitonin-salmon	This type of calcitonin has higher potency than mammalian calcitonin, and it acts for a longer time. Calcitonin does not induce long-term bone formation. Calcium supplements should always be given to prevent hyperparathyroidism

430

Table 6
(Continued)

Drug class	Drug mode of action	Specific drug	Drug common name	Indications for use and comments
Parathyroid hormone (PTH)	Reduces osteoblast apoptosis; prolongs osteoblast lifetime			PTH and PTH-related protein are responsible for skeletal physiology and mineral homeostasis. Major functions of this hormone include the regulation of acceptable level of ionized calcium in the plasma while consuming calcium-reduced diets. The PTH level changes with minute changes in the level of ionized calcium in the blood. PTH promotes bone resorption, release of calcium from skeletal reservoir, and induces renal conservation of calcium and excretion of phosphate. In addition, it indirectly affects the amount of intestinal calcium absorption by affecting the amount of the active form of vitamin D

For all antiosteoporosis drugs, calcium and vitamin D status needs to be optimal.

Therapy with omeprazole and other proton pump inhibitors that inhibit gastric secretion through increased gastric secretion. Calcitonin gene expression is affected by other factors: activation of cAMP and protein kinase C pathways, and glucocorticoid treatment increases transcription of the CT gene, whereas dihydroxy vitamin D3 inhibits transcription.

HRT: Compliance is one of the main issues. It is estimated that fewer than 20% of postmenopausal women take HRT. Estrogen is the cornerstone of preventative therapy for osteoporosis in menopausal women; it is effective in women with established osteoporosis. It is well-established that estrogen reduces bone loss, and the dose determines its effectiveness. The efficacy of combined therapy of medroxyprogesterone (contraceptive androgen) with estrogen has not been demonstrated, although the effect of progestins alone reduces bone loss.

Bisphosphonates: act on bone resorption in several ways; the physicochemical inhibition of crystal dissolution playing a smaller role than originally postulated. The main effects are considered to be at the tissue level; their main effect is to inhibit bone resorption and this results in a decrease in bone turnover. This is a result of a decrease in number and activity of osteoclasts. There are several major effects on osteoclasts, including inhibition of its recruitment, adhesion, and activity, and shortening its life span.

From references (8,34,66,78,79,124,127,130,133,136).

431

osteoporosis *(139–142)*. Chronic use at doses as low as 5 mg/d decrease BMD and increase fracture risk *(141)*. Fractures have been documented in approx 30% of individuals treated for an average of 5 yr. Chronic glucocorticoid administration can also result in collapse of large joints resulting from death of bone tissue *(137)*.

5.3. Transplantation-Induced Osteoporosis

Cytotoxic drugs, such as cyclophosphamide, methotrexate, and cyclosporine, disrupt DNA and protein synthesis in cells; the more rapidly dividing cells, such as those of the immune system and endothelial cells lining the digestive tract, are most affected. Thus, a predictable outcome of cytotoxic drug therapy is a significantly increased risk of infection and concomitant malabsorption of nutrients. Nausea and vomiting are also common side effects. Bone turnover can also be affected and result in overall decreased bone formation and/or frank loss of BMD *(101)*. Several studies have documented the rapid loss of BMD after heart transplantation. The combination of newer cytotoxic drugs, such as tacrolimus, and glucocorticoids decreases sex steroid synthesis that also adds to the loss of BMD in these patients. Increasing calcium and vitamin D intakes can partially offset the osteoporotic effects of cytotoxic drugs *(143)*.

5.4. Effect of Osteoporosis Drugs on Nutritional Status and Effects of Nutrients on Drugs Used to Treat Osteoporosis

Calcium supplementation does not completely stop bone loss in women who are postmenopausal but does slow the rate of loss by 30–50% *(144,145)*. Adequate calcium and vitamin D intakes are required for the efficacy of all drugs used to treat osteoporosis and reduce the risk of fracture *(11,34)*. Virtually all of the clinical studies undertaken for the approval of these drugs included the provision of calcium and/or vitamin D for all participants in the trials. It is well-recognized that without adequate calcium and/or vitamin D, the efficacy of these drugs would be diminished significantly *(146)*.

HRT has several effects on dietary habits. HRT is associated with fluid retention and modest, but consistent, weight gain. HRT may also enhance calcium absorption, thereby improving calcium balance. Nieves et al. *(147)* documented the importance of adequate calcium intake for the efficacy of both HRT and calcitonin in stopping bone loss. Bisphosphonates bind calcium and other minerals. These agents cannot be taken at the same time. GI tract disturbances are common with antiresorptives. These drugs do not affect the immune system's ability to fight infections.

6. CONCLUSIONS

There are few reviews of the nutritional effects of drugs used to treat immune system diseases. Four immune-related diseases, HIV, diabetes, RA, and osteoporosis, have been reviewed, with the emphasis on the drugs used to treat these diseases and the potential nutritional consequences of the disease and/or drug therapy. The extensive data in the tables clearly show that there are numerous side effects associated with most of the drugs reviewed. Common side effects include GI tract disturbances, weight gain, and liver effects. Immunosuppressive drugs, such as glucocorticoids, can also increase the risk of osteoporosis. Cytotoxic drugs are often antifolates and may increase homocysteine levels, further increasing the risk of vascular disease.

As the population ages, there will be an ever-increasing number of patients that are using drugs for the treatment of age- and immune-related diseases, such as type 2 diabetes and osteoporosis *(9,10,23,27,28,148)*. Nutritional consequences of drug therapy should be considered when dietary recommendations are made for these populations. The newer drugs to treat HIV and RA make it probable that patients will be using these drugs for long periods of time. Nutritional consequences of long-term use of some of these drugs have not been fully examined. Finally, in evaluating the effects of drug therapy on nutritional needs, it cannot be overlooked that most patients are using many drugs at the same time and that changes in drug therapies are common. Thus, a heightened awareness of the potential nutritional consequences of disease/drug/nutrient interactions is warranted.

7. "TAKE-HOME" MESSAGES

1. The therapies used for HIV, type 1 and 2 diabetes, RA, and osteoporosis usually adversely affect the patient's nutritional status.
2. Chronic treatments for most immune-related diseases with immunosuppressive agents, antiinflammatory drugs, and/or reduction in insulin secretion can often cause secondary osteoporosis, thus increasing the importance of optimal calcium, vitamin D, and other nutrients involved in bone health.
3. Immune system diseases often increase metabolic rate and temperature, include GI tract impairment of absorption and increased elimination, and cause liver and pancreas dysfunction and oxidative damage—all of which have direct adverse effects on nutritional status.
4. Regarding HIV, antiviral drugs have negative effects along the entire GI tract, reducing nutritional status. Additionally, oxidative damage, and decreased absorption have been associated with significantly increased requirements for most vitamins and certain minerals.
5. Diabetes is associated with increased oxidative stress and chronic inflammation. Insulin and other drugs often result in increased weight gain that further affects the secondary consequences of diabetes.
6. Chronic use of antiinflammatory drugs in the treatment of RA can result in secondary osteoporosis. There is often an increased need for antioxidants.
7. Treatments for osteoporosis are all predicated on the patient's consuming optimal levels of calcium, vitamin D, and other nutrients needed for bone health.
8. Bisphosphonates often adversely affect appetite.

REFERENCES

1. Ershler WB, Harman SM, Keller ET. Immunologic aspects of osteoporosis. Dev Comp Immunol 1997;21:487–499.
2. Beers MH, Berkow R. Osteoporosis. In: Beers MH, Berkow R (eds.). The Merck Manual of Diagnosis and Therapy. Merck Research Laboratory, Whitehouse Station, NJ, 1999, pp. 469–473.
3. Bhattoa HP, Kiss E, Bettembuk P, Balogh A. Bone mineral density, biochemical markers of bone turnover, and hormonal status in men with systemic lupus erythematosus. Rheumatol Int 2001;21: 97–102.
4. Bikle DD. Osteoporosis in gastrointestinal, pancreatic, and hepatic diseases. In: Marcus R, Feldman D, Kelsey J (eds.). Osteoporosis (volume II). Academic Press, New York, 2001, pp. 237–258.
5. Gennari C, Martini G, Nuti R. Secondary osteoporosis. Aging (Milano) 1998;10:214–224.

6. Goldring SR. Osteoporosis associated with rheumatologic disorders. In: Marcus R, Feldman D, Kelsey J (eds.). Osteoporosis (volume II). Academic Press, New York, 2001, pp. 351–362.

7. Leong GM, Center JR, Henderson NK, Eisman JA. Glucocorticoid-induced osteoporosis. In: Marcus R, Feldman D, Kelsey J (eds.). Osteoporosis (volume II). Academic Press, New York, 2001, pp. 169–193.

8. Budavari S, O'Neil MJ, Smith A, Heckelman PE, Kinneart JF. The Merck Index: An Encyclopedia of Chemicals, Drugs, and Biologicals (12th ed.). Merck Professional Handbook, Whitehouse Station, NJ, 1996.

9. Beers MH, Berkow R. Nutrition: general consideration. In: Beers MH, Berkow R (eds.). The Merck Manual of Diagnosis and Therapy. Merck Research Laboratory, Whitehouse Station, NJ, 1999, pp. 1–23.

10. Beers MH, Berkow R. Factors affecting drug response. In: Beers MH, Berkow R (eds.). The Merck Manual of Diagnosis and Therapy. Merck Research Laboratory, Whitehouse Station, NJ, 1999, pp. 2574–2587.

11. Becker KL. Principals and Practice of Endocrinology and Metabolism (3rd ed.). Lippincott Williams & Wilkins, Philadelphia, PA, 2001.

12. Bowman BA, Russell RM. Present Knowledge in Nutrition (8th ed.). ILSI, Washington, DC, 2001.

13. Committee on Nutrition Services for Medicare Beneficiaries. Nutrition support. In: Institute of Medicine Committee on Nutrition Services for Medicare Beneficiaries (ed.). The Role of Nutrition in Maintaining Health in the Nation's Elderly. National Academy Press, Washington, DC, 2002, pp. 173–212.

14. Alonso-Aperte E, Varela-Moreiras G. Drugs-nutrient interactions: a potential problem during adolescence. Eur J Clin Nutr 2000;54(Suppl 1):S69–S74.

15. Berg MJ, Rivey MP, Vern BA, Fischer LJ, Schottelius DD. Phenytoin and folic acid: individualized drug-drug interaction. Ther Drug Monit 1983;5:395–399.

16. Bernard SA, Bruera E. Drug interactions in palliative care. J Clin Oncol 2000;18:1780–1799.

17. Brown RO, Dickerson RN. Drug-nutrient interactions. Am J Manag Care 1999;5:345–352.

18. Gauthier I, Malone M, Lesar TS, Aronovitch S. Comparison of programs for preventing drug-nutrient interactions in hospitalized patients. Am J Health Syst Pharm 1997;54:405–411.

19. Maka DA, Murphy LK. Drug-nutrient interactions: a review. AACN Clin Issues 2000;11:580–589.

20. Murray JJ, Healy MD. Drug-mineral interactions: a new responsibility for the hospital dietitian. J Am Diet Assoc 1991;91:66–70, 73.

21. Roe DA. Drug and Nutrient Interaction (5th ed.). The American Dietetic Association, 1994.

22. Thomas JA. Drug-nutrient interactions. Nutr Rev 1995;53:271–282.

23. Thomas JA, Burns RA. Important drug-nutrient interactions in the elderly. Drugs Aging 1998;13: 199–209.

24. Trovato A, Nuhlicek DN, Midtling JE. Drug-nutrient interactions. Am Fam Physician 1991;44: 1651–1658.

25. Utermolen V. Diet, nutrition, and drug interactions. In: Shils ME, Olson JA, Shine M, Ross AC (eds.). Modern Nutrition in Health and Disease. Lippincott Williams & Wilkins, New York, 1999, pp. 1619–1641.

26. Parker P. Impact of nutritional status on immune integrity. In: Gershwin ME, German JB, Keen CL (eds.). Nutrition and Immunology Principals and Practice. Humana, Totowa, NJ, 2000, pp. 147–156.

27. Vellas BJ, Garry PJ. Aging. In: Bowman BA, Russell RM (eds.). Present Knowledge in Nutrition. ILSI, Washington, DC, 2001, pp. 439–446.

28. Meskin MS. Type 2 diabetes mellitus in the elderly. Nutr M D 2000;26:4.

29. Beisel WR. AIDS. In: Gershwin ME, German JB, Keen CL (eds.). Nutrition and Immunology Principals and Practice. Humana, Totowa, NJ, 2000, pp. 389–401.

30. Gerrior J, Wanke C. Nutrition and immunodeficiency syndromes. In: Coulston AM, Rock CL, Monsen ER (eds.). Nutrition in the Prevention and Treatment of Disease. Academic, New York, 2001, pp. 741–750.

31. Cunningham-Rundles S. Trace element and mineral nutrition in HIV infection and AIDS: implications for host defense. In: Bogden JD, Klevay LM (eds.). Clinical Nutrition of the Essential Trace Elements and Minerals. Humana, Totowa, NJ, 2000, pp. 333–351.

32. Beers MH, Berkow R. Human immunodeficiency virus infection. In: Beers MH, Berkow R (eds.). The Merck Manual of Diagnosis and Therapy. Merck Research Laboratory, Whitehouse Station, NJ, 1999, pp. 1312–1323.

33. Sinclair AJ, Barnett AH, Lunec J. Free radicals and antioxidant systems in health and disease. Br J Hosp Med 1990;43:334–344.
34. Sifton DW. Physicians' Desk Reference (55th ed.). Medical Economics Company, Inc., Montvale, NJ, 2001.
35. Baum C, Moxon D, Scott M. Gastrointestinal disease. In: Bowman BA, Russell RM (eds.). Present Knowledge in Nutrition. ILSI, Washington, DC, 2001, pp. 472–482.
36. Krensky AM, Storm TB, Bluestone JA. Immunomodulators: immunosuppressive agents, tolerogens, and immunomodulators. In: Hardman JG, Limbird LE, Gilman AG (eds.). The Pharmacological Basis of Therapeutics. McGraw-Hill, New York, 2001, pp. 1463–1484.
37. Migueles SA, Tuazon CU. Endocrine disorders in human immunodeficiency virus infection. In: Becker KL (ed.). Principles and Practice of Endocrinology and Metabolism. Lippincott Williams & Wilkins, Philadelphia, PA, 2001, pp. 1947–1958.
38. Kupka R, Fawzi W. Zinc nutrition and HIV infection. Nutr Rev 2002;60:69–79.
39. Tang AM, Graham NM, Chandra RK, Saah AJ. Low serum vitamin B-12 concentrations are associated with faster human immunodeficiency virus type 1 (HIV-1) disease progression. J Nutr 1997;127:345–351.
40. Beers MH, Berkow R. Disorders of carbohydrate metabolism. In: Beers MH, Berkow R (eds.). The Merck Manual of Diagnosis and Therapy. Merck Research Laboratory, Whitehouse Station, NJ, 1999, pp. 165–177.
41. Yoon JW, Jun HS. Cellular and molecular pathogenic mechanisms of insulin-dependent diabetes mellitus. Ann N Y Acad Sci 2001; 928:200–211.
42. Catanese VM, Kahn CR. Secondary form of diabetes mellitus. In: Becker KL (ed.). Principals and Practice of Endocrinology and Metabolism. Lippincott Williams & Wilkins, Philadelphia, PA, 2001, pp. 1327–1336.
43. Feldman EL, Stevens MJ, Russell JW, Greene DA. Diabetes neuropathy. In: Becker KL (ed.). Principles and Practice of Endocrinology and Metabolism. Lippincott Williams & Wilkins, New York, 2001, pp. 1391–1399.
44. Kahn CR. Etiology and pathogenesis of type 2 diabetes mellitus and related disorders. In: Becker KL (ed.). Principles and Practice of Endocrinology and Metabolism. Lippincott Williams & Wilkins, Philadelphia, PA, 2001, pp. 1315–1319.
45. Kahn CR. Glucose homeostasis and insulin action. In: Becker KL (ed.). Principles and Practice of Endocrinology and Metabolism. Lippincott Williams & Wilkins, New York, 2001, pp. 1303–1307.
46. Krolewski AS, Warram JH. Natural history of diabetes mellitus. In: Becker KL (ed.). Principles and Practice of Endocrinology and Metabolism. Lippincott Williams & Wilkins, New York, 2001, pp. 1320–1327.
47. Duncan BB, Schmidt MI. Chronic activation of the innate immune system may underlie the metabolic syndrome. Sao Paulo Med J 2001;119:122–127.
48. Vozarova B, Weyer C, Lindsay RS, Pratley RE, Bogardus C, Tataranni PA. High white blood cell count is associated with a worsening of insulin sensitivity and predicts the development of type 2 diabetes. Diabetes 2002;51:455–461.
49. Eizirik DL, Mandrup-Poulsen T. A choice of death—the signal-transduction of immune-mediated beta-cell apoptosis. Diabetologia 2001;44:2115–2133.
50. Eliopoulos GM. Diabetes and infection. In: Becker KL (ed.). Principles and Practice of Endocrinology and Metabolism. Lippincott Williams & Wilkins, New York, 2001, pp. 1424–1428.
51. Preuss HG. Effects of glucose/insulin perturbations on aging and chronic disorders of aging: the evidence. J Am Coll Nutr 1997;16:397–403.
52. Hehenberger K, King GL. Cardiovascular complications of diabetes mellitus. In: Becker KL (ed). Principles and Practice of Endocrinology and Metabolism. Lippincott Williams & Wilkins, New York, 2001, pp. 1380–1391.
53. Strain JJ. Disturbances of micronutrient and antioxidant status in diabetes. Proc Nutr Soc 1991;50: 591–604.
54. Devaraj S, Jialal I. Oxidative stress and antioxidants in type 2 diabetes. In: Bendich A, Deckelbaum RJ (eds.). Primary and Secondary Preventive Nutrition. Humana, Totowa, NJ, 2001, pp. 117–125.
55. Kukreja A, Cost G, Marker J, et al. Multiple immunoregulatory defects in type 1 diabetes. J Clin Invest 2002;109:131–140.

56. Nolsoe RL, Kristiansen OP, Larsen ZM, Johannesen J, Pociot F, Mandrup-Poulsen T. Complete mutation scan of the human Fas ligand gene: linkage studies in Type I diabetes mellitus families. Diabetologia 2002;45:134–139.

57. Jain SK, McVie R, Jaramillo JJ, Palmer M, Smith T. Effect of modest vitamin E supplementation on blood glycated hemoglobin and triglyceride levels and red cell indices in type I diabetic patients. J Am Coll Nutr 1996;15:458–461.

58. Kyurkchiev S, Ivanov G, Manolova V. Advanced glycosylated end products activate the functions of cell adhesion molecules on lymphoid cells. Cell Mol Life Sci 1997;53:911–916.

59. Lee KU. Oxidative stress markers in Korean subjects with insulin resistance syndrome. Diabetes Res Clin Pract 2001;54(Suppl 2):S29–S33.

60. Gale EA. The discovery of type 1 diabetes. Diabetes 2001;50:217–226.

61. Erbagci AB, Tarakcioglu M, Coskun Y, Sivasli E, Sibel NE. Mediators of inflammation in children with type I diabetes mellitus: cytokines in type I diabetic children. Clin Biochem 2001;34:645–650.

62. Cornish J, Callon KE, Reid IR. Insulin increases histomorphometric indices of bone formation in vivo. Calcif Tissue Int 1996;59:492–495.

63. Seeman E. Pathogenesis of bone fragility in women and men. Lancet 2002;359:1841–1850.

64. Albright A. Nutrition management for type I diabetes. In: Coulston AM, Rock CL, Monsen ER (eds.). Nutrition in the Prevention and Treatment of Disease. Academic, New York, 2001, pp. 429–440.

65. Davis SN, Granner DK. Insulin, oral hypoglycemic agents, and the pharmacology of the endocrine pancreas. In: Hardman JG, Limbird LE, Gilman AG (eds.). The Pharmacological Basis of Therapeutics. McGraw-Hill, New York, 2001, pp. 1679–1714.

66. Weir GC. Insulin therapy and its complications. In: Becker KL (ed.). Principles and Practice of Endocrinology and Metabolism. Lippincott Williams & Wilkins, New York, 2001, pp. 1348–1360.

67. Liu S, Manson JE, Buring JE, Stampfer MJ, Willett WC, Ridker PM. Relation between a diet with a high glycemic load and plasma concentrations of high-sensitivity C-reactive protein in middle-aged women. Am J Clin Nutr 2002;75:492–498.

68. Frier HI, Greene HL. Obesity and chronic disease impact of weight reduction. In: Bendich A, Deckelbaum RJ (eds.). Primary and Secondary Preventive Nutrition. Humana, Totowa, NJ, 2001, pp. 205–221.

69. Baldeon ME, Gaskins HR. Diabetes and immunity. In: Gershwin ME, German JB, Keen CL (eds.). Nutrition and Immunology Principles and Practice. Humana, Totowa, NJ, 2000, pp. 301–311.

70. de Luis DA, Fernandez N, Arranz M, Aller R, Izaola O. Total homocysteine and cognitive deterioration in people with type 2 diabetes. Diabetes Res Clin Pract 2002;55:185–190.

71. Defronao RH. Diabetic nephropathy. In: Becker KL (ed.). Principles and Practice of Endocrinology and Metabolism. Lippincott Williams & Wilkins, New York, 2001, pp. 1403–1418.

72. Eliopoulos GM. The diabetic foot. In: Becker KL (ed.). Principles and Practice of Endocrinology and Metabolism. Lippincott Williams & Wilkins, New York, 2001, pp. 1434–1438.

73. Mironova MA, Klein RL, Virella GT, Lopes-Virella MF. Anti-modified LDL antibodies, LDL-containing immune complexes, and susceptibility of LDL to in vitro oxidation in patients with type 2 diabetes. Diabetes 2000;49:1033–1041.

74. Pietropaolo M, Barinas-Mitchell E, Pietropaolo SL, Kuller LH, Trucco M. Evidence of islet cell autoimmunity in elderly patients with type 2 diabetes. Diabetes 2000;49:32–38.

75. Pozzilli P, Di Mario U. Autoimmune diabetes not requiring insulin at diagnosis (latent autoimmune diabetes of the adult.): definition, characterization, and potential prevention. Diabetes Care 2001;24:1460–1467.

76. Rand LI. Diabetes and the eye. In: Becker KL (ed.). Principles and Practice of Endocrinology and Metabolism. Lippincott Williams & Wilkins, New York, 2001, pp. 1418–1424.

77. Ternand C. A changing diet for patients with diabetes. Nutr M D 2000;27:6.

78. Hendler SS, Rorvik D. Physicians' Desk Reference for Nutritional Supplements. Medical Economics Company, Inc., Montvale, NJ, 2001.

79. Goldfine AB, Maratos-Flier E. Oral agents for the treatment of type 2 diabetes mellitus. In: Becker KL (ed.). Principles and Practice of Endocrinology and Metabolism. Lippincott Williams & Wilkins, Philadelphia, PA, 2001, pp. 1344–1348.

80. Moller DE. New drug targets for type 2 diabetes and the metabolic syndrome. Nature 2001;414:821–827.

81. Gordon FD, Falchuk KR. Gastrointestinal complications of diabetes. In: Becker KL(ed.). Principles and Practice of Endocrinology and Metabolism. Lippincott Williams & Wilkins, New York, 2001, pp. 1399–1403.

82. Buysschaert M, Bobbioni E, Starkie M, Frith L. Troglitazone in combination with sulphonylurea improves glycaemic control in type 2 diabetic patients inadequately controlled by sulphonylurea therapy alone. Troglitazone Study Group. Diabet Med 1999;16:147–153.

83. Cohen JA, Jeffers BW, Stabler S, Schrier RW, Estascio R. Increasing homocysteine levels and diabetic autonomic neuropathy. Auton Neurosci 2001;87:268–273.

84. Ambrosch A, Dierkes J, Lobmann R, et al. Relation between homocysteinaemia and diabetic neuropathy in patients with Type 2 diabetes mellitus. Diabet Med 2001;18:185–192.

85. Blom HJ. Diseases and drugs associated with hyperhomocysteinemia. In: Carmel R, Jacobsen DW (eds.). Homocysteine in Health and Disease. Cambridge University Press, New York, 2001, pp. 331–340.

86. Hovind P, Tarnow L, Rossing P, et al. Progression of diabetic nephropathy: role of plasma homocysteine and plasminogen activator inhibitor–1. Am J Kidney Dis 2001;38:1376–1380.

87. Mutus B, Rabini RA, Staffolani R, et al. Homocysteine-induced inhibition of nitric oxide production in platelets: a study on healthy and diabetic subjects. Diabetologia 2001;44:979–982.

88. Scaglione L, Gambino R, Rolfo E, et al. Plasma homocysteine, methylenetetrahydrofolate reductase gene polymorphism and carotid intima-media thickness in Italian type 2 diabetic patients. Eur J Clin Invest 2002;32:24–28.

89. Hoogeveen EK, Rothman KJ. Hyperhomocysteinemia, diabetes, and cardiovascular disease. In: Bendich A, Deckelbaum RJ (eds.). Primary and Secondary Preventive Nutrition. Humana, Totowa, NJ, 2001, 127–154.

90. Baynes JW. Role of oxidative stress in development of complications in diabetes. Diabetes 1991;40: 405–412.

91. Nath N, Chari SN, Rathi AB. Superoxide dismutase in diabetic polymorphonuclear leukocytes. Diabetes 1984;33:586–589.

92. Preuss HG. The insulin system: influence of antioxidants. J Am Coll Nutr 1998;17:101–102.

93. Paolisso G, D'Amore A, Galzerano D, et al. Daily vitamin E supplements improve metabolic control but not insulin secretion in elderly type II diabetic patients. Diabetes Care 1993;16:1433–1437.

94. Ceriello A, Giugliano D, Quatraro A, Donzella C, Dipalo G, Lefebvre PJ. Vitamin E reduction of protein glycosylation in diabetes. New prospect for prevention of diabetic complications? Diabetes Care 1991;14:68–72.

95. Anderson RA. Nutritional factors influencing the glucose/insulin system: chromium. J Am Coll Nutr 1997;16:404–410.

96. Anderson RA, Cheng N, Bryden NA, et al. Elevated intakes of supplemental chromium improve glucose and insulin variables in individuals with type 2 diabetes. Diabetes 1997;46:1786–1791.

97. Beers MH, Berkow R. Diffuse connective tissue disease. In: Beers MH, Berkow R (eds.). The Merck Manual of Diagnosis and Therapy. Merck Research Laboratory, Whitehouse Station, NJ, 1999, pp. 416–423.

98. Mongey AB, Hess EV. Drug and environmental effects on the induction of autoimmunity. J Lab Clin Med 1993;122:652–657.

99. Newkirk MM, LePage K, Niwa T, Rubin L. Advanced glycation endproducts (AGE) on IgG, a target for circulating antibodies in North American Indians with rheumatoid arthritis (RA). Cell Mol Biol (Noisy-le-grand) 1998;44:1129–1138.

100. Meyer O. Atherosclerosis and connective tissue diseases. Joint Bone Spine 2001;68:564–575.

101. Langford CA, Klippel JH, Balow JE, James SP, Sneller MC. Use of cytotoxic agents and cyclosporine in the treatment of autoimmune disease. Part 2: inflammatory bowel disease, systemic vasculitis, and therapeutic toxicity. Ann Intern Med 1998;129:49–58.

102. Balint G, Gergely P Jr. Clinical immunotoxicity of antirheumatic drugs. Inflamm Res 1996;45(Suppl 2):S91–S95.

103. Blanco R, Martinez-Taboada VM, Rodriguez-Valverde V, Sanchez-Andrade A, Gonzalez-Gay MA. Successful therapy with danazol in refractory autoimmune thrombocytopenia associated with rheumatic diseases. Br J Rheumatol 1997;36:1095–1099.

104. Axelrod L. Corticosteroid therapy. In: Becker KL (ed.). Principles and Practice of Endocrinology and Metabolism. Lippincott Williams & Wilkins, Philadelphia, PA, 2001, pp. 751–772.

105. Langford CA, Klippel JH, Balow JE, James SP, Sneller MC. Use of cytotoxic agents and cyclosporine in the treatment of autoimmune disease. Part 1: rheumatologic and renal diseases. Ann Intern Med 1998;128:1021–1028.

106. Morgan SL, Baggott JE. Role of dietary folate and oral folate supplements in the prevention of drug toxicity during anifolate therapy for nonneoplastic disease. In: Bendich A, Butterworth CE Jr (eds.). Micronutrients in Health and in Disease Prevention. Marcel Dekker, Inc., New York, 1991, pp. 333–358.

107. Rozin A, Schapira D, Braun-Moscovici Y, Nahir AM. Cotrimoxazole treatment for rheumatoid arthritis. Semin Arthritis Rheum 2001;31:133–141.

108. Enbrel: *www.enbrel.com*. 2002.

109. Chan LN. Drug-nutrient interactions in transplant recipients. J Parenter Enteral Nutr 2001;25: 132–141.

110. de Sousa M. Circulation and distribution of iron: a key to immune interaction. In: Cunningham-Rundles S (ed.). Nutrient Modulation of the Immune Response. Marcel Dekker, Inc., New York, 1993.

111. Galperin C, Fernandes G, Oliveira RM, Gershwin ME. Nutritional modulation of autoimmune diseases. In: Gershwin ME, German JB, Keen CL (eds.). Nutrition and Immunology Principles and Practice. Humana, Totowa, NJ, 2000, pp. 313–328.

112. Belluzzi A. Polyunsaturated fatty acids and autoimmune diseases. In: Bendich A, Deckelbaum RJ (eds.). Primary and Secondary Preventive Nutrition. Humana, Totowa, NJ, 2001, pp. 271–287.

113. Grodstein F, Colditz GA, Stampfer MJ. Post-menopausal hormone use and tooth loss: a prospective study. J Am Dent Assoc 1996;127:370–377.

114. Marcus R, Feldman D, Kelsey J. Osteoporosis (volume I) (2nd ed.). Academic, New York, 2001.

115. Marcus R, Feldman D, Kelsey J. Osteoporosis (volume II) (2nd ed.). Academic, New York, 2001.

116. Heaney RP. Osteoporosis: mineral, vitamins, and other micronutrients. In: Bendich A, Deckelbaum RJ (eds.). Preventive Nutrition: The Comprehensive Guide for Health Professionals. Humana, Totowa, NJ, 2001, pp. 271–292.

117. Orwoll ES. The prevention and therapy of osteoporsis in men. In: Orwoll ES (ed.). Osteoporosis in Men: The Effects of Gender on Skeletal Health. Academic, New York, 1999, pp. 553–569.

118. Andreassen H, Rungby J, Dahlerup JF, Mosekilde L. Inflammatory bowel disease and osteoporosis. Scand J Gastroenterol 1997;32:1247–1255.

119. Ebeling PR. Secondary causes of osteoporosis in men. In: Orwoll ES (ed.). Osteoporosis in Men: The Effects of Gender on Skeletal Health. Academic, New York, 1999, pp. 483–514.

120. Heller HJ, Sakhaee K. Anticonvulsant-induced bone disease: a plea for monitoring and treatment. Arch Neurol 2001;58:1352–1353.

121. Jamal SA, Browner WS, Bauer DC, Cummings SR. Warfarin use and risk for osteoporosis in elderly women. Study of Osteoporotic Fractures Research Group. Ann Intern Med 1998;128:829–832.

122. Kaye PS. Osteoporosis and fracture as a result of gastrointestinal and hepatic disorders. Practical Gastroenterol 2002;15–28.

123. Valmadrid C, Voorhees C, Litt B, Schneyer CR. Practice patterns of neurologists regarding bone and mineral effects of antiepileptic drug therapy. Arch Neurol 2001;58:1369–1374.

124. Lappe JM, Tinley ST. Prevention of osteoporosis in women treated for hereditary breast and ovarian carcinoma: a need that is overlooked. Cancer 1998;83:830–834.

125. Hertz M, Juji T, Tanaka SMS. A therapeutic RANKL vaccine induces neutralizing anti-RANKL antibodies and prevents bone loss in overiectomized mice. J Bone Miner Res 2001;16:S222.

126. Marcus R. Use of estrogen for the prevention and treatment of osteoporosis. In: Rosen CJ (ed.). Osteoporosis: Diagnostic and Therapeutic Principles. Humana, Totowa, NJ, 1996, 159–172.

127. Khosla S, Riggs BL. Treatment options for osteoporosis. Mayo Clin Proc 1995;70:978–982.

128. Guyatt GH. An introduction to clinical decision making in osteoporosis. In: Rosen CJ (ed.). Osteoporosis: Diagnostic and Therapeutic Principles. Humana, Totowa, NJ, 1996, pp. 145–149.

129. Risks and benefits of estrogen plus progestin in healthy postmenopausal women: principal results from the Women's Health Initiative randomized controlled trial. JAMA 2002;288:321–333.

130. Fleisch H. Basic biology of bisphosphonates. In: Marcus R, Feldman D, Kelsey J (eds.). Osteoporosis (volume I). Academic, New York, 2001, pp. 449–467.

131. Marcus R. Agents affecting calcification and bone turnover. In: Hardman JG, Limbird LE, Gilman AG (eds.). The Pharmacological Basis of Therapeutics. McGraw-Hill, New York, 2001, pp. 1715–1743.

132. Colman E, Hedin R, Swann J, Orloff D. A brief history of calcitonin. Lancet 2002;359:885–886.

133. Hoff AO, Cote GJ, Gagel RF. Calcitonin. In: Marcus R, Feldman D, Kelsey J (eds.). Osteoporosis (volume I). Academic, New York, 2001, pp. 247–255.

134. Gallagher JC, Fowler SE, Detter JR, Sherman SS. Combination treatment with estrogen and calcitriol in the prevention of age-related bone loss. J Clin Endocrinol Metab 2001;86:3618–3628.

135. Bilezikian JP, Silverberg SJ. The role of parathyroid hormone and vitamin D in the pathogenesis of osteoporosis. In: Marcus R, Feldman D, Kelsey J (eds.). Osteoporosis (volume II). Academic, New York, 2001, pp. 71–84.

136. Nissenson RA. Parathyroid hormone and parathyroid hormone-related protein. In: Marcus R, Feldman D, Kelsey J (eds.). Osteoporosis (volume I). Academic, New York, 2001, pp. 221–246.

137. Weinstein RS, Manolagas SC. Apoptosis and osteoporosis. Am J Med 2000;108:153–164.

138. Cassidy JT, Hillman LS. Abnormalities in skeletal growth in children with juvenile rheumatoid arthritis. Rheum Dis Clin N Am 1997;23:499–522.

139. Pollak RD, Karmeli F, Eliakim R, Ackerman Z, Tabb K, Rachmilewitz D. Femoral neck osteopenia in patients with inflammatory bowel disease. Am J Gastroenterol 1998;93:1483–1490.

140. Reid IR. Glucocorticoids and osteoporosis. In: Orwoll ES (ed.). Osteoporosis in Men: The Effects of Gender on Skeletal Health. Academic, New York, 1999, pp. 417–436.

141. Reid IR. Glucocorticoid-induced osteoporosis. Baillieres Best Pract Res Clin Endocrinol Metab 2000;14:279–298.

142. Silverberg MS, Steinhart AH. Bone density in inflammatory bowel disease. Clin Pers Gastroenterol 2000;117–124.

143. Stempfle HU, Werner C, Siebert U, et al. The role of tacrolimus (FK506)-based immunosuppression on bone mineral density and bone turnover after cardiac transplantation: a prospective, longitudinal, randomized, double-blind trial with calcitriol. Transplantation 2002;73:547–552.

144. Marcus R. Calcium as a primary treatment and prevention modality for osteoporosis. In: Rosen CJ (ed.). Osteoporosis: Diagnostic and Therapeutic Principles. Humana, Totowa, NJ, 1996, pp. 151–158.

145. Reid IR, Ames RW, Evans MC, Gamble GD, Sharpe SJ. Long-term effects of calcium supplementation on bone loss and fractures in postmenopausal women: a randomized controlled trial. Am J Med 1995;98:331–335.

146. Stock JL. Drug therapy. In: Rosen CJ, ed. Osteoporosis: Diagnostic and Therapeutic Principles. Humana, Totowa, NJ, 1996, pp. 173–187.

147. Nieves JW, Komar L, Cosman F, Lindsay R. Calcium potentiates the effect of estrogen and calcitonin on bone mass: review and analysis. Am J Clin Nutr 1998;67:18–24.

148. Coulston AM. Nutritional management for type 2 diabetes. In: Coulston AM, Rock CL, Monsen ER (eds.). Nutrition in the Prevention and Treatment of Disease. Academic, New York, 2001, pp. 441–452.

Appendix I

Abbreviations

ACF	aberrant crypt foci
ACTH	adrenocorticotrophin
ADCC	antibody-dependent cellular cytotoxicity
AGE	advanced glycation endproducts
AGP	α1-acid glycoprotein
AIDS	acquired immune deficiency syndrome
ALA	alpha linolenic acid
APP	acute-phase protein
APR	acute-phase response
BAL	bronchoalveolar lavage
BMD	bone mineral density
CD	clusters of differentiation
CDF	cation diffusion facilitator
CFU	colony-forming unit
CK	creatine kinase
CLA	conjugated linoleic acid
Con A	concanavalin A
COPD	chronic obstructive pulmonary disease
Cox	cyclo-oxygenase
CRP	C-reactive protein
CVD	cardiovascular disease
DEP	diesel exhaust particulate
DHA	docosahexaenoic acid
DMT	divalent metal transporter
DTH	delayed type hypersensitivity
ECP	eosinophil cationic protein
EFA	essential fatty acids
EPA	eicosapentaenoic acid
EPO	evening primrose oil
ESR	erythrocyte sedimentation rate
FEV_1	forced expiratory volume in 1 second
FFQ	food-frequency questionnaire
GALT	gut-associated lymphoid tissue
GCS	glutamylcysteine synthetase
GH	growth hormone

From: *Diet and Human Immune Function*
Edited by: D. A. Hughes, L. G. Darlington, and A. Bendich © Humana Press Inc., Totowa, NJ

GM-CSF	granulocyte-macrophage colony-stimulating factor
GPx	glutathione peroxidase
GSH	gluthathione
HIV	human immunodeficiency virus
HLA	human leukocyte antigens
HPA	hypothalamic-pituitary-adrenal (axis)
HSP	heat shock protein
IBD	inflammatory bowel disease
ICAM	intercellular adhesion molecule
IFN	interferon
Ig	immunoglobulin
IGF	insulin-like growth factor
IL	interleukin
IL-2R	interleukin-2 receptor
IRE	iron responsive elements
IRP	iron regulatory protein
LAB	lactic acid bacteria
LAK	lymphokine-activated killer (cell)
LDL	low-density lipoprotein
LFA	leukocyte function-associated antigen
LPR	lymphocyte proliferative responses
LPS	lipopolysaccharide
LT	leukotriene
MALT	mucosa-associated lymphoid tissue
MBP	major basic protein
MHC	major histocompatibility complex
MT	metallothionein
MUFA	monounsaturated fatty acid
NADPH	nicotinamide adenine dinucleotide phosphate
NF-κB	nuclear factor-kappa B (a transcription factor)
NK	natural killer
NO	nitric oxide
NOS	nitric oxide synthase
NSAIDs	nonsteroidal antiinflammatory drugs
OA	osteoarthritis
PBMN	peripheral blood mononuclear cells
PCM	protein calorie malnutrition
PCR	polymerase chain reaction
PG	prostaglandin
PHA	phytohemagglutinin
PKC	protein kinase C
PM	particulate matter
PMN	polymorphonuclear leukocytes
PPD	purified protein derivative (of *M. tuberculosis*)

PUFA	polyunsaturated fatty acid
PWM	pokeweed mitogen
RA	rheumatoid arthritis
RAR	retinoic acid receptor
RAREs	retinoic acid response elements
RBP	retinol-binding protein
RDA	recommended dietary allowance
RE	retinol equivalent
RES	reticuloendothelial system
RF	rheumatoid factor
ROI	reactive oxygen intermediates
ROS	reactive oxygen species
RSV	respiratory syncytial virus
RT-PCR	real-time polymerase chain reaction
RXR	retinoid-x receptor
SCID	severe combined immunodeficiency (syndrome)
Se	selenium
SLE	systemic lupus erythematosus
SOD	superoxide dismutase
TCR	T-cell receptor
TfR	transferrin receptor
TGF-ß	transforming growth factor-ß
Th	T-helper lymphocyte
TLC	total lymphocyte count
TNF-α	tumor necrosis factor-α
TR	thioredoxin reductase
TRx	thioredoxin
TTR	transthyretin
URTI	upper respiratory tract infection
UV	ultraviolet
UVR	ultraviolet radiation
VC	vitamin C
VE	vitamin E
WHO	World Health Organization
ZIP	zinc-regulated transporter, iron-regulated transporter-like protein
ZnT	zinc transporter

Appendix II   Glossary

Acquired immunity: an immune reaction involving *lymphocytes* that is specific to any given *antigen* and which gives rise to immunological *memory*.

Acute-phase proteins: liver-derived serum proteins produced during the early phase of an immune response.

Adaptive response: another term for *acquired immunity*.

Adhesion molecules: molecules expressed on the cell surface that are involved in the direct binding of one cell to another cell or to specific substrates (e.g., glycoproteins).

Adrenaline: synonym for epinephrine.

AIDS (acquired immunodeficiency syndrome): human disease caused by infection with the human immunodeficiency virus (*HIV*).

Allergen: an *antigen* that induces an allergic type 1 (*IgE*-mediated) hypersensitivity reaction, e.g., house dust mite, pollens, and dander.

Allergy: a synonym for *hypersensitivity*.

Antibody: a molecule produced by *B lymphocytes* in response to *antigen*, that binds specifically to the antigen which induced its formation.

Antigen: a molecule that elicits a specific immune response when introduced into the body. Most antigens are proteins, peptides, or polysaccharides. Large antigens bear small *epitopes* that can be recognized by specific *antibodies*, but *T lymphocytes* recognize only peptides derived from processed protein antigens (*see antigen-presenting cell*).

Antigen-presenting cell (APC): a cell (e.g., *monocyte, macrophage, Langerhans cell*, or *B cell*) that processes and presents antigen fragments on *major histocompatibility complex* (MHC) class II molecules to CD4+ T cells.

Apoptosis (programmed cell death): an active process requiring metabolic activity by the dying cell. Cells that die by apoptosis do not usually elicit the inflammatory responses associated with necrosis.

Arachidonic acid: an *essential fatty acid*, the precursor for the biosynthesis of *prostaglandins* and *leukotrienes*.

Atopy: clinical manifestation of a type 1 (IgE-mediated) *hypersensitivity* reaction, including asthma, eczema, allergic rhinitis (hay fever), and food allergy.

Autoimmune disease: a disease in which specific reactions of the immune system against self-tissues or antigens causes or contributes to the initiation or progression of the disease.

From: *Diet and Human Immune Function*
Edited by: D. A. Hughes, L. G. Darlington, and A. Bendich © Humana Press Inc., Totowa, NJ

Avidity: the strength of binding between an *antibody* and an *antigen*, expressed in arbitrary units.

B lymphocyte: a *lymphocyte* that bears *immunoglobulin* on its surface as a receptor for *antigen* and that can differentiate into a *plasma cell*.

Basophil: a *leukocyte* that has receptors for IgE antibodies and may contribute to allergic reactions.

CD antigens: "clusters of differentiation," a classification of cell-surface *antigens* based on their reactions with a panel of monoclonal antibodies. The CD nomenclature has been internationally adopted as a way of listing cell-surface molecules.

CD3: a CD antigen expressed on *T lymphocytes*.

CD4: a CD antigen expressed on *helper T lymphocytes*.

CD8: a CD antigen expressed on cytotoxic and *suppressor T lymphocytes*.

CD16: a CD antigen expressed on *NK cells*.

CD56: a CD antigen expressed on *NK cells*.

Cell-mediated immune response: *specific immunity* mediated by T cells that recognize *major histocompatibility complex*-bound *antigens* on contact with the cells bearing them.

Chemokines: a family of *cytokines* with cell-specific chemoattractant activity (*see chemotaxis*).

Chemotaxis: directed movement of cells in response to a concentration gradient of a chemical substance (chemotactic factor), such as *chemokines*, *complement* components, or *cytokines*.

Complement: a system of serum proteins and a group of membrane proteins that interact in a complex cascade reaction sequence. Involved in the control of *inflammation*, the destruction of cell membranes, and the activation of *phagocytes*.

Concanavalin A (Con A): *see mitogen*.

Cytokines: soluble intercellular messenger molecules produced by cells. They are important nonantigen-specific molecules that act locally. *Lymphocytes* produce many cytokines (*lymphokines*, such as *IL-2, IL-4,* and *IFN-γ*), others are produced by *mononuclear phagocytes* (*monokines*, such as *IL-1* and *TNF-α*).

Cytotoxic T lymphocyte (T_C cell): a T cell (usually *CD8+*) that directly lyses virus-infected cells.

Delayed type hypersensitivity (DTH) response: immune response involving memory of prior exposure to an antigen important in dealing with chronic infection, which has a characteristically slow appearance when a specific *antigen* (e.g., tuberculin as a test for tuberculosis) is injected into the skin.

Dendritic cell: important *antigen-presenting cell* found throughout the body, particularly at sites of contact with *antigen* (e.g., skin Langerhans cells and gut and lung dendritic cells).

Docosahexaenoic acid (DHA): an n–3 *PUFA*, found in oil-rich fish.

Eicosanoids: a generic term for several oxygenated fatty acids with potent biologic activities, includes *prostaglandins* and *leukotrienes*.

Eicosapentaenoic acid (EPA): an n–3 *PUFA*, found in oil-rich fish.

Eosinophil: a *granulocyte* containing granules of cationic proteins that can modulate an inflammatory reaction. Important in the control of parasitic infections and in atopic allergic reactions.

Epinephrine: synonym for adrenaline.

Epitope: an antigenic determinant—the part of the *antigen* with which an *antibody* or a T-cell receptor molecule interacts.

Essential fatty acids: fatty acids required for growth, reproduction, and good health in mammals: *arachidonic*, linolenic, and linoleic acids. These must be supplied in the diet as they cannot be synthesized endogenously in adequate quantities.

Helper T lymphocyte (Th cell): a thymus-derived *lymphocyte* (usually expressing the *CD4* molecule, i.e., CD4+) whose presence is needed to stimulate the production of *antibody* by B cells and for the normal development of *cell-mediated immune responses*. This help is mediated by *cytokine* production. Among the Th cells are Th1 cells, characterized by their production of *IL-2* and IFN-γ, which are involved in cell-mediated immune responses, and Th2 cells, which produce *IL-4* and *IL-10* and are involved in enhancing antibody production, particularly IgE responses involved in allergic responses.

HIV (human immunodeficiency virus): a virus that binds to *CD4* molecules on *helper T cells* and also on *monocytes*, allowing its entry into the cell, which may eventually lead to the cell's destruction and, thus, a progressive reduction in CD4+ cells (*see AIDS*).

Humoral immunity: *specific immunity* mediated by *antibodies*.

Hypersensitivity: a heightened reactivity to antigen that can result in tissue damage.

ICAM (intercellular adhesion molecule): a group of transmembrane proteins that are important *adhesion molecules*.

Immune response: the specific response to *antigen*. Includes the responses of *cell-mediated immunity* and *humoral immunity*.

Immunodeficiency: any condition in which a deficiency of *cell-mediated immunity* or *humoral immunity* exists.

Immunoglobulin (Ig): alternative name for the family of proteins that are *antibodies*. Families include IgA (the major Ig in secretions into the intestines, lungs, and saliva), IgE (the main Ig associated with allergic reactions), and IgG (the major Ig in the serum).

Inflammation: a tissue response to injury or other trauma characterized by pain, heat, redness, and swelling.

Innate immunity: natural nonspecific host defenses.

Interferons (IFNs): a group of mediators that increase the resistance of cells to viral infection and act as *cytokines*. IFN-γ is an important proinflammatory molecule.

Interleukins (ILs): molecules made by *leukocytes*, involved in signaling between cells of the immune system.

Interleukin-1 (IL-1): includes two related proteins, IL-1α and IL-1ß (also known as lymphotoxin), produced by *mononuclear phagocytes*. It is an inflammatory *cytokine* that induces fever, increases cell *adhesion molecule* expression, and causes neutrophilia (an increase in the number of *neutrophils* in the bloodstream).

Interleukin-2 (IL-2): a *cytokine* whose major function is in regulation of the immune response. Produced primarily by *helper T lymphocytes*. Required to initiate all T-cell responses and also enhances *NK cell* function.

Interleukin-4 (IL-4): a *cytokine* produced by activated T cells that activates B cells.

Interleukin-10 (IL-10): a *cytokine* that inhibits the release of cytokines and inhibits *MHC* class II molecule expression by *mononuclear phagocytes*, thus diminishing *delayed type hypersensitivity* responses.

Killer cell: term used for any cell that can exert a cytotoxic effect on target cells, including *NK cells*, cytotoxic T cells, *neutrophils*, and *macrophages*.

Leukocyte: the white blood cells and their precursors.

Leukotrienes: pharmacologically active substances generated by the action of lipoxygenase enzymes on the n–6 *PUFA*, *arachidonic acid*, which can be released from *mast cells*, *platelets*, and other *leukocytes*.

Ligand: term often used to describe a molecule that binds to another molecule or cell.

Lipopolysaccharide (LPS): a constituent part of the cell wall of all Gram-negative bacteria, consisting of a lipid core with a polysaccharide side chain. The LPS receptor is, therefore, an important recognition molecule on the surface of *macrophages*.

Lymphocyte: the cell type that carries receptors for, and recognizes, *antigen* and is, therefore, the mediator of *specific immunity*. There are two major forms of mature lymphocytes, the *B lymphocyte* and the *T lymphocyte*.

Lymphocyte transformation (activation): the change seen when *lymphocytes* are stimulated by a *mitogen* or an *antigen* to which they are primed. The cells enter the cell cycle sequence, divide, and differentiate into various functional types.

Lymphocyte transformation test: a test used to assess the ability of an individual's *lymphocytes* to respond to stimulation by *mitogens* or *antigens*.

Lymphokines: *cytokines* produced by activated *lymphocytes*, particularly T cells.

Macrophage: a large cell derived from *monocytes* that functions as a phagocytic cell, a cytotoxic killer cell, and an antigen-presenting cell.

Major histocompatibility complex (MHC): a set of genes found in all mammals that regulate the activation of T cells and that, by being markers of self, contribute to the tissue incompatibilities that cause graft rejection.

Mast cell: a tissue cell (similar to circulating *basophils*) that bears high affinity surface receptors for IgE. Plays an important role in allergic reactions.

Memory (immunologic): a characteristic of a specific immune response in which secondary exposure to a given *antigen* produces a faster and greater response.

Memory cell: T cells or B cells that mediate immunologic *memory*.

Monocyte: a large phagocytic cell that is the blood representative of the *mononuclear phagocyte* system. Monocytes remain in the blood for approx 24 h before migrating into the tissues, where they differentiate into *macrophages*.

Monokine: *cytokines* produced by *mononuclear phagocytes*, e.g., *IL-1* and *TNF-α*.

Mononuclear cells (peripheral blood mononuclear cells, PBMN): a vague term used to describe a mixture of *lymphocytes* and *mononuclear phagocytes*.

Mononuclear phagocytes: a system of phagocytic cells of which the mature functioning form is the *macrophage*.

N–3 or N–6: *see polyunsaturated fatty acid*.

Natural killer cell: *see* NK cell.

Neutrophil: the most numerous cell type in the bloodstream, a short-lived cell with a multilobed nucleus and a cytoplasm filled with granules. Actively phagocytic and has an efficient microbicidal capacity. The major cell type found in acute inflammatory lesions.

NF-κB: a transcription factor that binds to DNA and activates the expression of numerous genes, encoding proteins involved in immune responses, such as *cytokines* and *adhesion molecules*.

NK cell (natural killer cell): cytotoxic *lymphocytes* that lack the markers of T cells or B cells and contain prominent cytoplasmic granules. They bear the markers *CD16* and *CD56* and can kill virally infected cells and tumor cells by releasing perforins, proteins, which insert into the membrane of the target cell, resulting in its lysis.

Omega-3 or Omega-6: *see polyunsaturated fatty acid*.

Oxidative burst: the rapid generation of *reactive oxygen species (ROS)* in phagocytic cells after phagocytosis of foreign material.

Pathogen: an infectious disease-causing entity, e.g., certain viruses, bacteria, fungi, and parasites.

PHA (phytohemagglutinin): a strong *mitogen* for T cells, also causing agglutination (clumping) of red blood cells.

Phagocyte: a cell that can engulf, and often digest, large particles, such as bacteria, protozoa, and dead tissue cells.

Phagocytosis: "cell eating." The process of ingestion of cells or particles by a cell.

Plasma cell: a differentiated *B lymphocyte*, which is the major antibody-secreting cell type.

Platelet: a small nonnucleated "cell" found in the blood, important in blood coagulation, and can release inflammatory mediators such as *leukotrienes*.

Polymorphonuclear leukocyte (PMN): synonym for neutrophil, which, in its mature form, has a multilobed nucleus.

Polyunsaturated fatty acid (PUFA): fatty acids that contain adjacent carbon atoms linked by double bonds (in contrast to saturated fatty acids that contain no double bonds). Two major groups are the n–6 (also termed omega-6) fatty acids, where the first double bond from the methyl terminal end of the molecule is present on carbon atom 6 (e.g., *arachidonic acid*), and the n–3 fatty acids, where the first double bond is on carbon atom 3 (e.g., *DHA* and *EPA*). They mainly come from vegetables and fish.

Prostaglandins: biologically active group of compounds generated by the action of cyclooxygenase enzymes. They have several actions as inflammatory mediators, particularly those derived from the n–6 fatty acid, *arachidonic acid*, such as prostaglandin E_2 (PGE_2).

Reactive oxygen species (ROS): metabolites of molecular oxygen that are highly reactive and damaging to biochemicals. Produced during normal metabolism, but particularly by phagocytic cells, to destroy phagocytosed material.

Recommended dietary allowance (RDA): The amounts of a given nutrient considered adequate to meet the nutrient needs of practically all healthy people.

Respiratory burst: *see oxidative burst*.

Saturated fatty acids: fatty acids that have all the hydrogen they can hold on their chemical chains, i.e., no double bonds between adjacent carbon atoms (cf. *PUFA*). They mainly come from animal foods.

Specific immunity: a nonsusceptibility to reinfection by a pathogen that develops in an individual who survives a first encounter with the same pathogen.

Suppressor T lymphocyte: T cells that suppress immune responses. Can express the marker *CD8*.

T lymphocyte (T cell): a lymphocyte derived from the *thymus*, carrying an antigen-specific T-cell receptor and the marker *CD3*.

Th1 cell/Th2 cell: *see helper T lymphocyte*.

Thymus: the organ situated in the thorax where T cells mature and achieve immune competence.

Titer: a measure of the activity of a reagent obtained by serial dilution of the reactants and often expressed as arbitrary units. Widely used to measure the quantity of *antibody* in serum after a vaccination.

TNF (tumor necrosis factor)-α: an inflammatory *cytokine* produced by many types of *leukocyte*, named after its ability to kill tumor cells in tissue culture.

Tolerance: a situation where the *acquired immune* system does not respond to an *antigen*.

Appendix III

Related Books and Websites

BOOKS

1. Bendich, A., Deckelbaum, R.J. (Eds.). 2001. *Preventive Nutrition: The Comprehensive Guide for Health Professionals (2nd ed.)*. Humana, Totowa, NJ.
2. Bendich, A., Deckelbaum, R.J. (Eds.). 2001. *Primary and Secondary Preventive Nutrition*. Humana, Totowa, NJ.
3. Berdanier, C.D. (Ed.). 1996. *Nutrients and Gene Expression: Clinical Aspects*. CRC, Boca Raton, FL.
4. Berdanier, C.D., Failla, M.L. 1998. *Advanced Nutrition: Micronutrients*. CRC, Boca Raton, FL.
5. Bogden, J.D. 2000. *Clinical Nutrition of the Essential Trace Elements and Minerals*. Humana, Totowa, NJ.
6. Brody, T. 1998. *Nutritional Biochemistry (2nd ed.)*. Academic, San Diego, CA.
7. Cadenas, E., Packer, L. (Eds.). 1996. *Handbook of Antioxidants*. Marcel Dekker, New York.
8. Calder, P.C., Field, C.J., Gill, H.S. (Eds.). 2002. *Nutrition and Immune Function*. CABI Publishing, Oxon.
9. Chow, C.K. (Ed.). 1999. *Fatty Acids in Foods and Their Health Implications (2nd ed.)*. Marcel Dekker, New York.
10. Combs, G.F., Jr. 1998. *Vitamins: Fundamental Aspects in Nutrition and Health (2nd ed.)*. Academic, San Diego, CA.
11. Driskell, J. 1999. *Sports Nutrition*. CRC, Boca Raton, FL.
12. Eitenmiller, R.R., Landen, W.O., Jr. (Eds.). 1999. *Vitamin Analysis for the Health and Food Sciences*. CRC, Boca Raton, FL.
13. Garewal, H.S. (Ed.). 1997. *Antioxidants and Disease Prevention*. CRC, Boca Raton, FL.
14. Gershwin, M., Keen, C.L., German, J.B. (Eds.). 1999. *Nutrition and Immunology: Principles and Practice*. Humana, Totowa, NJ.
15. Gibson, G.R., Roberfroid, M.B. 1999. *Colonic Microbiota, Nutrition and Health*. Kluwer Academic, Boston, MA.
16. Heimburger, D.C., Weinsier, R.L. 1997. *Handbook of Clinical Nutrition (3rd ed.)*. Mosby, Inc., St. Louis, MO.
17. Hoffman-Goetz, L. (Ed.). 1996. *Exercise and Immune Function*. CRC, Boca Raton, FL.
18. Klein, J., Horejsi, V. 1997. *Immunology*. Blackwell Science, Oxford.

From: *Diet and Human Immune Function*
Edited by: D. A. Hughes, L. G. Darlington, and A. Bendich © Humana Press Inc., Totowa, NJ

19. Janeway, C.A., Travers, P., Walport, M., Shlomchik, M. 2001. *Immunobiology: The Immune System in Health and Disease.* Garland Science Publishing, New York.

20. Mann, J., Truswell, A.S., Truswell, S. (Eds.). 1998. *Essentials of Human Nutrition.* Oxford University Press, New York.

21. Mcardle, W.D., Katch, F.I., Katch, V.L. 1999. *Sports and Exercise Nutrition.* Lippincott Williams & Wilkins, Philadelphia.

22. Miller, T.L., Gorbach, S.L. (Eds.). 1999. *Nutrition Aspects of HIV Infection.* Oxford University Press, New York.

23. Morrison, G., Hark, L. 1999. *Medical Nutrition and Disease (2nd ed.).* Blackwell Science, Inc., Malden, MA.

24. Nairn, R., Helbert, M. 2002. *Immunology for Medical Students.* Mosby International, London.

25. Nieman, D.C., Pedersen, B.K. (Eds.). 2000. *Nutrition and Exercise Immunology.* CRC, Boca Raton, FL.

26. Oberleas, D., Harland, B.F., Bobilya D.J. 1999. *Minerals: Nutrition and Metabolism.* Vantage, New York.

27. O'Dell, B.L., Sunde, R.A. 1997. *Handbook of Nutritionally Essential Mineral Elements (Vol. 2).* Marcel Dekker Inc, New York.

28. Papas, A. (Ed). 1998. *Antioxidant Status, Diet, Nutrition, and Health.* CRC, Boca Raton, FL.

29. Playfair, J.H.L., Chain, B.M. 2001. *Immunology at a Glance (7th ed.).* Blackwell Publishing, Oxford.

30. Roitt, I., Delves, P.J. 2001. *Roitt's Essential Immunology.* Blackwell Science, Oxford.

31. Roitt, I., Brostoff, J., Male, D. 2001. *Immunology (6th ed.).* Mosby International, London.

32. Sadler, M.J., Strain, J.J., Caballero, B. (Eds.). 1998. *Encyclopedia of Human Nutrition.* Academic Inc, San Diego, CA.

33. Shils, M., Olson, J.A., Shike, M. (Eds.). 1998. *Modern Nutrition in Health and Disease (9th ed.).* Williams & Wilkins, Baltimore, MD.

34. Simopoulos, AP. 1997. *Nutrition and Fitness.* Karger, S., AG, Basel, Switzerland.

35. Stipanuk, M. (Ed.). 1999. *Biochemical and Physiological Aspects of Human Nutrition.* W.B. Saunders, Philadelphia, PA.

36. Taylor, C.E. (Ed.). 1997. *Nutritional Abnormalities in Infectious Diseases: Effects on Tuberculosis and AIDS.* Haworth, New York.

37. Tsang, R.C., Nichols, B.L., Zlotkin, S.H., et al. (Eds.). 1997. *Nutrition During Infancy: Principles and Practice (2nd ed.).* Digital Educational Publishing, Cincinnati, OH.

38. Veith, W.J. (Ed.). 1999. *Diet and Health (2nd ed.).* CRC, Boca Raton, FL.

39. Wardley, B., Puntis, J.W.L., Taitz, L.S. 1997. *Handbook of Child Nutrition (2nd ed.).* Oxford University Press, New York.

40. Watson, R.R. (Ed.). 1998. *Nutrients and Foods in AIDS.* CRC, Boca Raton, FL.

41. Watson, R.R., Mufti, S.I. (Eds.). 1996. *Nutrition and Cancer Prevention.* CRC, Boca Raton, FL.

42. Willett, W. 1998. *Nutritional Epidemiology (2nd ed.).* Oxford University Press, New York.

43. Wolinsky, I. (Ed.). 1998. *Nutrition in Exercise and Sport (3rd ed.).* CRC, Boca Raton, FL.

44. Wolinsky, I., Klimis-Tavantzis, D. (Eds.). 1996. *Nutritional Concerns of Women.* CRC, Boca Raton, FL.

45. World Health Organization. 1996. *WHO Publication: Trace Elements in Human Nutrition and Health.* WHO Publications Center USA, Albany, NY.
46. Ziegler, E.E., Filer, L.J., Jr. (Eds.). 1996. *Present Knowledge in Nutrition.* ILSI, Washington, DC.

WEBSITES

http://www.ifst.org/

The Institute of Food Science & Technology (IFST) is based in the United Kingdom, with members throughout the world, with the purpose of serving the public interest in the application of science and technology for food safety and nutrition, as well as furthering the profession of food science and technology. Eligibility for membership can be found at the IFST home page; an index and a search engine are available.

http://www.nysaes.cornell.edu/cifs/start.html

The Cornell Institute of Food Science at Cornell University home page provides information on graduate and undergraduate courses, as well as research and extension programs. Links to related sites and newsgroups can be found.

http://www.blonz.com

Created by Ed Blonz, PhD, "The Blonz Guide" focuses on the fields of nutrition, foods, food science, and health, supplying links and search engines to find quality sources, news, publication, and entertainment sites.

http://www.hnrc.tufts.edu/

The Jean Mayer United States Department of Agriculture (USDA) Human Nutrition Research Center on Aging (HNRC) at Tufts University. This research center is one of six mission-oriented centers aimed at studying the relationship between human nutrition and health, operated by Tufts University under the USDA. Research programs; seminar and conference information; publications; nutrition, aging, medical, and science resources; and related links are available.

http://www.fao.org/

The Food and Agriculture Organization (FAO) is the largest autonomous agency within the United Nations, founded "with a mandate to raise levels of nutrition and standards of living, to improve agricultural productivity, and to better the condition of rural population," emphasizing sustainable agriculture and rural development.

http://www.eatright.org/

The American Dietetic Association is the largest group of food and nutrition professionals in the United States; members are primarily registered dietitians (RDs) and dietetic technicians, registered (DTRs). Programs and services include promoting nutrition information for the public; sponsoring national events, media, and marketing programs, and publications (*The American Dietetic Association*); and lobbying for federal legislation. Also available through the Web site are member services, nutrition resources, news, classifieds, and government affairs. Assistance in finding a dietitian, marketplace news, and links to related sites can also be found.

http://www.asns.org

The American Society for Nutritional Sciences (ASNS) located in Bethesda, MD, is a research society facilitating, for example, animal and human nutrition studies, official publication (*The Journal of Nutrition*, available through nutrition.org), annual meetings, education and training opportunities, and professional networking. Categories for membership include regular, associate, student, and emeritus.

http://www.faseb.org

The Federation of American Societies for Experimental Biology (FASEB) is a coalition of member societies with the purpose of enhancing the profession of biomedical and life scientists, emphasizing public policy issues. FASEB offers logistic and operational support, as well as sponsors scientific conferences and publications (*The FASEB Journal*).

http://ific.org/

The International Food Information Council (IFIC) is a nonprofit organization whose purpose is to provide access to health and nutrition resources, data, and information based on science to professionals, educators, journalists, government officials, and others to facilitate the communication of health and nutrition information to consumers.

http://www.foodsciencecentral.com/

The International Food Information Service (IFIS) is a leading information, product, and service provider for professionals in food science, food technology, and nutrition. IFIS publishing offers a range of scientific databases, including FSTA—Food Science and Technology Abstracts. IFIS GmbH offers research, educational training, and seminars.

http://www.ift.org/

The Institute of Food Technologists (IFT) is a membership organization advancing the science and technology of food through the sharing of information; publications include *Food Technology* and *Journal of Food Science*; events include the Annual Meeting and Food Expo. Members may choose to join a specialized division of expertise (there are 23 divisions); IFT student associations and committees are also available for membership.

http://www.veris-online.org/

The VERIS Research Information Service is a nonprofit corporation, focusing on antioxidants, providing professionals with reliable sources on the role of nutrition in health. Data in VERIS publications, distributed without fee to those who qualify, is based on technical peer-reviewed journals. Quarterly written reports and newsletters, research summaries, annual abstract books, vitamin E fact book, and educational programs are among the available VERIS publications and communications. Links to helpful Web resources are also accessible.

http://www.osteo.org/

The National Institutes of Health Osteoporosis and Related Bone Diseases–National Resource Center's (NIH ORBD-NRC) mission is to "provide patients, health professionals, and the public with an important link to resources and information on metabolic bone diseases, including osteoporosis, Paget's disease of the bone, osteogenesis imperfecta, and hyperparathyroidism. The center is operated by the National Osteoporosis Foundation, in collaboration with The Paget Foundation and the Osteogenesis Imperfecta Foundation.

http://www.calciuminfo.com

This is an online information source created, copyrighted, and maintained by GlaxoSmithKline Consumer Healthcare Research and Development. The nutritional and physiologic role of calcium is presented in formats designed for healthcare professionals, consumers, and kids. References and related links, educational games for kids, calcium tutorials, and a calcium calculator are easily accessible.

http://www-sci.lib.uci.edu/~martindale/Nutrition.html

Martindale's Health Science Guide–2003: "The Virtual Nutrition Center," provides a large volume of information. The Nutrition Overview lists resources, such as travel warnings and immunization, online nutrition calculators, nutrition journals, literature and patent searches, conferences, and dictionaries. Nutrition Interactive allows access to databases, courses, and tutorials. All sections are accessed through a single site, use caution when printing!

http://www.usda.gov

The USDA provides a broad scope of service to the nation's farmers and ranchers. In addition, the USDA ensures open markets for agricultural products, food safety, environmental protection, conservation of forests and rural land, and the research of human nutrition. Affiliated agencies, services, and programs are accessible through this Web site.

http://www.fns.usda.gov/fns/

The Food and Nutrition Service (FNS) administers the USDA's 15 food assistance programs for children and needy families with the mission to reduce hunger and food insecurity. Details of nutrition assistance programs and related links can be found.

http://www.who.int/nut/

The World Health Organization (WHO) has regarded nutrition to be fundamentally important for overall health and sustainable development. The global priority of nutritional issues, activities, mandates, resources, and research are presented in detail.

http://www.nutrition.org.uk/

The British Nutrition Foundation (BHF) promotes the nutritional well-being of society through the impartial interpretation and effective dissemination of scientifically based nutritional knowledge and advice. It works in partnership with academic and research institutes, the food industry, educators, and government. The Foundation influences all in the food chain, government, the professions, and the media. The Foundation is a charitable organization that raises funds from the food industry, government, and several other sources.

http://www.ifr.ac.uk/

The Institute of Food Research (IFR) is the United Kingdom's only integrated basic science provider focused on food and is publicly funded to conduct independent basic and strategic research in food safety, nutrition, and food materials science. The site provides information on current research topics and contains a range of information sheets on food-related topics.

http://12.17.12.70/aai/default.asp/

The American Association of Immunologists (AAI) is the largest professional association of immunologists in the world. *The Journal of Immunology* is the official journal of the AAI.

http://www.immunology.org/

The British Society for Immunology (BSI) advances the science of immunology through the publication of its journals, the organization of scientific meetings, and its work with schools and the general public.

http://www.efis.org/

The European Federation of Immunological Societies (EFIS) is the federation of 27 immunology societies in 31 countries in Europe. Altogether, members of immunology societies that belong to EFIS exceed 16,000 immunologists.

http://www.qimr.edu.au/iuis/

The International Union of Immunological Societies (IUIS) is an umbrella organization for many of the regional and national societies of immunology throughout the world. International Congresses of Immunology are held every 3 yr under the auspices of IUIS.

http://www.academicinfo.net/

Academic Info's aim is to provide underrepresented students, educators, and librarians with an easy-to-use online subject directory to access quality, relevant, and current Internet resources on each academic discipline.

http://www.food.gov.uk/

The Food Standards Agency is an independent U.K. food safety watchdog set up by an Act of Parliament in 2000 to protect the public's health and consumer interests in relation to food. The Web site contains current news and feature articles.

http://bcs.whfreeman.com/immunology5e/

Immunology online provides multiple links to Web sites on several immunology-related topics.

Index

About the Editors

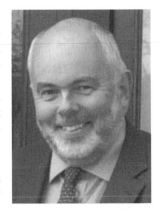

Dr. David Aled Hughes is a Principal Research Scientist within the Nutrition Division at the Institute of Food Research, Norwich. He is currently Scientist-in-Charge of the Institute's Human Nutrition Unit, where dietary intervention studies on healthy volunteers are undertaken, and Chair of the Institute's Human Research Governance Committee. He is a Registered Nutritionist with the Nutrition Society, holds an Honorary Readership at the University of East Anglia, Norwich and is currently Honorary Secretary of the Nutritional Immunology Group of the British Society for Immunology.

Dr. Hughes has 25 years experience as a cellular immunologist, formerly in respiratory medicine, and for the last decade in nutrition research. His primary interest is in understanding the mechanisms by which dietary components modulate human immune function, particularly in the context of the development of immune-related conditions such as heart disease and cancer. He has written several reviews and book chapters in the area of nutritional immunology and has given numerous invited lectures at international conferences. He is an Editor of *Nutritional Genomics and Functional Food* and a member of the Editorial Advisory Board for *Nutrition: The International Journal.*

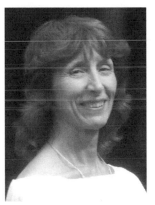

Dr. Gail Darlington is a senior specialist in General Internal Medicine and Rheumatology at Epsom and St Helier University Hospitals NHS Trust in the United Kingdom where she is also Lead Clinician for Research and heads a large clinical research team investigating rheumatoid arthritis, osteoporosis, diabetes, stroke, depression, cannabis toxicity, and Huntington's disease.

Dr. Darlington was a PPP Foundation Research Fellow at Jesus College, Cambridge, and is a member of several European research groups. She is Lead Clinician of a clinical/scientific research team and is co-author of *Pills, Potions and Poisons* with Professor Trevor Stone of the University of Glasgow—a book designed to make drugs more understandable to the reader.

Dr. Darlington was one of the first British specialists to undertake research into the role of dietary manipulation in the management of rheumatoid arthritis and to try to establish a dialogue between doctors (who have tended to be sceptical about dietary treatment) and patients (who have tended to believe, sometimes too trustingly, in the benefits of dietary manipulation). The absence of such dialogue in the past has led to a stand-off between patients and doctors, which has resulted in many patients being vulnerable to unsound advice from unscrupulous advisers. The book *Diet and Arthritis,* written by Dr. Darlington and Linda Gamlin, has proved to be extremely valuable to patients needing reliable scientific advice on this subject.

Dr. Darlington has a major interest in making scientific information about food available to as many people as possible, and she is well known for her radio and television appearances on this subject.

About the Editors *(cont'd)*

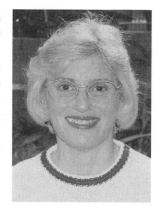

Dr. Adrianne Bendich is Clinical Director of Calcium Research at GlaxoSmithKline Consumer Healthcare, where she is responsible for leading the innovation and medical programs in support of TUMS and Os-Cal. Dr. Bendich has primary responsibility for the direction of GSK's support for the Women's Health Initiative intervention study. Prior to joining GlaxoSmithKline, Dr. Bendich was at Roche Vitamins Inc., and was involved with the groundbreaking clinical studies proving that folic acid-containing multivitamins significantly reduce major classes of birth defects. Dr. Bendich has co-authored more than 100 major clinical research studies in the area of preventive nutrition. Dr. Bendich is recognized as a leading authority on anti-oxidants, nutrition, immunity, and pregnancy outcomes, vitamin safety, and the cost-effectiveness of vitamin/mineral supplementation.

Dr. Bendich is the editor of nine books, including *Preventive Nutrition: The Comprehensive Guide for Health Professionals,* and is Series Editor of *Nutrition and Health* for Humana Press. She also serves as Associate Editor for *Nutrition: The International Journal of Applied and Basic Nutritional Sciences,* and Dr. Bendich is on the Editorial Board of the *Journal of Women's Health and Gender-Based Medicine,* as well as a member of the Board of Directors of the American College of Nutrition.

Dr. Bendich was the recipient of the Roche Research Award, a *Tribute to Women and Industry* Awardee, and a recipient of the Burroughs Wellcome Visiting Professorship in Basic Medical Sciences, 2000–2001. Dr. Bendich holds academic appointments as Adjunct Professor in the Department of Preventive Medicine and Community Health at UMDNJ, Institute of Nutrition, Columbia University P&S, and Adjunct Research Professor, Rutgers University, Newark Campus. She is listed in Who's Who in American Women.